MICROSCOPIC ANATOMY

AN ATLAS OF
LIGHT AND ELECTRON MICROSCOPY

PIETRO MOTTA

Professor and Chairman, Department of Anatomy
FACULTY OF MEDICINE, UNIVERSITY OF ROME «LA SAPIENZA», ITALY

MICROSCOPIC ANATOMY

AN ATLAS OF
LIGHT AND ELECTRON MICROSCOPY

Foreword by
KEITH R. PORTER
Wilson Elkins Distinguished Professor
and Chairman
Department of Biological Sciences
The University of Maryland
Baltimore County, U.S.A.

185 plates with 212 figures in color and 332 in black and white

English Translation of the Third Edition

PICCIN

First Italian Edition, 1972
Spanish Edition, 1974
Portuguese Edition, 1974
Second Italian Edition, 1977
Third Italian Edition, 1984
French Edition, 1989

ISBN 88-299-0082-6

Published in Italy

© 1990 by PICCIN NUOVA LIBRARIA S.p.A., Padua

In Loving Memory
of My Father

FOREWORD

The author of this extraordinary book is well known for his contributions to the histological literature, especially books designed to provide instruction to students and their instructors. It is no exaggeration to say that he excells himself in this 3rd edition of «Anatomia Microscopica». Fortunately for the students and professors of microscopic anatomy, this edition has been translated into very readable English and thus made available to a wider readership. For several reasons, it is a book to be treasured.

The abundance, quality and selection of the illustrations is outstanding and must surely excite the interest of even the most lethargic student. Each chapter is illustrated by both light and electron micrographs. Thus, the reader can easily make the transition between the more familiar light images and the higher-resolution electron micrographs. The former are especially elegant, indeed it is doubtful whether any text is illustrated by a finer collection of colored plates. The quality of the engravings and the color printing are superb. Added to that, the author, with a longtime esperience in teaching histology, has made a valuable choice of micrographs and has organized their presentation in a most logical fashion. Again, I must say that this book is a gem among books of this type.

Each chapter is introduced by a few pages of text, succinctly stated, plus carefully selected diagrams and graphics. These few pages are followed by more numerous pages of illustrations with entirely adequate legend. The translation is characterized for its precision and simple style. The author and the publisher deserve congratulations for putting together this exquisite offering to the histological literature. It should enjoy a long life and go down as a milestone in the evolution of such books.

Keith R. Porter

PREFACE TO THE THIRD EDITION

The aim of this atlas is to prepare students more thoroughly for examinations in histology and microscopic anatomy. All of the illustrations are collected in one volume. The chapters open with a brief discussion of the topic, which is aimed at providing the reader with a comprehensive view of the cell, tissues and organs. I have been encouraged by the favorable reception given to the two previous editions to issue a third without essential changes in the original format.

The present edition differs from its predecessors in having some textual changes and in the addition of many new figures obtained by more recent techniques in microscopy. From an original 139 the total number of plates is now 185. A number of diagrams have been added to the text to help in interpreting the figures. I have replaced certain illustrations with others prepared for this volume in my laboratory or kindly supplied by colleagues, whose names are acknowledged in the relevant captions.

I thank Dr. M. Piccin especially for his generosity in making this revised edition possible, and Mr. T. De Meda both for his patience and the thoroughness of his help during the revision process.

Some colored SEM pictures have been included in the present edition of the book. I am pleased to thank Dr. S.A. Nottola for her artistic work on them. Thanks are also due to Dr. R.A. Collinssplatt for having provided the English version of the manuscript. I am also grateful to Dr. H. Bell and Prof. M. Bonneville of the Department of Molecular, Cellular and Developmental Biology of the University of Colorado at Boulder for their kind editorial advice. Finally, my thanks go to Drs. S.V. Greene, D.W. Finn, Mrs. S. Fraccaro and Mrs. M. Coraiola for their patience in helping me to re-read and re-check the proofs of the manuscript during the various stages of its production.

I hope that colleagues and students will feel as free to criticize and make suggestions for this edition as they did for two predecessors. Such commentary can only serve to improve the atlas by fitting it to current conditions and, above all, to the needs of students, for whom it is chiefly intended.

Rome, 28 May 1989   **Pietro Motta**

CONTENTS

PART I

THE CELL

PART II

TISSUES

CATALOGUE OF PLATES [1]

MICROSCOPIC ANATOMY

AN ATLAS OF
LIGHT AND ELECTRON MICROSCOPY

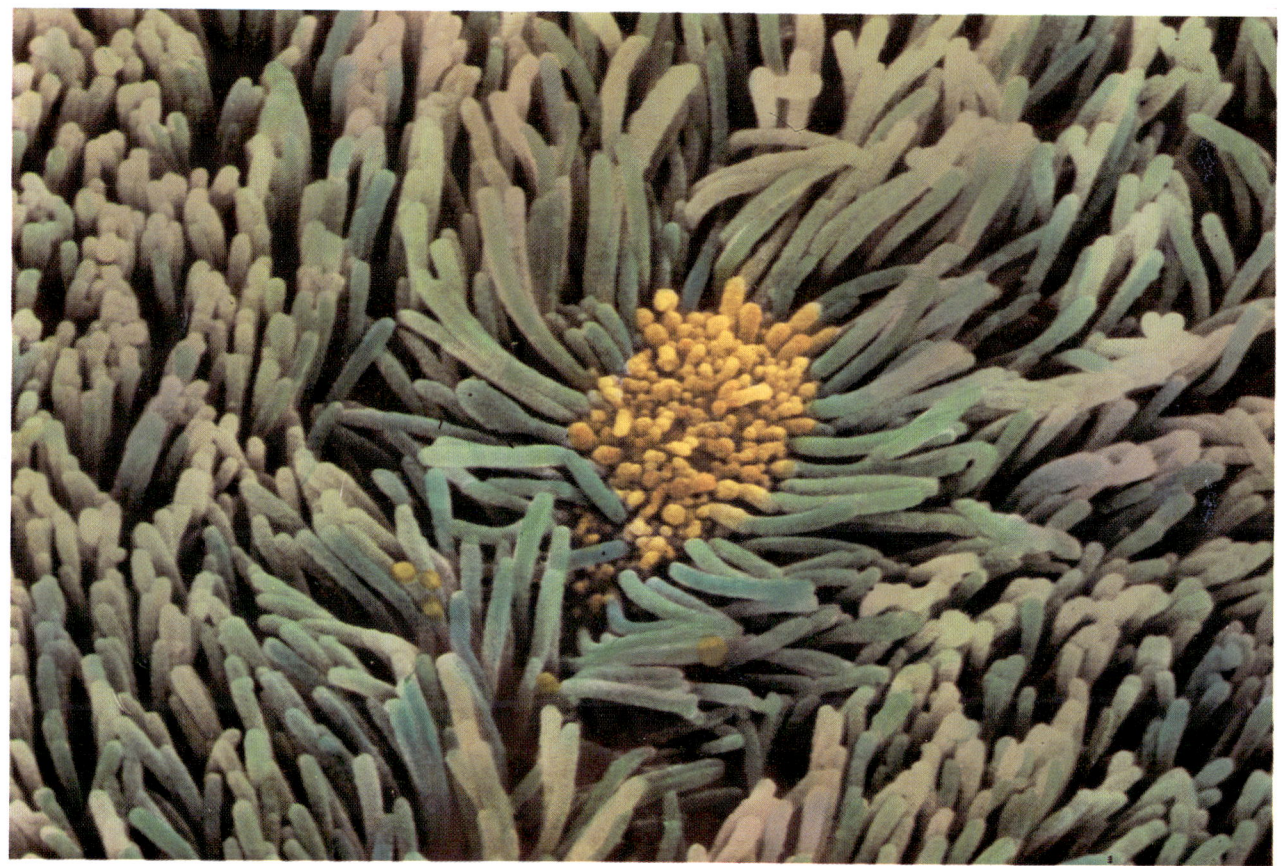

Colored scanning electron microscopy of cell surface with cilia (green) and microvilli (yellow) from rat trachea. (9,300 x).

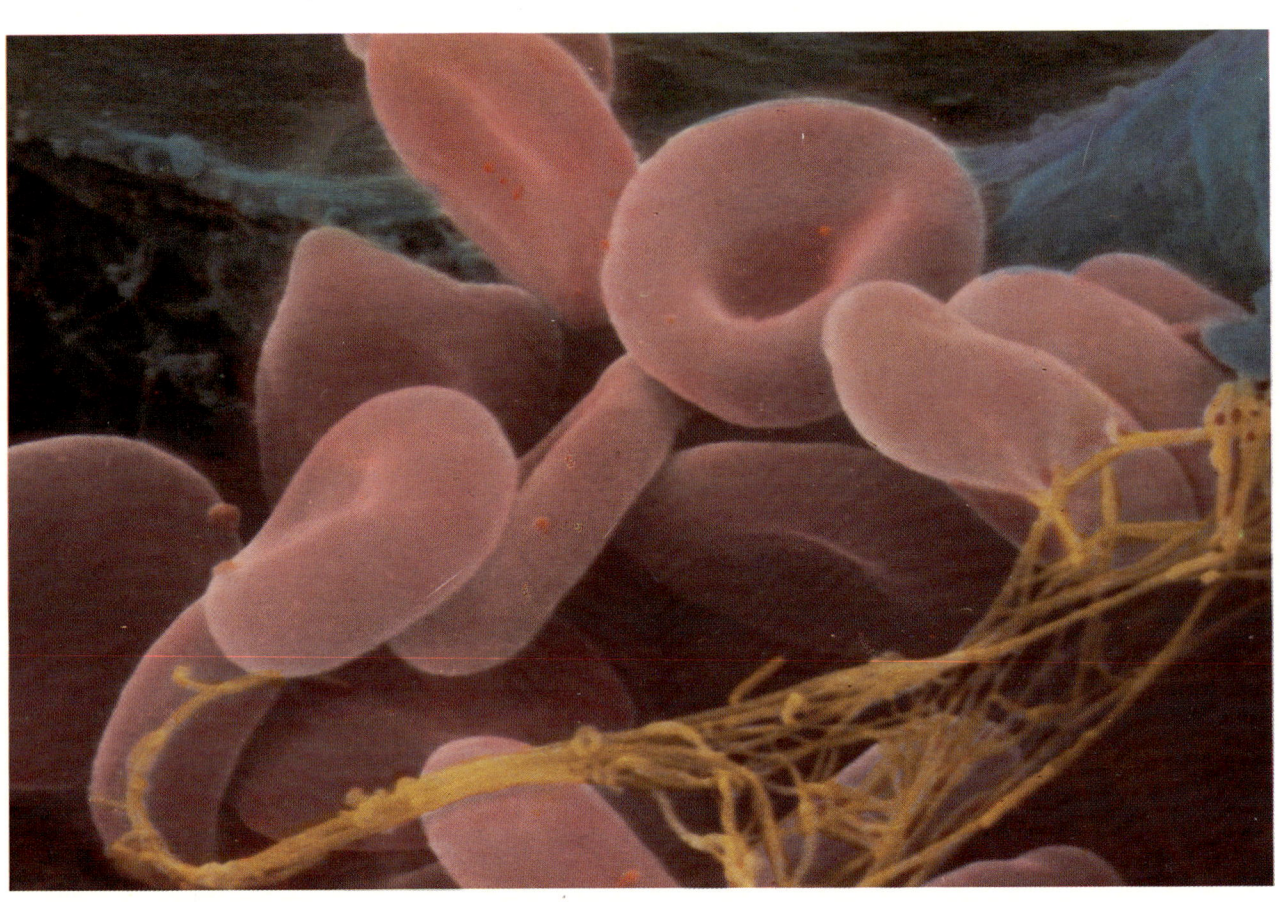

Red blood cells in a portion of a blood clot appear intermingled with fibrin threads. (Colored SEM; 10,300 x).

PART ONE

THE CELL

The cell is an indivisible biological unit capable of self-replication and metabolic autoregulation. Each cell is composed of the nucleus and its surrounding cytoplasm, and is enclosed by a cell membrane. The shape and size of the cell vary according to its specific functions. Cells that are free of attachment to other cells tend to be spherical in shape. Their diameter varies widely, ranging from 5-6 um for lymphocytes to 100 and 200 um for neurons and oocytes. Both the nucleus and cytoplasm contain organelles. The specific function of the cell depends on these organelles; each is discussed in succeeding sections of this chapter.

The units of measurements used in this book are the micrometer (um), formerly called the micron (u), the nanometer (nm), and the Angstrom unit (A). lu = 0,001 mm, 1 nm = 0,001 um, 1 A = 0,0001 um. The micrometer (um) and the manometer (nm) are the most commonly employed units of measure for cells and their components. This system has been recommended by the Systeme International d'Unites (SI).

The abbreviations used in the plates are LM, light micrograph; EM, electron micrograph; H & E, hematoxylin and eosin.

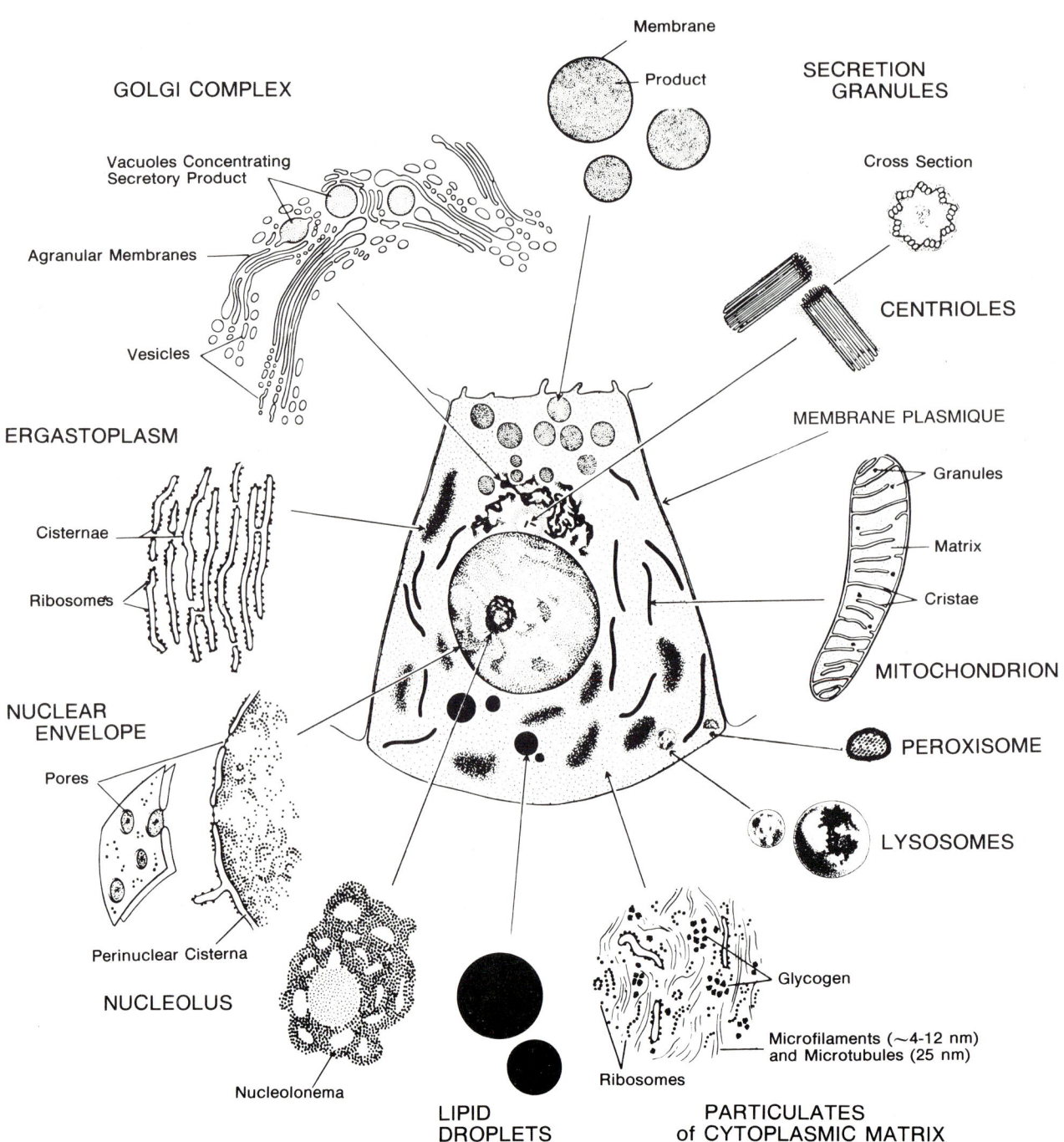

Diagram of the cell, showing organelles and inclusions as they appear by light microscopy. These same organelles as seen by electron microscopy are represented around the periphery of the cell. By courtesy of D. W. Fawcett, in: W. Bloom and P. W. Fawcett: A Textbook of Histology 10th ed. W.B. Saunders Co. Philadelphia/London/Toronto, 1975.

NUCLEUS AND CYTOPLASM

THE NUCLEUS

The nucleus, through its involvement in protein synthesis, plays a critical role in the regulation of cell processes, and it controls the transmission of hereditary characteristics. However, certain cell types, such as the erythrocyte, lack a nucleus when mature; other cell types, such as the hepatocyte, may have two or more nuclei; still others, such as skeletal muscle, regularly have many nuclei.

The most important component of the nucleus is DNA, which is responsible for specifying the proteins synthesized by the cells, and thus the structural and functional features of the organism.

The ratio between the nuclear and cytoplasmic volume usually is constant. Mitosis follows an increase in cytoplasmic volume. During mitosis the nucleus passes through a series of morphological stages that distinguish it from the nucleus during interphase, and are the manifestation of an orderly process that gives rise to two viable daughter cells.

The nucleus during interphase

During interphase the following nuclear structures may be seen: the *nucleoplasm, chromatin, the nucleolus, the nuclear envelope* and, sometimes, *accessory structures* (Plates 1.1, 1.2, 1.3, 1.5, 1.8).

The nucleoplasm or nuclear matrix, like the cytoplasmic matrix, appears translucent in the light microscope. With the electron microscope it is seen as an ultrafine network of filaments. The nucleoplasm is colloid in nature, having an aqueous phase in which are dispersed protein macromolecules. These macromolecules often are enzymes, as well as metabolites and ions.

The term chromatin refers to chromosomes as they exist during interphase, when specific regions are uncoiled and being actively transcribed into RNA. The chromosomes are made up of DNA, which constitutes the genetic code, with associated proteins. Most of the DNA in the cell is in the form of chromatin, and it is here that the various types of RNA are synthesized: *messenger, transfer and ribosomal RNA (mRNA, tRNA and rRNA,* respectively). In the interphase nucleus the part of the chromatin that is visible is that which is genetically and therefore metabolically inactive, the *heterochromatin.* The active region, the *euchromatin,* is dispersed in the nucleoplasm and during interphase appears largely as electron-lucent areas.

The nucleolus is a round body that often appears as an irregularly twisted ball of yarn (the *nucleonema*). Its position within the nucleus varies with the cell type. The number of nucleoli per cell usually equals the number of sets of chromosomes (e.g., two in a diploid cell). The size of the nucleolus can vary considerably. It is particularly large in cells actively involved in protein synthesis, for example, neurons, oocytes and tumor cells. The nucleolus, which is not membrane-bound, is composed mainly of RNA and basic proteins. In the electron microscopic image, it is in part fibrous, the *pars fibrosa,* and in part granular, the *pars granulosa.* These granules and ultrafine filaments contain mainly ribonucleic proteins, which are thought to be precursors of ribosomes (Plates 1.2, 1.3, 1.13).

Filaments of DNA, the so-called *nucleolar-associated chromatin*, also are present in the nucleolus. The ribosomal RNA is synthesized in this region of the nucleolus and is processed and temporarily stored in the pars fibrosa and pars granulosa before being transferred to the cytoplasm.

The nucleolus disappears at the beginning of mitosis (Plate 1.7).

During interphase, accessory structures of the nucleus may be present. These include *lipids, proteins, and glycogen*. Accessory structures often have a characteristic morphology (*crystals, filaments, spheroid bodies*, etc.), and their presence probably is related to the special function of the particular cell type (Plate 1.31 C,D).

Frequently there is a dense layer of uniform thickness adhering to the inner surface of the nuclear envelope. This layer, termed the *zonula nucleum limitans* or *lamina fibrosa*, is believed to be composed of protein that stabilizes nuclear morphology during interphase (Plate 1.8).

During interphase, the nuclei of many female cells show a small dense Barr body, the inactive form of one of the sex chromosomes. The *Barr body* usually is associated with the internal surface of the nuclear envelope or with the nucleolus (Plate 1.10 A).

The nucleus during cell division

During mitosis, the nuclear envelope, which is a specialized part of the endoplasmic reticulum, and the nucleolus disappear. The chromosomes condense to form coils of constant shape and size that are characteristic for each species. The chromatin stains deeply, and the chromosomes are clearly seen (Plates 1.4, 1.5, 1.6, 1.7). These changes take place gradually in the nucleus as mitosis progresses, and various stages have been described: *prophase, metaphase, anaphase, telophase*. During metaphase the chromosomes can be observed most clearly (Plates 1.5, 1.10, 1.11, 1.12).

Every human cell has 46 chromosomes (*the diploid number*) consisting of paired sets. Mature germ cells are the exception to the rule, having only 23 chromosomes (*the haploid number*) consisting of one set. Of the diploid number of chromosomes, two are sex chromosomes (*hete-rochromosomes*) and the other 44 are somatic chromosomes (*autosomes*). Chromosomes are observed to have arms of various lengths, which take up basic stains readily, and a small spherical region (*centromere* or *kinetochore*), which resists stain. The centromere has a diameter of 300-500 nm, and is seen as a narrow region (*primary constriction*) between the two arms of the chromosome (Plate 1.10).

Chromosomes can be distinguished according to the position of the centromere, which is the same in both chromosomes of a pair (except in the case of the male sex chromosome). The *telocentric* chromosome has the centromere at one end, the *metacentric* type has the centromere at the center (two arms of equal length), and the *subtelocentric* has two unequal arms. During mitosis each chromosome splits lengthwise into two parts, the *chromatids*. At metaphase the chromatids remain attached to the centromere, the region where the mitotic spindle fibers are joined to the chromosome. At anaphase the centromere splits lengthwise, and the two daughter chromosomes move to opposite poles of the spindle. The female sex chromosomes are called the XX pair. As mentioned previously, the inactive form of one of the pairs sometimes can be seen in the nucleus during interphase as a dense mass in the nucleus during interphase (*Barr body*). Male sex chromosomes consist of an X and a Y chromosome, the X being larger in comparison to the Y (Plates 1.10, 1.11, 1.12).

THE CYTOPLASM

The finely granular portion of the cytoplasm is termed the *hyaloplasm* or *cytoplasmic matrix*, and contains the organelles and cell inclusions. Enveloping the cytoplasm is the *plasma membrane* or *plasmalemma* (Plates 1.1, 1.2, 1.3, 1.5).

The plasma membrane

The plasma membrane is composed of a bilayer of lipid molecules in which are embedded globular protein molecules of various complexity. The lipid bilayer acts as a fluid matrix in which

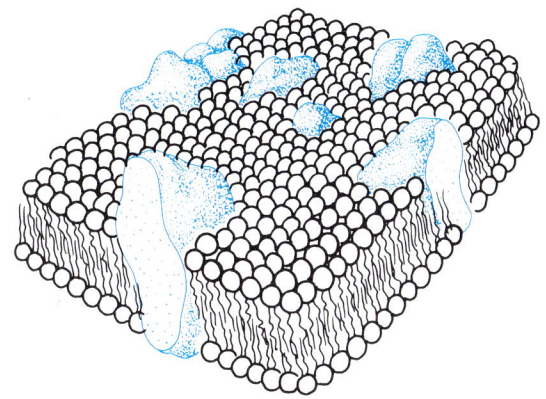

The fluid mosaic model of membrane structure, in which lipids and globular proteins are arranged in a mosaic fashion in a fluid matrix. The circles represent the hydrophilic regions and the wavy lines represent the hydrophobic regions of the lipid molecules. The irregular masses represent globular proteins embedded in the lipid bilayer. Portions of these molecules may extend above and below the outer and inner surface of the membrane. Modified from S.J. Singer and G.L. Nicolson, Science, 175:720, 1972.

the proteins, like icebergs floating atop the sea, can move laterally. The consequence of this movement is a modification in the macromolecular and functional arrangement of the limiting membrane of the cell. Thus the plasma membrane is not a static but a dynamic structure. Singer and Nicolson termed this arrangement of protein and lipid molecules the *fluid mosaic model* of the cell membrane.

When examined by an electron microscope the plasma membrane is seen to consist of two layers 2-2.5 nm thick separated by an electron-lucent space of 2.5-3.5 nm. The membrane appears to be three-layered because osmium tetroxide stains the lipids in the region of the hydrophilic groups at its outer and inner surface. The characteristic three-layered structure, often referred to as *Robertson's unit membrane,* has served as a model for the structural plan of biological membranes (Plate 1.14). More recent studies have shown that the proteins of the cell membrane may be catagorized into two broad types, *peripheral* (or *extrinsic*) and *integral* (or *intrinsic*). The peripheral proteins are bound loosely to the areas toward the surface of the membrane and are more easily separated by extraction. Integral proteins are found within the fluid matrix and are therefore more tenaciously bound to the lipid layer. They usually contain hydrophobic regions

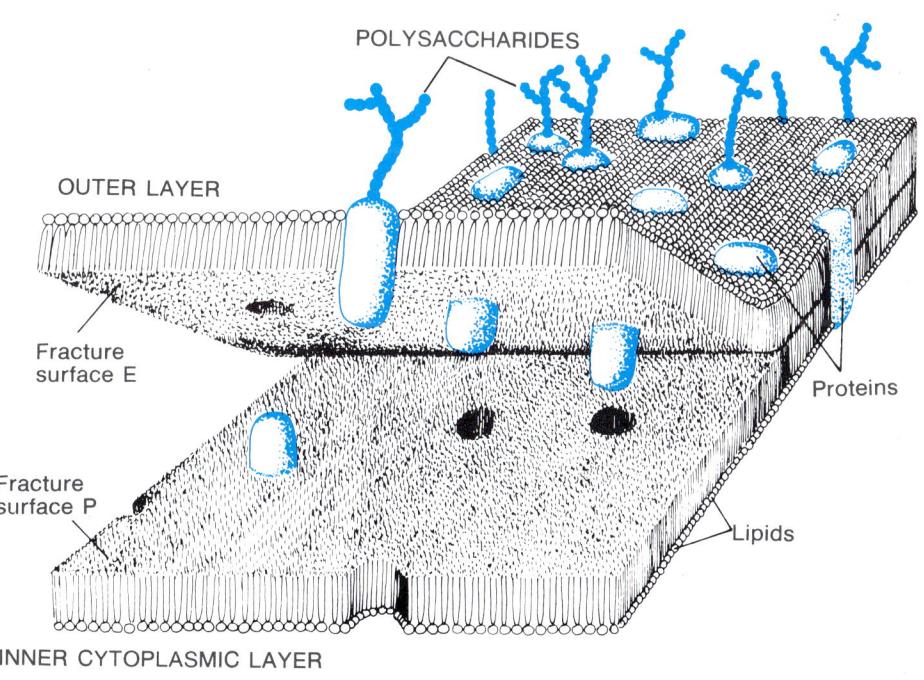

Schematic illustration of the "freeze fracture" technique. The area of the membrane shown at the top right is an intact portion in which the proteins and glycoproteins are embedded in the lipid bilayer. When the membrane is frozen and subsequently fractured, the two lipid layers are separated along a plane between the hydrophobic parts of the lipid molecules. This fracture exposes the integral proteins embedded in the hydrophobic region of the membrane. The proteins are not fractured. In the electron microscope the proteins are seen as small protuberances or, in places where they have been pulled out of the membrane, as corresponding depressions. Modified from B. Satir. Scientific American, 223:29, 1975. In: V. Monesi. *Istologia.* 2nd edition. Piccin Editore, Padua, 1980.

that span the membrane.

Carbohydrates also may be found on the outer surface of membranes, and are combined with either proteins or lipids to form glycoproteins or glycolipids. The *glycocalyx* is the carbohydrate-rich coat that is present in most cell types. Because of their complex macromolecular structure, these molecules possess distinctive antigenic sites and thus play a key role in cell interactions and in communication among cells.

The cell matrix

In the light microscope the cytoplasm may appear homogenous. At the level of resolution attainable by the electron microscope the cytoplasm contains a fine network of fibers, filaments and tubules that form the *cytoskeleton*. With the high voltage electron microscope a complex web of thin strands 5-6 nm thick also can be seen, the *microtrabecular lattice* of Porter and Wolosewick. The microtrabeculae of this network constitute the gel phase of the cytoplasmic ground substance. Other constituents of the cell, such as *microfilaments, microtubules, endoplasmic reticulum and ribosomes* are associated with the lattice. The microtrabecular network is believed capable of contracting and expanding, and can apparently direct and transport organelles and inclusions into various areas of the cytoplasm according to the requirements of the cell (Plates 1.3, 1.15).

The endoplasmic reticulum

The membranes within the cytoplasm that form the endoplasmic reticulum may have originated during evolution by progressive infolding

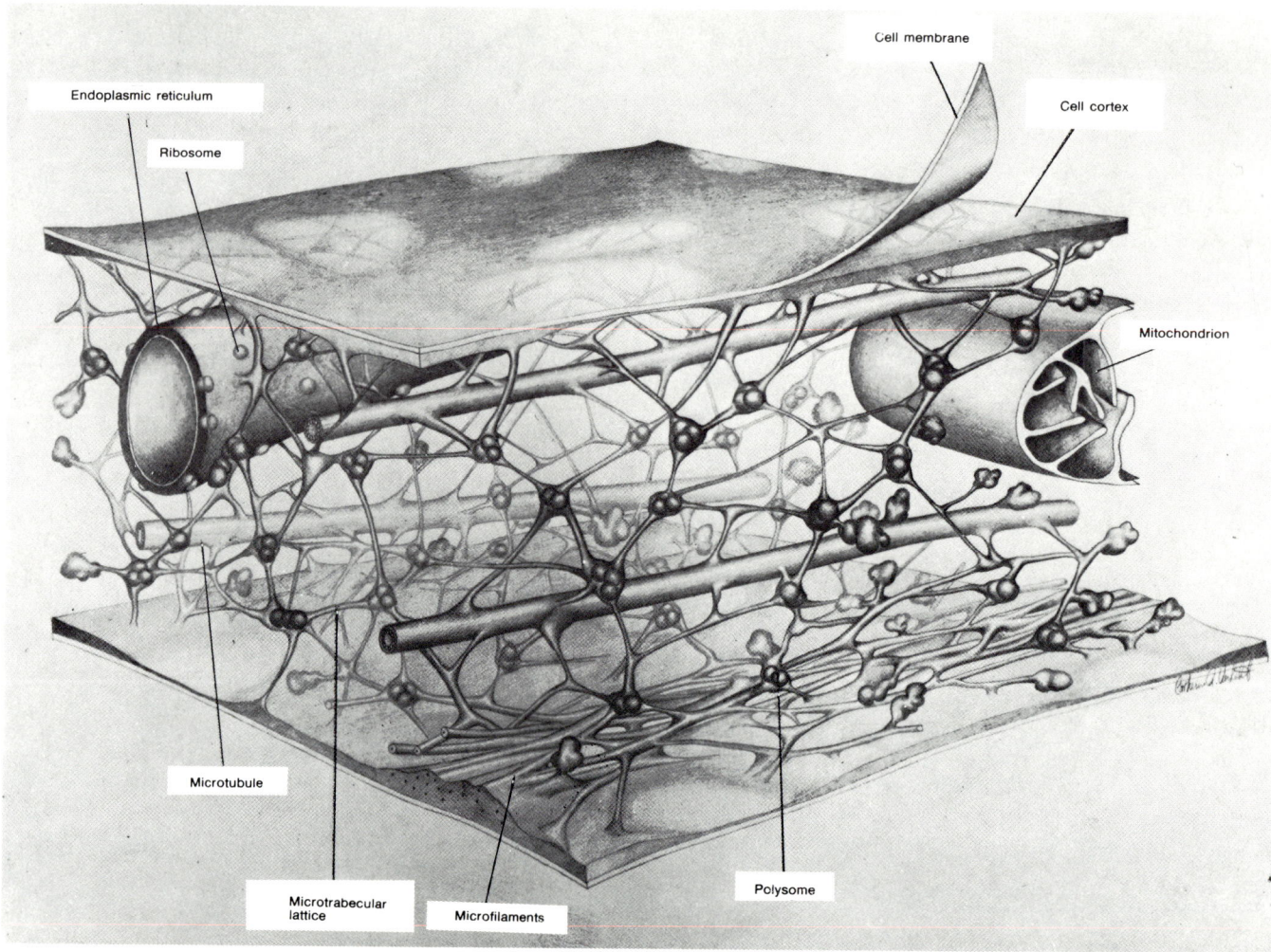

A three-dimensional model of the microtrabecular lattice in the cytoplasm of a cultured cell observed "in toto" with the high voltage electron microscope. The microtrabeculae are attached to the microtubules and to the membranes of the endoplasmic reticulum. They appear as a continuation of the microfilaments adhering to the plasmalemma. The polysomes are fixed at the nodal points of the microtrabecular network and thus their position in the cytoplasm is thought to be conditioned by the microtrabecular lattice. By permission of K.R. Porter and J. Wolosewick.

of the cell membrane. The architecture and molecular composition of the endoplasmic reticulum are the same as those of the plasma membrane. The extensiveness and appearance of the endoplasmic reticulum vary from one type of cell to another and within the same cell according to its activity. In certain phases of cell activity there are dense granules (the *ribosomes*) that adhere to the surface of these membranes. Ribosomes are ubiquitous particles, seen by the electron microscope as electron-dense granules of constant size (15-20 nm) whose chemical composition is ribonucleic protein. The endoplasmic reticulum is characterized by the presence (*rough endoplasmic reticulum*) or absence (*smooth endoplasmic reticulum*) of attached ribosomes. Ribosomes in the cytoplasm occur either in isolation or in groups linked together by filaments of mRNA. The *polyribosomes* or *polysomes* often appear as rosettes and spirals. In general, polysomes are considered to be involved in the synthesis of the structural proteins retained within the cell. Ribosomes attached to the endoplasmic reticulum are involved in the synthesis of either proteins that remain within the membrane or secretory proteins that are transferred across the membrane into the lumen of the endoplasmic reticulum. In some cells the rough endoplasmic reticulum is the predominant form seen (Plates 1.16, 1.17, 1.19).

In certain images there is continuity between the smooth and the rough endoplasmic reticulum. Such images are interpreted as demonstrating the smooth endoplasmic reticulum is formed by the rough endoplasmic reticulum. The smooth endoplasmic reticulum differs from the rough not only in its absence of ribosomes but also in having biochemical functions that are related to the composition of the membrane. For example, the smooth endoplasmic reticulum of liver cells contains enzymes for the detoxification of drugs. Occasionally the smooth endoplasmic reticulum has the appearance of tubules in an anastomosing network that opens into cisternae or small vesicles. In skeletal and cardiac muscle the smooth endoplasmic reticulum (*sarcoplasmic reticulum*) is especially complex. In the absorptive cells of the small intestine the smooth endoplasmic reticulum resynthesizes lipids from absorbed monoglycerides and fatty acids. In cells producing steroid hormones smooth endoplasmic reticulum abounds, and many of the enzymes responsible

for certain steps in steroid synthesis are associated with its membranes. Examples of such cells are those of the corpus luteum, interstitial cells of the testis and thecal cells of the ovary, and cells of the adrenal cortex (Plate 1.18, 1.22).

The Golgi complex

The Golgi complex is a special system of smooth-surfaced cytoplasmic membranes often located near the nucleus of the cell. Although its membranes are slightly thicker than those of the endoplasmic reticulum, their structure conforms to that described in the fluid mosaic model of membranes. The Golgi complex consists of parallel arrays of membranes forming saccules flattened in the middle (*lamellae*) and expanding at their extremity (*cisternae*). Numerous layers of saccules can be seen, which vary from 2 to 6 or more. Numerous vesicles also are located in the region of the Golgi complex, which vary in diameter from 20-60 nm. Some of these vesicles are formed from the membranes of the adjacent endoplasmic reticulum and carry the secretory product to the convex surface of the outer saccules of the complex (the *proximal* or *forming face* of the Golgi complex) (Plates 1.20, 1.21, 1.22).

In secretory cells the saccules of the concave inner surface of the Golgi complex gradually become expanded cisternae from which are detached or "pinched off" dense vacuoles containing secretory material (the *distal* or *maturing face* of the Golgi complex). Thus, in cells that secrete protein, the Golgi complex is that cellular component in which material that has been synthesized in the rough endoplasmic reticulum is segregated and concentrated. The secretory granule, when mature, is transported to the cell surface for extrusion (*exocytosis*) (Plate 1.20).

In cells that elaborate glycoprotein the Golgi complex is the site at which certain carbohydrates are added to the protein element produced in the rough endoplasmic reticulum. The Golgi complex thus takes part not only in the formation and transport of material destined for secretion (enzymes, hormones, etc.), but also plays an important role in the assembly of the plasma membrane, complete with its glycocalyx. The Golgi complex also is the site for the formation of lysosomes which are then segregated in a special part of the forming face of the membrane complex. Because of its close relationship with the endoplasmic reticulum, this portion of the Golgi complex is called the *Golgi* associated *endoplasmic reticulum* from which *lysosomes* form (GERL) (Novikoff).

The nuclear envelope

The membranes of the endoplasmic reticulum form a continuous boundary (the nuclear envelope) for the structures in the nucleus during interphase. During this period the nuclear and cytoplasmic compartments are segregated. The membranes of the endoplasmic reticulum separate from the nucleus during mitosis and the nuclear envelope breaks down and becomes dispersed in the cytoplasm. The nuclear and cytoplasmic zones of the cell thus are no longer distinct, and the condensed chromosomes migrate from one area of the cell to another.

The nuclear envelope consists of two membranes, each 5-7 nm thick. They are separated by a space of 20-60 nm wide, the *perinuclear cistern* (Plate 1.7, inset). The layer of the nuclear envelope facing the cytoplasm often has ribosomes on its outer surface. The layer facing the nucleoplasm is smooth and regular and is in close association with the condensed chromosomal material (Plates 1.2, 1.8, 1.19).

The two layers of the nuclear envelope fuse at irregular intervals to form pores of 50-80 nm in diameter (*nuclear pores*). Communication between the nucleus and cytoplasm occurs through these pores. Their number varies with the stage of development and the activity of the cell. Each nuclear pore has a complex octagonal structure. The pores are capable of opening and closing and thus act as regulators for the passage of materials between the nucleus and cytoplasm (Plates 1.8, 1.13 D).

In many cells that are active metabolically there can be seen arrays of membrane layers that have an arrangement similar to that of the nuclear envelope. These *annulate lamellae* consist of a set of double parallel membranes penetrated by small pores at regular intervals (Plate 1.18 A). Annulate lamellae are thought to be transient structures originating from layers of membrane shed by the nuclear envelope for incorporation into the membranes of the rough endoplasmic reticulum.

Mitochondria

The cellular organelles of eucaryotic cells that are the site of aerobic synthesis of ATP, and therefore contain the major respiratory enzymes, are the mitochondria. They vary in number, shape and size (diameter 0.5 um, length 2-5 um) according to the type and functional activity of the cell. In cells in which the need for energy in the cytoplasm is high, mitochondria are more numerous. Each mitochondrion has an outer limiting membrane separated from an internal membrane by a space of 8-10 nm. The internal membrane sometimes possesses numerous infoldings that project into the mitochondrion to form characteristic shelves, called cristae, which, depending upon the type of cell, vary in number, arrangement and shape (lamellae, tubules, villi, vesicles, etc.). The space between cristae contains fine granular material, the mitochondrial matrix (Plates 1.17, 1.23, 1.24, 1.25). As with other membranous organelles, mitochondrial membranes have the trilaminar lipoprotein structure (Plate 1.24).

Mitochondria are unusual among cytoplasmic organelles in that they are formed from preexisting mitochondria. In the mitochondrial matrix are granules of RNA and fine filaments of DNA. Together these two nucleic acids govern the synthesis of specific mitochondrial proteins.

In the mitochondrial matrix can be seen dense granules with a diameter of 30-50 nm which are localized accumulations of calcium ions (*matrix granules*). Mitochondria can contain a great variety of inclusions (lipids, glycogen, protein crystalloids, etc.) which are associated with special activity or pathology of the cell (Plate 1.17).

On the internal surface facing the matrix are mushroom-shaped particles (*inner membrane subunits*). Each particle consists of a spherical headpiece 9-10 nm in diameter and is attached to the internal membrane of the mitochondrion by means of a small stalk about 5 nm in length (Fernandez-Moran). These subunits have been shown to be the ATPase of oxidative phosphorylation (Plate 1.25).

Peroxisomes

Peroxisomes are ovoid organelles with a diameter of 0.2-0.6 um and are enclosed by a smooth membrane (Plate 1.31). They contain fine granular material that sometimes condenses to form a crystalline inclusion (*nucleoid*). The most common enzyme found in peroxisomes is catalase. Other enzymes found commonly in peroxisomes are glycolate oxidase and flavin oxidase.

Smaller peroxisomes (diameter 0.15-0.25 um) called *microperoxisomes* have been described in various types of cells. These peroxisomes are without nucleoids but possess high peroxidase activity. Peroxisomes and microperoxisomes are often associated with smooth endoplasmic reticulum, and it has been suggested that the smooth endoplasmic reticulum is the site of origin for these organelles. Because peroxisomes resemble lysosomes in their morphology, special cytochemical techniques often are required to identify these organelles conclusively.

Lysosomes

Lysosomes are polymorphous cell organelles with a diameter of 0.3-0.6 um. They contain a number of acid hydrolases capable of digesting protein, lipids and other substances. De Duve has defined these organelles as a sort of intracellular digestive system. *Primary lysosomes* contain the latent enzymes. *Secondary lysosomes* or *digestive vacuoles* are those lysosomes that have fused with the phagocytic vacuole and are actively engaged in the digestive process (Plate 1.26). *Phagosomes* or *heterophagosomes* digest exogenous material, whereas *autophagosomes* (autophagic *vacuoles*) are directed to breaking down normally occurring constituents of the cell, such as mitochondria, for recycling.

Filaments and microtubules

In the cytoplasm of all eucaryotic cells exist thin filaments 6-7 nm in diameter and of indefinite length, the *microfilaments* (Plates 1.15, 1.27 C). These filaments, consisting of actin, are capable of providing a supporting structure for the cell. In addition, in conjunction with the thick filaments of myosin, they play a role in contraction (e.g., in smooth and striated muscle).

Intermediate filaments, approximately 7 nm thick (e.g., various keratin filaments of epithelial cells, glial filaments of glial cells, neurofilaments of many neurons, desmin filaments in muscle cells, and *vimentin filaments* in mesenchymal cells) are structural in nature, providing strength to the cytoplasm.

Microtubules, which have a diameter of about 25 nm and are of indeterminate length, constitute a second major type of filamentous structure found in the cytoplasm. The microtubule is a cylindrical structure formed by 13 protofilaments of tubulin dimers with an electron-lucent center. Microtubules are found in all cells, and play a major role in both the regulation of cell shape and in the direction and orientation of cytoplasmic movements (Plate 1.27).

Centrioles

The centriole is a cylindrical structure 300-500 nm long and 150-200 nm in diameter, with an electron-lucent center. It is often found in association with the Golgi complex. Nine sets of tubule triplets can be seen in the cross-sectional view of a centriole (Plate 1.28). Thin filaments attached to each of the 9 sets of tubules converge like the spokes of a wheel towards the center of the centriole. Centrioles are associated either directly or indirectly with the formation of cilia and flagella (see below), and the formation of the mitotic spindle (Plate 1.27). Centrioles are formed from *microtubule organizing centers* (MTOC) that initiate the formation of tubulin dimers into specific microtubular orientations.

Inclusions in the cytoplasm

In the cytoplasm of many types of cells exist a variety of droplets or secretion granules, aggregations of substances (proteins, lipids and glycogen), and various pigments (*ferritin, melanin, lipofuscin, lipochrome, bilirubin, crystalline inclusions*) (Plates 1.17, 1.18 B, 1.23, 1.26 A, 1.30, 1.31).

DIFFERENTIATED CELL SURFACES

Cilia and flagella

Cilia (shorter appendages) and flagella (longer appendages) are motile organelles projecting from the cell surfaces (Plates 1.32 A,B, 1.33, 1.34). They are produced from basal bodies, which resemble centrioles and are located at the periphery of the cell. In addition to those at the periphery, each cell usually contains two centrioles perpendicular to each other and located near the Golgi (Plate 1.28).

Arrays of cilia are capable of coordinated movement, and can be described as movable bundles of microtubules. The number of cilia varies with the cell type; in tracheal epithelium there may exist as many as 200 or 250 per cell. Cilia measure from 5-10 um in length and have a diameter of 0.2 um. In the cilium are nine doublets of peripheral microtubules, with one pair in the core (the 9 + 2 pattern or axoneme). Except in rare cases this arrangement is constant in all animal and plant cells. At the base of the cilium the nine doublets are attached to the basal body in which the central pair is absent. In some instances *ciliary rootlets* (striated fibers 50-70 nm in diameter) may extend from the base of the centriole into the cytoplasm.

Flagella of sperm have the same 9 + 2 pattern as cilia, but are longer (70-100 um) and have a dense fibrous sheath surrounding the axoneme for much of its length. Mitochondria form a sheath covering the midpiece of the tail (Plate 1.34).

In living organisms the movement of cilia and flagella is based on a sliding action of the microtuble doublets. As well as tubulin, the specific protein of microtubules, cilia and flagella contain a special protein dynein that possesses ATPase activity.

The cilium appears to be a feature of a wide variety of connective and epithelial cells, as well as neurons, and may occur as a single small projection from the free surface of the cell. The function of such single cilia, though undefined, is connected with the activity of the centriole (Plates 1.28, 1.29).

Microvilli

Microvilli are specialized finger-like projections of the plasma membrane (Plates 1.4, 1.35, 1.36, 1.37, 1.38). They increase substantially the surface area of the cell, with the result that the transfer of materials across epithelia is more efficient. The absorptive cells of the epithelium in the small intestine possess numerous microvilli, which appear as regular cylindrical projections on the free surface of the cell. The cell membrane is covered by a complex cell coat (*glycocalyx*). In the intestine, microvilli reach 1 um in length and about 0.1 um in diameter. Internally, microvilli enclose a bundle of filaments that extend into a circumferential band of filaments lying in the apical cytoplasm. The two arrays of filaments interact to form the so-called *terminal web*. The web is made of filaments and is thought to allow movement of the microvilli. The filaments in the absorptive epithelium of the intestine are made up of actin, whereas the terminal web into which they extend probably contains myosin as well as actin and other intermediate filaments of the cytoskeleton, such as keratin filaments (tonofilaments). These microvilli therefore are capable of contraction. The microvilli of the proximal convoluted tubules of the kidney, although of the same diameter as those of the intestine, are longer and can measure up to 1.5-3 um. Such a regular arrangement of microvilli, when observed in the light microscope, was formerly called a *striated* or *brush border*. Microvilli also occur on the surface of liver cells facing the bile canaliculus.

In certain cells that function mainly to protect from mechanical damage (covering epithelium of the cornea, vagina, esophagus, etc.) the cell surface is raised in processes called *microplicae,* 0.1-0.2 um thick and 0.4-0.5 um long. When sectioned, microplicae resemble microvilli, but when observed on the surface of the organ they form crests and furrows. Mucous cells or glands may also be present, and the mucus probably acts as an anti-friction lubricant on the free surface of epithelium (Plate 1.40 C). The cell membrane of the epithelium opposite that on which the microvilli and microplicae occur may be infolded to form deep cylindrical invaginations which often are regular in appearance. Like other foldings of the cell surface these invaginations also increase the surface area of the cell and expand the area for exchange of materials (Plate 1.43).

Stereocilia

Stereocilia, like microvilli, are evaginations of the cell membrane but they are much longer (Plate 1.32). Although called stereocilia, they have a core of actin filaments rather than microtubules, and hence they more closely resemble microvilli than cilia. Stereocilia are found in certain epithelia of the male reproductive system (epididymis and vas deferens). In these tissues the cells have a tuft of stereocilia. In fixed preparations the stereocilia may entwine with those from other cells to form a web.

Evaginations and invaginations of the cell surface

Infoldings and protuberances of various shape and size can be seen on the cell surface. The infoldings include vesicular invaginations such as phagocytic vesicles, micropinocytotic vesicles, and coated pits. Such structures are transient and are associated with uptake mechanisms, such as endocytosis, of particles and liquids (*phagocytosis* and *pinocytosis,* respectively), and with specific uptake of proteins (*coated pits*). In cultured cells the lamellipodia are involved in phagocytosis.

Pseudopodia and ruffled membranes are associated with movement and cell migration in cultured cells and migratory cells such as macrophages. Filopodia are long projections which function as anchors for dividing cells in culture (Plates 1.4, 1.6, 1.39, 1.40).

Surface coats of the plasma membrane

Glycoproteins and glycolipids are an integral part of the cell membrane. In most cells the membrane is covered on its outer surface with a layer of various thickness and consistency, made of polysaccharides extending from the membrane proteins and glycolipids. This layer is called the glycocalyx or surface coat. It constitutes a part of the cell membrane.

With special staining techniques the glyco-calyx can be visualized by the electron microscope. It appears as a fine filamentous material. In some instances the glycocalyx can be rather thick and vary in its carbohydrate composition, but it is usually negatively charged and thus has an effect on transport across the plasma membrane (Plates 1.42, 1.43).

At the basal surface of epithelia, at the outer surface of muscle cells, and where nerve tissue faces connective tissue an extracellular layer called the basal lamina is a constant feature. In the electron microscope an electron-lucent region is seen immediately surrounding the cells, and then a fine fibrous layer which separates these three types of tissue from connective tissue may be seen. The basal lamina is a complex of proteins and polysaccharides that plays a role in exchanges between the tissues separated by it. In normal tissue the basal lamina marks the boundary among tissue types.

Intercellular Junctions

The area of contact between epithelial cells is designed to form a barrier that is highly selective in the passage of liquids and dissolved substances between the cells. The areas specialized for this role form the so-called junctional complex. This complex consists of three types of attachment, the *zonula occludens* or *tight junction,* which seals the cells together and impedes transport between the cells. In the *zonula adherens* or *intermediate junction,* the cell membranes maintain separate identities, with a space of 20 nm between them. On the cytoplasmic side of each of the two membranes the actin filaments of the cytoskeleton run in a circumferential bundle. In the *macula adherens (desmosome)* the cytoplasmic surfaces of adjacent membranes have a dense pad (the plaque) into which bundles of tonofilaments (intermediate filaments) attach. The membranes of the desmosome are separated by an intercellular space (25-30 nm wide), which is filled with a dense fibrous structure consisting of glycoprotein and probably acting as a cement. Hence, it is more common in epithelium but is found also in other tissues (muscle and nerve tissue) where it can vary slightly from the basic form (Plates 1.44, 1.45).

Junctions are considered to keep the cells together and, in the case of the tight junction, to make the cell barrier impermeable. Another connecting structure between cells is the so-called *gap junction* or *communicating junction,* which ultimately results in undelayed transmission of stimuli between adjacent cells, and therefore coordinates cell activity. In these junctions the parallel plasma membranes are 2 nm apart, the gap being traversed by a regular pattern of tube-like protein structures (channels) 1 nm in diameter. Molecules and ions can pass through these gaps as a part of intercellular communication (Plates 1.45 B,C).

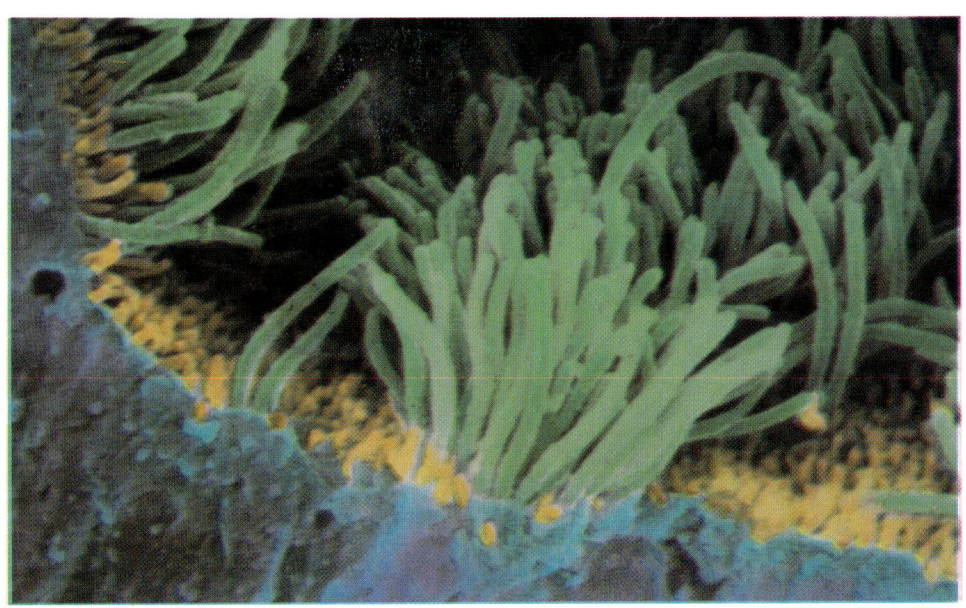

Ciliated cells of rat trachea. The cilia (green) and the microvilli (yellow) are often present over the apical surface of the same cells (blue). (Colored SEM; 6,700 x).

Plate 1.1   11

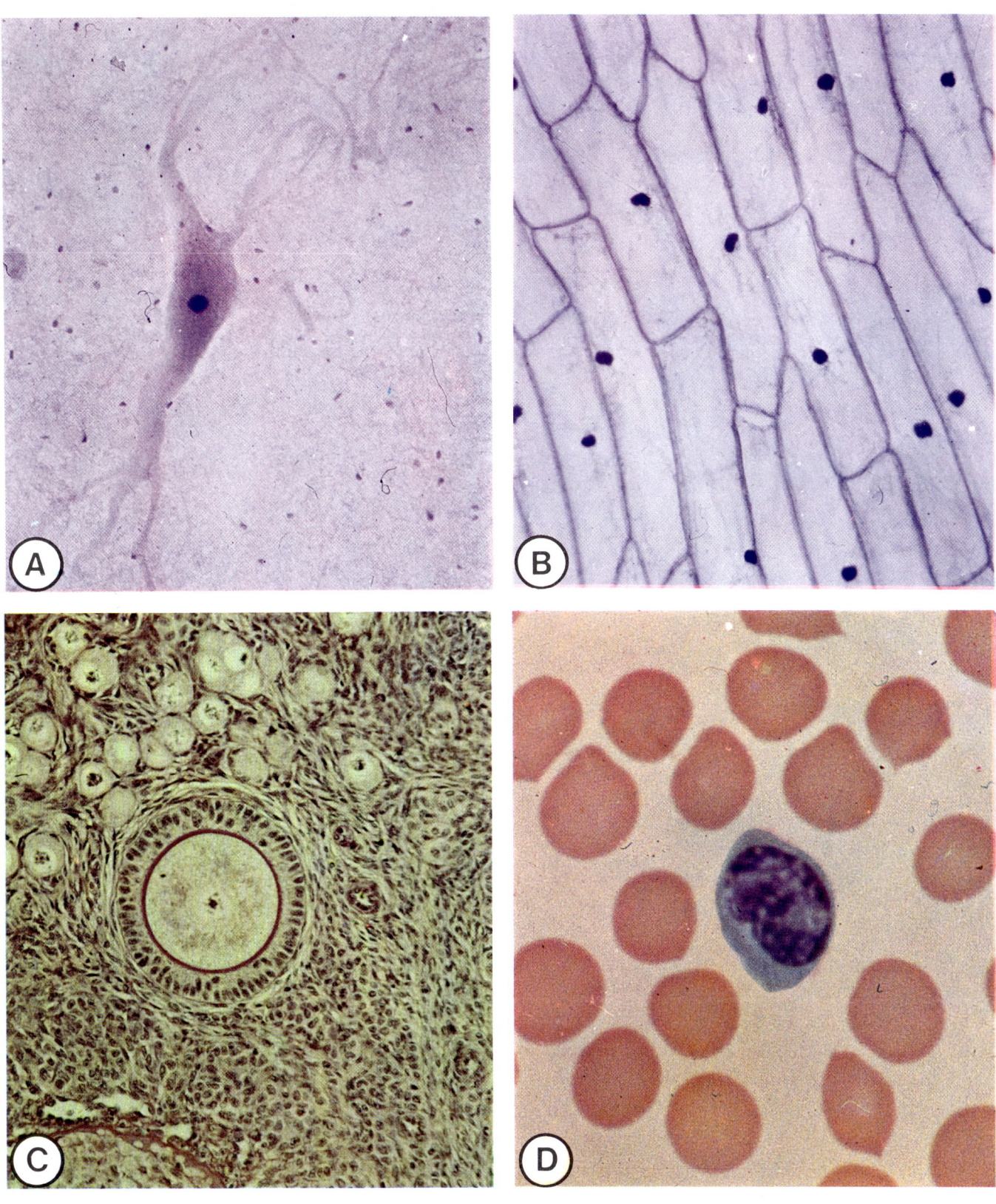

A   **Isolated nerve ganglion cell of bovine autonomic nervous system (ammoniacal carmine, x425).**

B   **Plant cells (carmine, x450).** Note the regular outline of the cell wall and the extensive cytoplasm with small nucleus.

C   **Rabbit oocyte with zona pellucida (in red) surrounded by follicle cells (PAS-hemalum, x250).** The oocyte is one of the largest cells in the body.

D   **Human blood smear (May-Grunwald-Giemsa, x1,500).** In the middle of the field is a lymphocyte with a large nucleus and narrow basophilic cytoplasm, surrounded by numerous erythrocytes. The lymphocyte is one of the smallest cells.

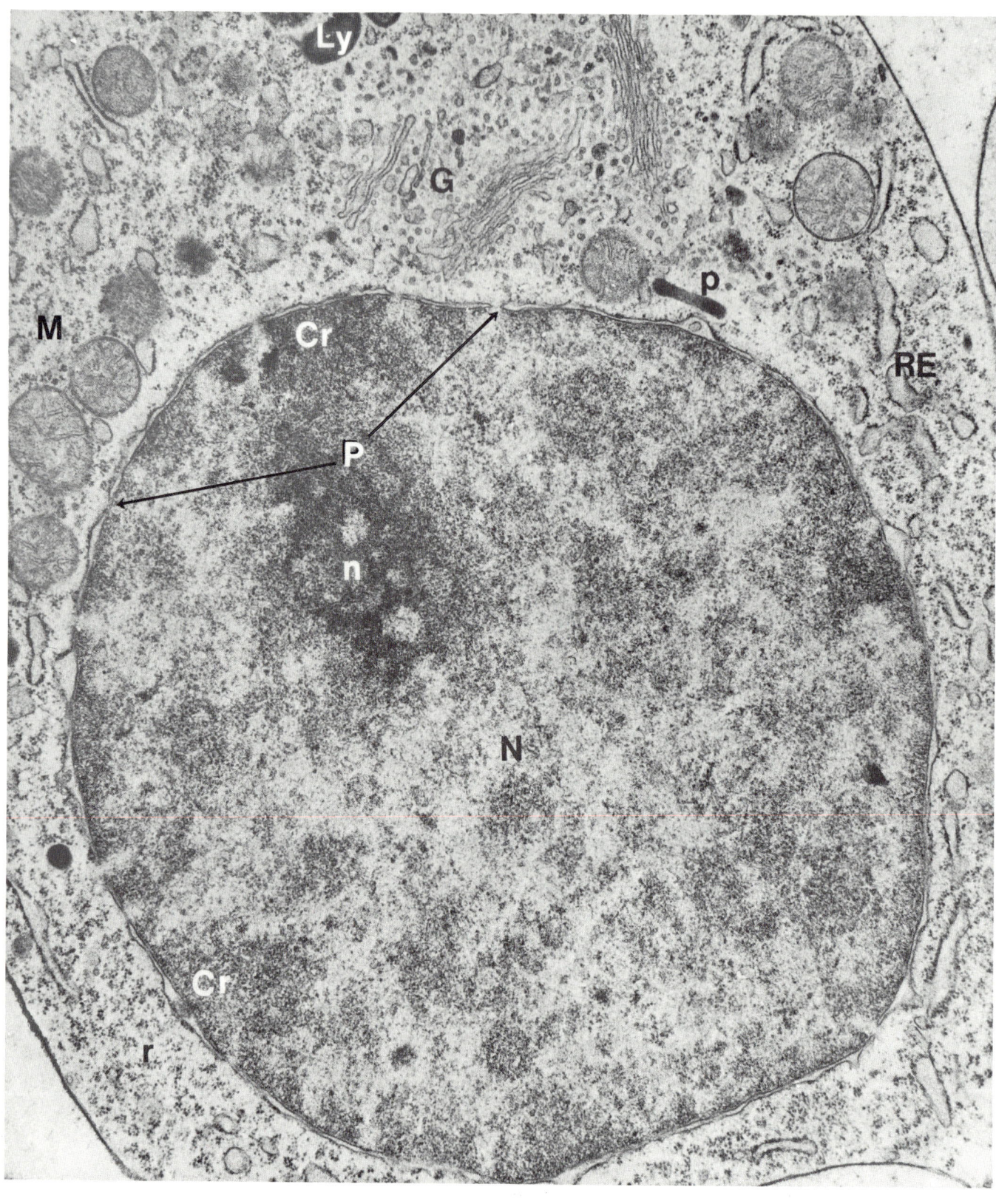

General view of a typical mammalian cell (EM, x22,000). N = nucleus with chromatin uniformly dispersed in the center and condensed (**Cr**) at the periphery. **n** = nucleolus. The internal and external membranes can be seen in the nuclear envelope, together with pores (**P →**). In the cytoplasm there are abundant mitochondria (**M**) with typical cristae. The Golgi complex (**G**) is made up of a parallel array of saccules and of vesicles. Endoplasmic reticulum (**RE**), free ribosomes (**r**), a lysosome (**Ly**) and a pigment granule (**p**) are present.

Plate 1.3   **13**

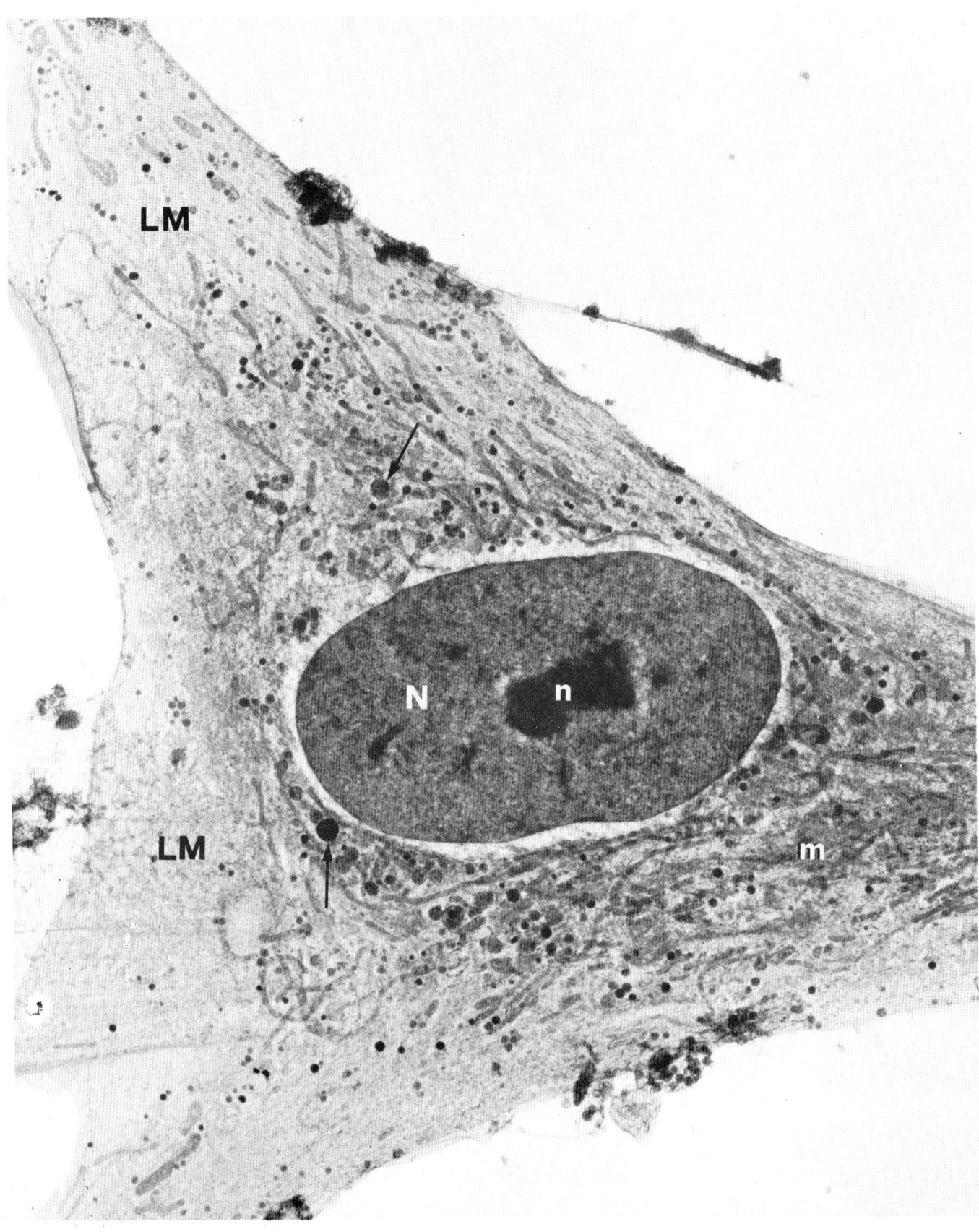

Isolated human diploid cell (high voltage EM observed "in toto," x5,200). In the center of the nucleus (**N**) a nucleolus (**n**) is clearly visible. Abundant elongated mitochondria (**m**) with pigment granules (arrows) lie in the cytoplasmic matrix containing filaments of the microtrabecular lattice (**LM**). Original micrograph by J. Wolosewick.

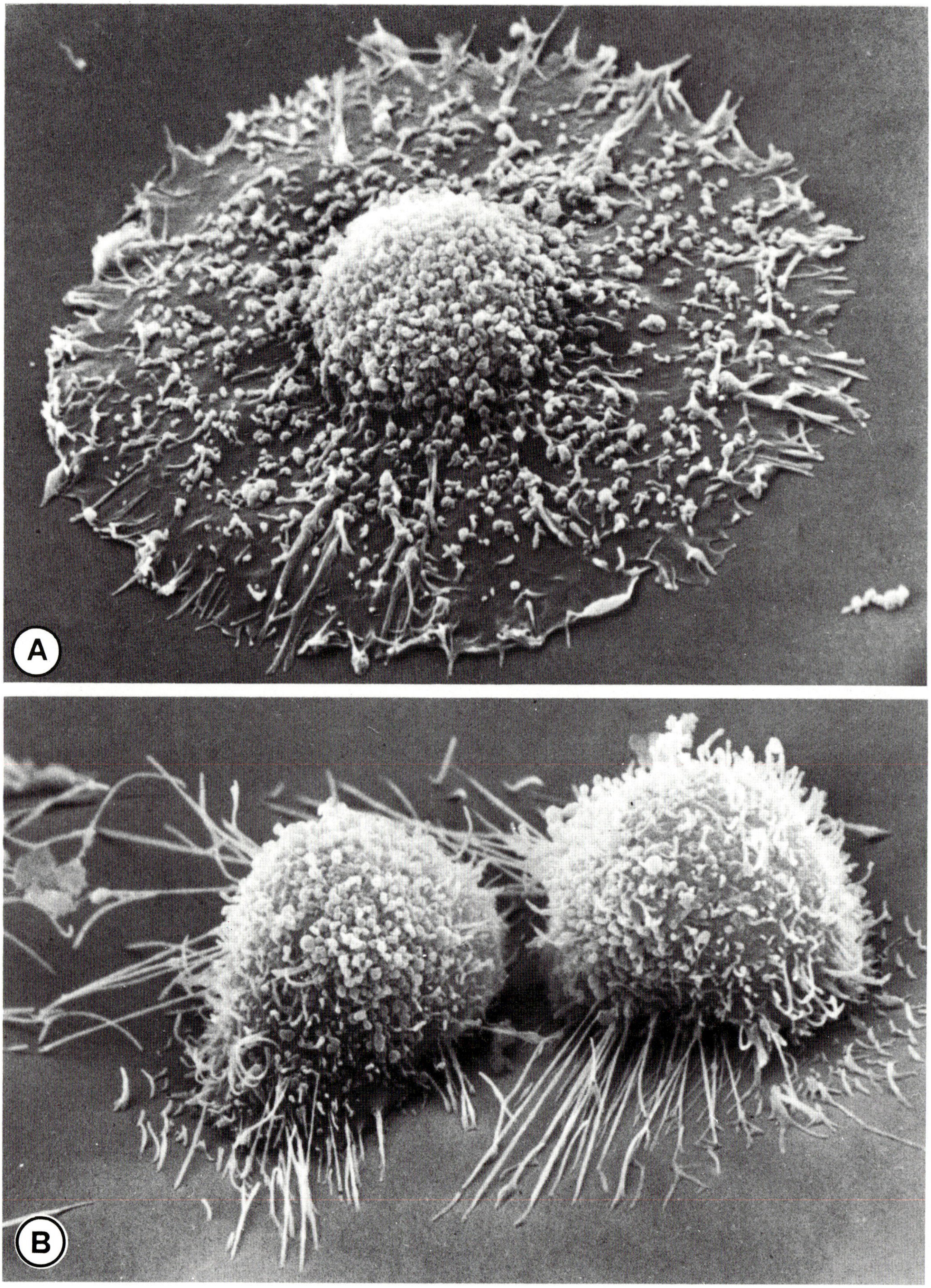

Plate 1.4

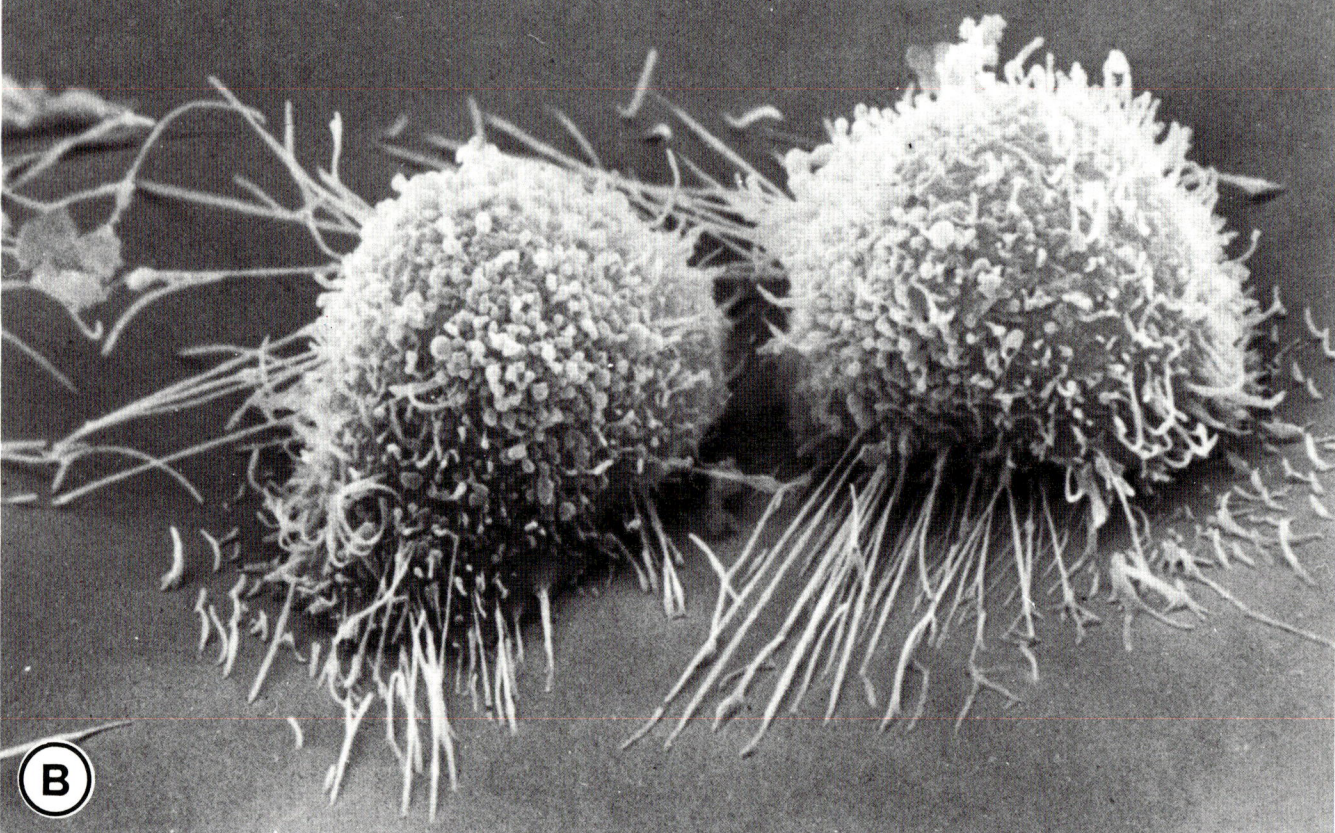

Cultured cells from hamster ovary

A   **Cell in interphase (scanning EM, x8,300).** In the region of the nucleus the cell is dome-shaped, with minute blebs and microvilli projecting from it. Similar projections are seen on the flattened peripheral regions of the cell.

B   **Cells in mitosis (scanning EM, x8,200).** The surface of the cells is rich in blebs and microvilli. By courtesy of M. Gershenbaum.

Plate 1.5   **15**

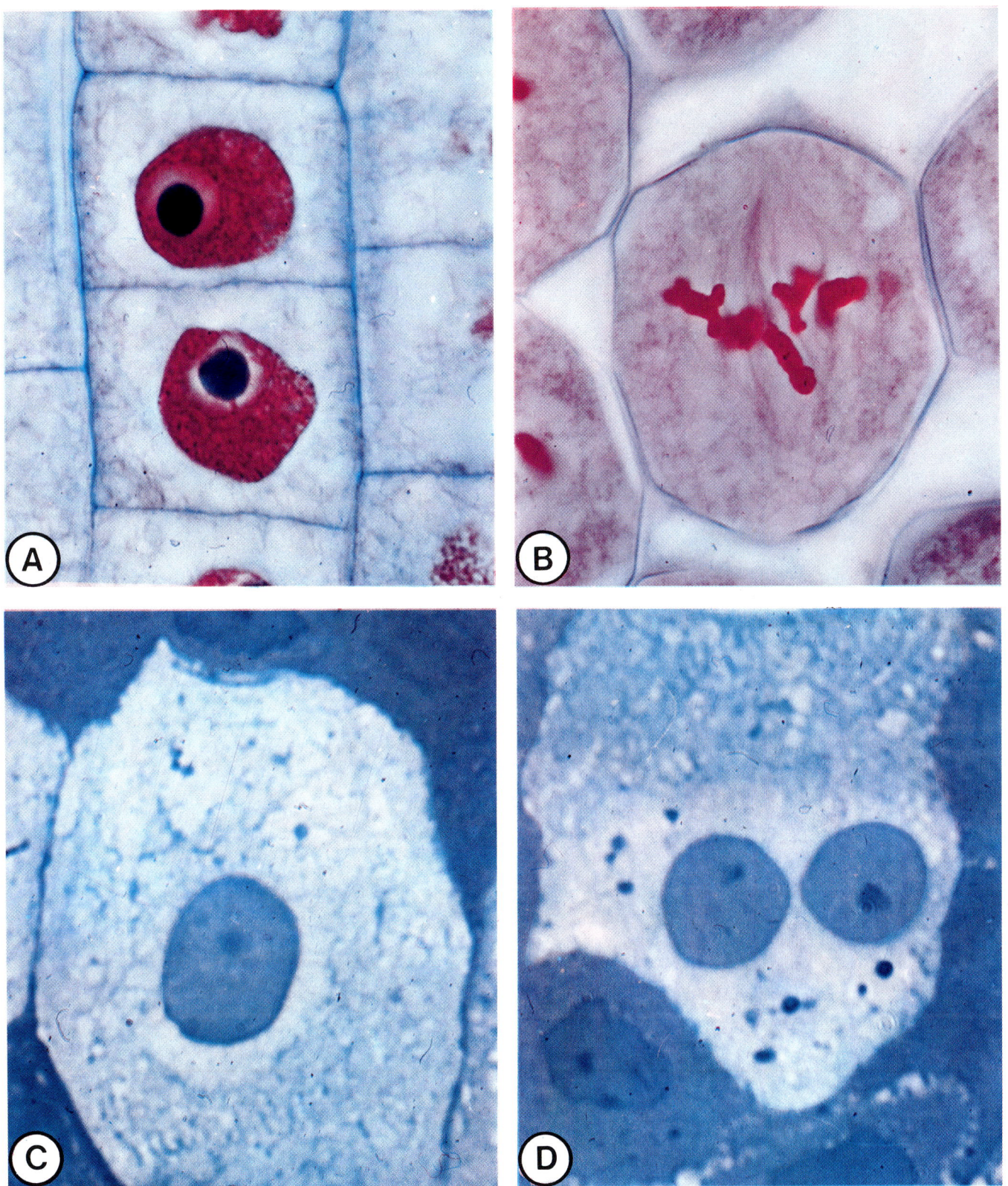

A   **Plant cells in interphase (Feulgen & toluidine blue, x800).** The nucleolus is dark blue, the nucleus red, the cytoplasm medium light blue, and the cell wall, outlining the cells, is pale blue.

B   **Plant cell in mitosis (metaphase) (Feulgen & toluidine blue, x800).** Chromosomes (red) are attached to fibers of the mitotic spindle.

C   **Adluminal cells from transitional epithelium (urothelium) of the rat urinary bladder. (methylene blue, x1,700).**

D   **Binucleate cell from the luminal layer of transitional epithelium of rat urinary bladder (methylene blue, x1,700). Semithin section.** By courtesy of E. Nesci.

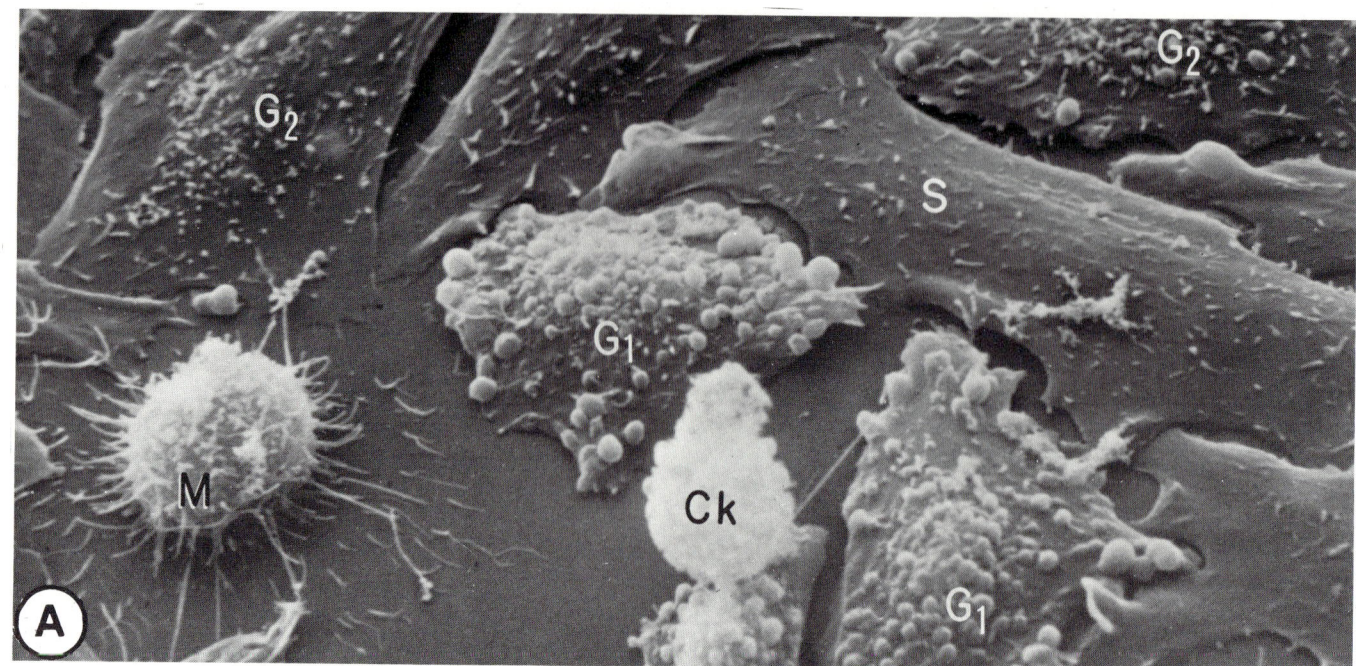

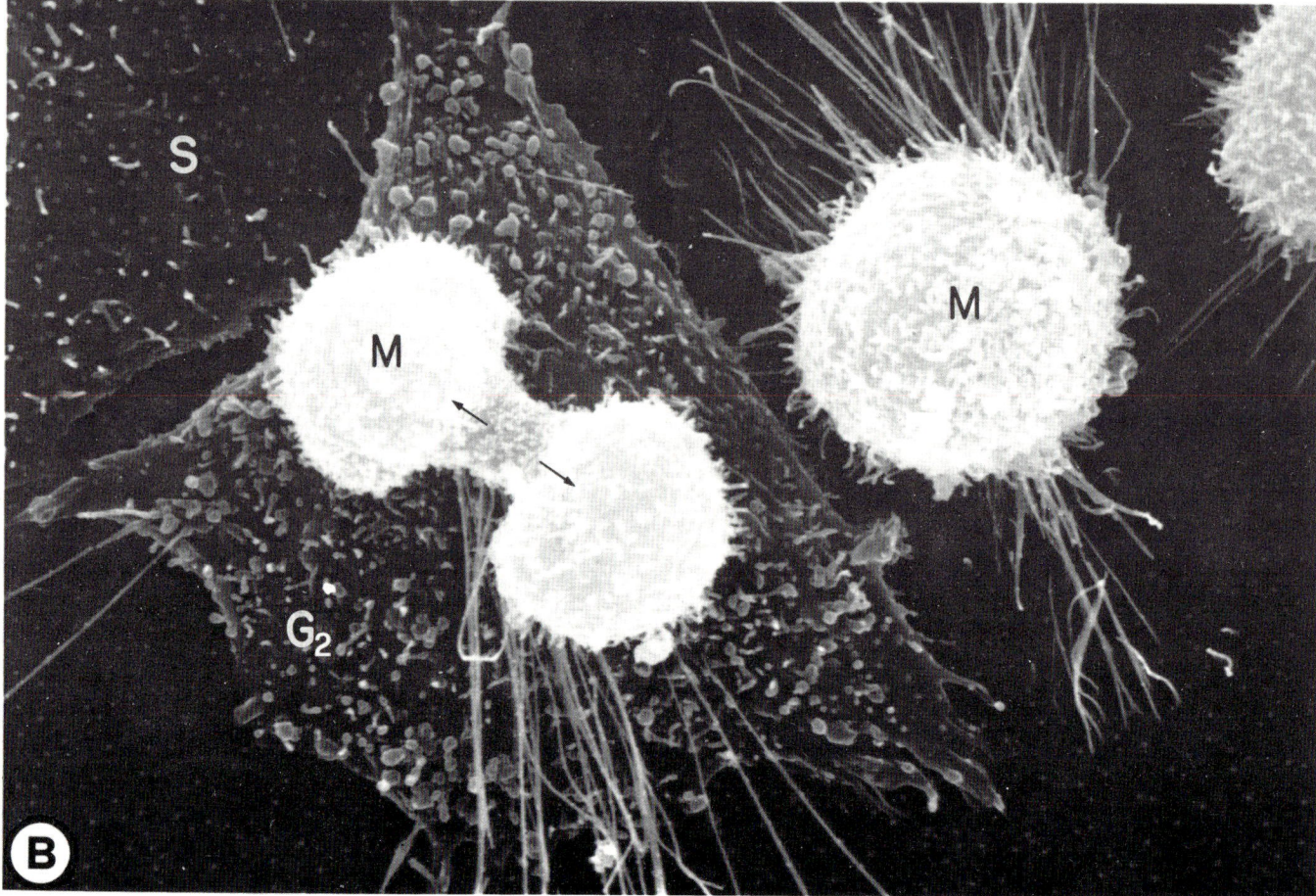

A   **Cells in various phases of the cell cycle (scanning EM, x200).** During mitosis **(M)** the cells are attached to the culture
    substratum by thin filopodia. Blebs are abundant during the **G1** phase. In the **S** phase the cells have a moderately smooth
    surface. Microvilli reappear in the **G2** phase. The cell marked **Ck** is in the last phase of mitosis. By courtesy of K.R. Porter,
    T.T. Puck, H.H. Hsie and D. Kelly. Cell 2:145, 1974.
B   **Cells in culture (scanning EM, x4,100).** Some cells are in mitosis **(M)** and have microvilli and typical long filopodia. S and G2
    indicate two cells in the **S** and **G2** phases of the cell cycle. The cell in the middle is in the last stage of mitosis (*cytokinesis*) and
    is about to split into two daughter cells (→).

Plate 1.7   **17**

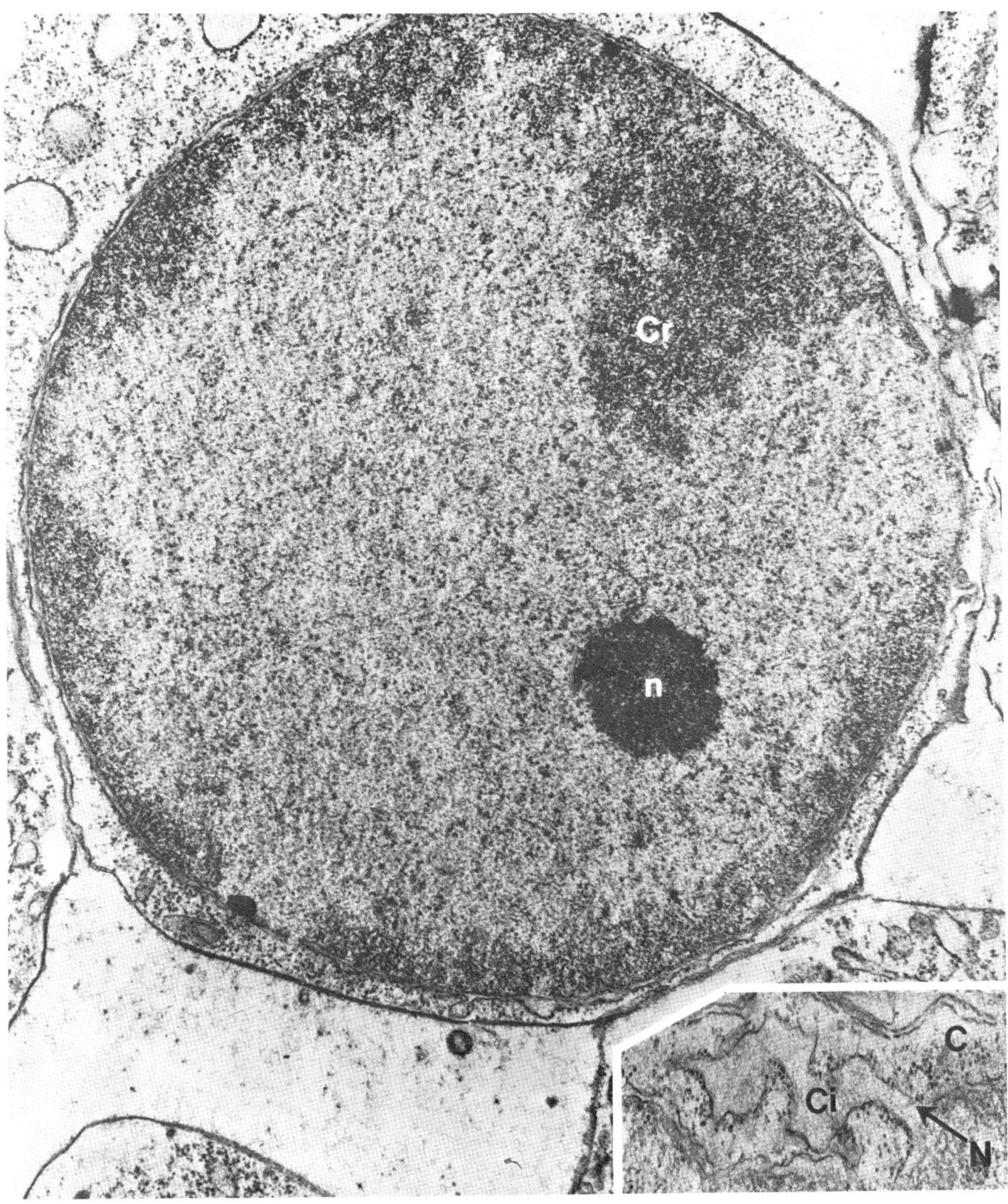

Nucleus and perinuclear cistern (EM, x25,000). The nucleus is a dynamic structure which undergoes continual change. The picture shows the nucleus of a perfectly regular mouse epithelium cell about to undergo mitosis (early prophase). The nuclear envelope is still visible but is about to disappear. The chromatin **(Cr)** inside the nucleus will be condensing to form the chromosomes. The nucleolus **(n)**, now reduced to a dense mass, will also disappear during mitosis.

Inset, bottom right: a nuclear envelope raised to form a spacious cistern (→) connected to the membrane system of the endoplasmic reticulum (x45,000). N = nucleus. **Ci** = perinuclear cistern continuous with the cytoplasmic membranes **(C)**. From P. Motta. Z. Zellforsch. 68:308, 1965.

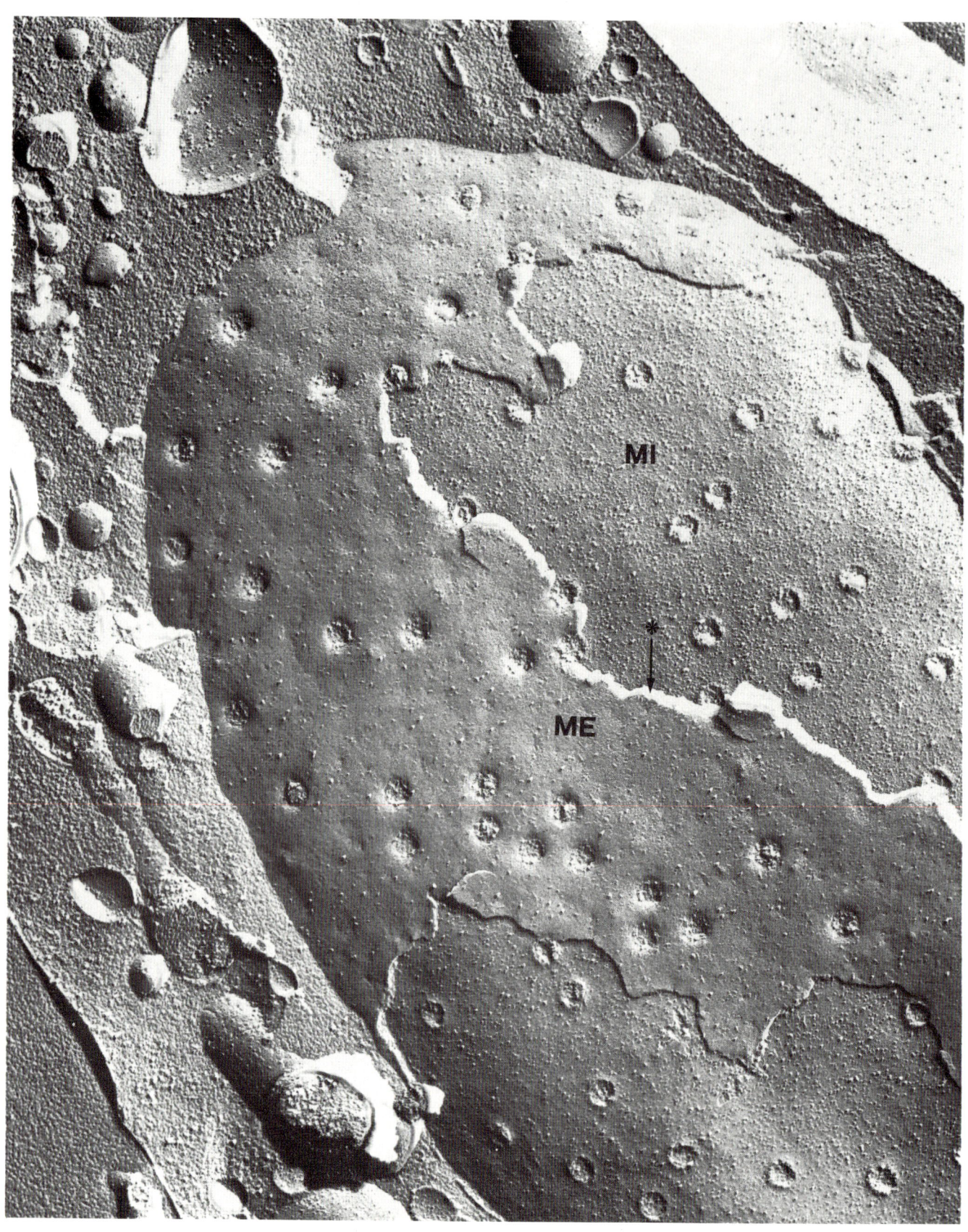

Interphase nucleus with pores of the nuclear envelope (EM, freeze fracture, x54,000). Both the internal **(MI)** and the external **(ME)** membranes of the nuclear envelope can be seen. The fracture plane includes the inner compartment of the envelope (*→). Around the nucleus a fringe of cytoplasm is visible. By courtesy of L.A. Staehelin.

Plate 1.9   19

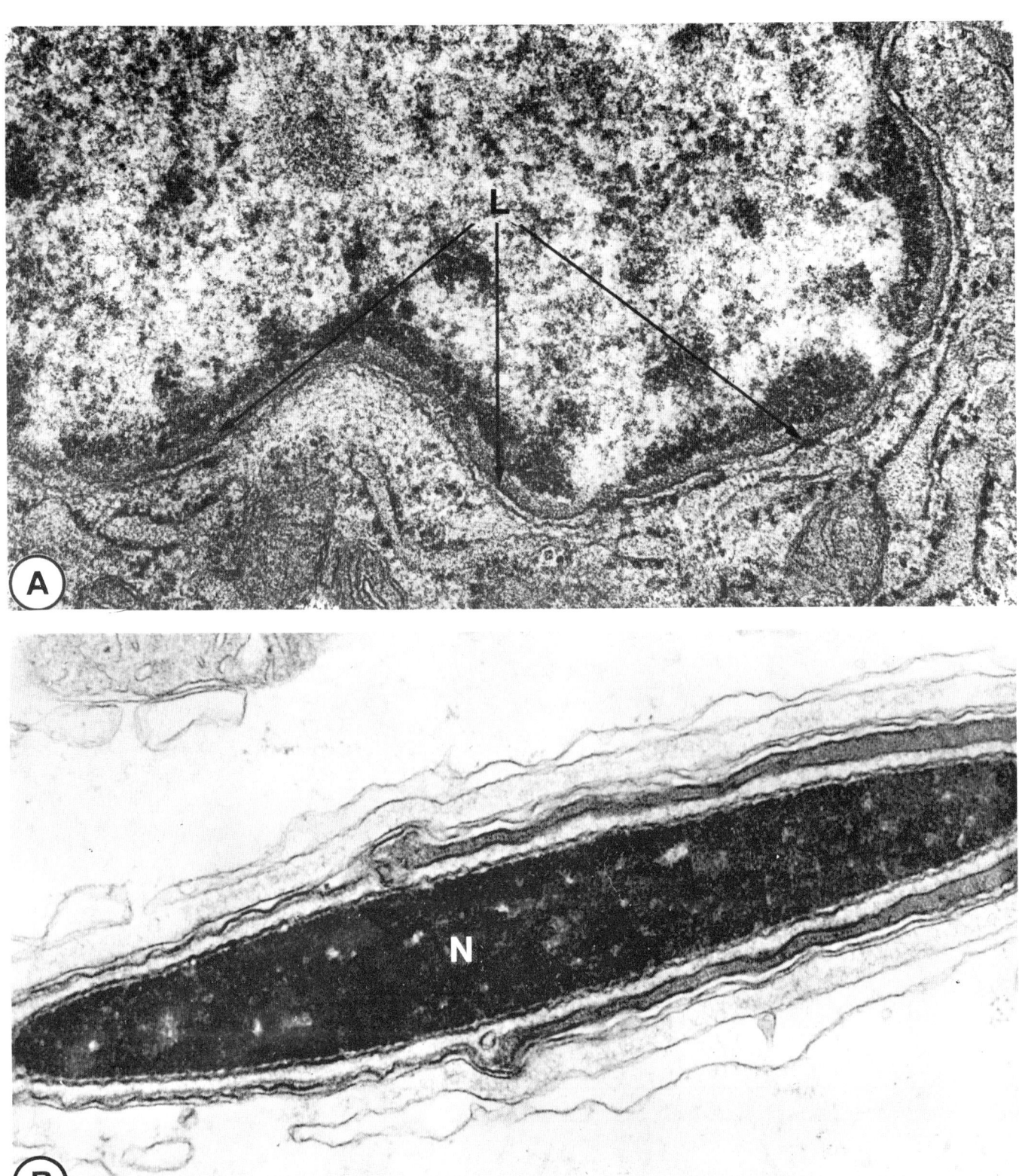

A   **Nucleus of human plasma cell (EM, x65,000).** The nucleus has an irregular outline. The internal layer of the nuclear envelope has a dense lamina (*zonula nucleus limitans*) (**L→**). The lamina is present in many cells, and plays a supporting role. By courtesy of G.F. Patrizi.

B   **Head of mouse sperm (EM, x40,000).** The head of the spermatozoon is a typical example of a highly modified nucleus. The chromatin is highly condensed, and the nuclear material (**N**) is enclosed by a nuclear envelope.There is no nucleolus.

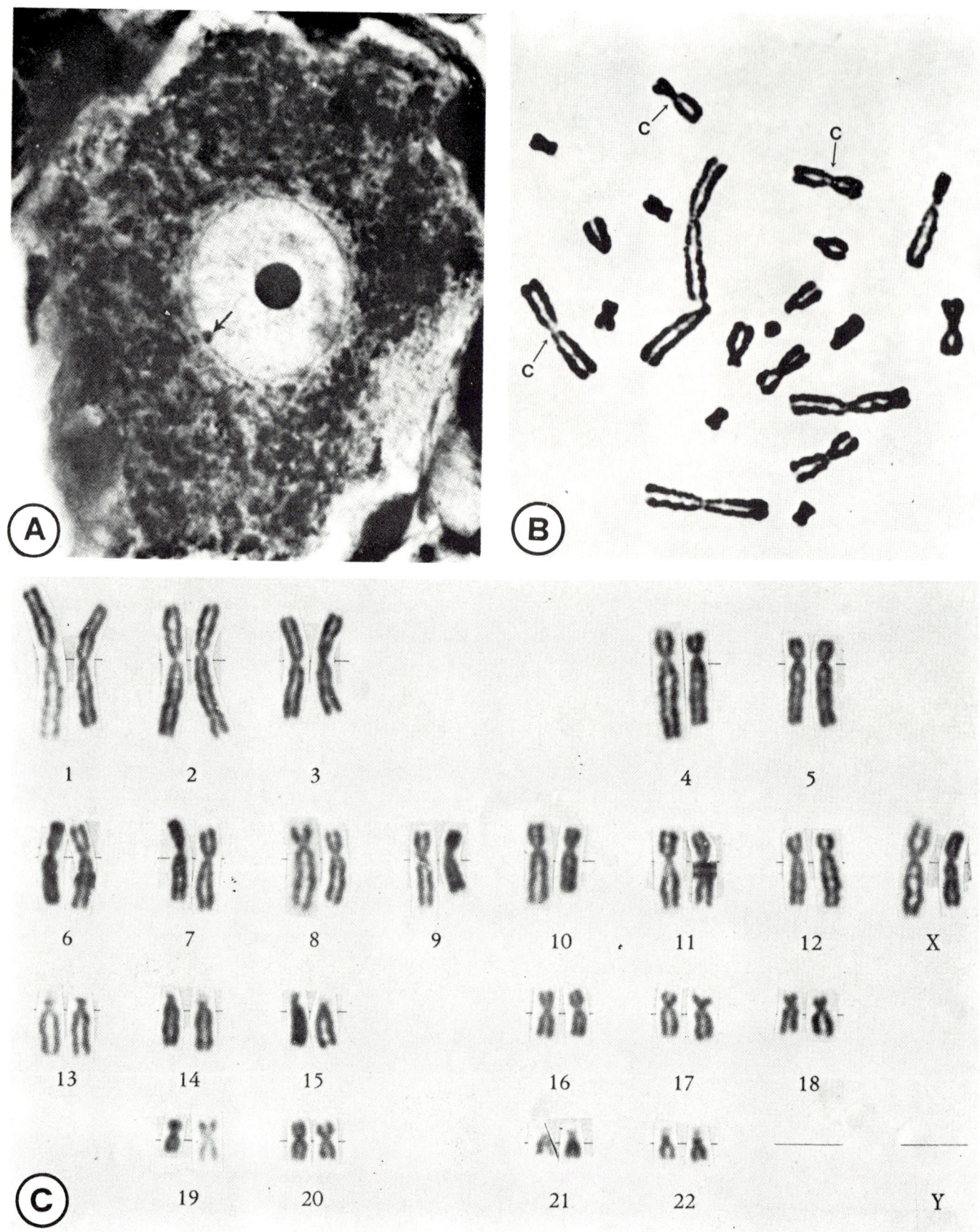

A   **Sex chromatin (iron hematoxylin, x350).** The "Barr body" or sex chromatin in a female cell of a spinal ganglion. It is attached (→) to the internal layer of the nuclear envelope. From M.L. Barr. In: V. Monesi. *Istologia*. Piccin Editore, Padua, 1980.

B   **Metaphase chromosomes in male hamster germ cell (2n = 22) (orcein, x1,700).** The chromosomes isolated from a cell in metaphase show the typical constriction (centromere) (**C→**). By courtesy of V. Monesi.

C   **Karyotype of human female (XX) (Giemsa, x1,320).** Original photograph by R. M. Gualtieri and C.R.S. Motta.

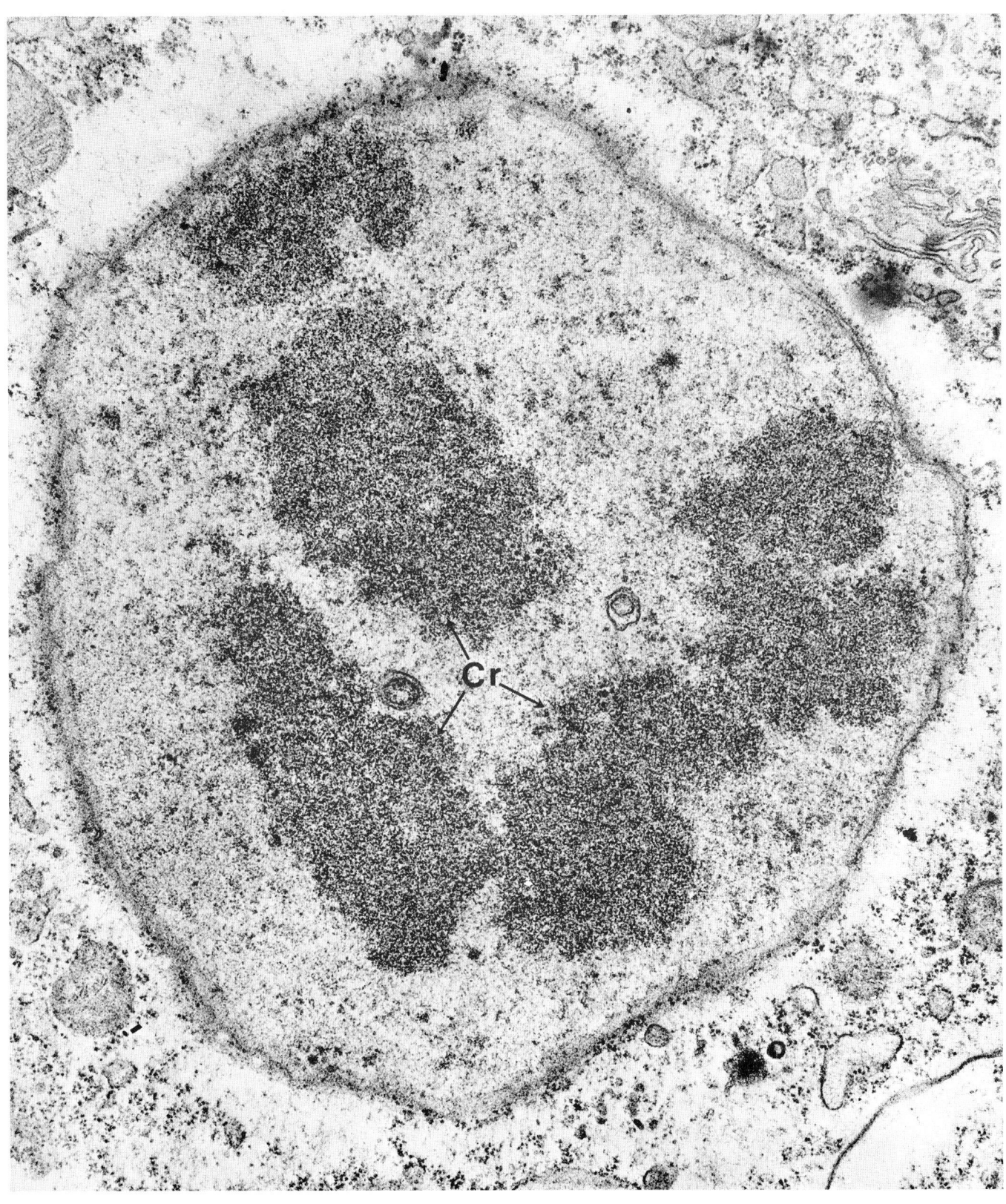

Chromosomes in mouse epithelial cell (EM, x19,500). The nucleus of this epthelial cell was photographed in mitosis between late prophase and the beginning of metaphase. The nuclear envelope will soon disappear. The chromatin has condensed to form opaque masses, the condensing chromosomes. The nucleolus is no longer a component of the nucleus, having totally disappeared. Note the zone of low density around the nucleus.

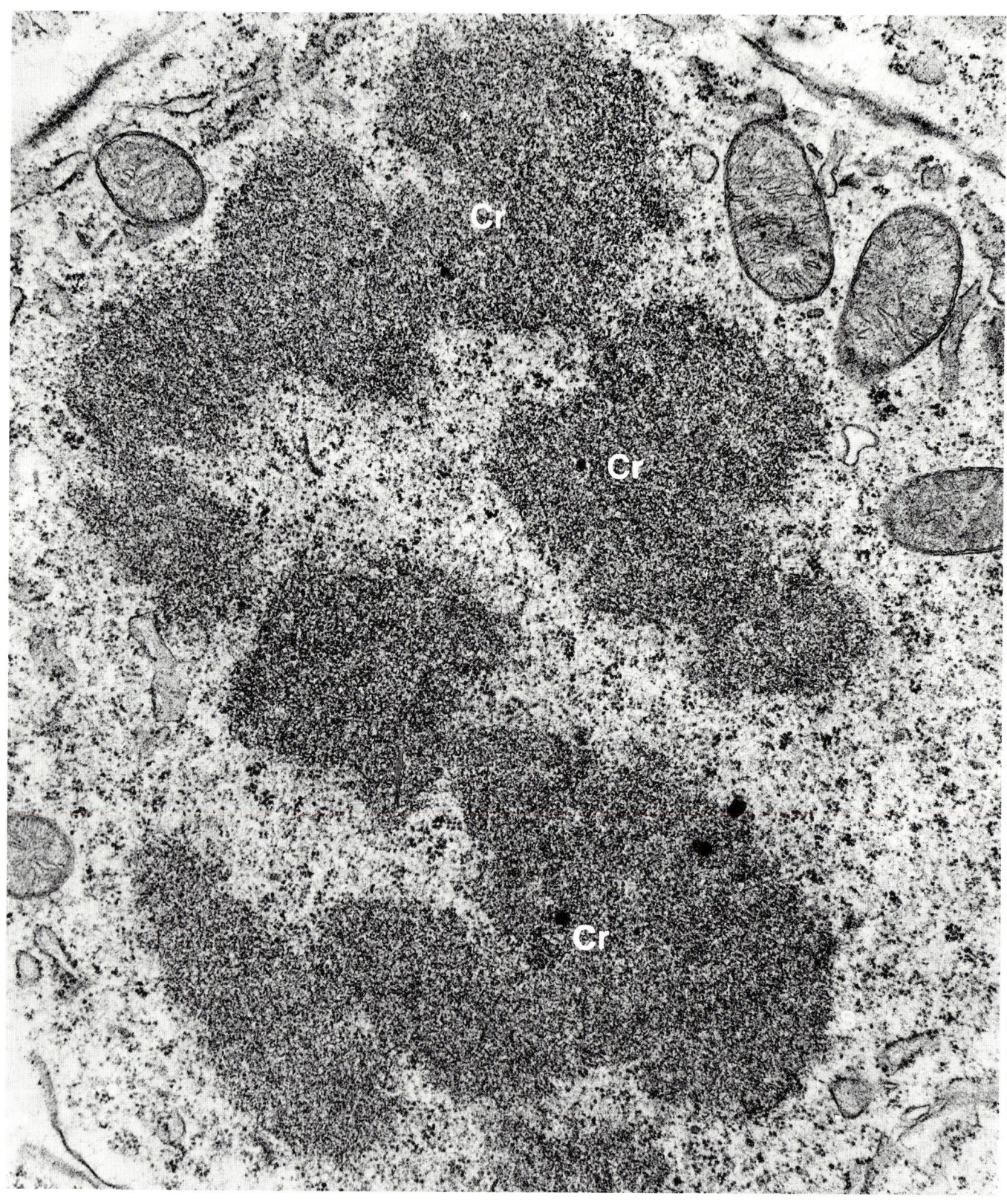

Early metaphase chromosomes in mouse epithelial cell (EM), × 25,000). chromatin has condensed into chromosomes **(Cr).** The nuclear envelope no longer intervenes between the chromosomes and the mitochondria of the cytoplasm. Few structural details of the chromosomes can be distinguished in thin sections by the electron microscope. They appear as thin filaments and highly concentrated small granules.

Plate 1.13   23

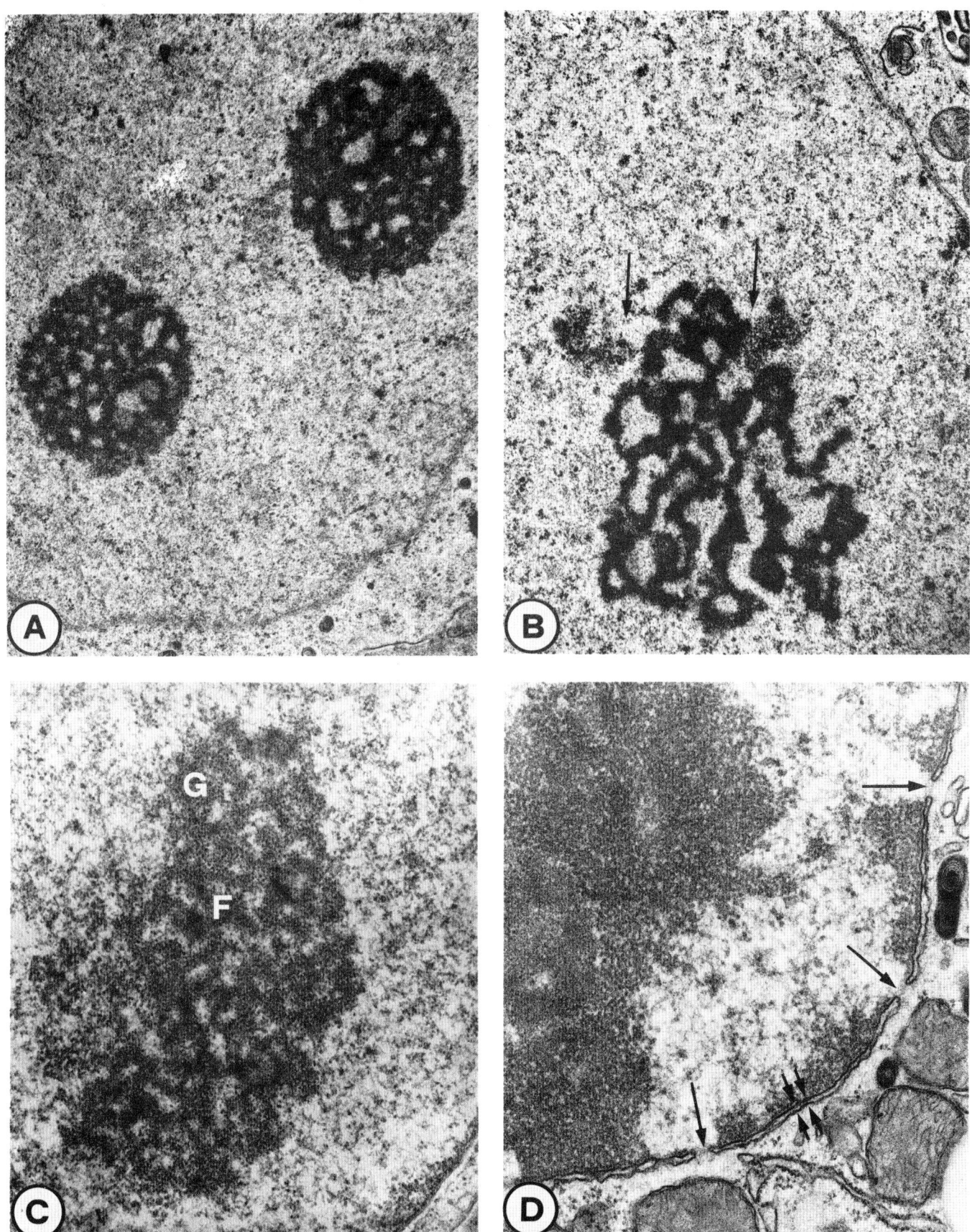

A **Nucleus with two nucleoli in human female germ cell (EM, x14,300).** Note the reticular structure of the nucleolus
    (nucleolonema), and the extreme density of the nucleolus as compared with the surrounding nuclear matrix.

B **Nucleolus of human luteal cell (EM, x16,250).** Small masses of chromatin (arrows) are associated with the nucleolus.

C **Nucleolus of rat liver cell (EM, x27,000).** The filamentous (F) and granular (G) components are apparent.

D **Nucleolus, pores and nuclear envelope of rat cell (EM, x25,000). The nucleolus and the condensed chromatin
    that is in contact with the internal layer of the nuclear envelope can be seen. The pores of the nuclear envelope (→) are visible,
    as are the two layers of the envelope enclosing a narrow perinuclear cistern (→←).**

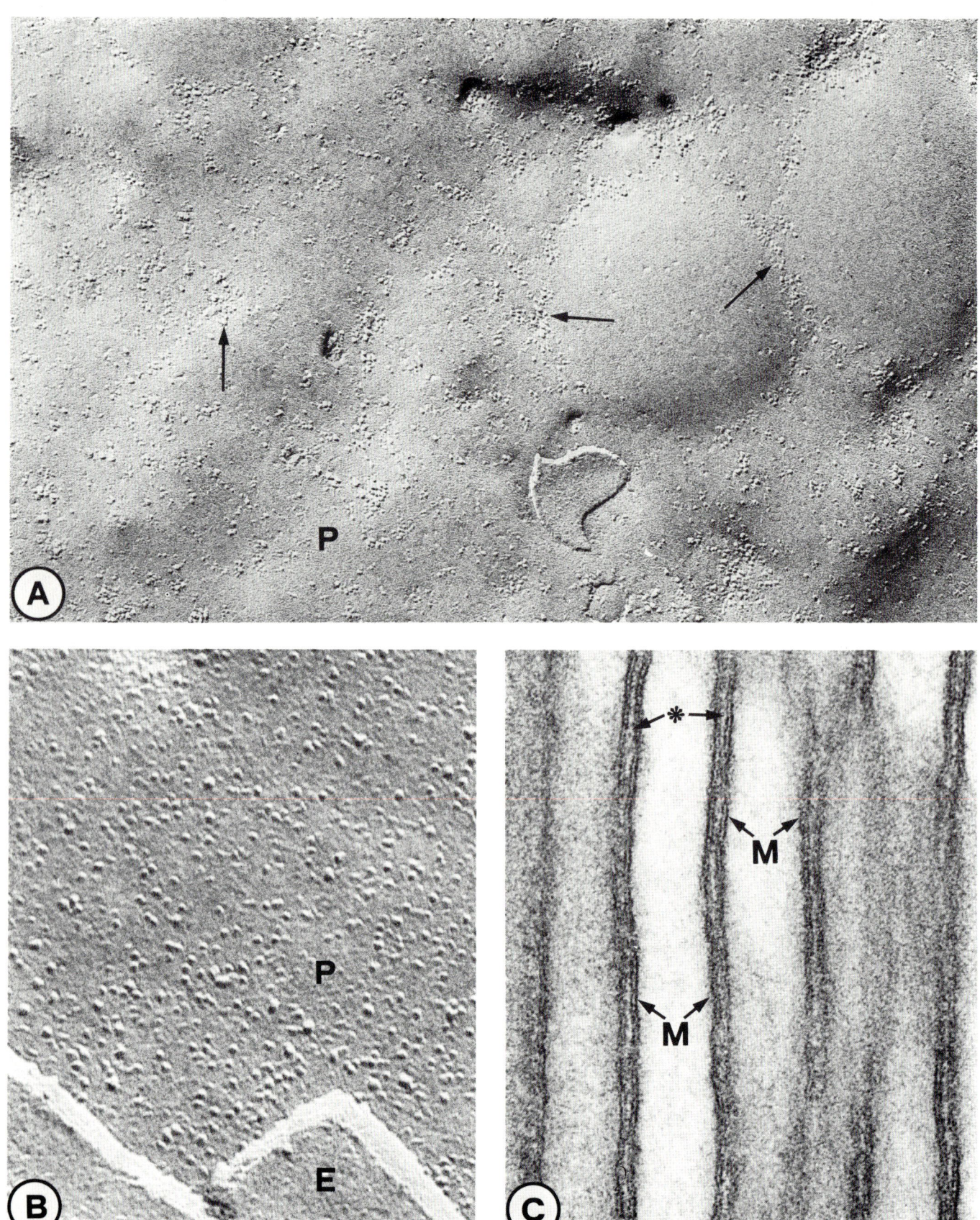

A **Plasma membrane of an epithelial cell (EM, freeze fracture, x63,000).** The fracture shows the protoplasmic surface of the plasmalemma (P face). The particles scattered on this face (→) are large membranous proteins embedded in the lipid bilayer.

B **Plasma membrane of an epithelial cell (EM, freeze fracture, x160,000).** The fracture shows the P face of the membrane. The small protuberances on side P are proteins of the membrane. A small area of the external face **(E)** of the plasmalemma can be seen.

C **Plasma membranes of adjacent microvilli (EM, x160,000).** Note the trilaminar structure of the plasma membranes (**M** →) separated by narrow intercellular spaces (*→). Original micrographs by G. Familiari.

Plate 1.15   **25**

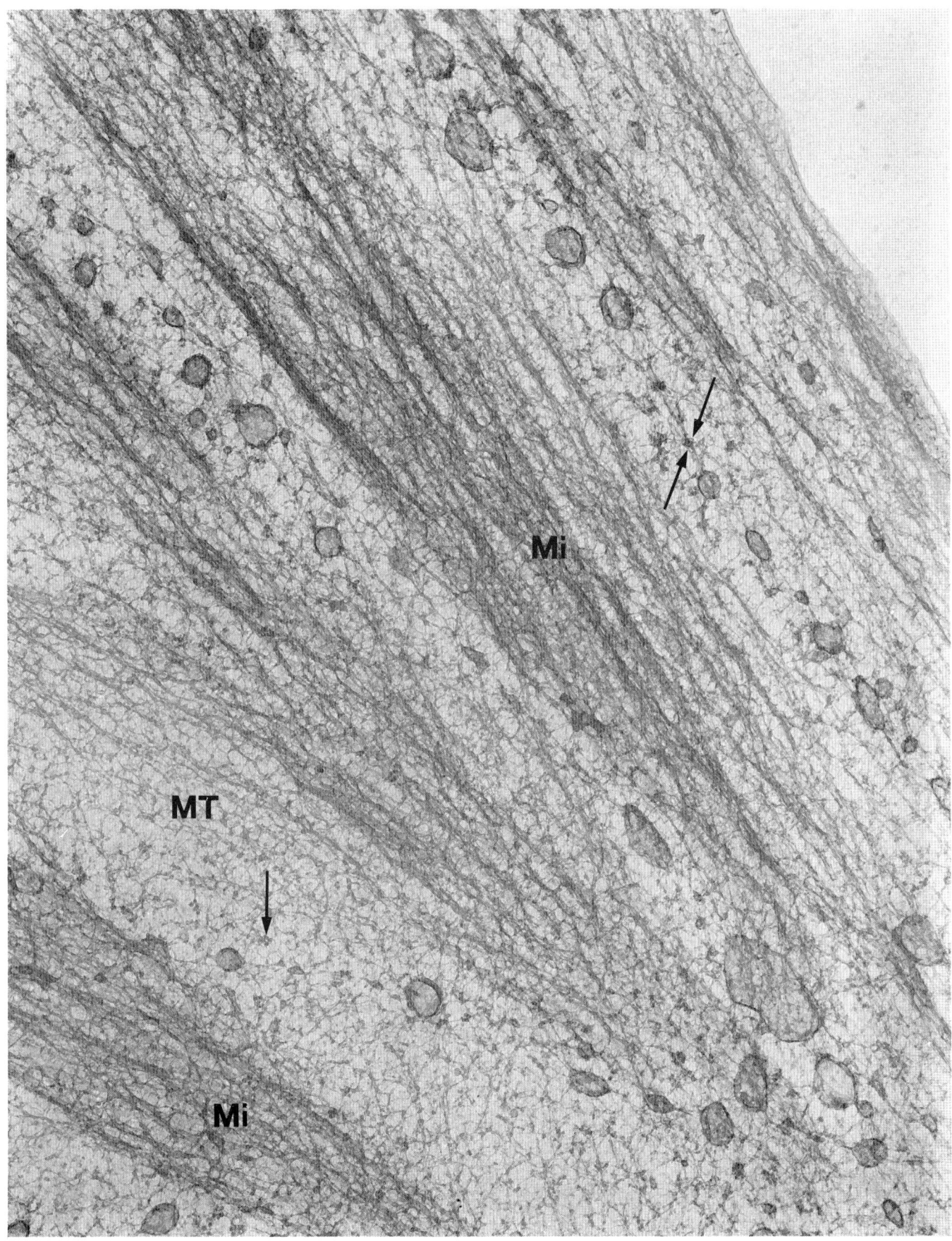

Microtrabecular lattice of mammalian cell cultured in vitro (high voltage EM, x50,000). At this magnification the lattice is seen to consist of a fine web of filaments (*microtrabeculae*) (**MT**). This lattice acts as a supporting structure for the cell, maintaining the position as well as directing the movement of cellular organelles. Bundles of microfilaments (**Mi**) running lengthwise are associated with the microtrabecular network. Numerous polysomes are contained at the nodal points of the microtrabeculae (→). By courtesy of K.R. Porter.

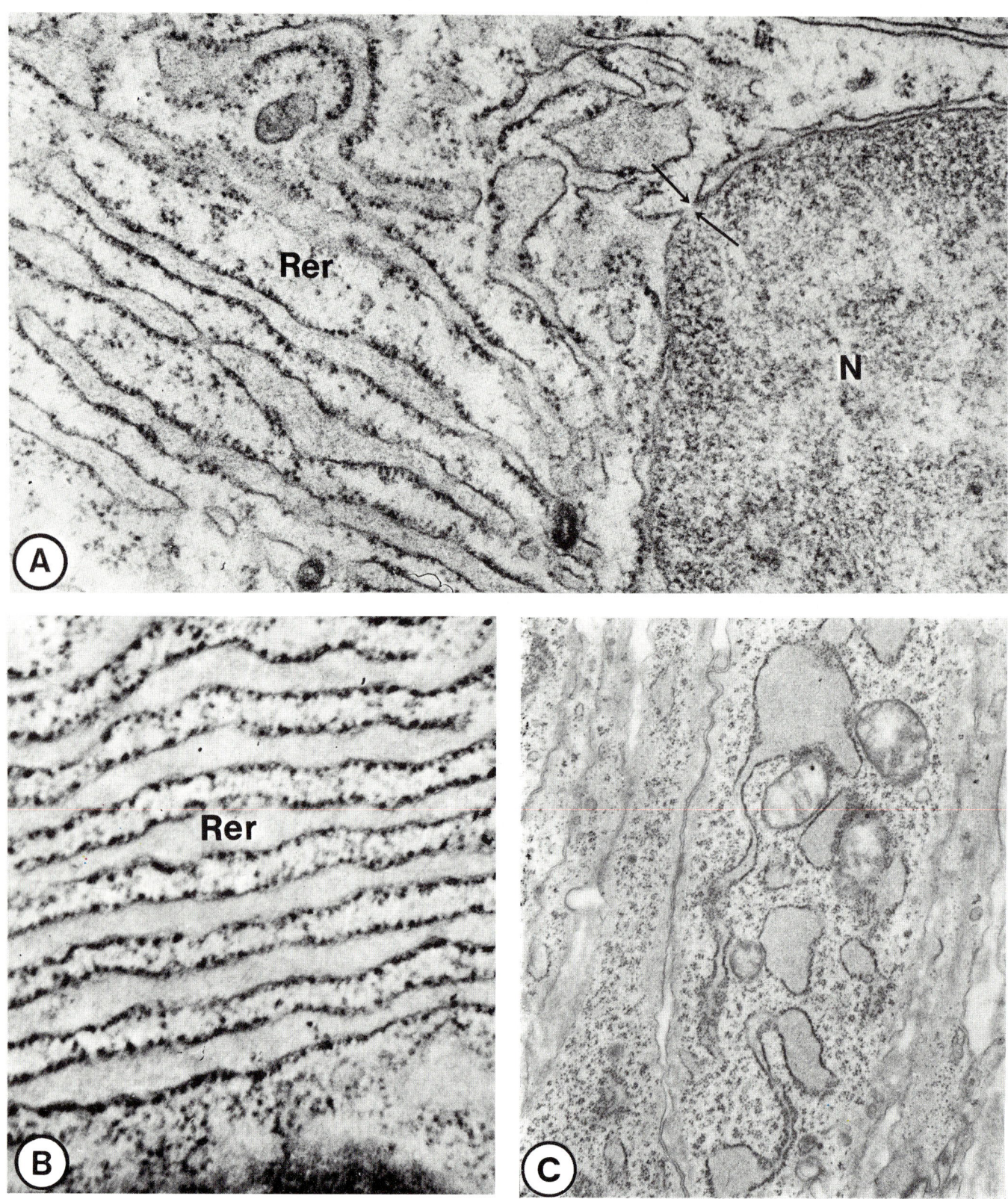

A **Rough endoplasmic reticulum in a protein-secreting cell of rat connective tissue (EM, x42,000).** Adhering to the membranes of the endoplasmic reticulum (**Rer**) there are numerous ribosomes. The cisternae of the endoplasmic reticulum contain material denser than the surrounding cytoplasm, which is the synthetic product. Note the continuity between the endoplasmic reticulum and the nuclear envelope (→). N = nucleus.

B **Endoplasmic reticulum of a rabbit plasma cell (EM, x60,000).** The membranes (**Rer**) are regularly aligned and are studded with ribosomes.

C **Cisternae of the rough endoplasmic reticulum of fibroblast (EM, x16,500).** The dilated cisternae of the endoplasmic reticulum contain protein material. There appear to be a number of free ribosomes in the cytoplasm.

Plate 1.17 27

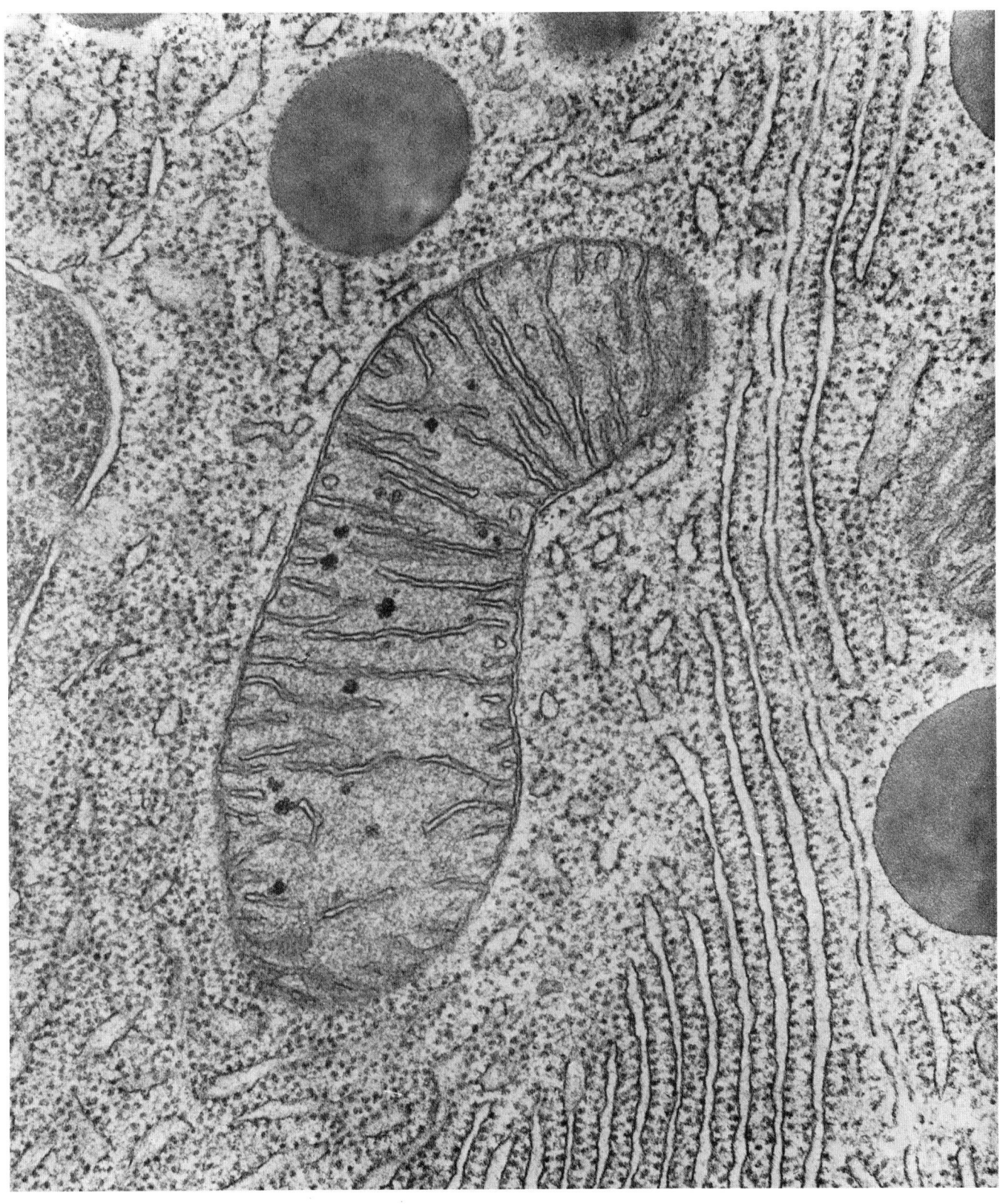

Rough endoplasmic reticulum and mitochondria of pancreatic acinar cell (EM, x77,500). The organelle in the center of the field shows the typical mitochondrial structure. Dense granules lie among the cristae. The spherical bodies in the cytoplasm are lipid droplets. By courtesy of K.R. Porter.

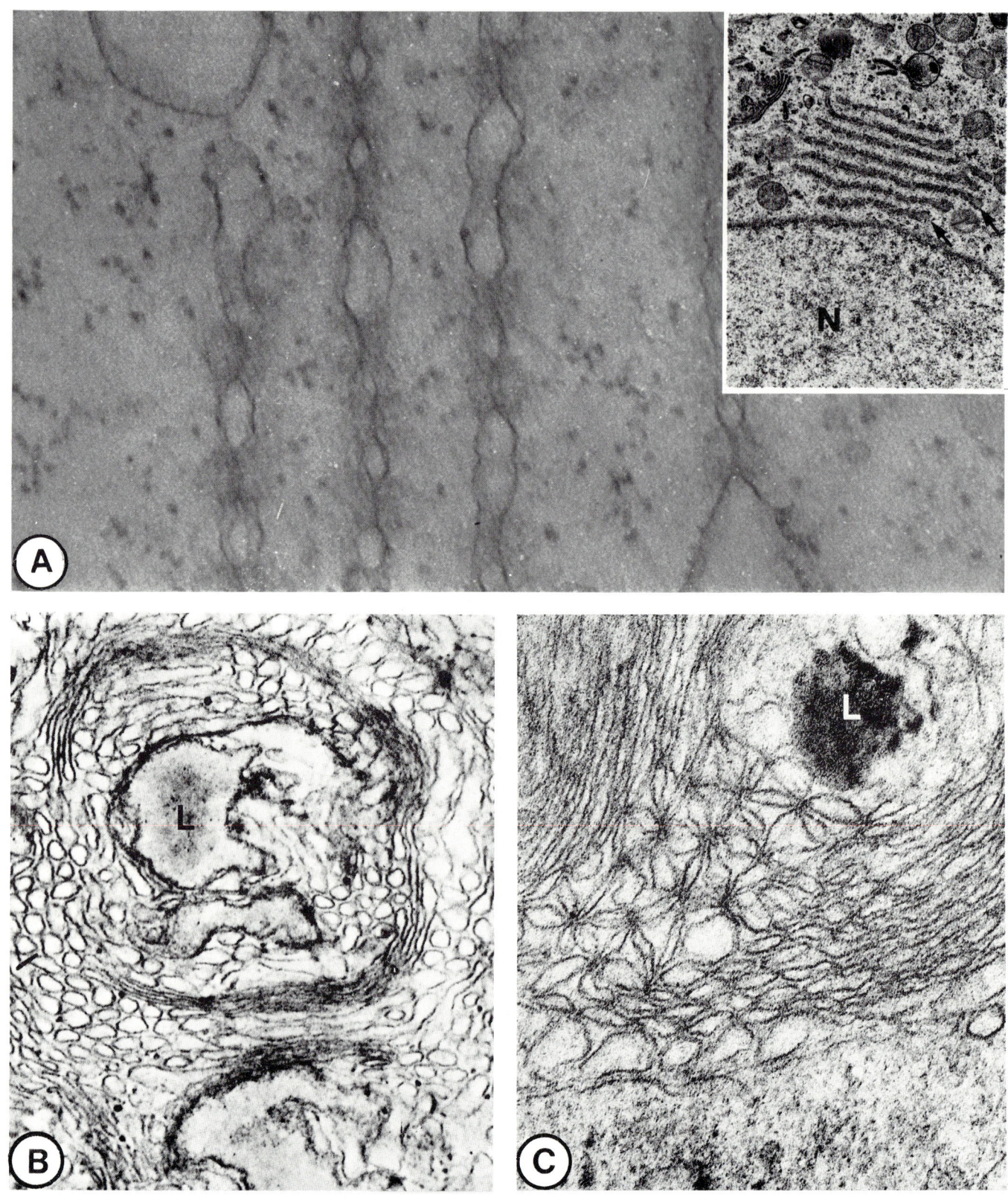

A   **Annulate lamellae in the cytoplasm of salamander oocyte EM, x73,000).** The membranes of the annulate lamellae are similar
    to those of the nuclear envelope and also to the endoplasmic reticulum, from which they may be derived. By courtesy of S.
    Wischnitzer. Int. Rev. Cytol. 27:265, 1970. **Inset: seven annulate lamellae aligned parallel (→) to the nuclear envelope
    (x10,000). N** = nucleus.

B   **Smooth endoplasmic reticulum of steroid-secreting cell from rabbit ovary (EM, x40,000).** Note typical honeycomb
    arrangement of the smooth endoplasmic reticulum surrounding the lipid inclusions (L). From P. Motta. Biol. Lat. 19:107,
    1966.

C   **Membranes of the smooth endoplasmic reticulum (EM, x60,000).** Parallel arrays of membranes are seen. **L** = lipid
    droplet.

Plate 1.19   **29**

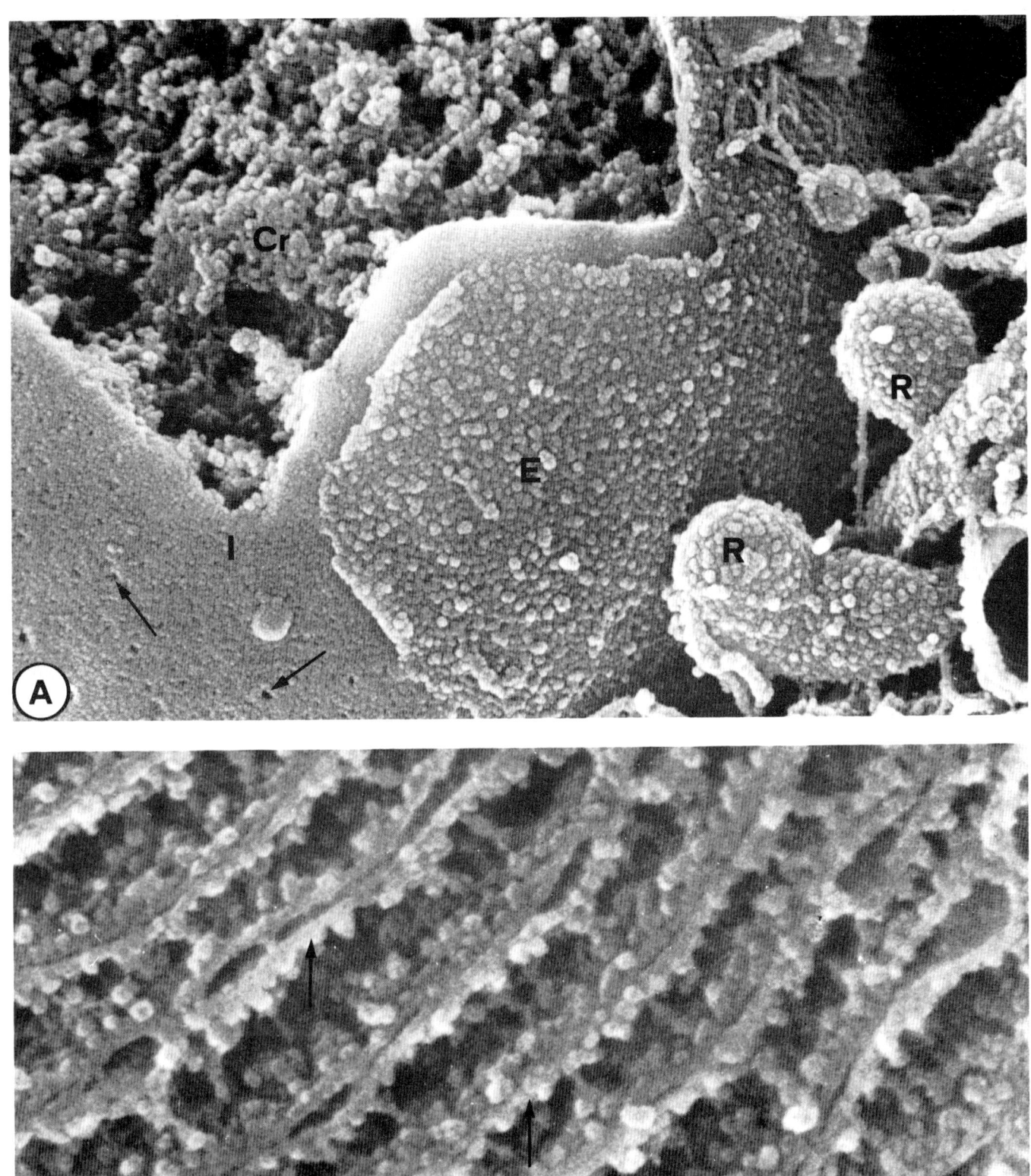

A   **Nucleus, nuclear envelope and rough endoplasmic reticulum (scanning EM, x48,000).** The internal layer **(I)** of the nuclear
    envelope has a smooth surface with small pores (→). The external layer **(E)** has an abundance of ribosomes. In the adjacent
    cytoplasm are elements of the rough endoplasmic reticulum **(R)** with a structure similar to that of the external layer of the
    nuclear envelope. The nucleus contains small globular material which may be chromatin **(Cr)**.

B   **Rough endoplasmic reticulum (scanning EM, x86,000).** Ribosomes (→) are located on the cytoplasmic surface of the
    membranes. By courtesy of K. Tanaka. In: T. Fujita, K. Tanaka and J. Tokunaga. *Scanning Electron Microscopic Atlas of
    Cells and Tissues.* Igaku-Shoin Ltd., Tokyo/New York, 1981.

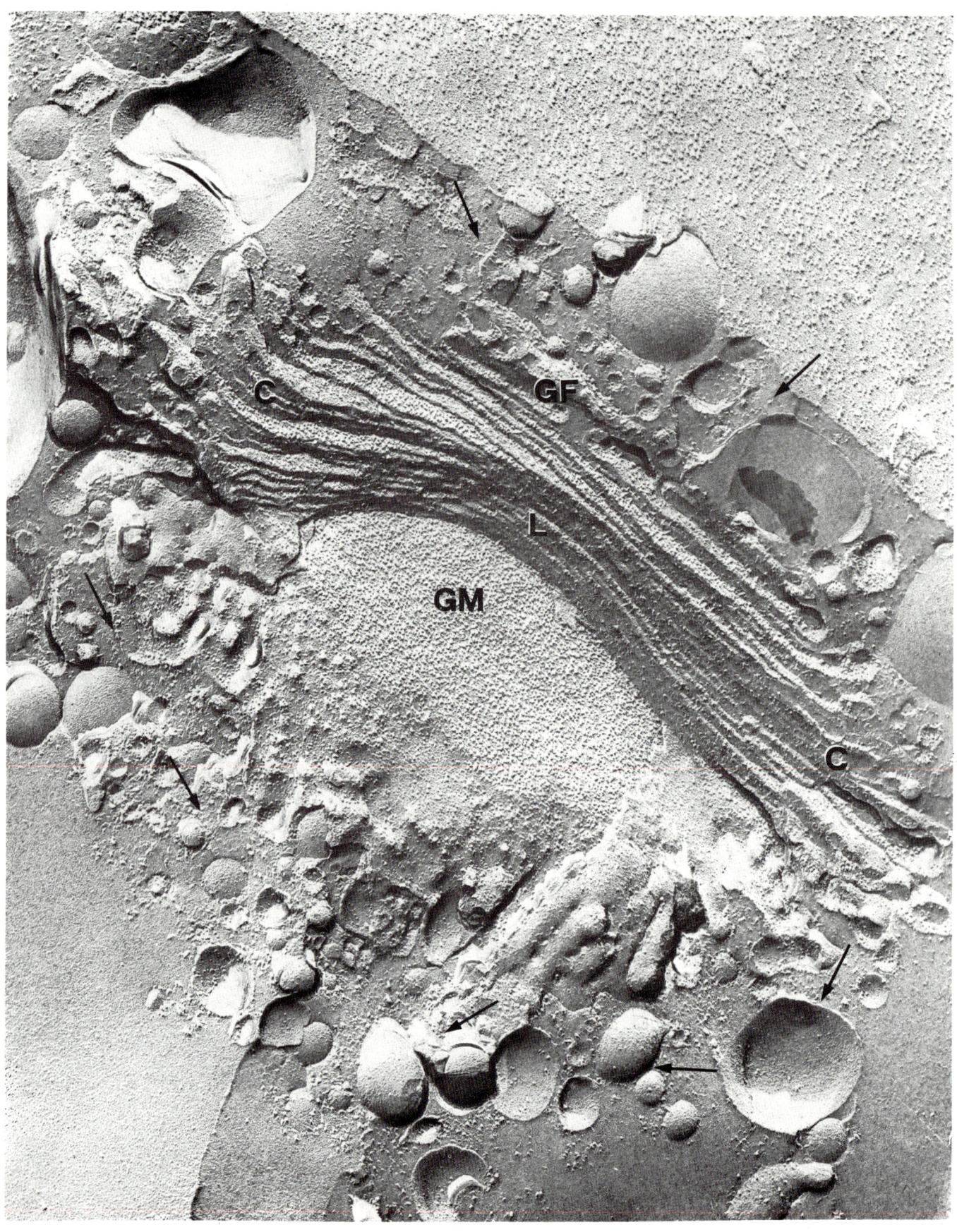

Active Golgi complex in plant cell (EM, freeze-fracture, x45,000). The Golgi complex appears in this cell as a series of stacked lamellae **(L)**, flat in the center and expanding at the periphery into saccules (cisternae) **(C)**. A number of vesicles originating from the endoplasmic reticulum are found on the forming (convex) face of the complex **(GF)**. Larger vesicles or vacuoles are detaching from the maturing (concave) face of the Golgi complex **(GM)** to form secretion granules. The arrows indicate the probable pathway for the movement of materials from the forming face to the maturing face of the Golgi complex. By courtesy of L.A. Staehelin.

Plate 1.21   **31**

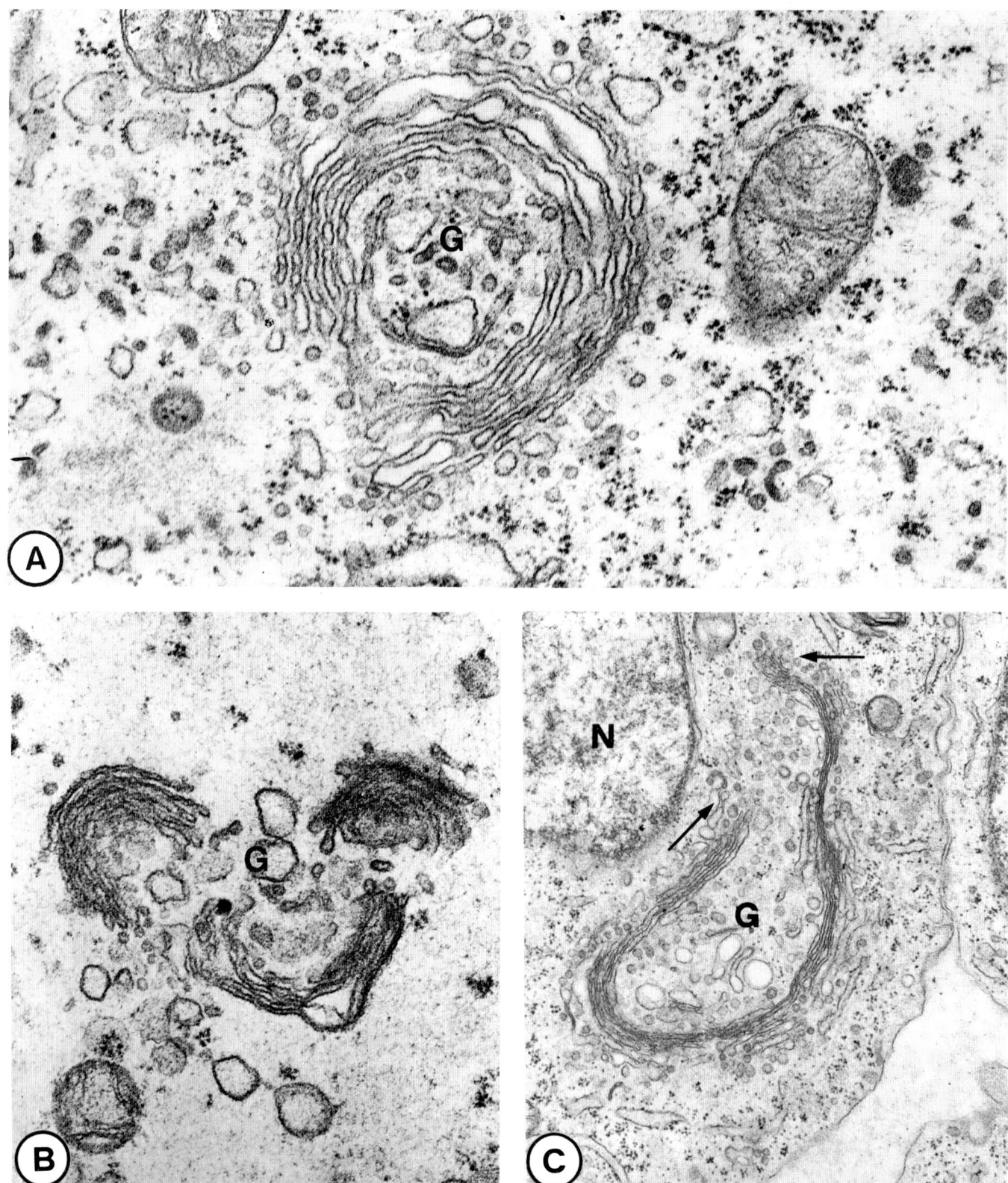

A   **Golgi area in mouse oocyte (EM, x40,000).** The Golgi complex can be seen to be composed of a set of membrane-limited saccules and a number of vesicles. In this section the Golgi (**G**) has a horseshoe shape. Around the complex are mitochondria and rosettes of ribosomes.

B   **Golgi areas in mouse oocyte (EM, x33,000).** Here the Golgi complex (**G**) appears as three groups of concentric stacks of saccules associated with vesicles. The number of saccules and vesicles in the complex can vary greatly from one cell to another, and within the same cell according to the phase of its activity.

C   **Golgi area in epithelial cell (EM, x22,500).** The complex (**G**) is next to the nucleus (**N**). At the periphery of the lamellae are small vesicles (→).

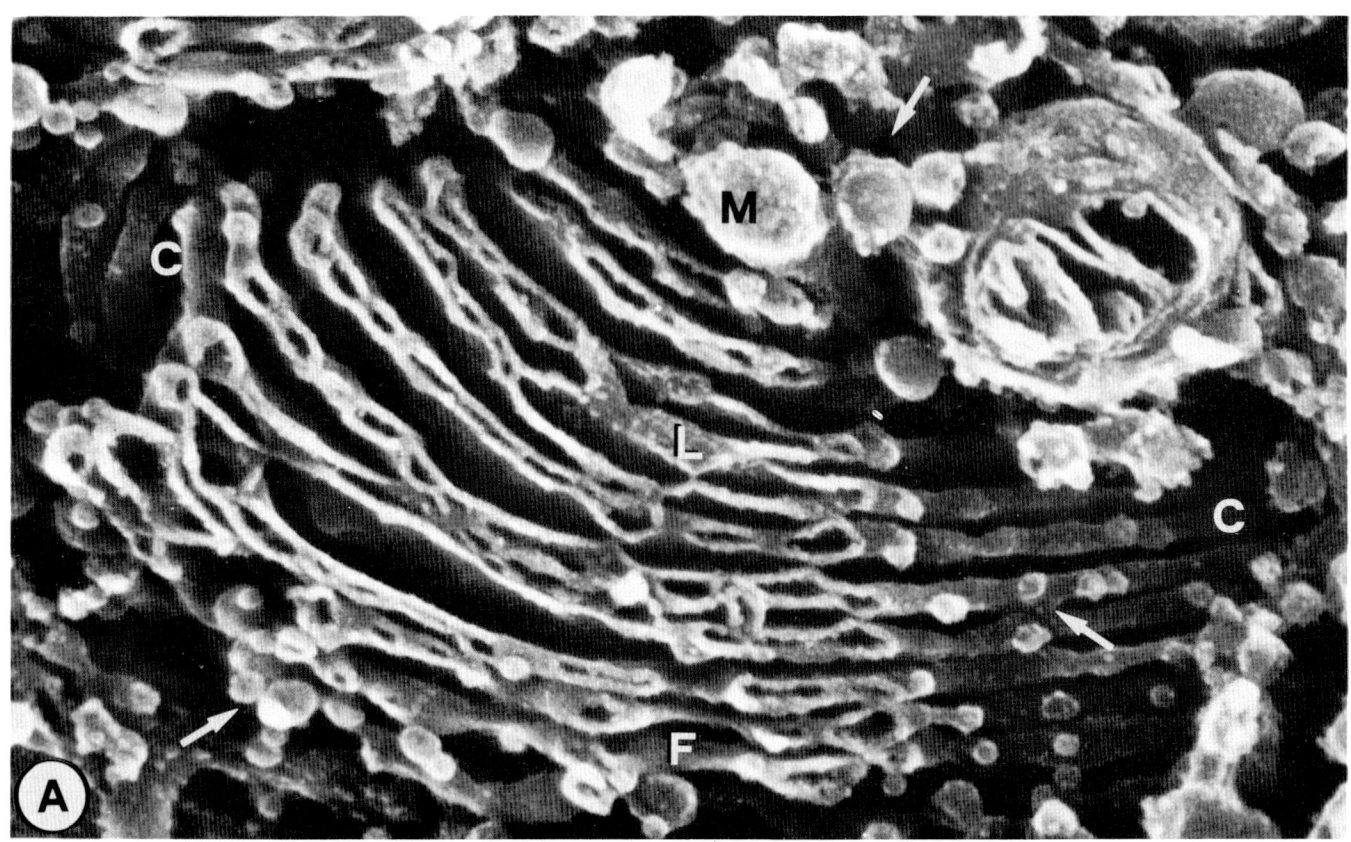

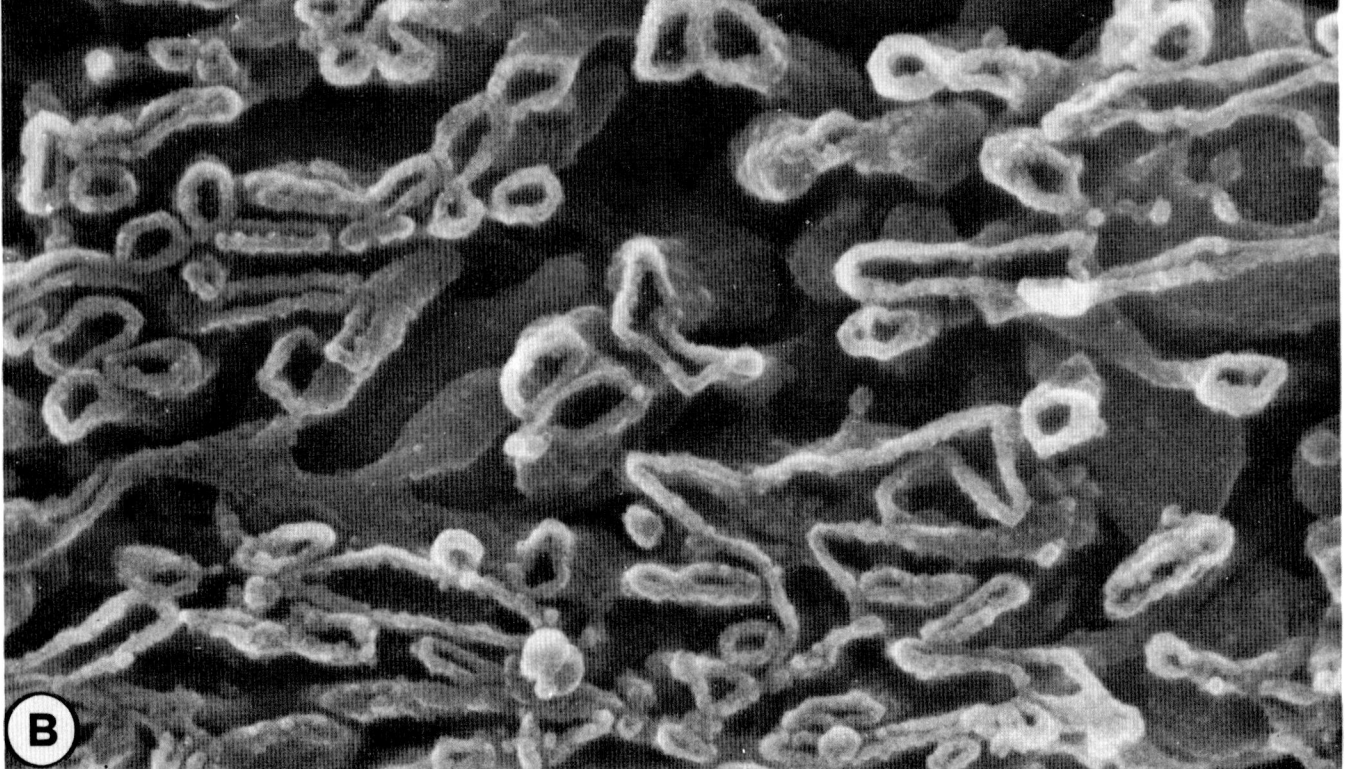

A   **Golgi complex of rat epididymal cell (scanning EM, x70,000). L** = lamellae. **C** = cisternae. On the maturing face **(M)** and forming face **(F)** of the complex are vesicles and vacuoles (→).

B   **Smooth endoplasmic reticulum of the vas deferens from rat (scanning EM, x90,000).** The membranes form an anastomosing network of sacs. By courtesy of K. Tanaka.

Plate 1.23   33

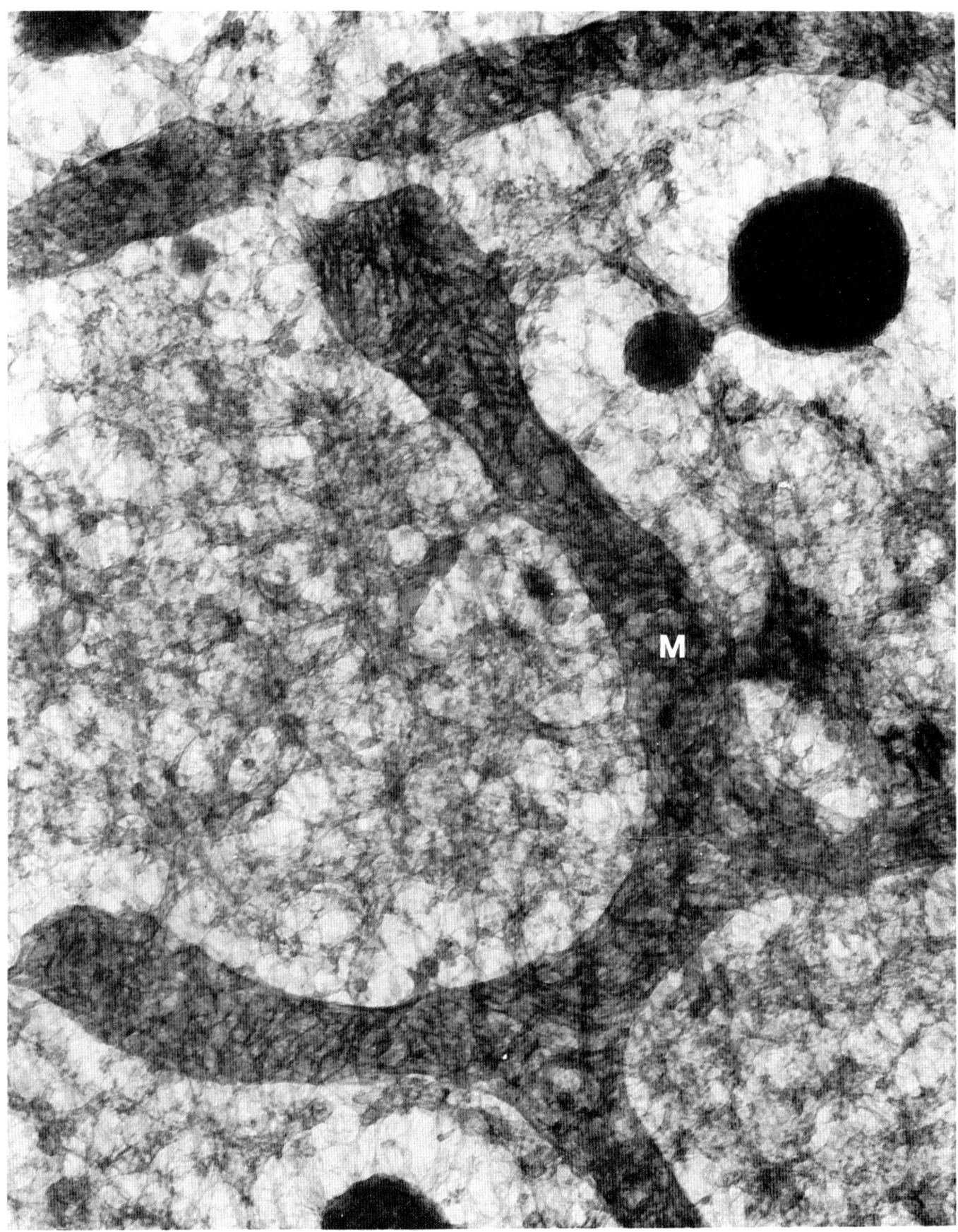

Branched mitochondrion from cultured cell observed "in toto" (high voltage EM, x83,000). The mitochondrion **(M)** is branched and is surrounded by the cytoplasmic ground substance which includes the microtrabecular lattice (top right). By courtesy of J. Wolosewick and K.R. Porter.

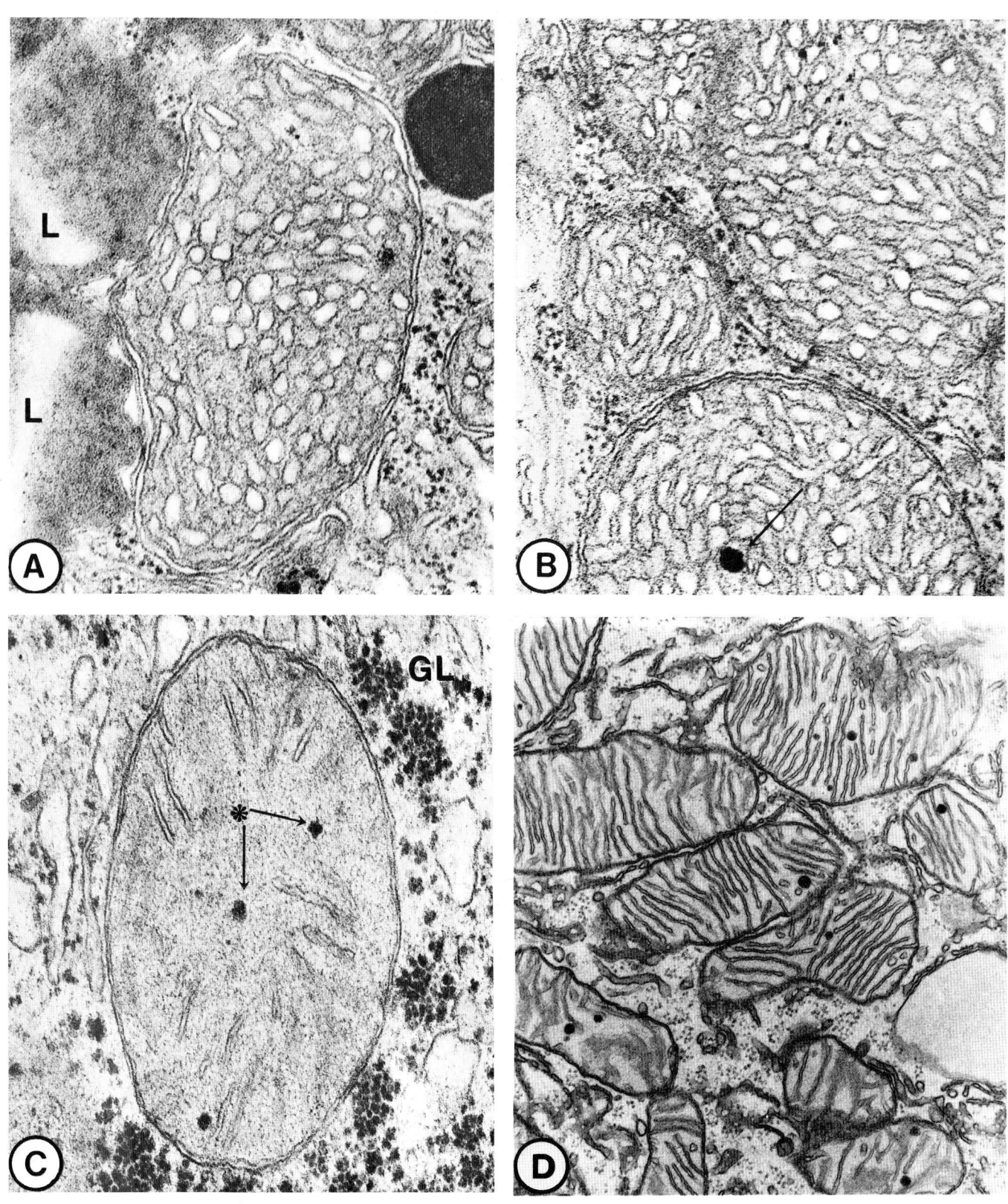

A **Mitochondrion with villiform cristae from an endocrine cell of mouse ovary (EM, x60,000).** The tubular cristae are seen in cross section. **L** = lipid droplets.

B **Mitochondrion from steroid-secreting cell of mouse ovary (EM, x65,000).** Note the complicated arrangement of the tubular cristae. Among the cristae in the mitochondrial matrix is a dense granule (→).

C **Mitochondrion of rat liver cell (EM, x52,000).** Liver cell mitochondria have the shape of short rods and possess only relatively few cristae. Intramitochondrial granules (*→) are present. **GL** = glycogen granules in the cytoplasm.

D **Mitochondria with lamellar cristae from rat kidney cell (EM, x28,000).** Among the numerous cristae some dense granules can be seen.

Plate 1.25   35

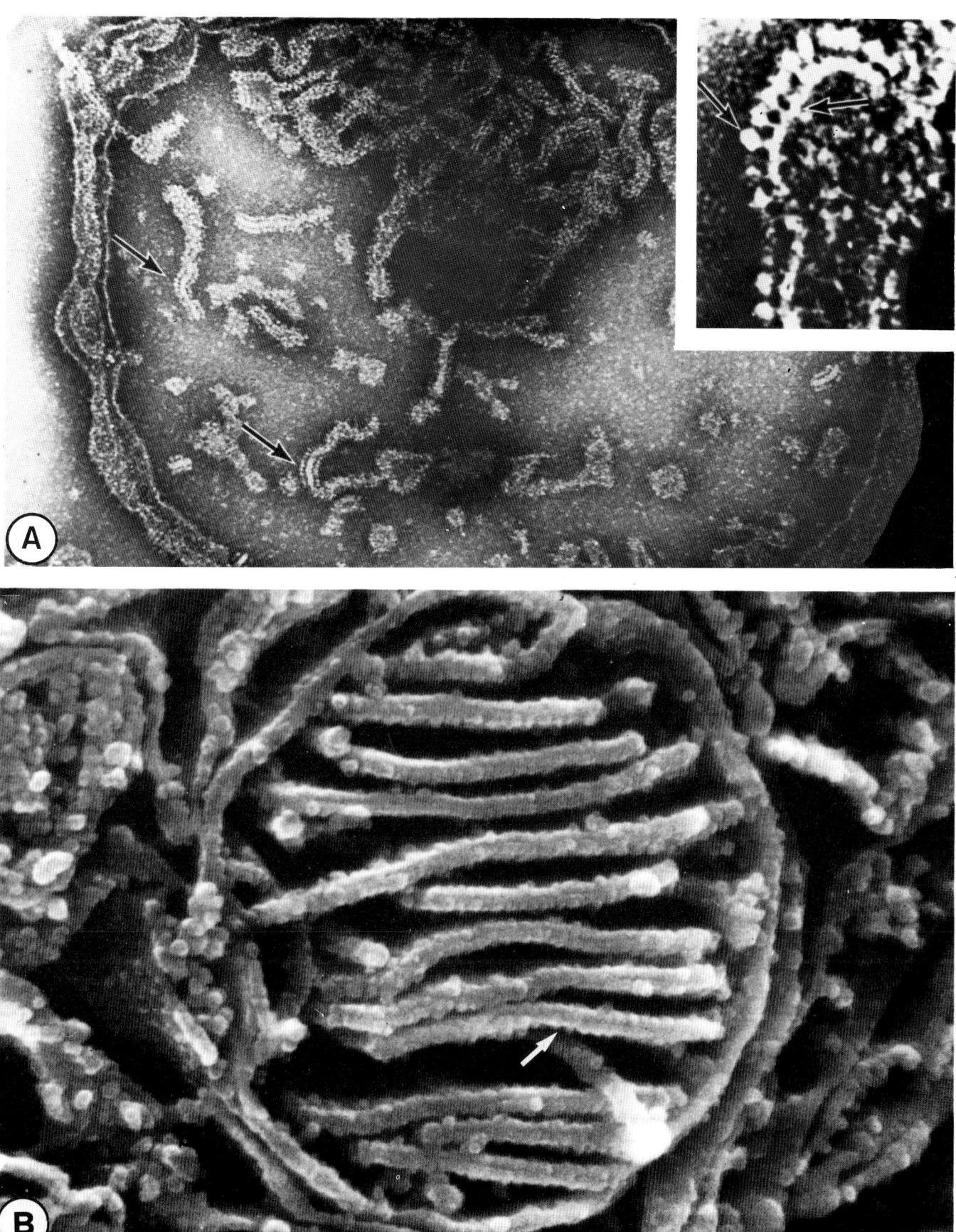

A   **Mitochondrion after exposure to hypotonic solution (negative staining with phosphotungstic acid, EM, x95,000).** A number of isolated cristae can be seen in the swollen matrix. **Inset: crista with a number of elementary particles (× 500,000).** Each of the particles is attached to the membrane of the crista by a stalk (→). By courtesy of H. Fernandez-Moran.

B   **Mitochondrion of rat epididymal cell (scanning EM, x70,000).** On the surface of the cristae are small protuberances, probably elementary particles (→). By courtesy of K. Tanaka.

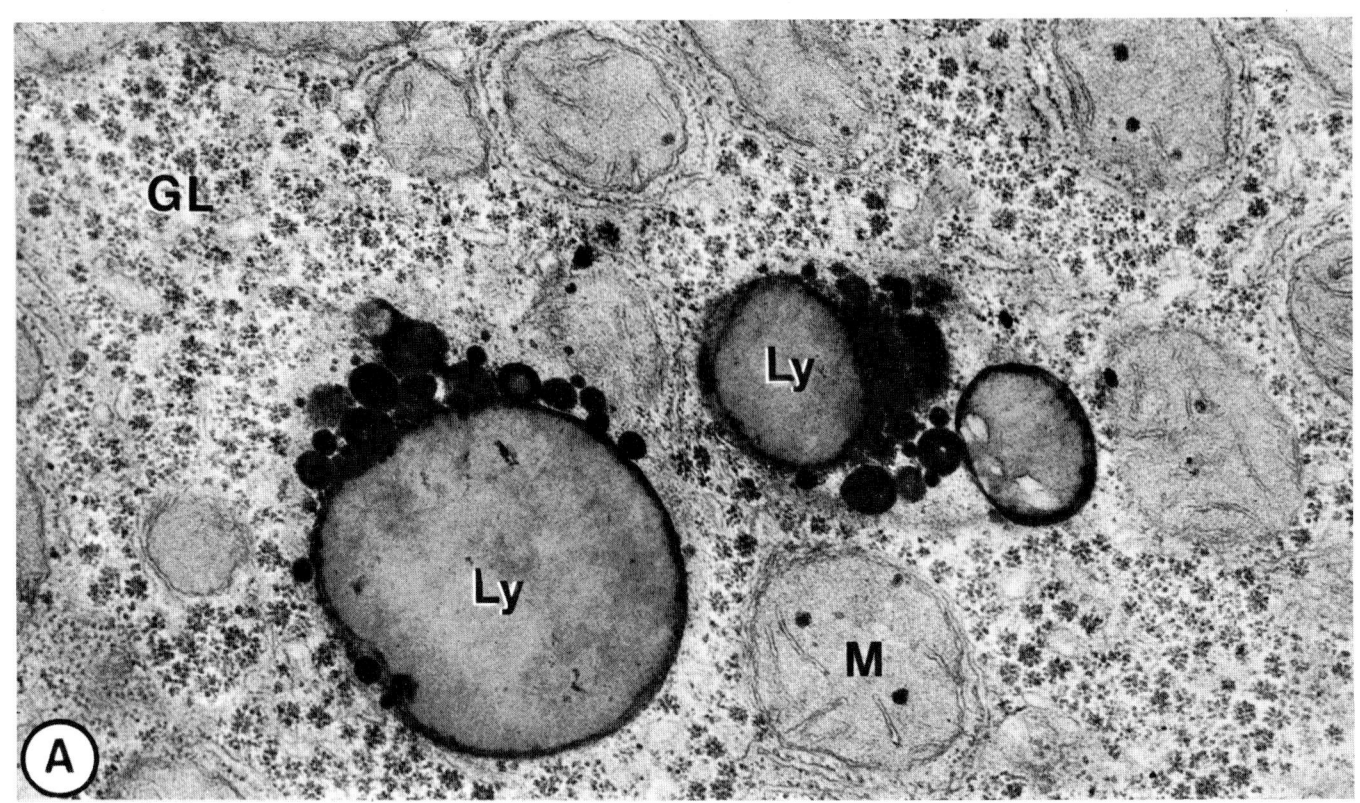

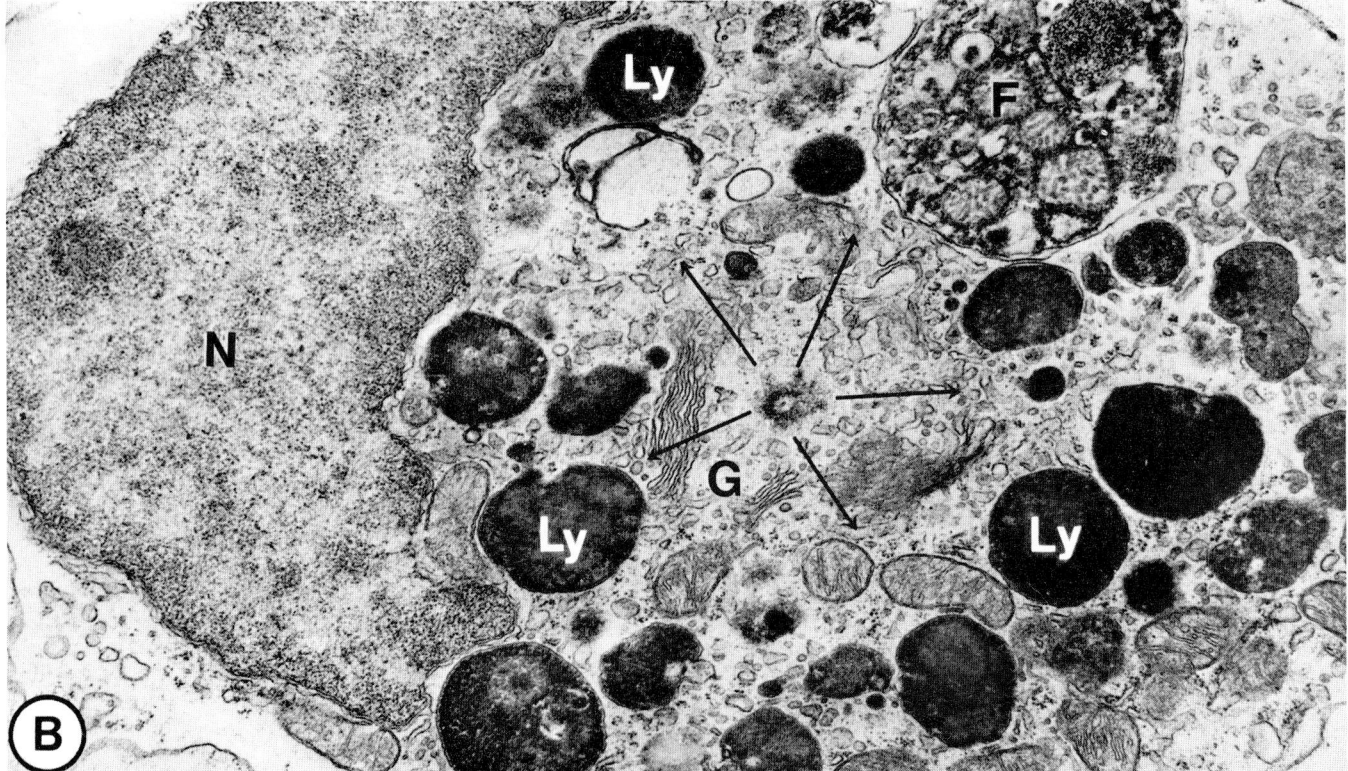

A **Lipofuscin pigments in human liver cell (EM, x50,000). Among glycogen rosettes (GL)** and mitochondria (M) in the cytoplasm, deposits of lipofuscin pigment can be seen. The pigments are probably residues undigested by the lysosomes **(Ly).** By courtesy of C. Inferrera.

B **Lysosomes and phagocytosis in macrophage from rat lymph node (EM, x29,000).** Large, dense bodies of lysosomes (Ly) are present around a Golgi complex (**G →**)which has a centriole in the center. An amorphous mass of material (top right) is partly digested and included in a large heterophagic vacuole **(F)**. The nucleus (N) has an irregular shape.

Plate 1.27   37

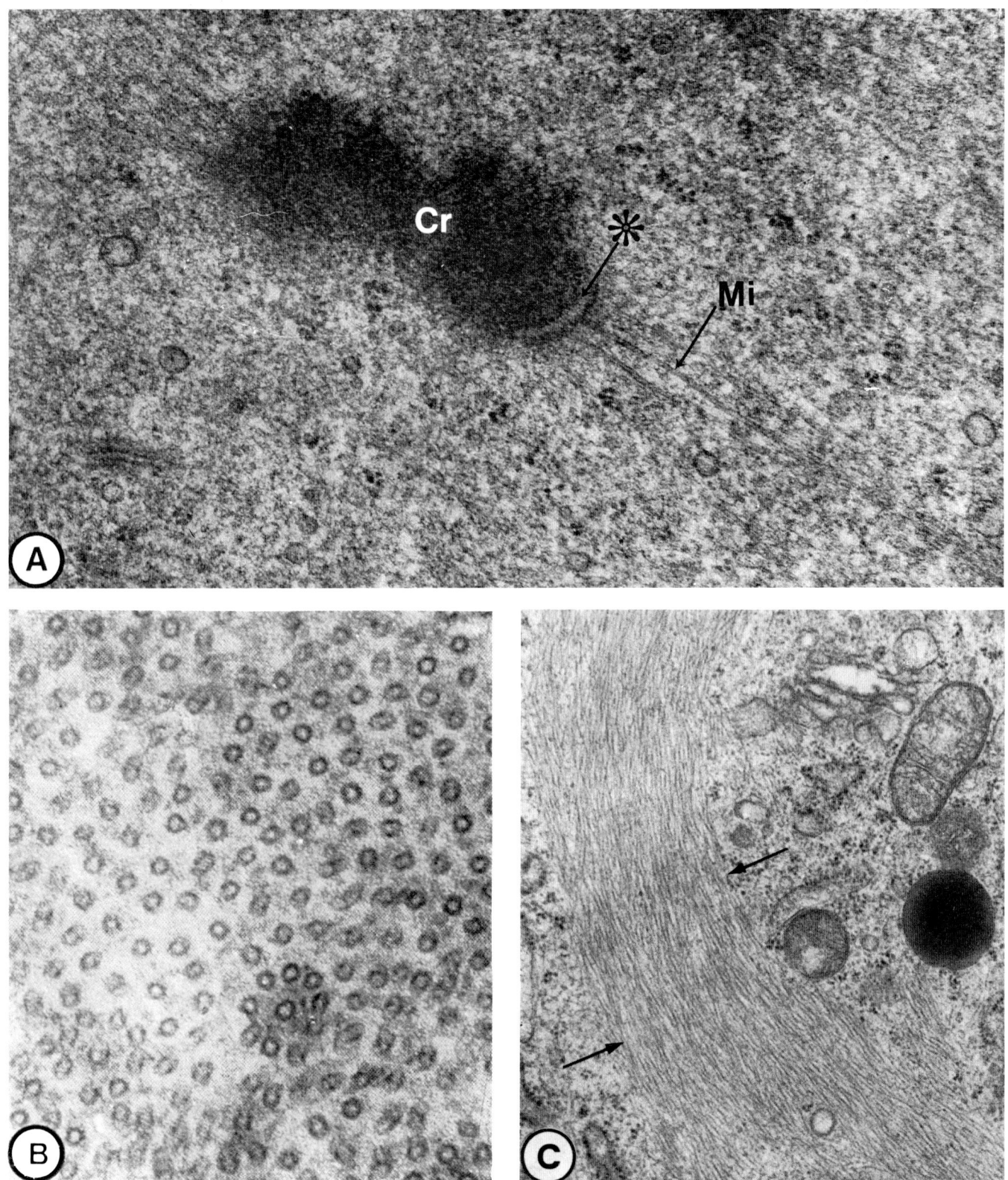

A **Chromosomes, centromere and spindle fibers from mouse oocyte (EM, x60,000).** A centromere (*) unites some chromatin
   (Cr) to the microtubules **(Mi→)** of the mitotic spindle. Original by M. Stefanini.

B **Microtubules of mouse oocyte (EM, x140,000).** Cross sections of a number of microtubules can be seen in the cytoplasm. By
   courtesy of M. Stefanini, C. Oura and L. Zamboni.

C **Microfilaments in epithelial cell (EM, x35,000). Parallel bundles of microfilaments (→) are features of many cells.**

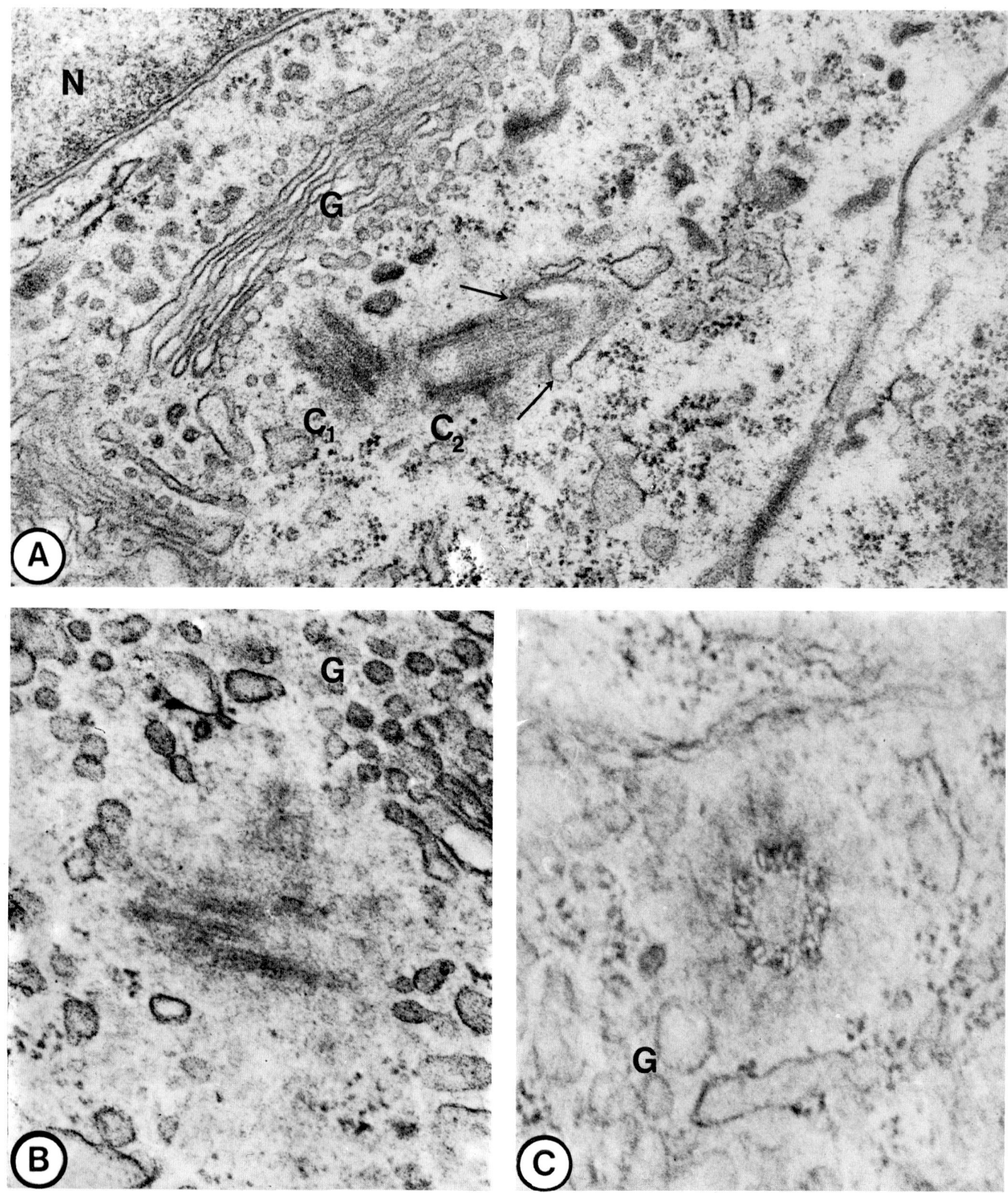

A   **Centrioles and ciliogenesis in mouse ovary follicular cell (EM, x60,000). N** = nucleus. **G** = Golgi complex. Two centrioles
     (centrosome) are sectioned lengthwise (C1, C2) and lie almost at right angles to each other. The distal centriole is interacting
     with a cytoplasmic vesicle and is about to form a cilium (→). From P. Motta, Z. Takeva and D. Palermo. Acta Anat. 78:591,
     1970.

B   **Centriole in longitudinal section (EM, x76,000).** The close proximity between the centriole and the Golgi complex (G) can be
     seen.

C   **Centriole in cross section (EM, x82,000).** Note the ring formation of the peripheral tubules. **G** = vesicles of Golgi
     complex.

Plate 1.29 39

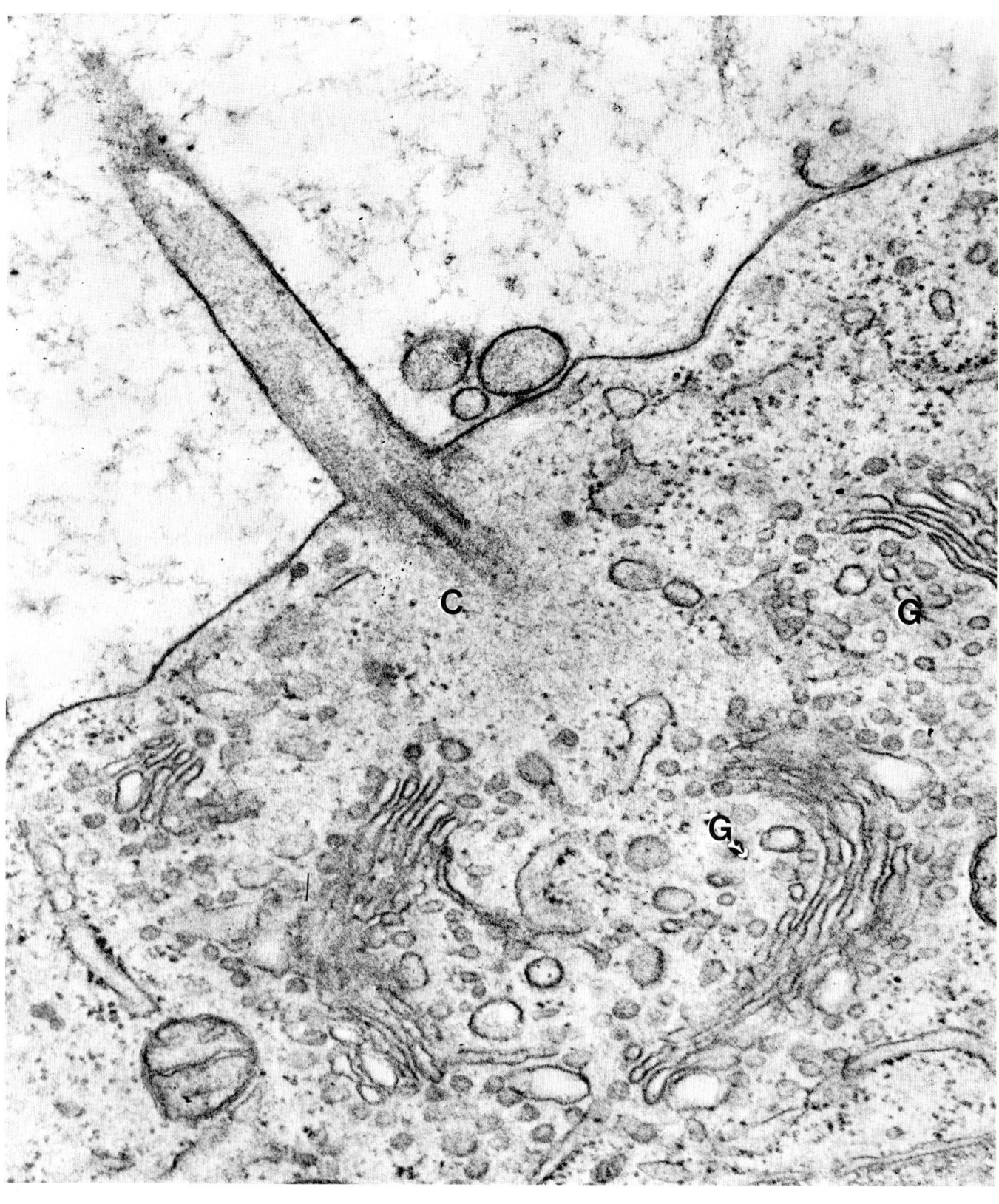

Cilium, centriole and Golgi area in the follicular epithelial cell from rabbit ovary (EM, x62,000). A typical Golgi complex (**G**) can be seen in the cytoplasm near the base of a cilium sectioned lengthwise (**C**). The basal body is seen above the label **C**. Many epithelial cells possess cilia. The basal body forms the cilium. The function of the cilia in this tissue is uncertain. From P. Motta. Boll. Soc. Ital. Biol. Sper. 41:31, 1965.

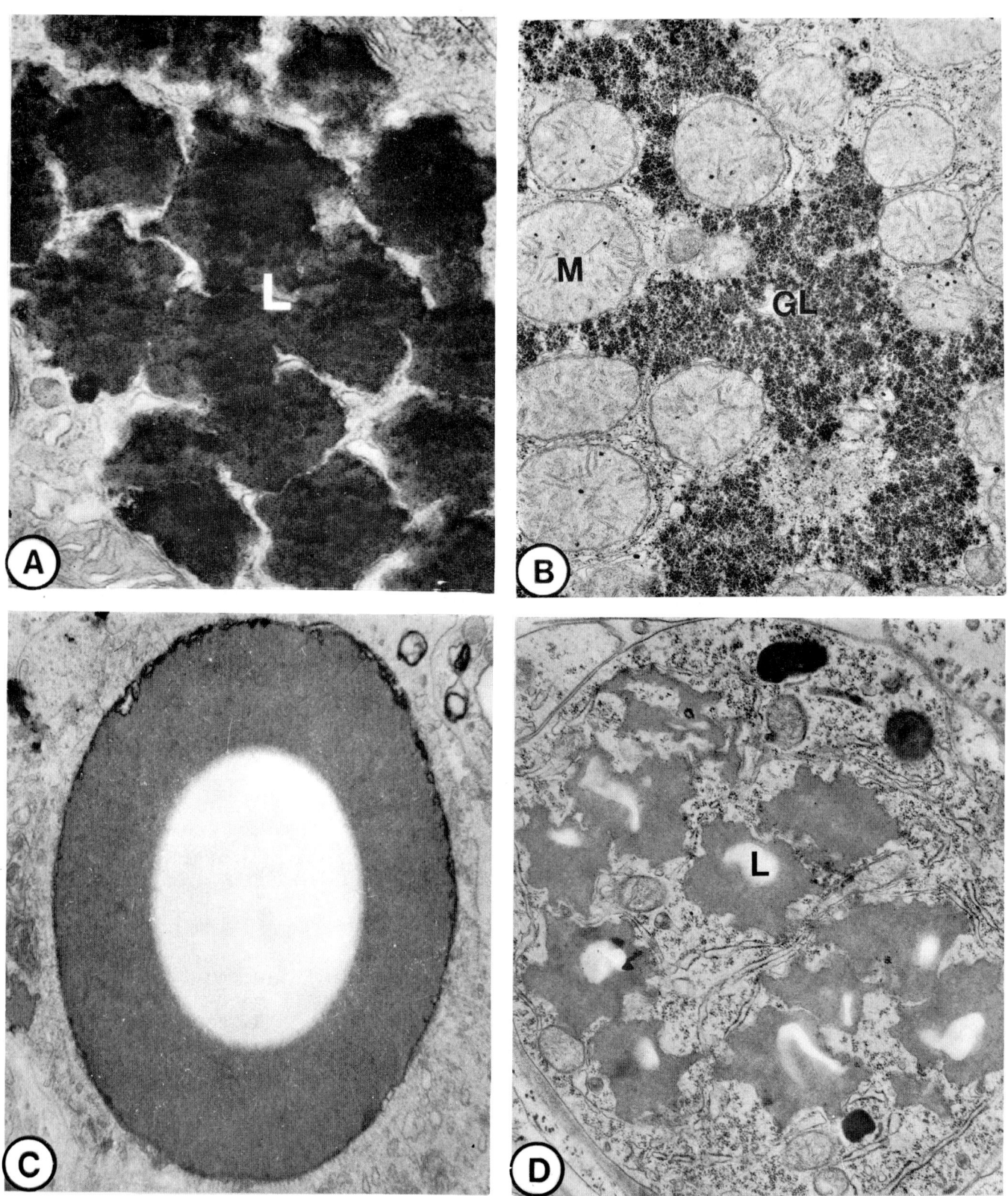

A   Cytoplasmic lipid inclusion (EM, x30,000). The lipid droplets **(L)**, which were fixed with osmium tetroxide, are dense to the electron beam. They may vary greatly in volume and have irregular outlines.

B   Glycogen in mouse liver cell (EM, x28,000). Glycogen appears in the cytoplasm as dense granules **(GL)** which have a greater diameter than ribosomes (20-25 nm). **M** = mitochondria.

C,D   Cytoplasmic inclusions, probably lipoproteins (EM, x46,000, x18,000). The central translucent area of the lipid inclusions **(L)** is probably caused by partial extraction during fixation of the material.

Plate 1.31   **41**

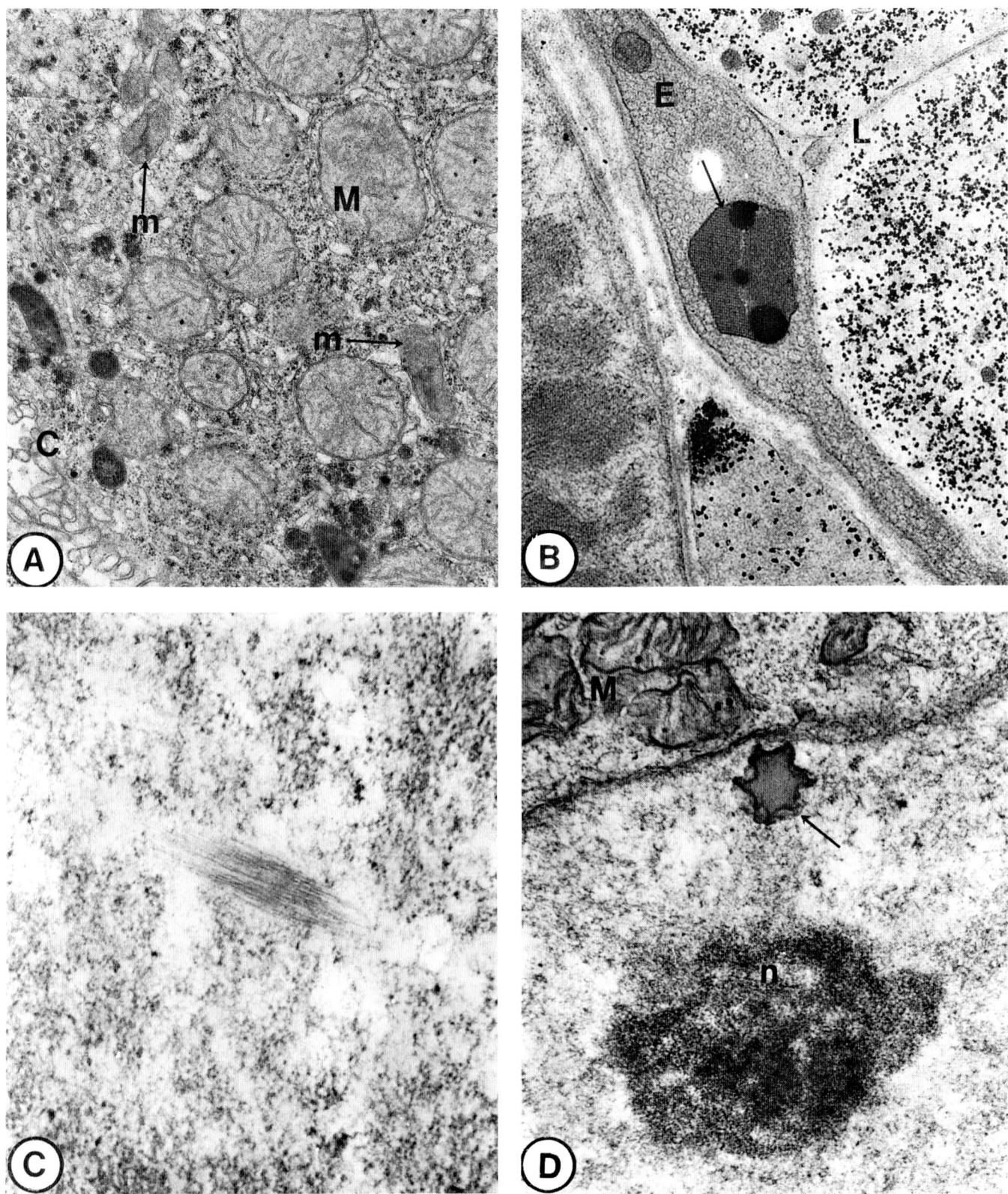

A   **Peroxisomes in rat liver (EM, x25,000).** Two peroxisomes **(m→)** can be seen in the cytoplasm of the hepatocyte near the bile canaliculus **(C)**. They are irregular in shape, membrane-bound, and contain dense material. Numerous mitochondria **(M)** are seen in the field.

B   **Crystalline inclusion in endothelial cell from human muscle (EM, Thiery's method, x30,000).   E** = cytoplasm of the endothelial cell with a large crystalline inclusion **(→). L** = lumen of the capillary with portions of leukocytes. By courtesy of F. Inferrera.

C   **Nuclear inclusion in nerve cell from rabbit cerebral cortex (EM, x30,000).** The inclusion is apparently made up of filaments. Such filaments often are found in certain neurons of the central nervous system. By courtesy of A. Santoro.

D   **Nuclear lipid inclusion in hepatoblast from chick embryo (EM, x28,000).** An irregular lipid inclusion **(→)** is visible next to a large nucleolus **(n)** within the nucleus. **M** = mitochondria of the surrounding cytoplasm.

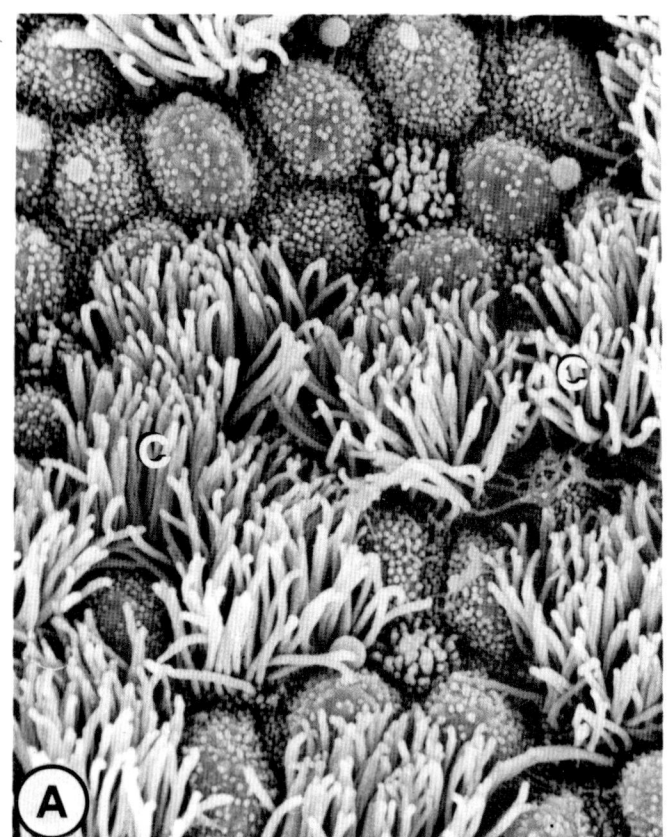

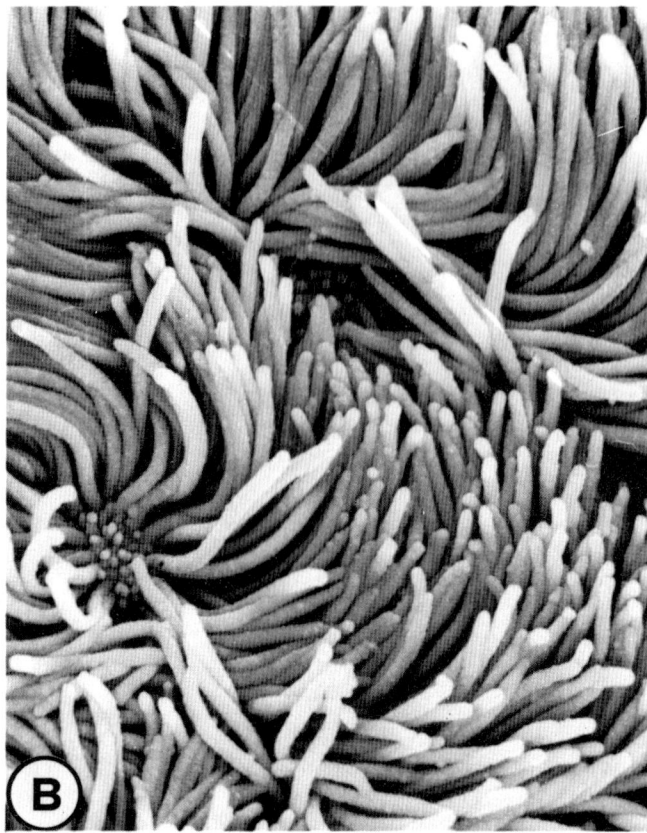

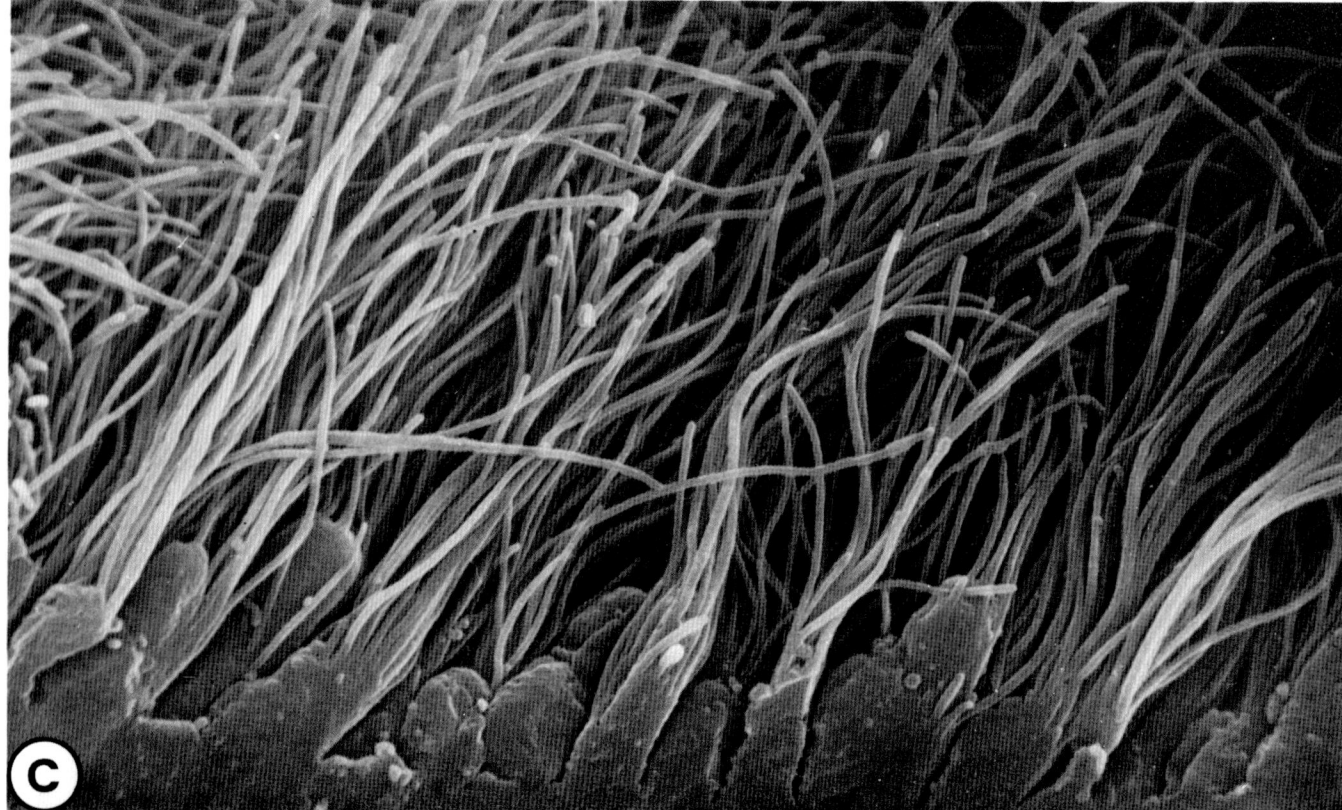

A   **Cells with cilia from rat tracheal mucosa (scanning EM, x5,800).** Cells with microvilli are interspersed with cells having cilia (C).

B   **Motile cilia from rat trachea (scanning EM, x11,500).** Note the uniform structure of these cell processes.

C   **Stereocilia from monkey epididymis (scanning EM, x12,200).** Bundles of stereocilia protrude from the apex of each cell. In thickness stereocilia resemble long microvilli; unlike cilia, however, they are not motile. By courtesy of M. Murakami.

Plate 1.33   **43**

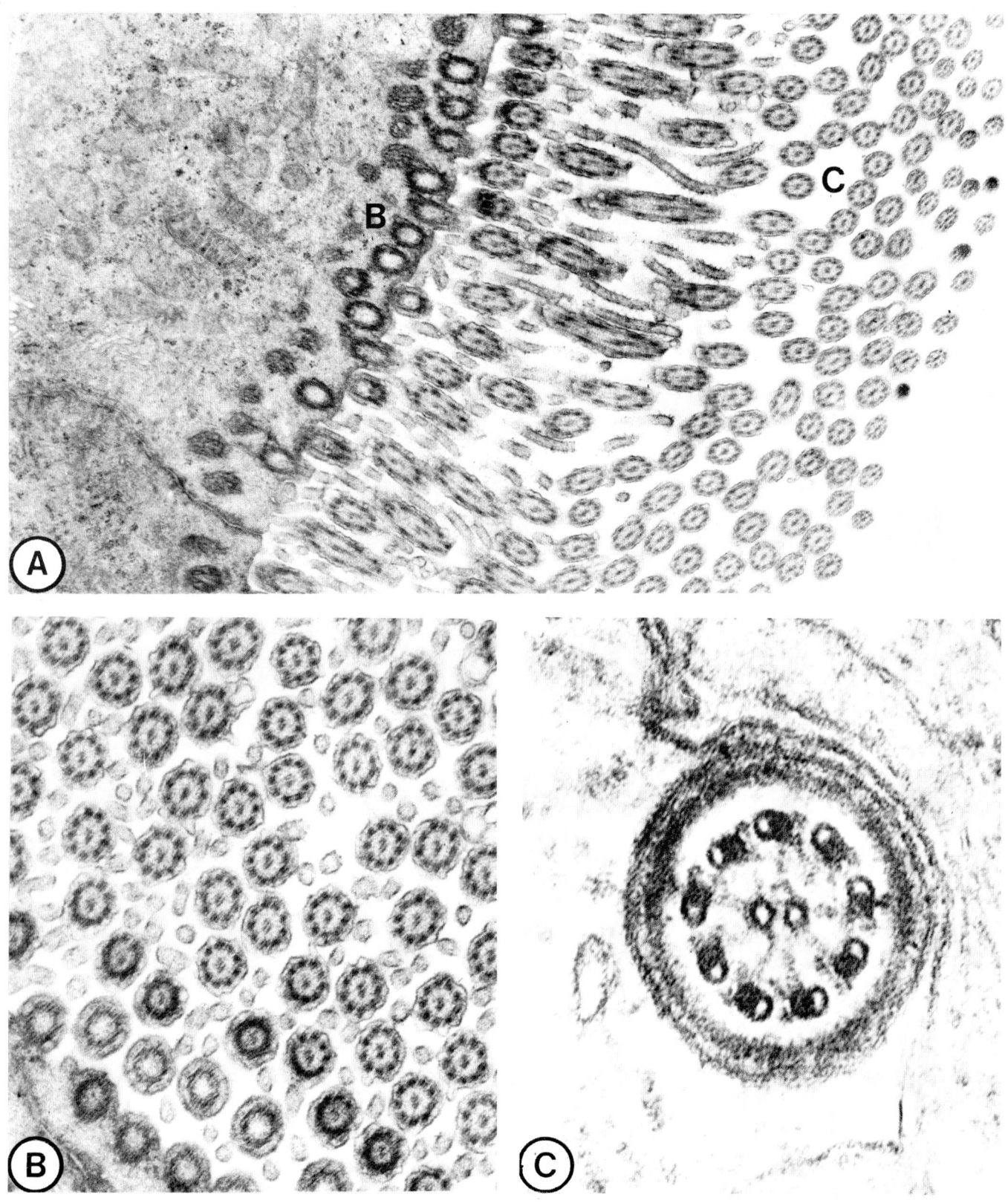

A   **Cilia from mouse oviduct (EM, x20,000).** Profiles of cilia (C) are seen in tangential cross section. At left are basal bodies **(B)** beneath the cell surface where the cilia merge into the basal corpuscles.

B   **Cilia in cross section (EM, x25,000).** The array of microtubules inside each cilium forms nine doublets at the periphery surrounding a central pair (9 + 2 pattern).

C   **Flagellum of mouse spermatozoon in cross section (EM, x180,000).** The outer doublets and central pair of microtubules in the end piece of the flagellum display the typical 9 + 2 pattern.

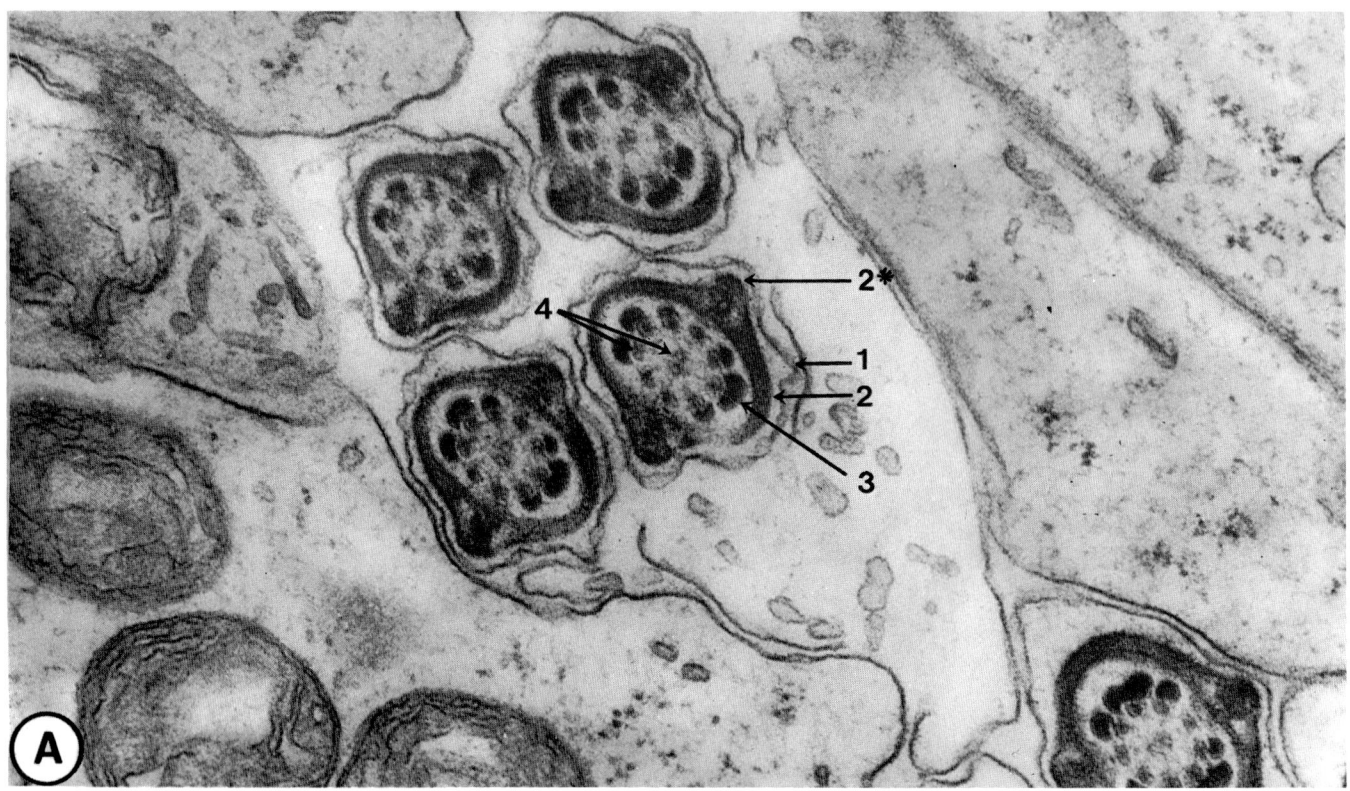

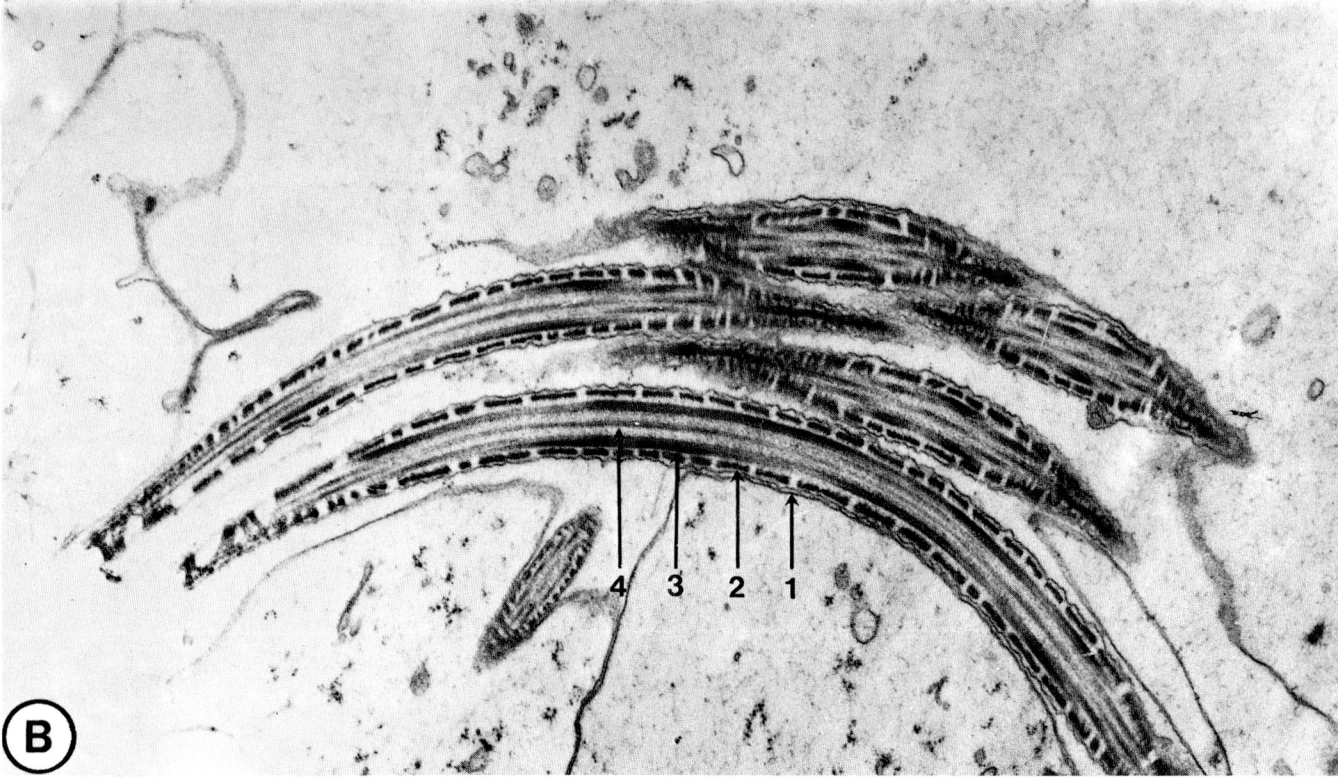

A **Flagella of mouse sperm in cross section (EM, x52,000).** The sperm flagellae are sectioned at the main piece. **1** = cell membrane of tail. **2** = thick fibrous sheath, which at opposite sides is thickened to form a ridge along the tail (2*). **3** = external fibers made of dense material next to the peripheral and central filament ciliary doublets (microtubules) **(4)**.

B **Oblique section of mouse sperm flagella (EM, x32,000).** The numbers indicate the same components as in the preceding figure. Note that the thick fibrous sheath **(2)** appears discontinuous.

Plate 1.35   **45**

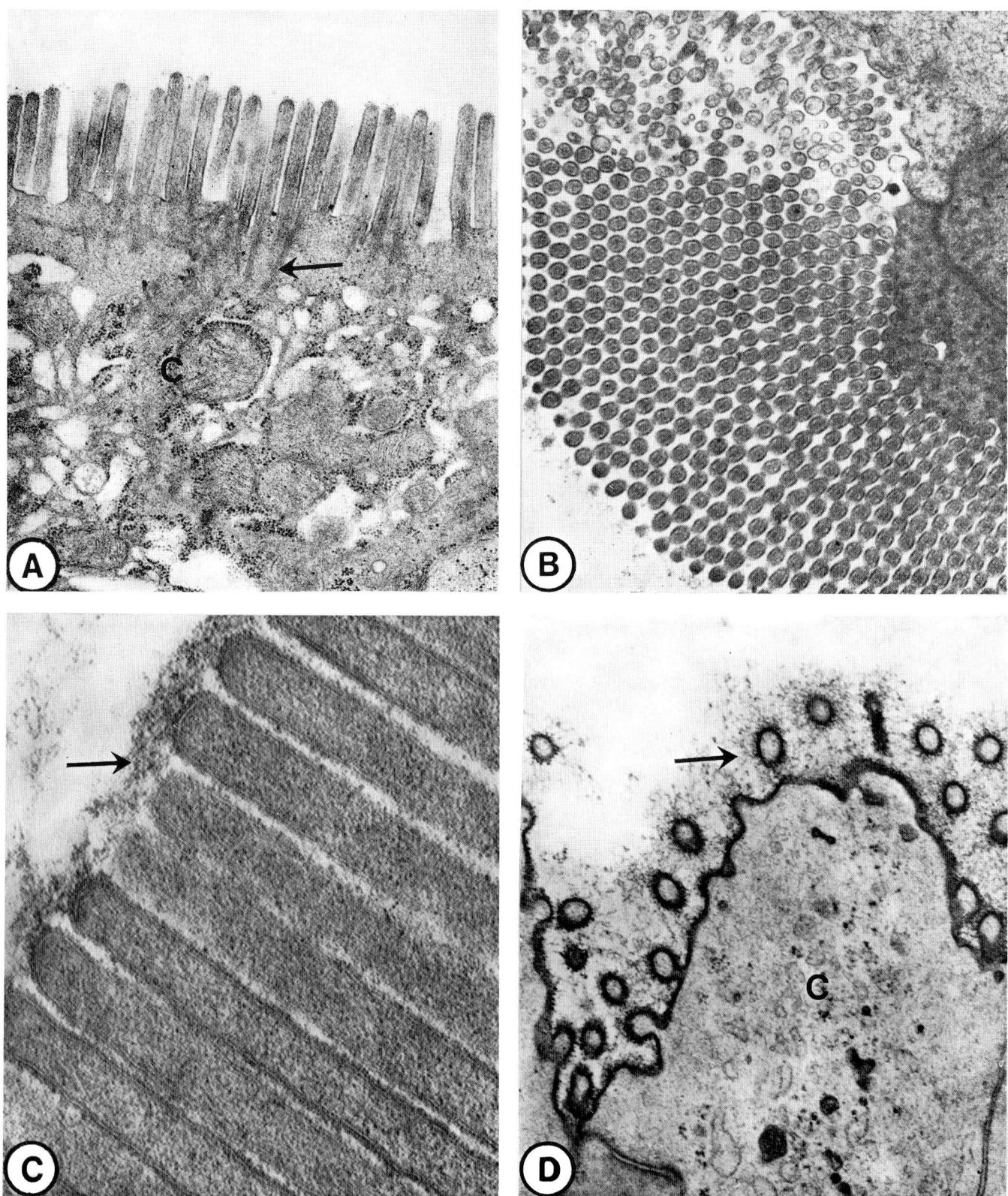

A   **Longitudinal section of microvilli in epithelium from rabbit intestine (EM, x22,000).** The free surface of these cells is covered with a regular array of finger-like projections, the microvilli (striated border). Running lengthwise in each microvillus are thin filaments extending into the cortical cyotplasm to form the "terminal web" of microfilaments (→).

B   **Cross section of microvilli of epithelium from rabbit intestine (EM, x20,000).** Top: the cells are visible.

C   **Microvilli and glycocalyx in rabbit intestinal epithelium (EM, x76,000).** The surface of the microvilli is covered with a layer of proteoglycan, the external limiting layer (glycocalyx) (→).

D   **Microvilli and glycocalyx from epithelium of mouse oviduct (EM, x38,000).** The short microvilli of the secretory cells (C) are shown mainly in cross section. The glycocalyx is visible surrounding the profiles of the microvilli (→).

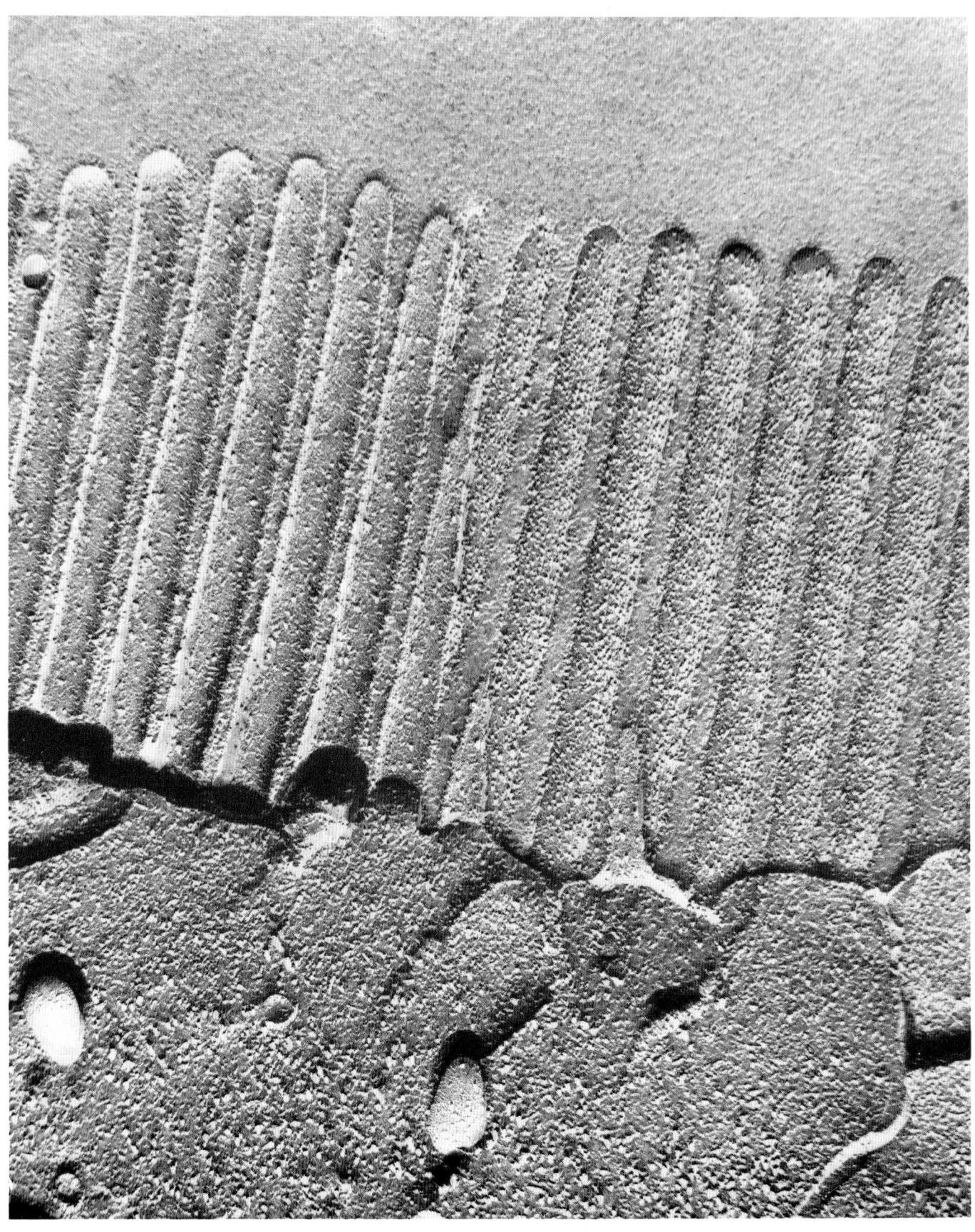

Microvilli of absorptive epithelium from rat small intestine (EM, freeze fracture, x56,000). The microvilli, fractured lengthwise, are seen projecting from the cell surface. At the right-hand side of the figure bundles of actin filaments running longitudinally may be detected. Original by L. A. Staehelin.

Plate 1.37   **47**

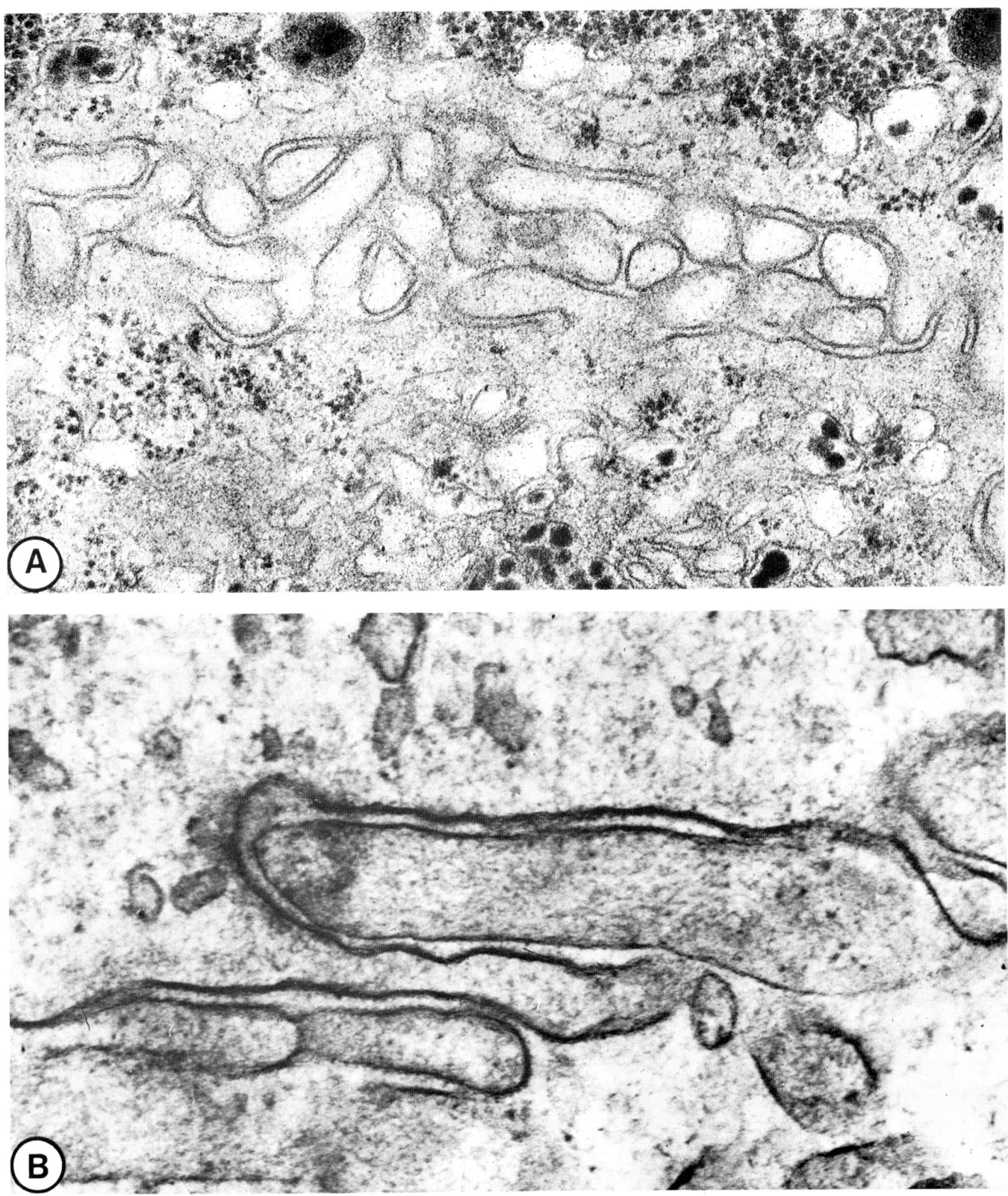

A   **Microvilli from guinea-pig liver cells (EM, x68,000).** In the middle are a number of microvilli projecting from adjacent liver cells into the bile canaliculus. Being sectioned tangentially, the lumen of the canaliculus is not easily visible.

B   **Microvilli and cytoplasmic processes from follicle cell of rabbit oocyte (EM, x80,000).** The follicular cell (right) and the oocyte (left) interlock by means of their projecting microvilli.

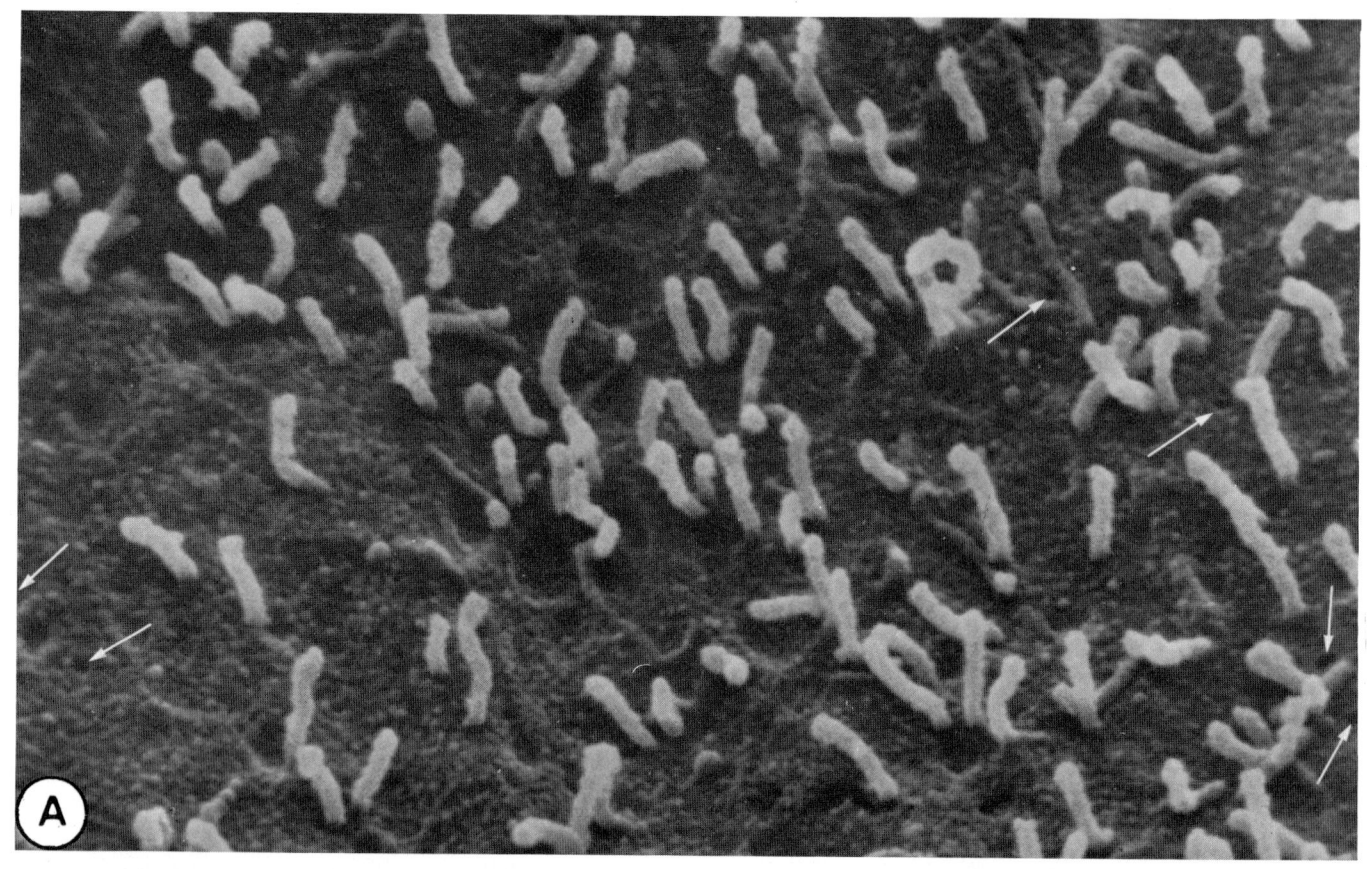

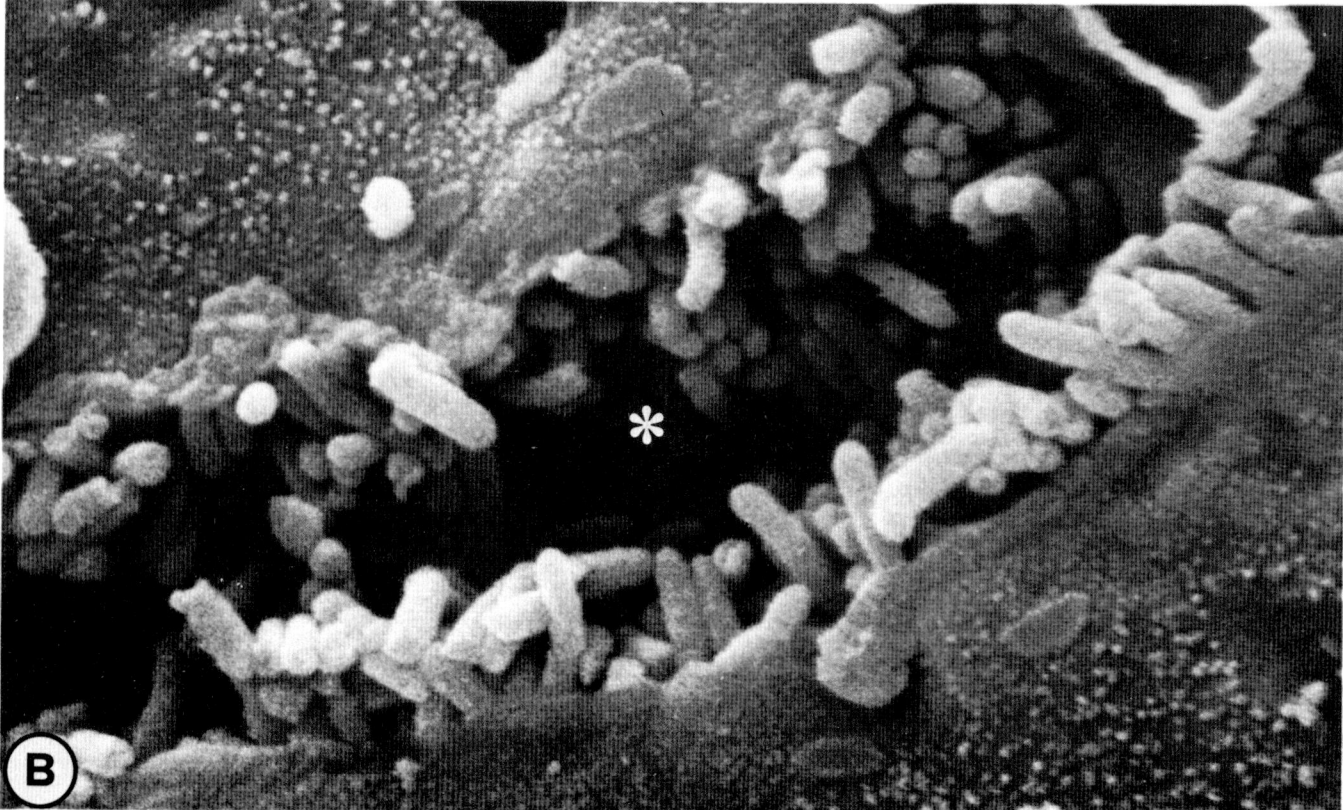

A **Microvilli in mesothelium from rat peritoneum (scanning EM, x12,000).** Thin microvilli are scattered over an area of the cell membrane where small pinocytotic infoldings (caveolae) can be seen (→). From P.M. Motta. Int. Rev. Cytol. Suppl. 6:347, 1977.

B **Microvilli of rat liver cell (scanning EM, x23,000).** The microvilli are abundant and cover the walls of a bile canaliculus (*). From P.M. Motta, M. Muto and T. Fujita. The Liver. *An Atlas of Scanning Electron Microscopy.* Igaku-Shoin Ltd. Tokyo/New York, 1978.

Plate 1.39   **49**

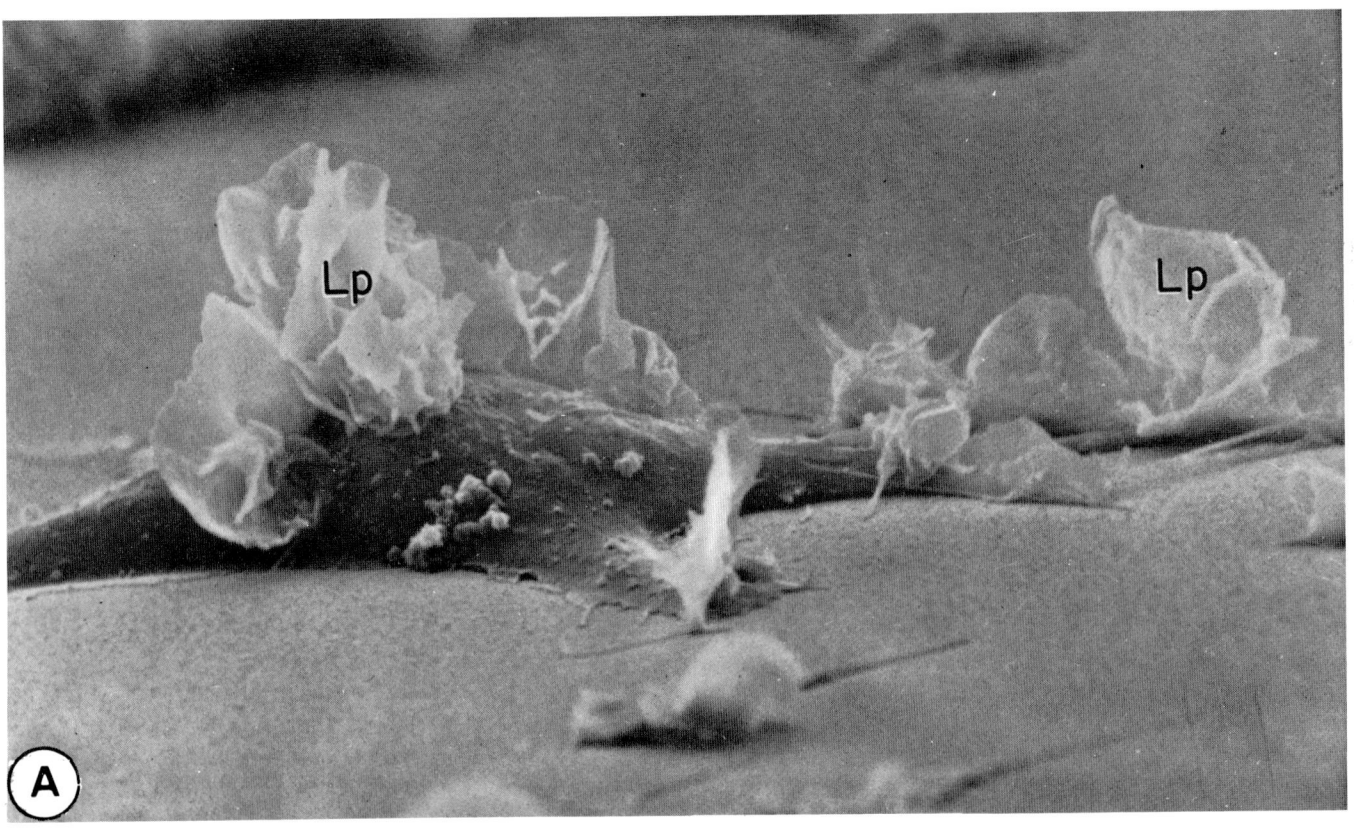

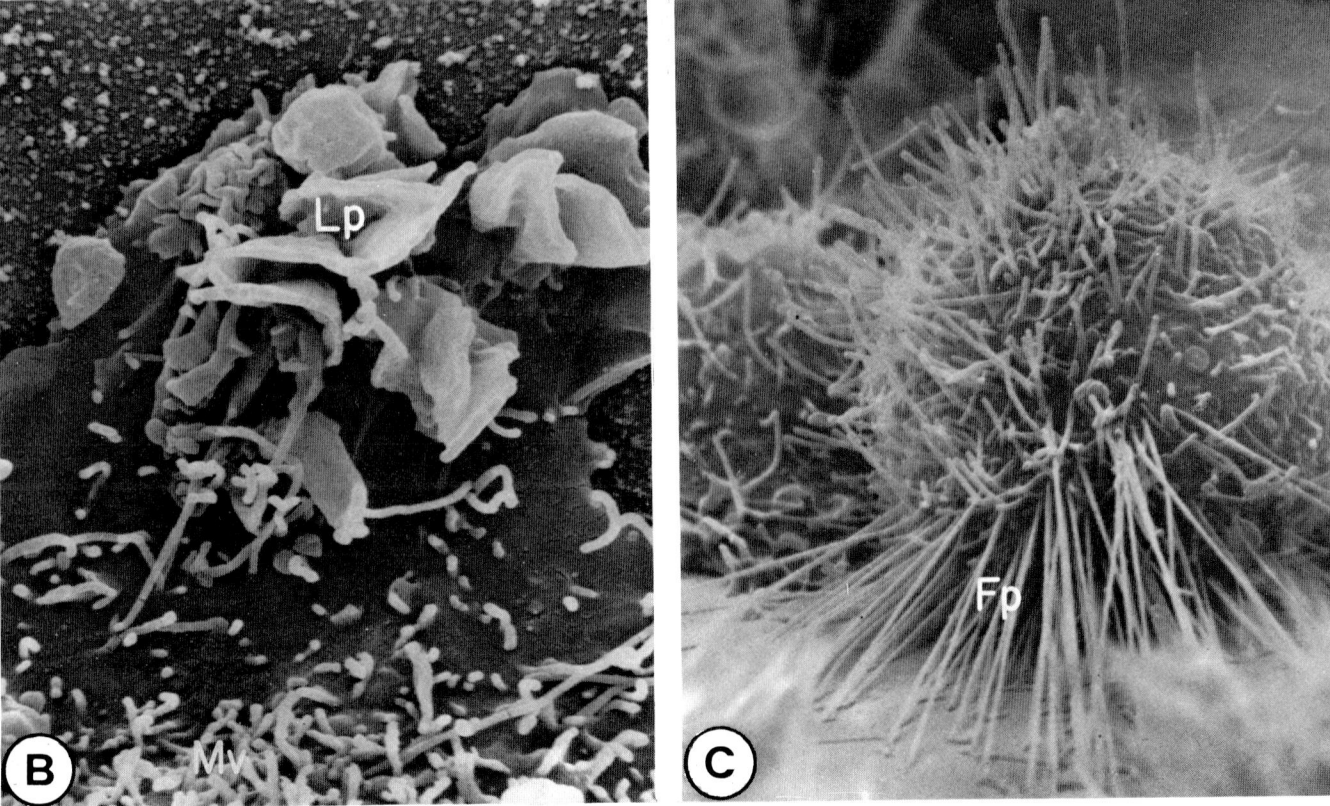

A   **Lamellar outgrowths in mouse macrophage (scanning EM, x3,500).** These lamellipodia **(Lp)** probably have a role in pinocytosis and phagocytosis.

B   **Lamellar outgrowths and microvilli on rat tumor cell (scanning EM, x6,000).** Lamellar outgrowths **(Lp)** are highly motile, forming rapidly and moving from the periphery to the center of the cell for uptake of small quantities of fluid. Bottom: microvilli **(Mv).**

C   **Filopodia and microvilli in cultured mouse cell (scanning EM, x4,200).** The cell is in metaphase and has extended from its base long thin filopodia, which adhere to the substratum and are typical of cells in mitosis. These processes are longer and thinner than the microvilli on the rest of the cell surface. Tendrils are typical of cells in mitosis. By courtesy of V. Fonte, N. Weller and K.R. Porter. 31st Ann. Proc. Electron Microscope Soc. Amer., p 608, 1973.

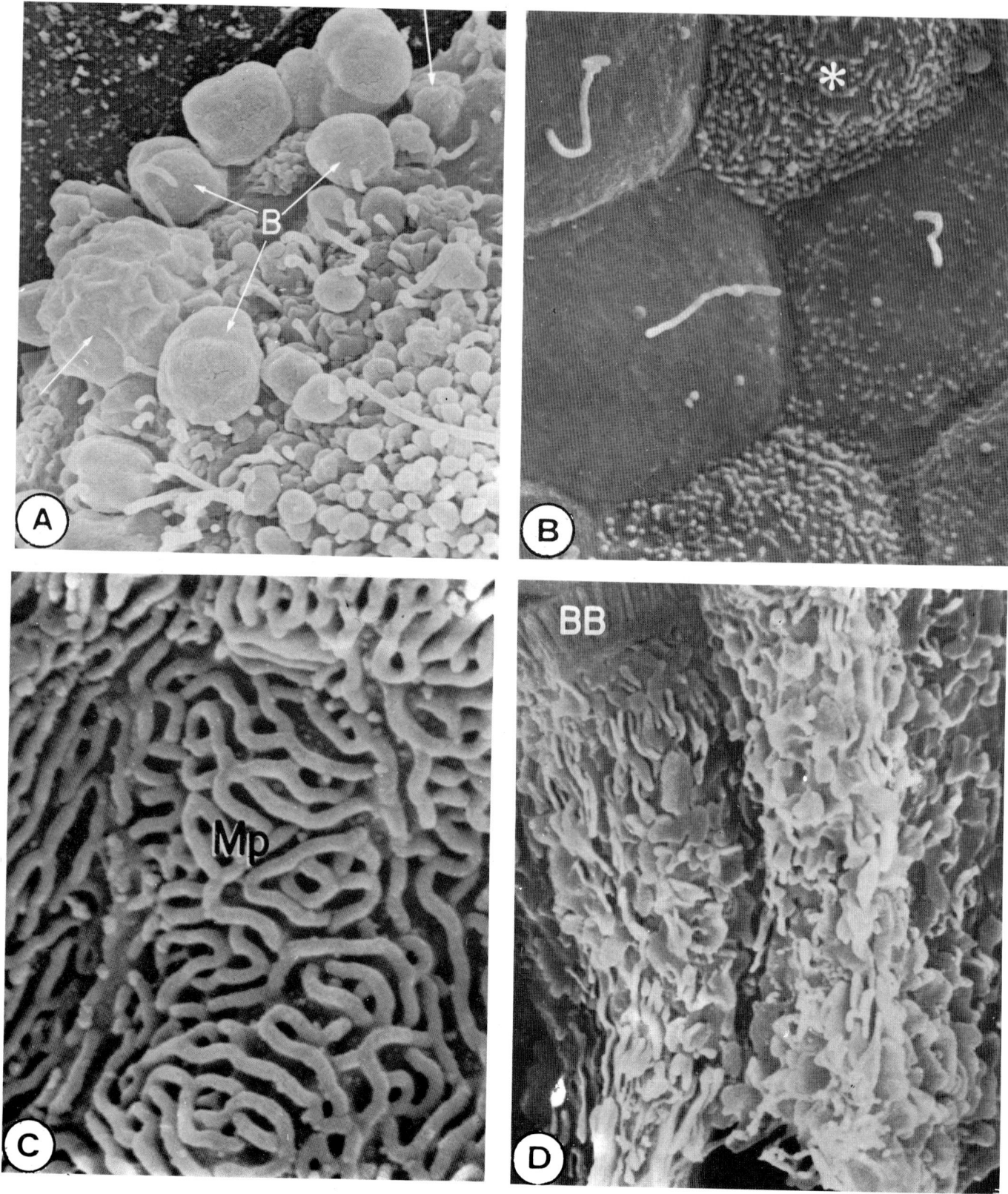

A   **Blebs on surface of rat tumor cell (scanning EM, x8,500).** The blebs (B) are spheroid processes of the cell membrane. In this
     figure some of the processes have shrunken (→).
B   **Single cilia projecting from monkey kidney cells (scanning EM, x8,000).** The smooth free surface of some cells has a single
     cilium while the adjacent cells have short microvilli (*). Original micrograph by P.M. Andrews.
C   **Microplicae of epithelium from monkey tongue mucosa (scanning EM, x14,000).** Microplicae (Mp) are uniform processes of
     the cell surface forming a labyrinth. They are a typical feature of cells whose free surfaces slide over one another.
D   **Microvilli and lamellar outgrowths of absorptive cells from rat intestine (scanning EM, x4,500).** Abundant microvilli are
     aligned on the free surface of the cells to form a striated or brush border (**BB**). The lateral surfaces of the absorptive cells
     have abundant outgrowths which, together with similar structures on adjacent cells, form a labyrinth of intercellular
     spaces.

Plate 1.41   **51**

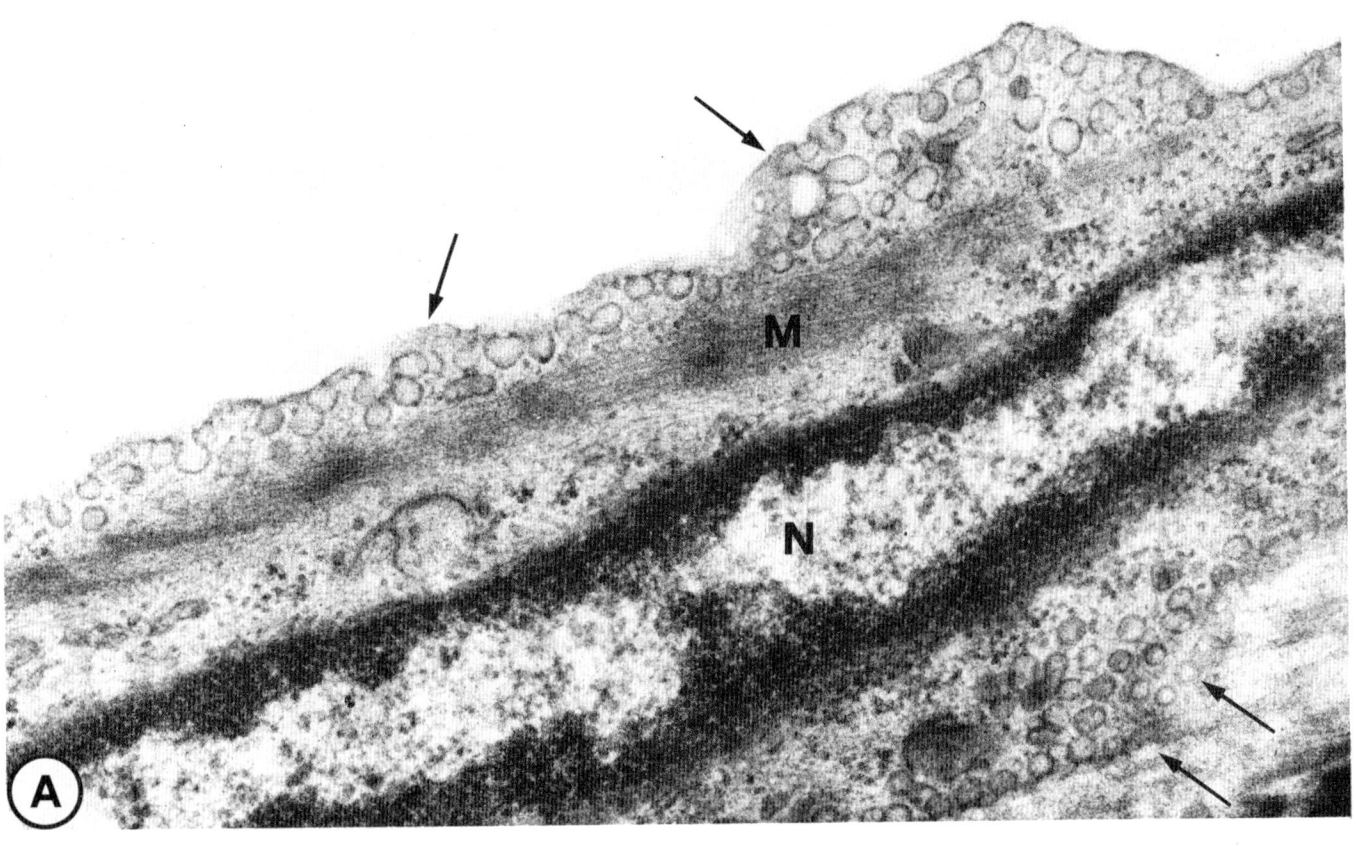

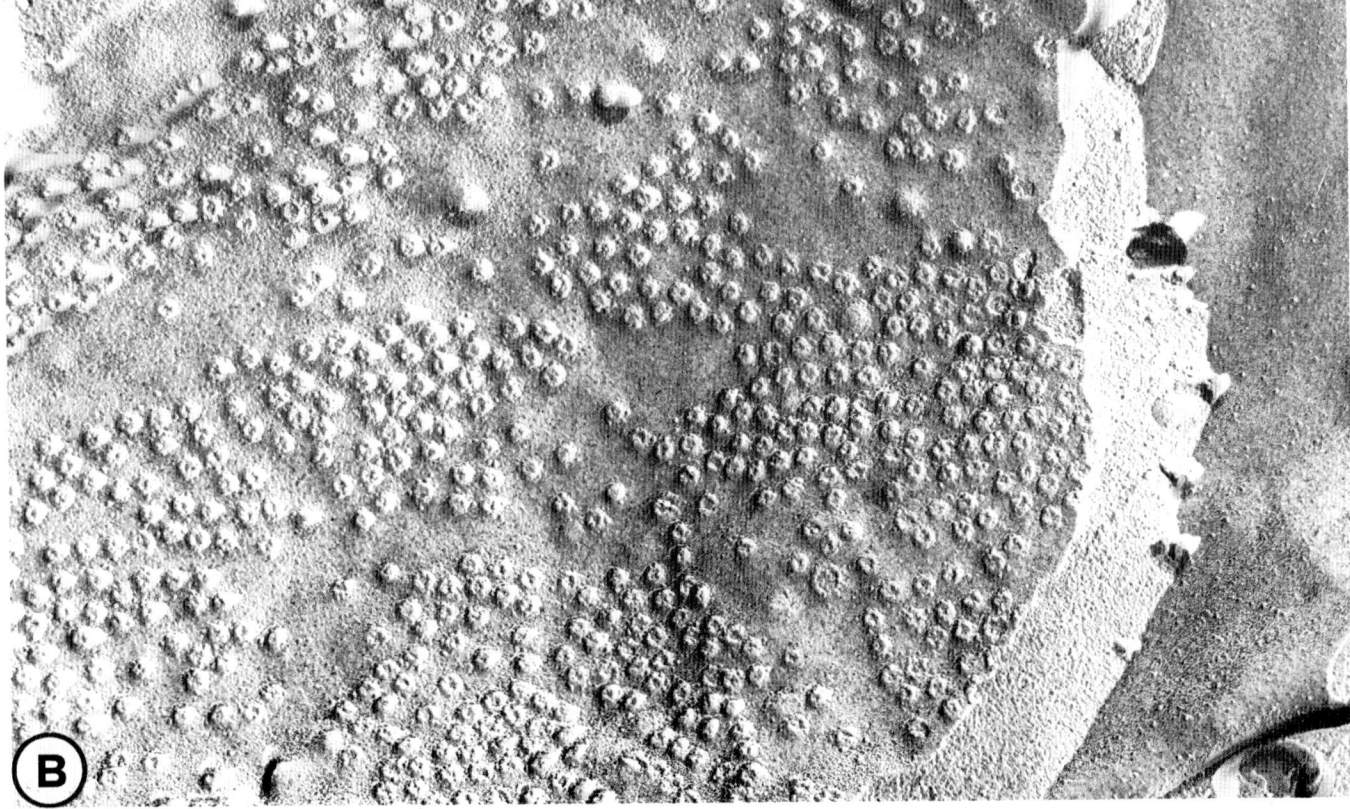

A **Pinocytotic vesicles in endothelium from rat femoral artery (scanning EM, x45,000).** The cell membrane of both the luminal side and the basal side of the endothelial cell is infolded to form many pinocytotic vesicles (→). **M** = bundle of filaments. **N** = nucleus of the endothelial cell.

B **Pinocytosis in endothelium of capillary from mouse ovary (EM, freeze fracture, x40,000).** The fracture plane lies on the surface of the vascular endothelium facing the lumen and shows many pinocytotic vesicles. Original micrograph by G. Macchiarelli and G. Familiari.

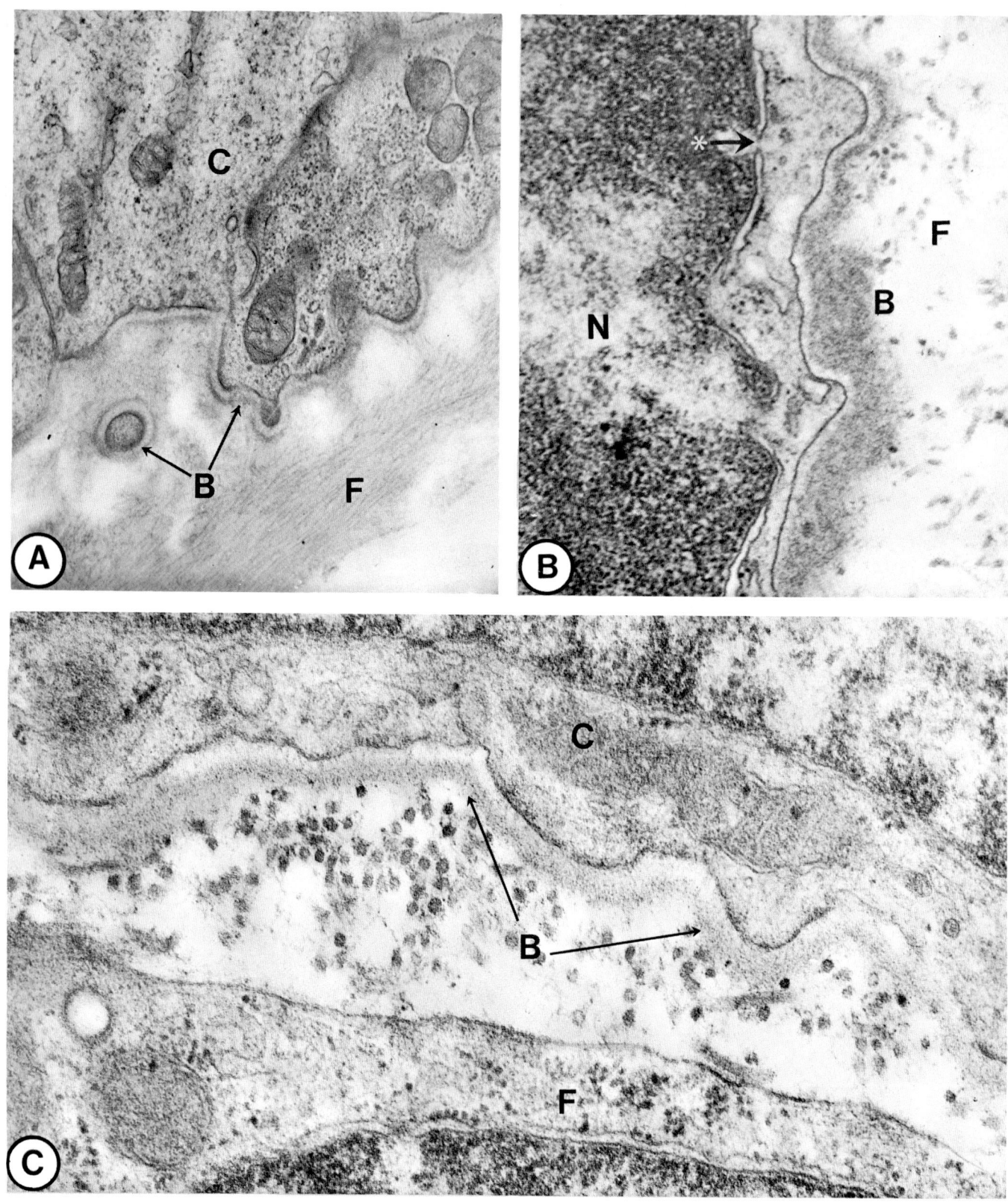

A   **Epithelial lining of human oviduct (EM, x50,000).** The basal lamina **(B→)** underlies the basal surface of the epithelial cells **(C)** adjacent to the connective tissue. A bundle of filaments **(F)** can be seen in the connective tissue.

B   **Basal lamina in epithelium from mouse spleen capillary (EM, x70,000).** The cell membrane is separated from the surrounding connective tissue (right) by the filamentous basal lamina **(B)**. Fibers **(F)** of reticular connective tissue can be seen at right. N = nucleus with nuclear envelope pore (*→).

C   **Basal lamina from serosa of rat intestine (EM, x80,000).** C = cytoplasm of mesothelial cell next to underlying connective tissue. **(B→)** = basal lamina with underlying connective tissue fibers. **F** = fibrocyte.

Plate 1.43   53

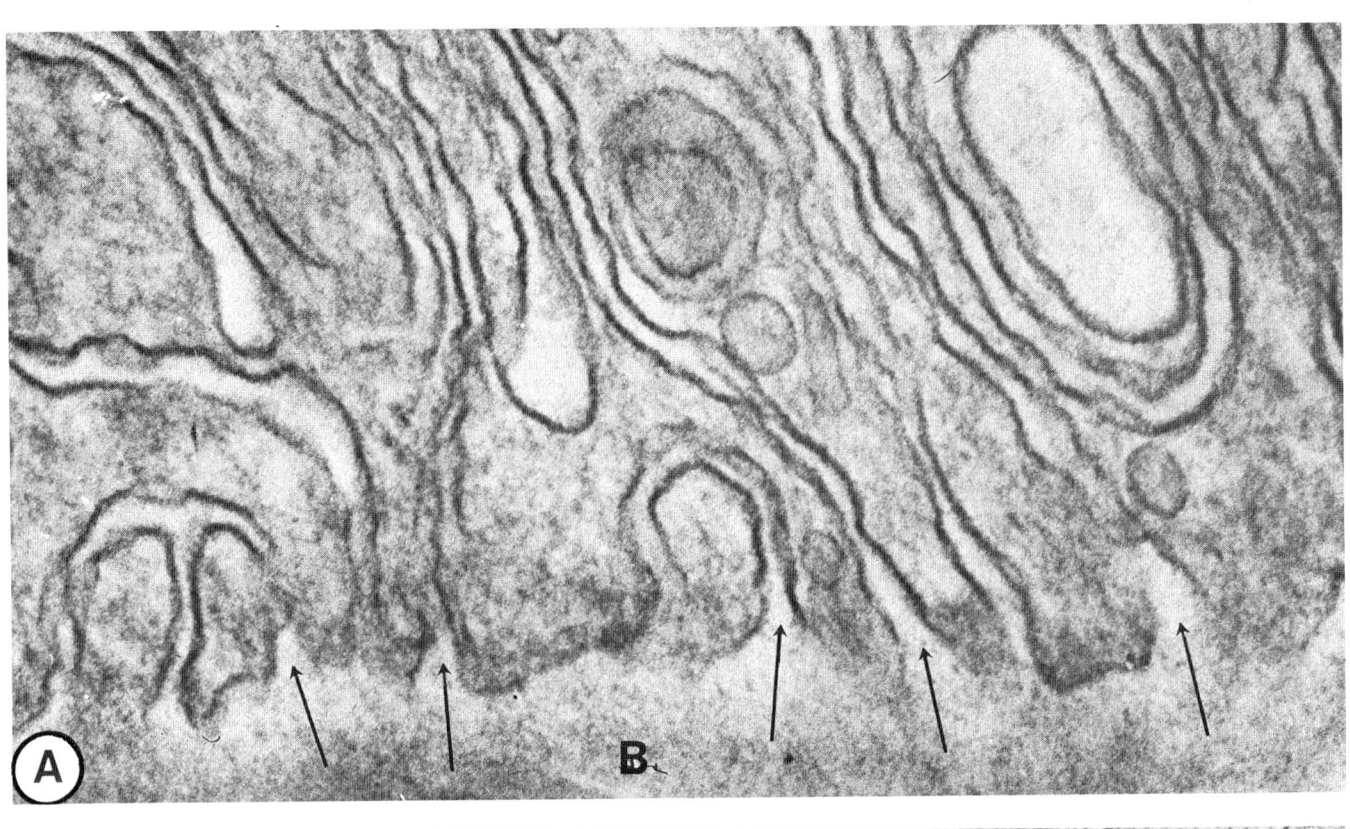

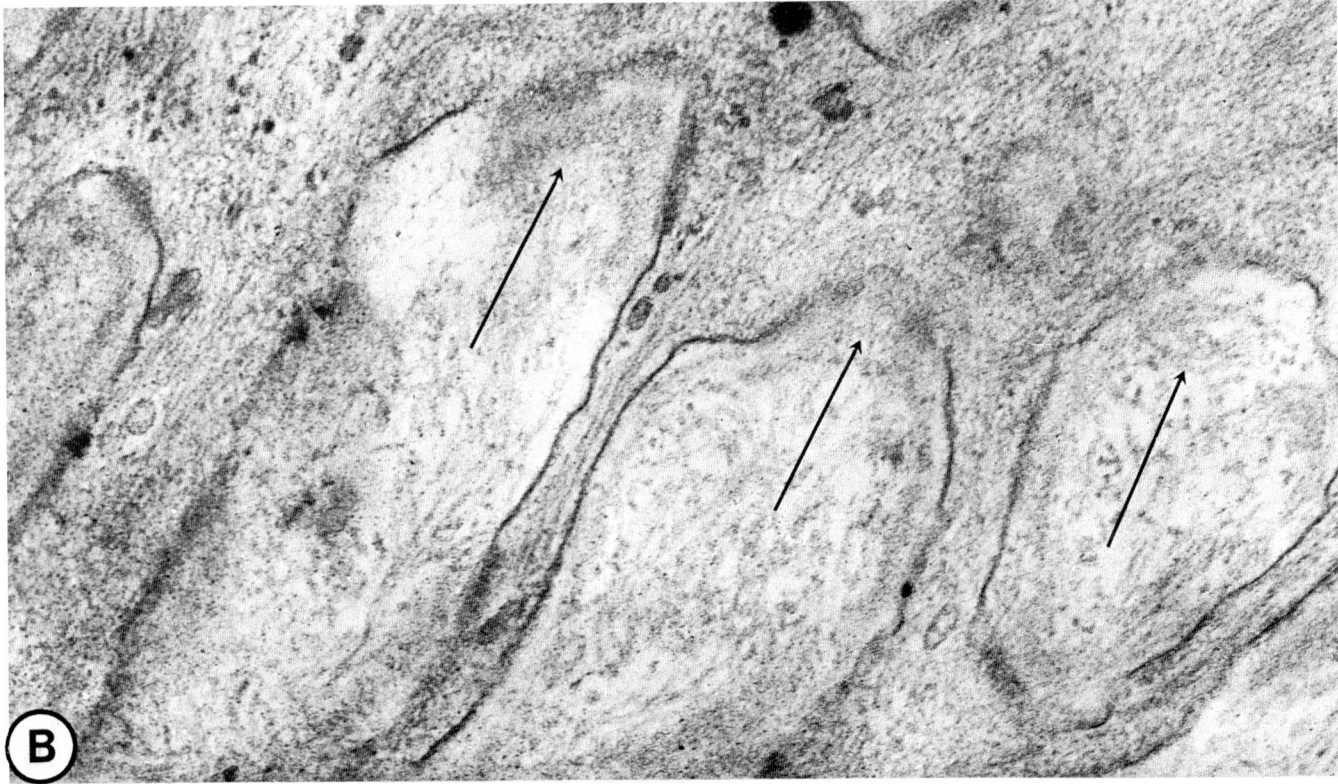

A **Invaginations of plasma membrane of pigmented epithelium of rabbit retina (EM, x70,000).** The basal regions of the epithelial cells are visible adjacent to the basal lamina (B). The cell membrane is folded to form a number of deep invaginations (→).

B **Infoldings in basal region of amniotic epithelium (human) (EM, x60,000).** The plasma membrane, together with its underlying basal lamina, is folded to form large irregular invaginations (→). By courtesy of A. Santoro.

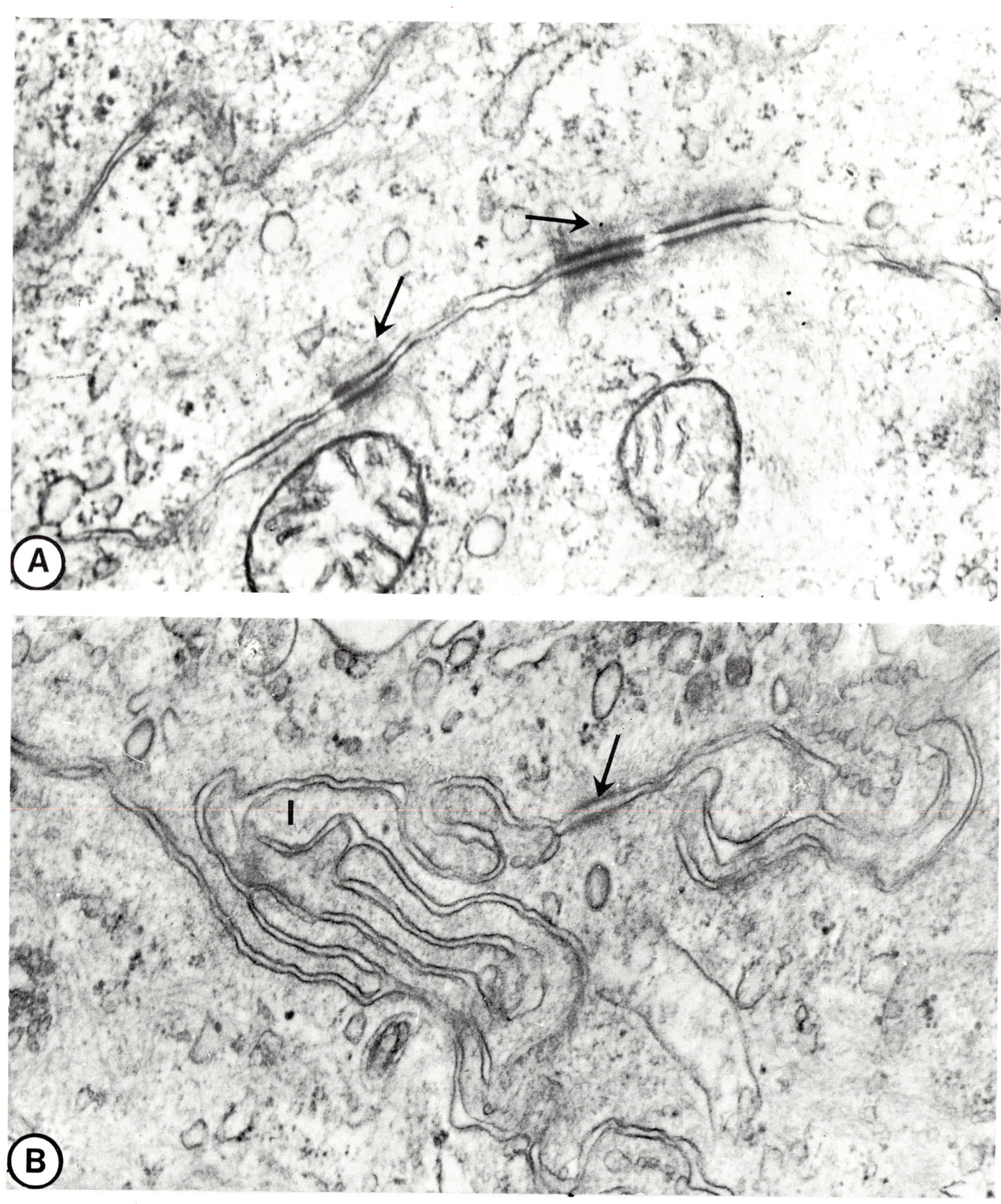

A **Desmosomes between amniotic cells of chick embryo (EM, x500,000).** The cell membranes of the two adjacent cells are close together and run parallel to each other. At certain points (→) desmosomes are present.

B **Interdigitation and junctions between amniotic cells of chick embryo (EM, x50,000). I** = interdigitation of two contiguous cell elements. (→) = desmosome (zonula adherens). This sort of relationship is common between epithelial cells but is also found in other tissues. By courtesy of M. P. Franceschini and A. Santoro.

Plate 1.45   55

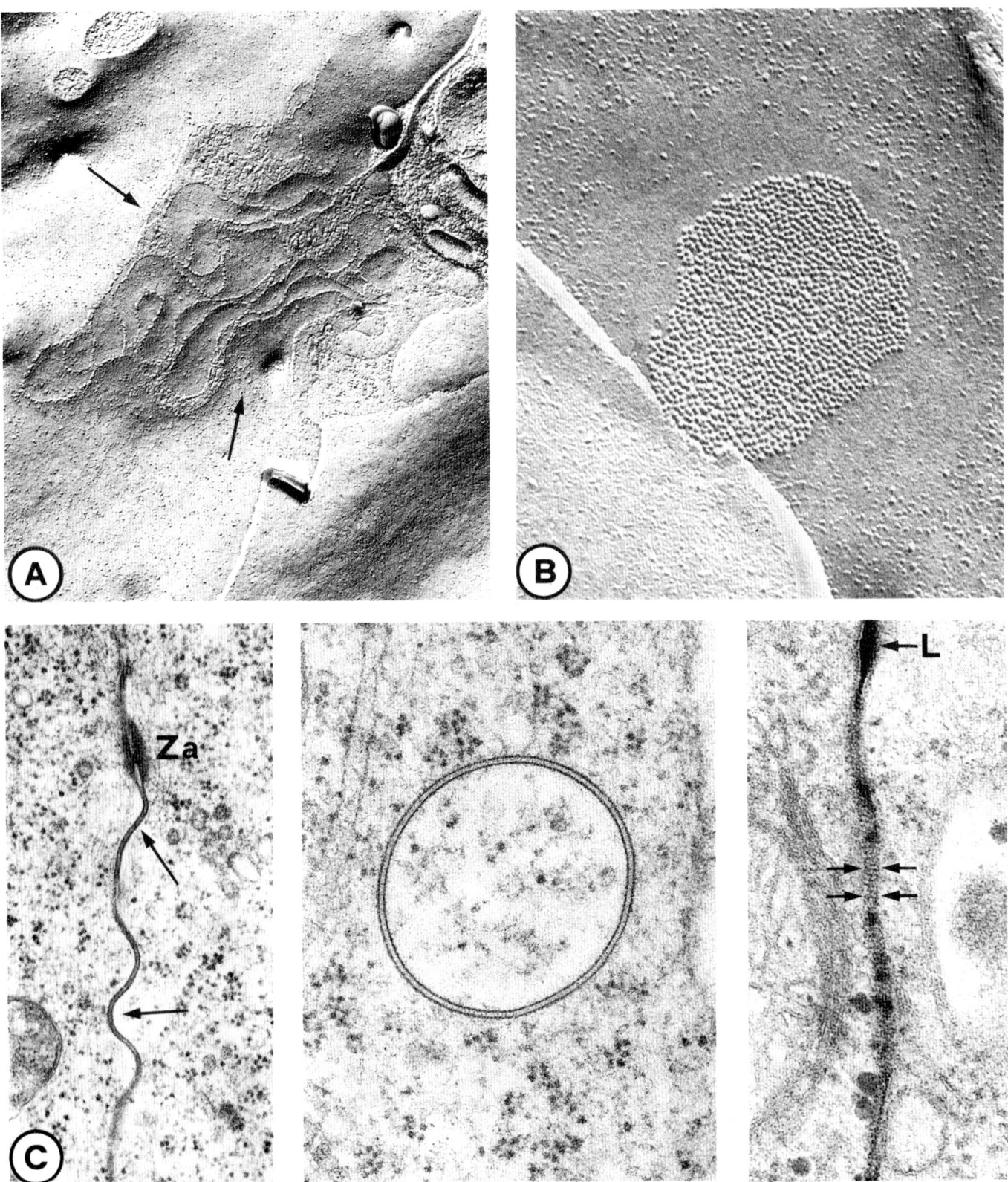

A   **Tight junction (zonula occludens) between epithelial cells (EM, freeze fracture, x45,000).** Intermembranous particles that are aligned in rows (→) form the tight junction which seals the adjacent epithelial cells together.

B   **Gap junction between epithelial cells (EM, freeze fracture, x100,000).** The junction in the face view appears as a plate made up of regular arrays of particles. Every particle contains a minute channel through which the cells in contact exchange ions and metabolites.

C   **Gap junctions between epithelial cells (EM, x37,000, x70,000, x110,000).** In these junctions the cell membranes are close together but separated by a thin intercellular space 2 nm in width. In the left-hand figure the desmosome (zonula adherens) (**Za**) lies very near the gap junction (→). In the center figure a ring-like gap junction is visible. In the right-hand figure lanthanum has been introduced into the intercellular space (**L**→) and outlines the minute channels of communication between the closely connected membranes of the gap junction (→←). By courtesy of G. Familiari and F. Barberini.

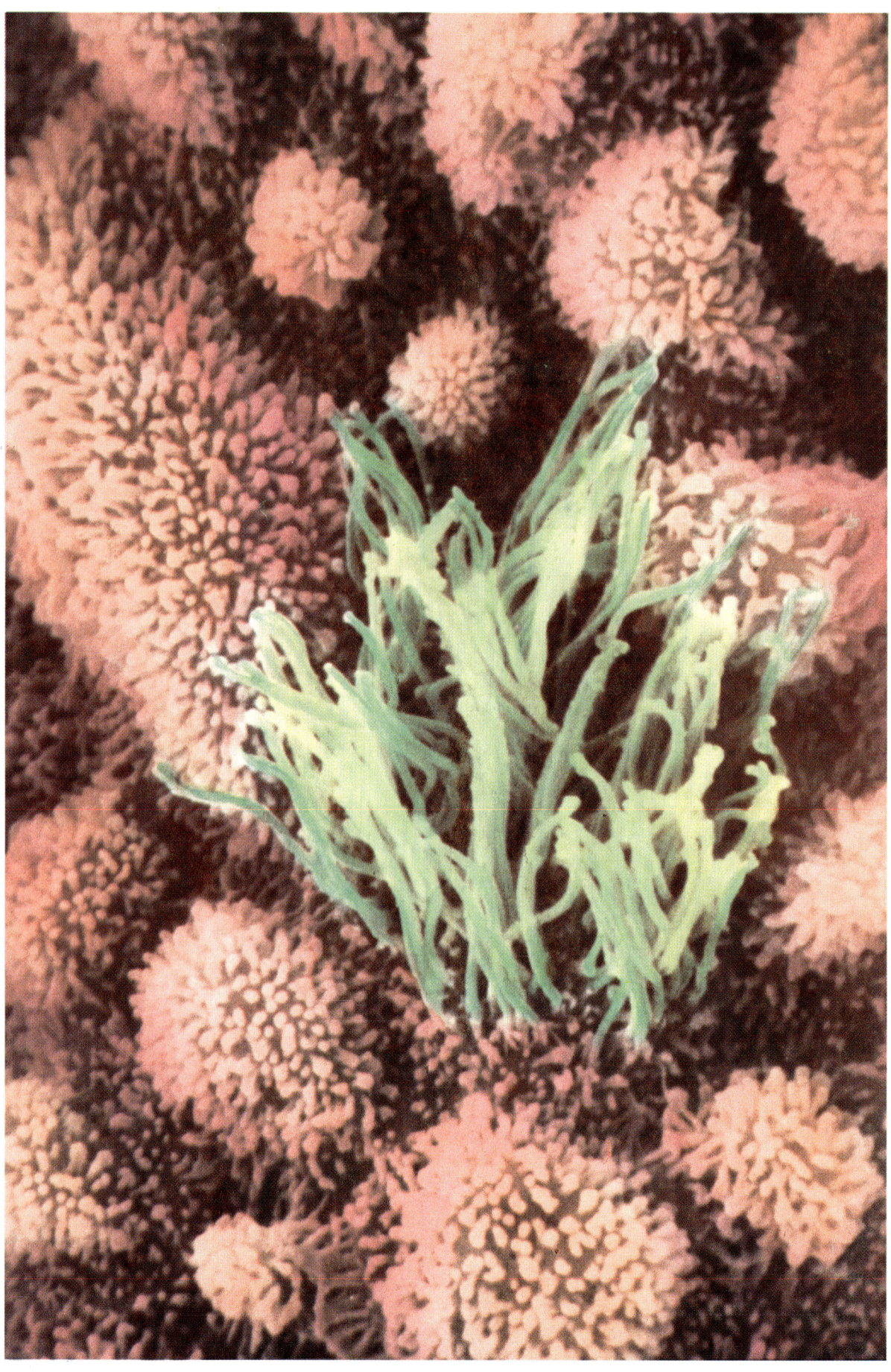

Epithelial tissue. The ciliated and microvillous cells form the epithelial layer of the uterine mucosa (endometrium) of a rat. (Colored SEM; 7,500 x).

PART II

TISSUES

A tissue can be defined as a complex of cells that have the same origin and are differentiated morphologically to perform the same functions. All the organs of the body are composed of four fundamental types of tissue: *epithelium, connective tissue, muscular tissue and nervous tissue.* A fifth type of tissue, though less easily categorized according to traditional histology, is the germinal tissue. Gametes from both sexes unite in the process of fertilization and, with successive divisions, produce the embryonic layers from which all other tissues are derived.

CHAPTER

2

EPITHELIUM

An epithelium is composed of cells in direct contact with one another without the presence of intercellular substances. The cells are differentiated morphologically to act as protective coverings, to produce secretions, to carry out sensory functions, and to effect transport between compartments. Thus the tissues can be classified into subgroups of *covering, secretory, sensory and transporting epithelium.*

Covering epithelium

Covering epithelia are formed of one or more layers of cells resting on a *basal* or *basement membrane*, which itself rests on underlying connective tissue. This type of epithelium forms the outer layer that covers the outer surface of the human body (the *epidermis*), the inner surface of hollow organs that communicate with the outside (*mucosal surface*) and the lining of the body cavities (*serosal surface*) which are not in communication with the outside. Blood and lymph vessels do not enter epithelia; rather, they are supplied with nutrients by diffusion of substances transported from the blood vessels across the connective tissue and epithelial basal lamina.

Epithelial cells generally are polyhedral in shape. Covering epithelia have the capacity to reproduce readily, and thus can replace those cells that become damaged or worn out. They often contain granules of pigment in varying quantities. Because these cells lack substances to bind them together they form various types of intercellular junctions (*zonula occludens, zonula adherens, macula adherens*).

The free surface of epithelia may be adapted for movement and absorption, since they can have numerous cilia, stereocilia, microvilli and both phagocytotic and pinocytotic invaginations. In certain epithelia with a pronounced protective function the surface can be built up into microplicae. The basal surface that adheres to the basal lamina often is highly folded, forming deep and sometimes regular invaginations.

A covering epithelium is classified according to the shape and number of cell layers of which it is composed. The primary classifications include *simple squamous epithelium, cuboidal epithelium, columnar epithelium* (*simple or stratified*) or *pseudostratified,* i.e., nuclei at differerent levels, and *transitional epithelium* (cells of variable shape) (Plates 2.1, 2.2, 2.3).

Secretory epithelium

Secretory epithelium is made up of cells whose function is to produce and discharge synthesized material from the cell. The substances are specific to the cell type (Plates 2.4, 2.5). Secretions are discharged directly or via a duct to an external or internal surface of the body (*exocrine secretion*), or are discharged directly into the blood system (*endocrine secretion*). Secretory epithelia carry out the basic function of exocrine and endocrine glands.

Three phases can be distinguished in the secretion of polypeptides, proteoglycans or glycoproteins: an *excitatory phase*, a *synthetic phase* and an *extrusion phase*. Each of these is characterized by particular changes in the cell. Excitation involves activation of the plasma membranes in response to neural or hormonal stimulation. In the extrusion phase the product is released by exocytosis of secretory granules. In the synthetic phase the secretory granules are reformed.

In special cases (*holocrine secretion*) the entire cell is shed in effecting liberation of the secretory product. A second special case is *merocrine secretion*, in which only a part of the cytoplasm is discharged and the cell remains intact and regenerates the lost cytoplasm.

Sensory epithelium

Sensory epithelium includes neurons associated with epithelial cells that surround and support them. The sensory epithelia are specialized by their morphology and function to receive certain stimuli. These cells resemble receptor neurons and are in functional contact with the nervous system (Plates 2.6, 2.7). Thus the cells of this type are linked to nerve processes with which they form special contacts called the *cytoneural junction*. In general these cells act as transducers conveying external stimuli to the nervous system.

A typical sensory epithelial cell consists of 1) a surface or receptor area formed by long cytoplasmic protrusions very often derived from cilia, 2) an area of intermediate cytoplasm rich in mitochondria which supply the energy for transduction, and 3) a base or junctional area that contains the nucleus and is connected to one or more of the cytoneural junctions. When the quantities of outside energy, usually in minute amounts, reach the excitation threshold, they initiate a complex chemical change in the membrane that transforms and amplifies the external signal and thus leads to the formation of a nerve impulse that is transmitted along the nerve fibers.

Examples of sensory epithelial cells include those in the taste bud, which are spindle-shaped and are surrounded by support cells (Plate 2.6 A). Another example is the internal and external hair cells of the inner ear. These cells are prismatic and columnar in shape, and they too are interspersed between special supporting cells. Together the acoustic and supporting cells comprise the spiral *organ of Corti* (Plates 2.6 B,C,D, 2.7 A). *Ciliated cells of the utricle and of the saccule* of the inner ear also are interspersed between support cells. These cells are in the shape of a prism or a flask and form the *static maculae* of the membranous labyrinth (Plate 2.7 B). Flask-shaped hair cells (*ampulla cells*) also are interspersed between support cells. They are found in the ampullae of the semicircular canals, each constituting a *crista ampullaris*.

Transporting epithelium

Another important function of epithelia is to monitor exchanges between compartments. These transporting epithelia, which are exemplified by the epithelium lining the intestines, will be discussed in chapter 8.

Plate 2.1   **61**

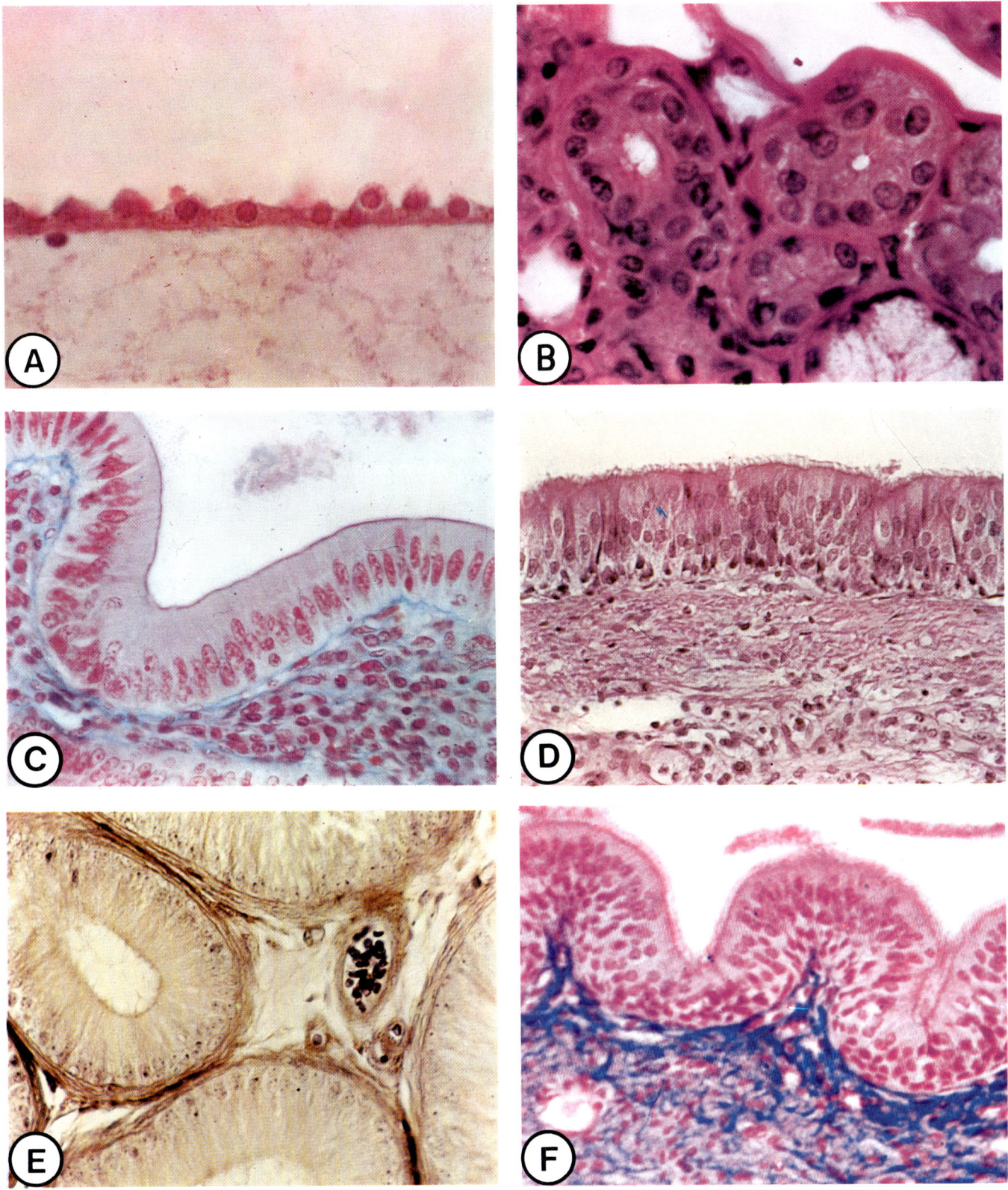

A   Simple squamous epithelium from the membranous labyrinth of human fetus (H & E, x330).
B   Cuboidal epithelium of ducts of salivary gland (H & E, x410).
C   Brush border of columnar epithelium of intestinal mucosa (azan-Mallory, x370).
D   Ciliated columnar epithelium of oviduct (H & E, x330).
E   Columnar epithelium with stereocilia from wall of ductuli efferentes of epididymis (iron-hematoxylin, x370).
F   Pseudostratified columnar epithelium with cilia from respiratory mucosa (azan-Mallory, x330).

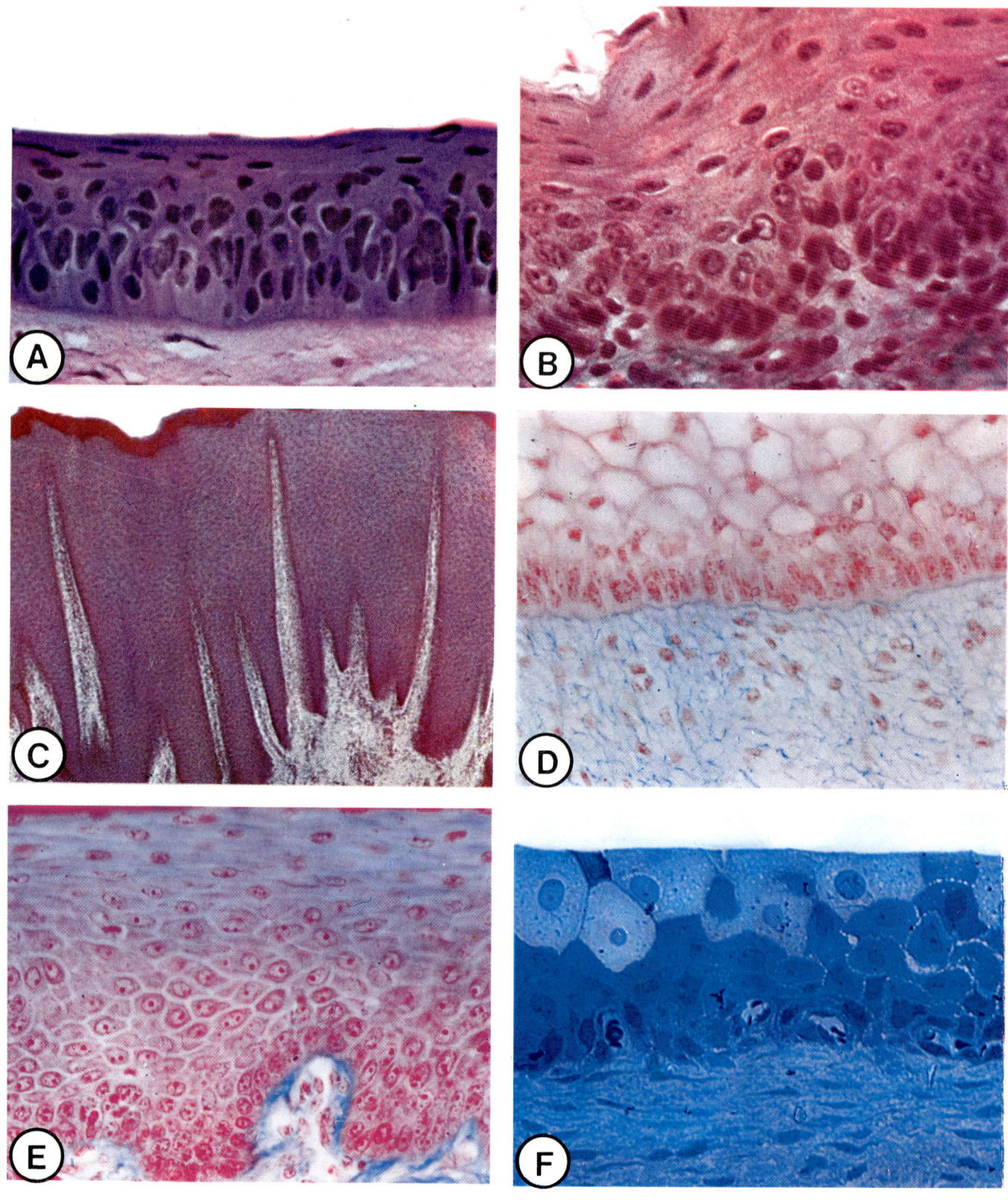

A   Stratified squamous epithelium of pig cornea (H & E, x320).
B   Stratified squamous epithelium of human esophagus (azan-Mallory, x370).
C   Keratinized stratified squamous epithelium from skin of calf lip (H & E, x75).
D   Basal lamina of stratified squamous epithelium of human fetal epidermis (azan-Mallory, x320).
E   Keratinized squamous epithelium of human epidermis (azan-Mallory, x350)
F   Transitional epithelium of rat urinary bladder (Methylene blue, x370).

Plate 2.3 63

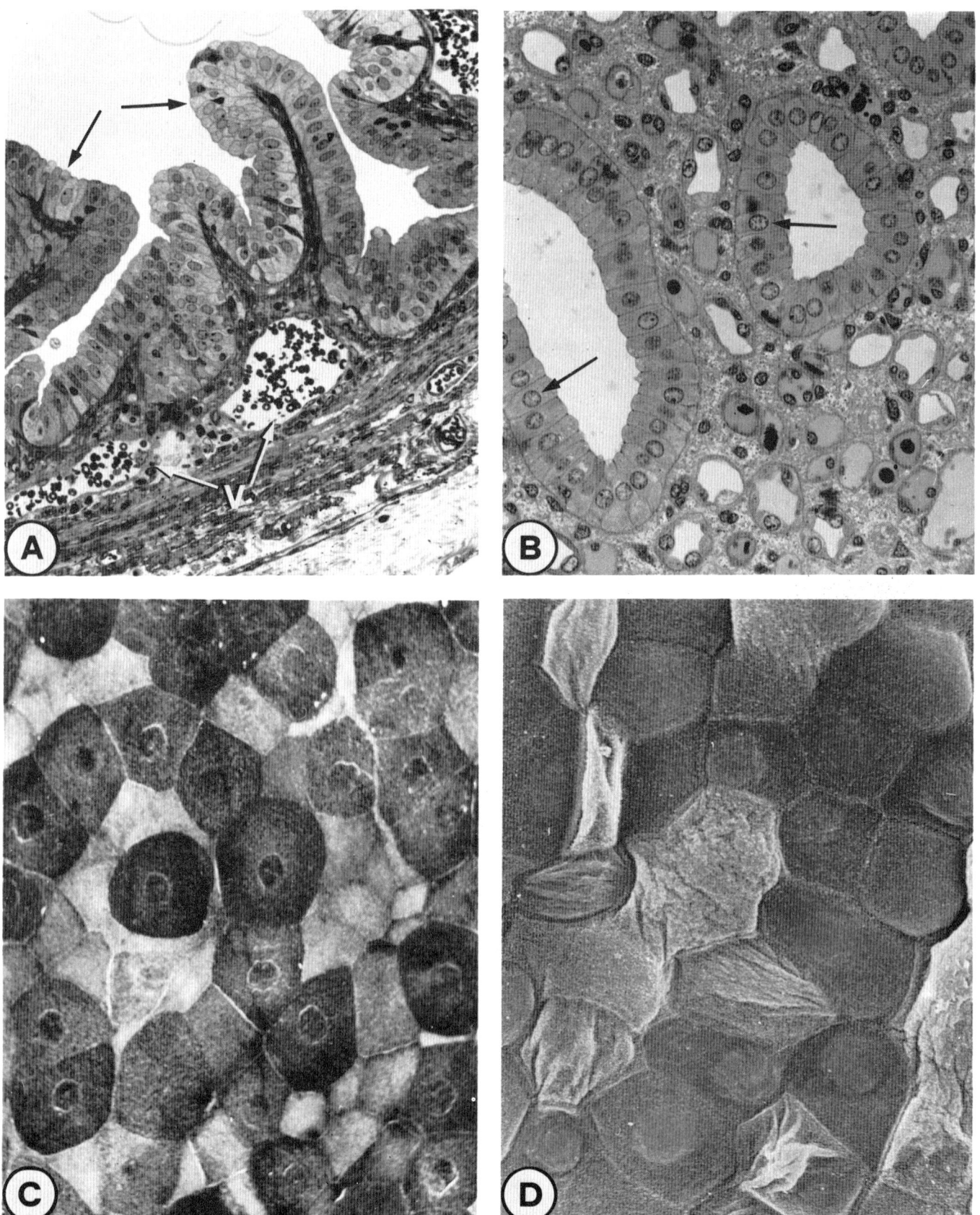

A Semithin section of epithelium lining the gallbladder of cat (toluidine blue, x760). The columnar epithelial cells ($\rightarrow$) rest on the highly folded lamina propria. V = blood vessels containing abundant red cells. Original micrograph by M. Castellucci.

B Semithin section of simple columnar epithelium of papillary ducts from pig kidney (toluidine blue, x810). Note that the nuclei are positioned in the central region ($\rightarrow$) of each of the cells. Courtesy of M. Castellucci.

C Epithelial covering of human cornea (EM, x2,900). The outlines of the polygonal cells are clearly visible with centrally located nuclei. Original by M. Ripani.

D Epithelial lining of the renal calyx of rat (scanning EM, x3,200). The contraction of the wall has caused the surface of some of the cells to appear wrinkled. Original microgrpah by F. Carpino.

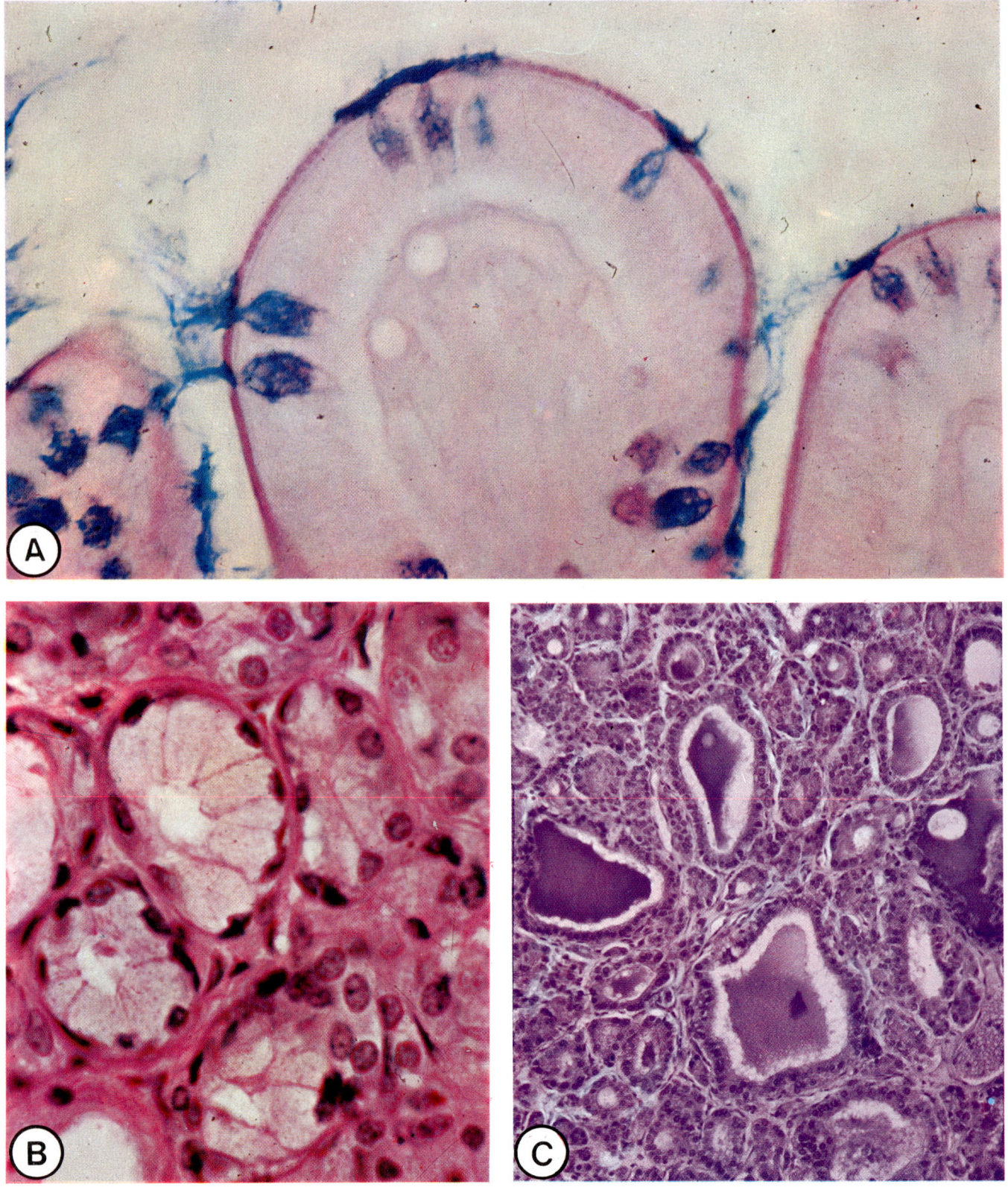

A **Goblet cells from apex of villus in chick intestine (Gendre Alcian blue, PAS, x420).** The goblet cells, stained dark blue, lie in the intestinal epithelium. The brush border is stained red. Goblet cells function as unicellular glands. By courtesy of E. Nesci and D. Palermo. Biol. Lat. 29:619, 1966.

B **Human seromucous exocrine gland (sublingual salivary gland) (H & E, x480).** The mucus-secreting cells of the glandular units are lightly stained and have a flattened nucleus in the basal region.

C **Follicles from rabbit thyroid (endocrine gland) (H & E, x220).** Secretory cells of the thyroid gland form follicles, each having a central cavity in which the secretory product is stored before release into the bloodstream.

Plate 2.5   **65**

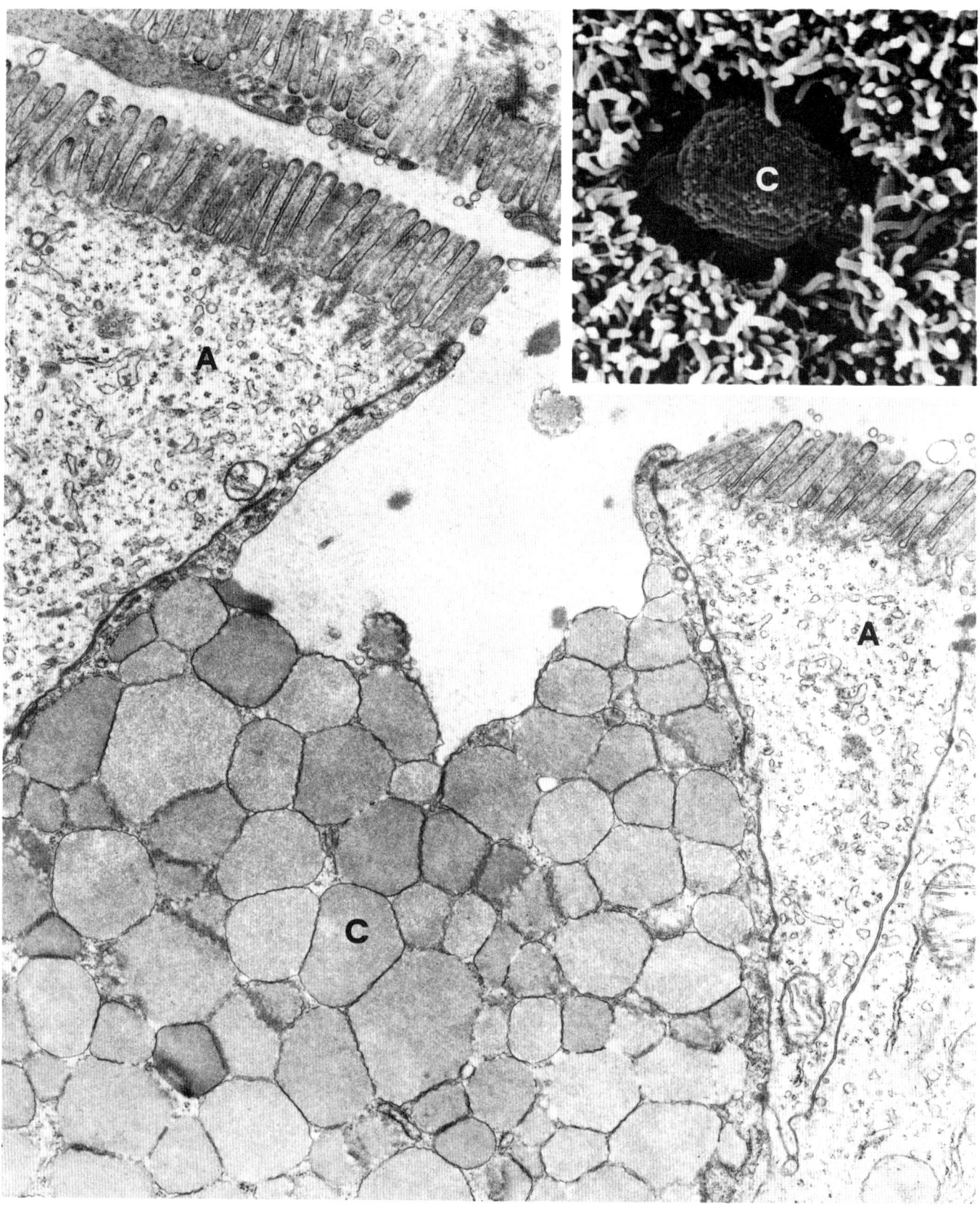

Mucus-secreting goblet cell from rat small intestine (EM, x12,500). The cell has numerous secretory granules **(C)** in its apical region and is wedged between two absorptive cells **(A),** which have a border of microvilli. Original by J. Van Blerkom. **Inset: apical surface of a goblet cell (C) from monkey large intestine (Scanning EM, x6,500).** This secretory cell is surrounded by the microvilli of neighboring absorptive cells.

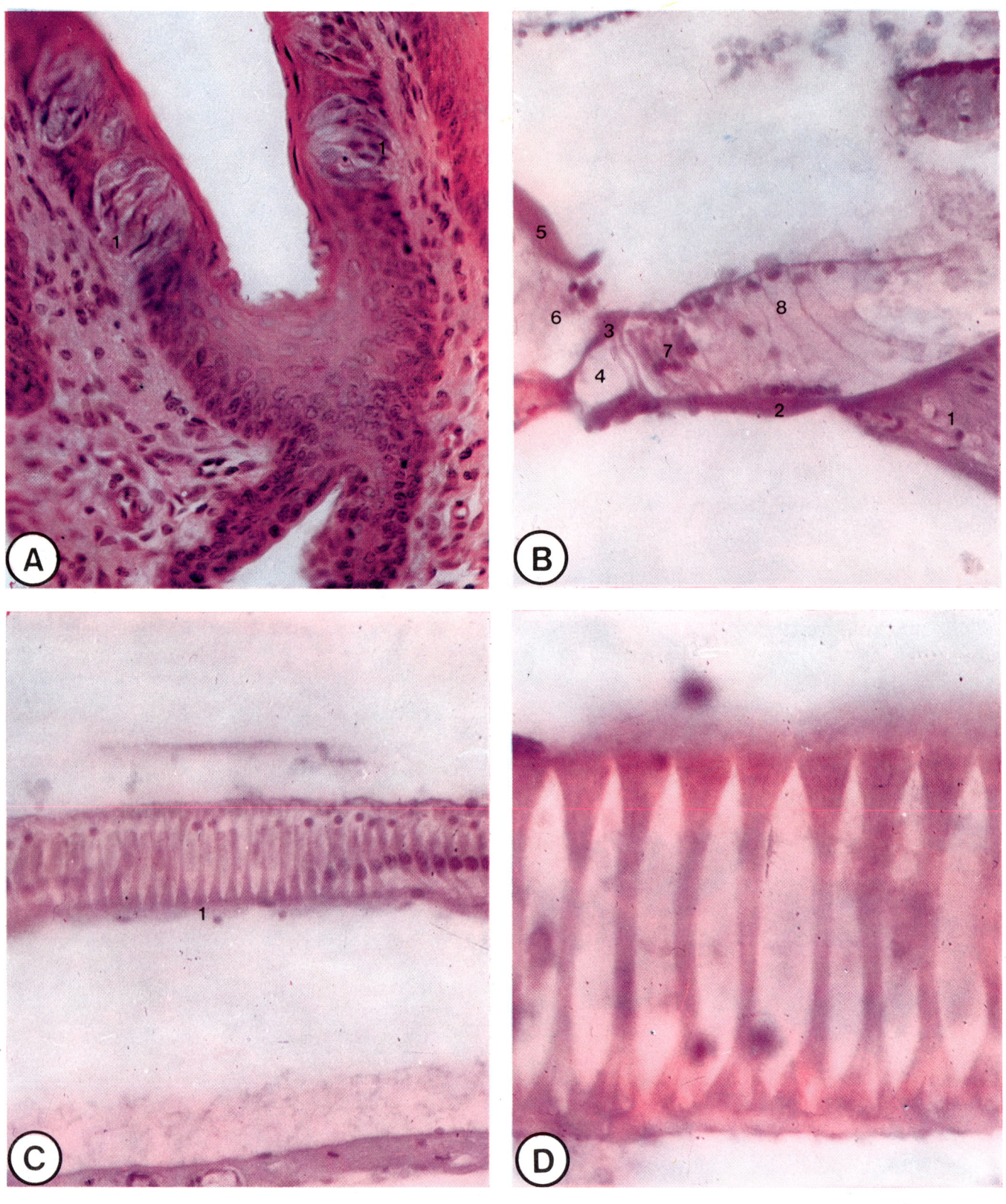

A   **Taste buds from mouse tongue mucosa (H & E, x320).** Each taste bud **(1),** oval in shape, is composed of taste cells (sensory epithelium) and prismatic supporting cells around a narrow duct.

B   **Organ of Corti from bat (H & E, x450).** **1** = spiral ligament. **2** = basilar membrane. **3** = inner and outer pillar cells surrounding the tunnel of Corti **(4).** **5** = tectorial membrane. **6** = inner hair cells. **7** = outer hair cells. **8** = cells of Hensen.

C   **Tunnel of organ of Corti from a bat (H & E, x320).** Sectioned parallel to the main axis of the tunnel. **1** = interspersed outer pillar cells and outer hair cells resting on the basal membrane. Above, scala vestibuli; below, scala tympani.

D   **Outer pillar cells and hair cells in organ of Corti of bat (H & E, x900).** Outer hair cells (translucent) and outer pillar cells (dark) alternate in a columnar pattern. By courtesy of E. Borghesan.

Plate 2.7   **67**

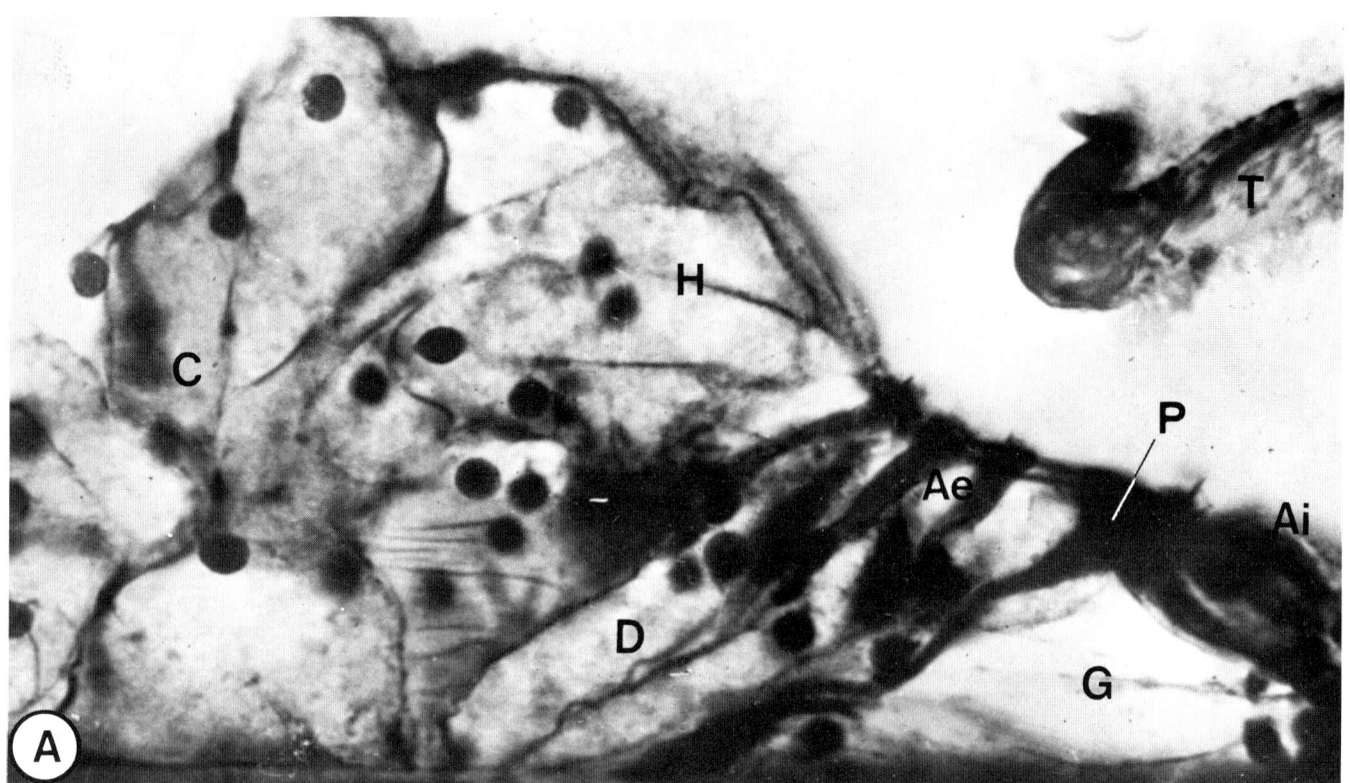

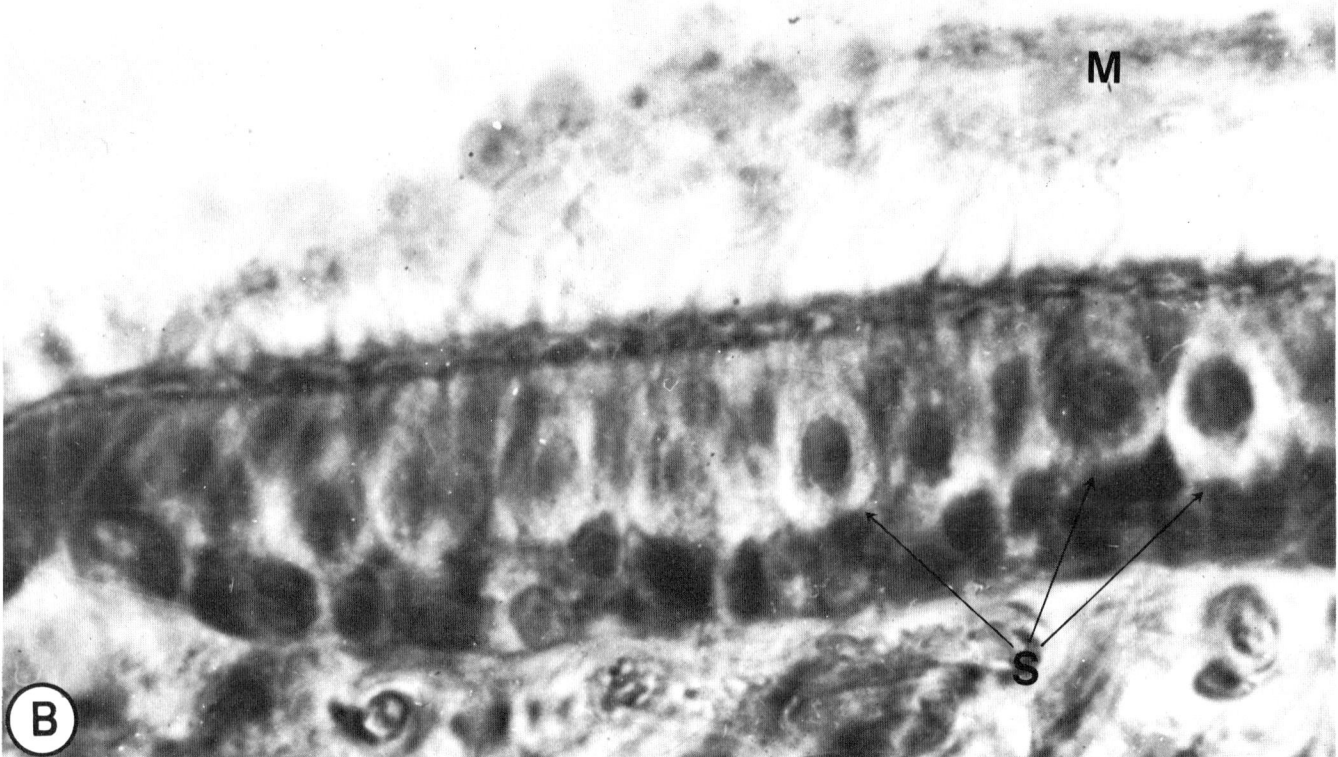

A   **Rabbit organ of Corti (H & E, x1,100). T** = tectorial membrane. **G** = internal spiral tunnel. **P** = pillar cells (inner and outer). **H** = cells of Hensen. **D** = cells of Deiters. **C** = cells of Claudius. The inner and outer hair cells **(Ai, Ae)** have modified cilia that act as receptors.

B   **Macula from rabbit saccule (H & E, x1,100).** The epithelium is made of columnar receptor cells. On the surface of the macula the otolith membrane **(M)** can be seen. By courtesy of E. Borghesan.

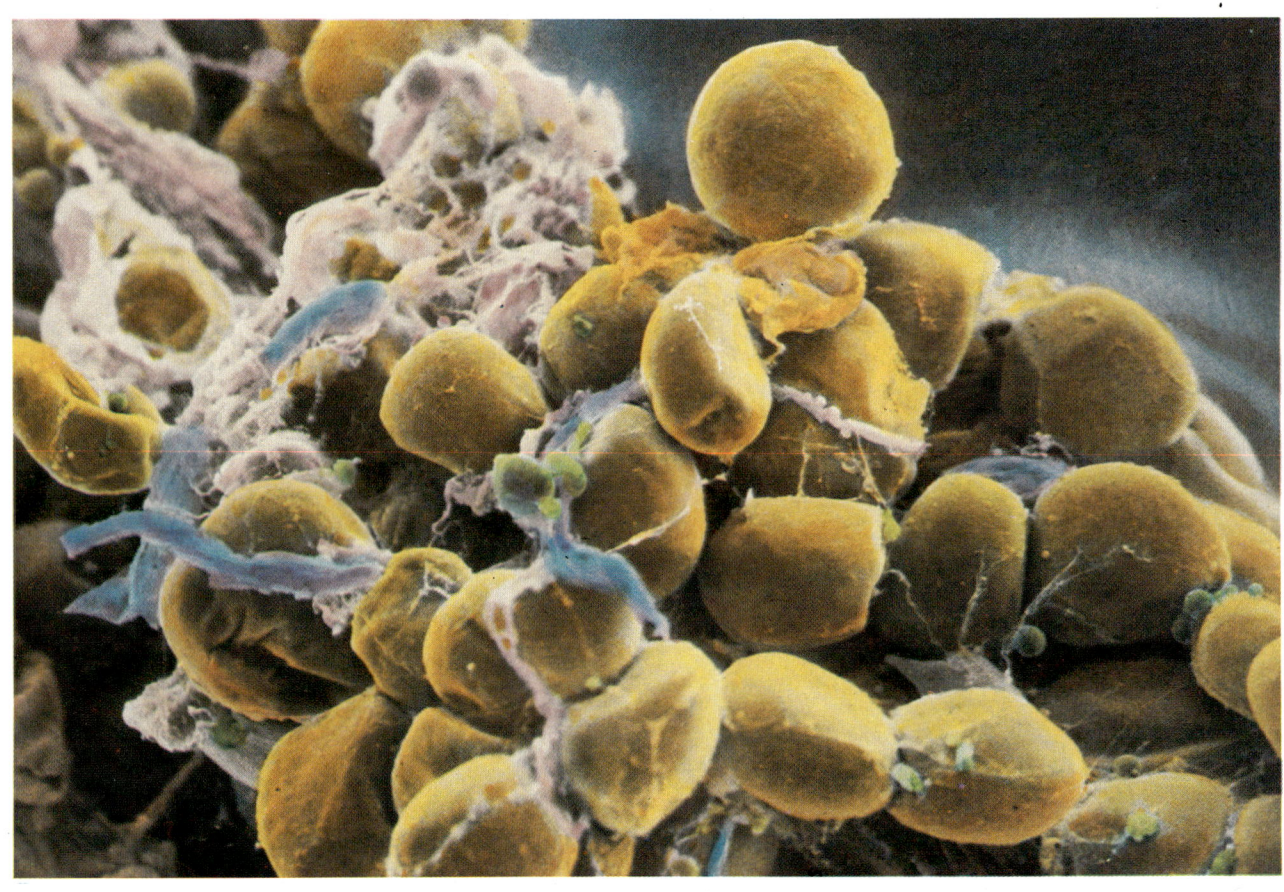

Connective tissue. Adipose cells supported by strands of collagen fibers and covered by a delicate network of reticular fibrils. Capillaries and nerve fibers are associated with the adipose tissue. (Mouse. Colored SEM; 680 x).

CONNECTIVE TISSUE

The cells comprising the connective tissues vary greatly in shape. They are separated from one another by intercellular substance which appears amorphous and fibrous. This matrix, which is organic, non-living material produced by the connective tissue cells, is the predominant supporting element of cells and therefore has a mechanical function. Connective tissue binds together the different parts of the organism, supporting the other tissues, and filling the spaces between different parts of an organ and between different tissues. It forms a sheath around nerve bundles and around blood and lymph vessels. Moreover, all exchange of materials between the blood and the cells occurs via the connective tissue. Also, many of the defenses of the organism against foreign antigens occur in certain types of connective tissue.

Mesenchyme, the embryonic connective tissue, is capable of forming all the various types of connective tissue.

Ground substance

A specific ground substance exists for each type of connective tissue. In certain connective tissues the ground substance forms the bulk of the tissue. This substance reacts weakly with acidic stains. It is often translucent when viewed by the light microscope, and its consistency varies with its functional state. It is metachromatic and reacts positively to PAS. It is composed of water, salts and a mixture of proteoglycans, especially glycosaminoglycans bound to proteins. Glycosaminoglycans (GAG) may be sulfated (chondroitin sulfates A, B and C; keratosulfate and heparin) or non-sulfated (hyaluronic acid). The viscosity of the ground substance can be modified by spreading factors such as the enzyme hyaluronidase and by hormones.

Connective tissue fibers

Fibers are embedded in the ground substance and are composed of dense scleroprotein. Filaments combine to form *protofibrils,* and the protofibrils merge to form larger bundles, the *fibers.* Three types of fibers are classified by biochemical and morphological criteria: *collagen, reticular fibers* and *elastic fibers.*

Collagen fibers are ribbon-like and are especially numerous in tendons and ligaments. They have no specific length and usually do not exceed 200 nm in thickness and width. They resist tension strongly, yield gelatin when boiled, and will dissolve in strong acids or alkali. They are digested by pepsin but not by trypsin. They stain red with hematoxylin and eosin (H & E) and blue with Mallory's stain. The fibers are composed of small units of collagen fibrils (*tropocollagen*) 280-300 nm long and 1.5 nm wide. The fibrils are arranged such that when viewed at high magnification a typical banding pattern can be seen, having regular intervals of 60-70 nm (Plates 3.3 A, 3.4, 3.5).

Reticular fibers are visible at the level of the light microscope only by stains containing silver. Reticular fibers are found in the basal lamina as short fibers or fibrils that form a complex network. They have low elasticity, resist concentrated acids and alkali, stain blue with Mallory's, green with Masson stain, and black with silver. By electron microscopy they show the same banding pattern as collagen fibers (60-70 nm). The difference between collagen and reticular fibers is thought to depend on the number and arrangement of the collagen protofibrils and on properties of the mucopolysaccharides that bind the fibrils rather than on a difference in the type of protein (Plate 3.5 C).

Elastic fibers are threads of variable thickness, from 200 nm to 12 um. The elastin making up the fibers is joined together to form a cross-link network. It is composed of elastin filaments bound by an amorphous substance (*tropoelastin*), which can be digested by the enzyme elastase. The fibers are highly elastic. They are easily digested with trypsin but not at all with pepsin. They stain yellow with van Gieson stain, dark red with resorcin fuschin. There is no banding pattern present (Plate 3.2 C).

Connective tissue with little ground substance

Connective tissues with little ground substance include a category of tissues that are mainly cellular, such as the notochord of vertebrate embryos. The embryonic mesenchyme (Plate 3.2 A) constitutes the mesoderm and thus gives rise to the connective tissue, muscle and many epithelia.

Endothelium and mesothelium are two types of epithelium derived from mesenchyme. They form the lining of the body cavities and the vascular system, both closed cavities within the body. Circulating fluids such as blood and lymph are contained in the vessels. Morphologically, endothelia are frequently simple squamous epithelia, but their shape may vary according to the particular vessels in which they occur.

The endothelial cells of some highly permeable capillaries have a cytoplasm that contains many pores, such as in the capillaries of the kidney glomerulus and many endocrine glands. Their plasma membranes may be infolded to form numerous pinocytotic vesicles (Plates 1.41, 4.1).

Connective tissue with abundant ground substance

Classification of connective tissue depends not only on the composition of the ground substance, but also on the quantity and quality of the fibers. The cells that compose it differ in their morphology and arrangement. Connective tissues with abundant ground substance include connective tissue proper, cartilage, bone and dentin.

Connective tissue proper

Connective tissue proper is composed of cells having various shapes, which can be grouped into a) *fixed cells (fibrocytes, adipose cells)* (Plates 3.4 A,B, 3.5, 3.10), and b) *mobile* (or *potentially mobile) cells (lymphocytes, granular basophils or mast cells, plasma cells, macrophages, polymorphonuclear leukocytes)* (Plates 3.2 E, 3.3, 3.7 A,C,D, 3.8 A,B, 3.9 A,B).

If the amorphous ground substance and cellular elements predominate, then the connective tissue has a loose consistency, whereas if the fibrous part is abundant, the connective tissue is dense and compact. In the embryo the *loose connective tissue* is in the form of mesenchyme and the so-called *mucous connective tissue* (*Wharton's jelly* in the umbilical cord). In the adult, on the other hand, a greater variety of loose connective tissue exists (*reticular, lymphoid* and *adipose tissue*). Dense connective tissue is rich in collagen and elastic fibers usually having a parallel arrangement. Dense connective tissue is found in tendon, ligament, fascia and vessel walls (*elastic tissue*) (Plate 3.2).

Cartilage

Cartilage is a specialized connective tissue lacking vessels and containing a ground substance made up mainly of chondroitin sulfate in which are embedded many fibers (Plates 3.6, 3.7 B). Isolated or small groups of cartilage cells (*chondrocytes*) are contained in hollow cavities in the matrix. Although there is only a small amount of matrix in *cellular cartilage*, which is the embryonic form of cartilage, in adults three types of cartilage can be distinguished according to the composition of the matrix.

Hyaline cartilage is bluish-white in color, translucent, and contains abundant ground substance (chondromucoid) and numerous collagen fibers which are not visible in the light microscope (Plate 3.6 D,E,F). *Elastic cartilage* has a yellowish color and contains collagen fibers and networks of elastic fibers (Plates 3.6 B). *Fibrous cartilage* is whitish and typically contains cartilage cells nestled at intervals among entwined collagen fibers (Plate 3.6 C). The fibers are not as difficult to observe as those of elastic cartilage.

Bone

Bone is a complex connective tissue of cells lying in lacunae within a mineralized matrix. The particular mineral composition of bone matrix, hydroxyapatite, is a calcium phosphate salt and gives great strength to this tissue (Plate 3.11).

Different types of bone are distinguished according to the number and arrangement of the collagen fibers forming them. One type is *lamellar bone*, in which the piles of collagen fibers are so arranged that they run in different directions in each succeeding lamella. When the osseous lamellae are not precisely organized but form irregular spicules, the tissue is called *spongy bone*, whereas when the lamellae form a tightly organized structure, the result is *compact bone*.

In compact bone a number of lamellae are organized around a central cavity containing blood vessels. The central cavity is called the *Haversian canal*, and the cavity plus the lamellae are referred to as the *osteon* or *Haversian system*, the primary unit of compact bone. Haversian canals have their main axes along the main axis of the bone, the spaces between the osteons being filled by interstitial lamellae. Transverse channels (*Volkmann's canals*) interconnect and bring blood vessels into the Haversian systems.

Perforating (Sharpey's) fibers are bundles of collagen fibers found in areas of bone where tendons and ligaments, of which these fibers are a

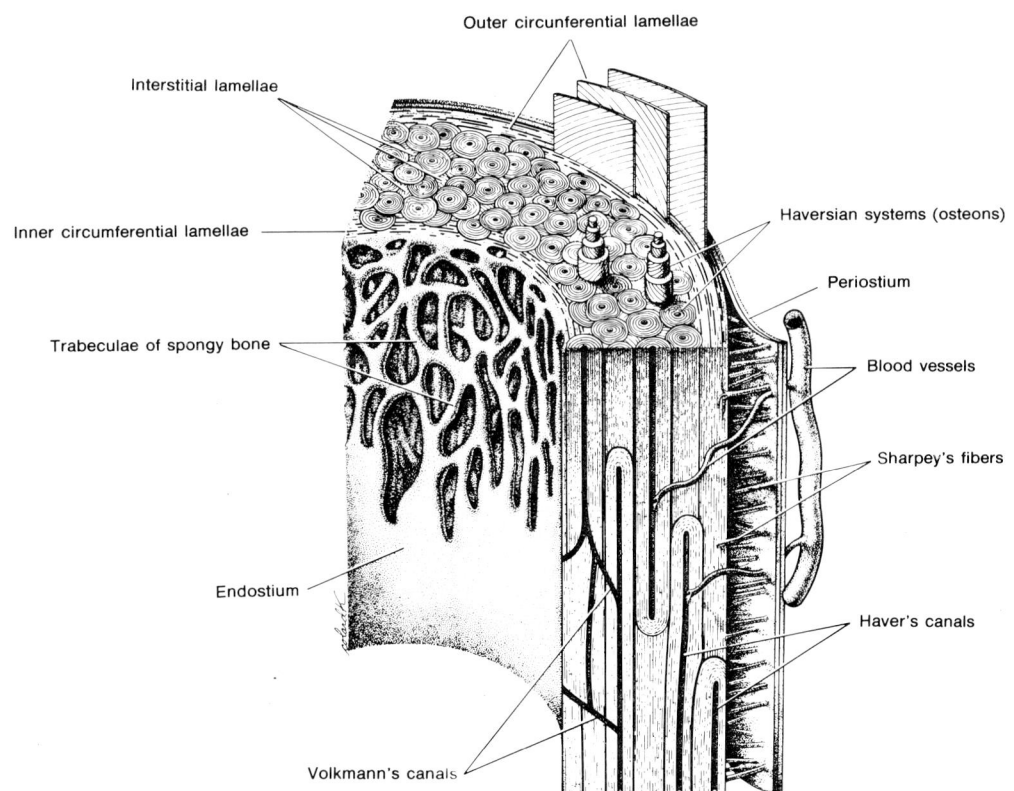

Diaphyseal segment of a long bone showing the arrangement of the Haversian systems, the interstitial lamellae and the outer and inner circumferential lamellae. From A. Benninghoff and K. Goerttler. *Textbook of Functional Anatomy* Vol. 1. Piccin Editore, Padua, 1980.

continuation, join the bone.

Bone tissue can form directly from mesenchyme (*direct ossification*) or indirectly by the replacement of cartilage (*indirect ossification*). The cells of bone tissue (osteocytes) are stellate and have long, thin branching processes that form gap junctions with adjacent cells. The intercellular matrix contains intercommunicating cavities and canaliculi (*bone lacunae*) in which the bone cells and their processes lie.

Dentin

Dentin, like bone, is a tissue made of bundles of collagen fibers bound by a cementing substance. Dentin cells (*odontoblasts*) are prismatic and are arranged in a single layer. From one side of the cell a thin, extra-long cytoplasmic process forms (*dentinal fiber*), and is ensheathed in a canaliculus which it fills. From the opposite side of the cell short branched processes form which insinuate themselves into the underlying connective tissue (*pulp*) (Plate 3.12).

Blood and lymph

Blood and lymph can be considered to be connective tissue having a fluid matrix (Plates 3.13, 3.14). Blood is composed of a liquid part (plasma) and formed elements, including red corpuscles (*erythrocytes*), white corpuscles (*leukocytes*) and platelets. Lymph is a yellowish transparent liquid containing only leukocytes.

Erythrocytes are specialized cells that transport oxygen. They are without a nucleus and have the shape of a biconcave disk. On the average they are 7.7 um in diameter and 2 um thick. In the blood of a normal adult human male there are from 5 to 6 million red cells per mm3, and in a female from 4 to 5 million per mm3. In order to pass through the extremely narrow lumen of certain capillaries, erythrocytes can bend dramatically (Plates 3.9 A,C, 3.13, 3.14 B).

Reticulocytes are erythrocytes that are not fully mature. They are distinguished by having less hemoglobin than mature erythrocytes, and in their cytoplasm residues of polysomes or other organelles can be found (Plates 3.8 C, 3.14 A).

Leukocytes are cells capable of ameboid activity. These cells can be found in connective tissue proper, having migrated from the circulatory system to the tissue spaces by transversing temporary openings in the blood vessel walls (*diapedesis*). In normal conditions there are 5,000 to 9,000 leukocytes in one mm3 of blood (Plates 3.13, 3.14).

Leukocytes can be divided into two main groups.

Granulocytes are characterized by the types of granules found within them. They include *eosinophils, basophils* and *polymorphonuclear leukocytes (neutrophils). Agranular leukocytes* include *monocytes* and *lymphocytes.*

Neutrophils are polymorphonuclear leukocytes with a diameter of 10 to 14 um, having a multilobular nucleus and a cytoplasm rich in small granules (Plates 3.9 B, 3.13 C, 3.14). *Eosinophilic granulocytes* are cells with a diameter of 12-16 um, and have a nucleus with two or three lobes and a cytoplasm containing many acidophilic or eosinophilic granules. Basophil granulocytes are cells with a diameter of 10-13 um, have an S-shaped nucleus and an abundance of basophilic granules.

Lymphocytes, small, medium and *large,* belong to the category of mononuclear leukocytes (Plate 3.13 B). The small and medium lymphocytes have a diameter ranging from 4-10 um; large lymphocytes are rarely greater than 10 to 15 um. These latter are roundish and have a nucleus with a regular profile (Plates 3.9 A, 3.13 A).

Monocytes are large cells, with a diameter from 12-20 um, and a basophilic cytoplasm containing a round or oval nucleus usually having an indentation on one side (Plates 3.8 A, 3.13 E). Monocytes in the circulation are precursors of the macrophages present in the tissues.

Platelets originate by the fragmentation of the cytoplasm of megakaryocytes. They are disk-shaped and measure 1-3 um in diameter. A central densely staining region (*centromere*) can be distinguished from a lightly staining peripheral ring (*hyalomere*). In human adults there are 200,000 to 300,000 platelets per mm3 of blood (Plates 3.9 C, 3.13 F, 3.14 F).

Plate 3.1   73

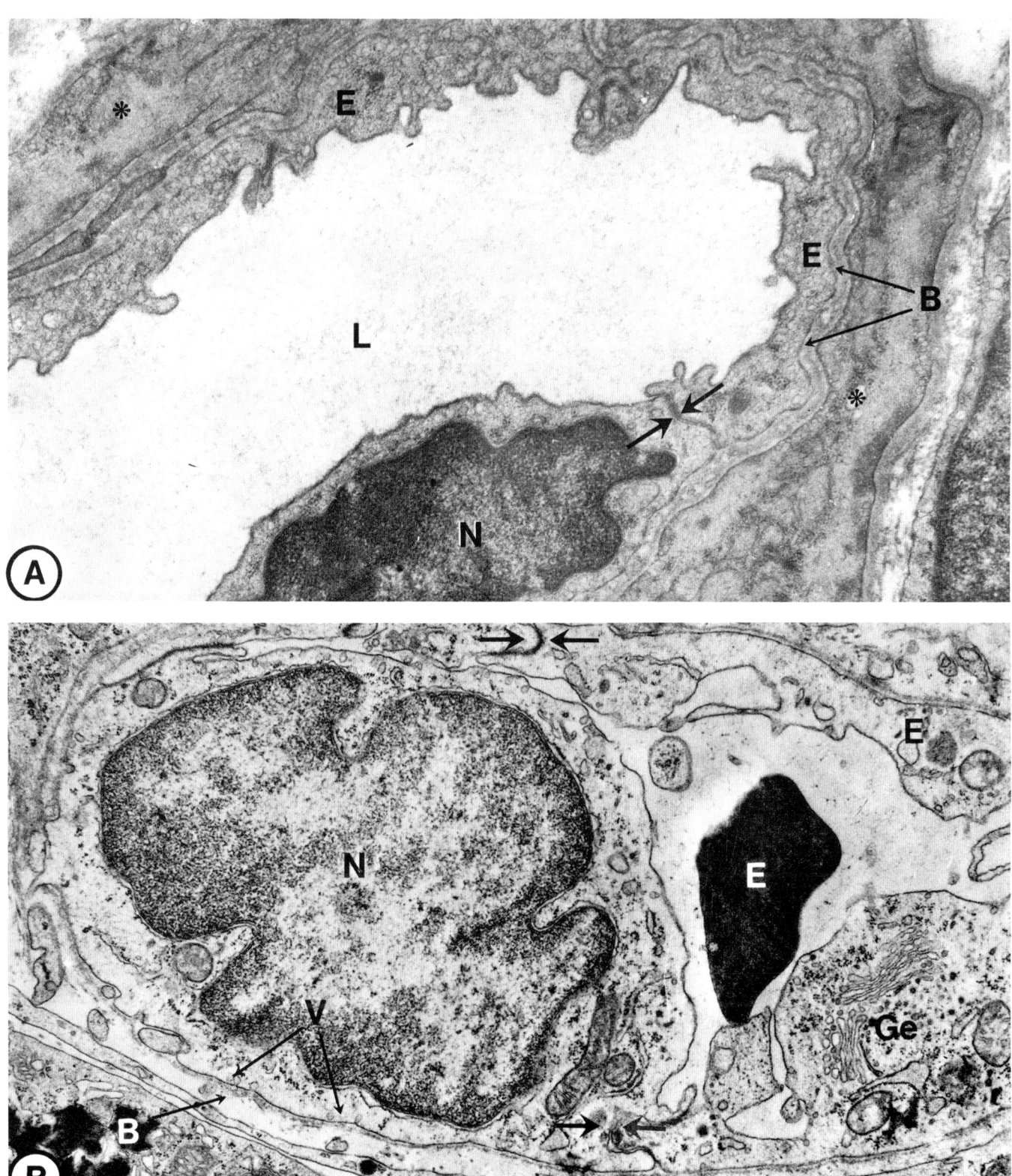

A **Endothelium from arteriole of mouse muscle (EM, x24,000).** The thin layer of endothelial cytoplasm becomes thicker in the nuclear region **(N)** of the cell and protrudes into the lumen **(L)** of the vessel. The plasma membrane is folded to form irregular microvilli. Endothelial cells have typical junctions (→). Pinocytotic vesicles are abundant in the cytoplasm. **(B→)** = basal lamina * = smooth muscle cells of the vessel wall.

B **Endothelial cells from capillary of mouse (EM, x37,000).** One endothelial cell is sectioned through the nucleus **(N)**, which is large with an irregular outline. In the cytoplasm of an adjacent cell (black **E**) a small Golgi complex can be seen **(Ge)**. Mitochondria and pinocytotic vesicles are clearly visible **(V→)**. **(B→)** = basal lamina. White **E** = erythrocyte in the narrow lumen of the capillary. (→←) = junction area.

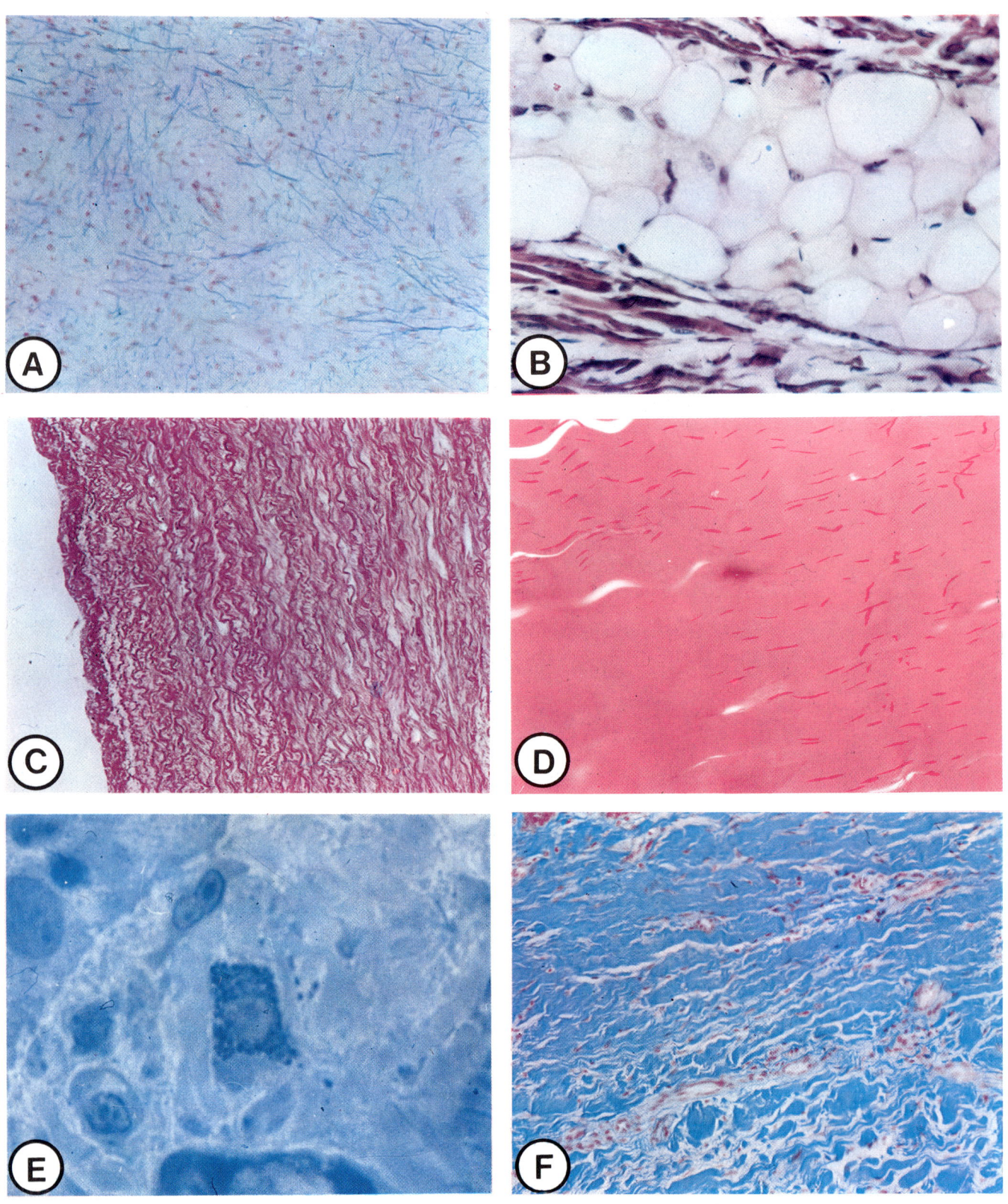

A   Connective tissue of human embryo (azan-Mallory, x150).

B   Human adipose tissue (H & E, x620).

C   Elastic tissue from tunica media of human aorta (Resorcin-fuschsin, x80).

D   Dense connective tissue from calf tendon (H & E, x150).

E   Semithin section including mast cell (center) from lamina propria of mouse tongue mucosa (methylene blue, x800).

F   Dense connective tissue from dermis of human scalp (azan-Mallory, x80).

Plate 3.3   **75**

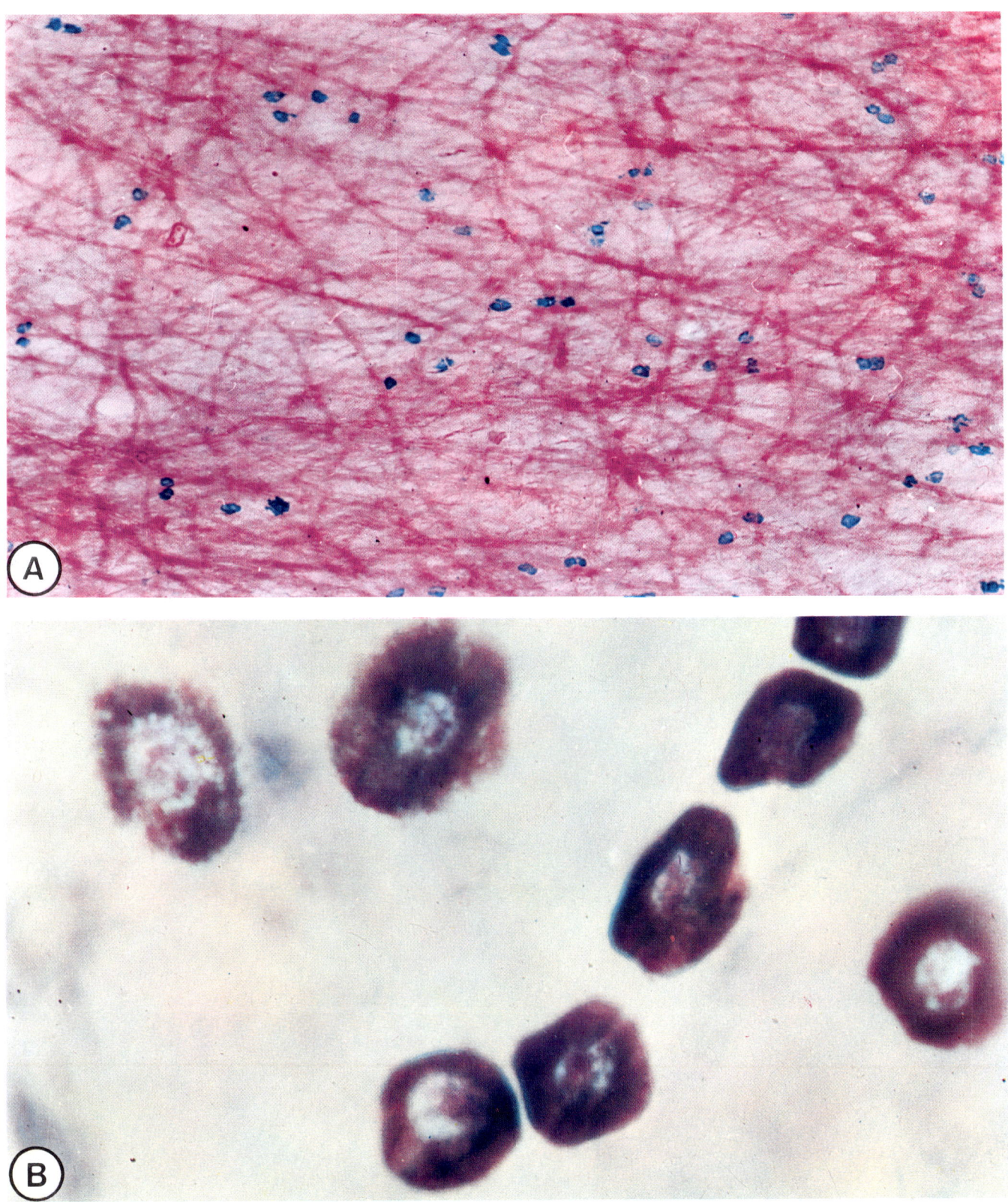

A   **Loose connective tissue from rat mesentery (Alcian blue and PAS, x550).** PAS has stained the collagen fibers red. The mast cells are stained blue.

B   **Mast cells from rat mesentery (toluidine blue, x1,200).** By courtesy of G. Quintarelli.

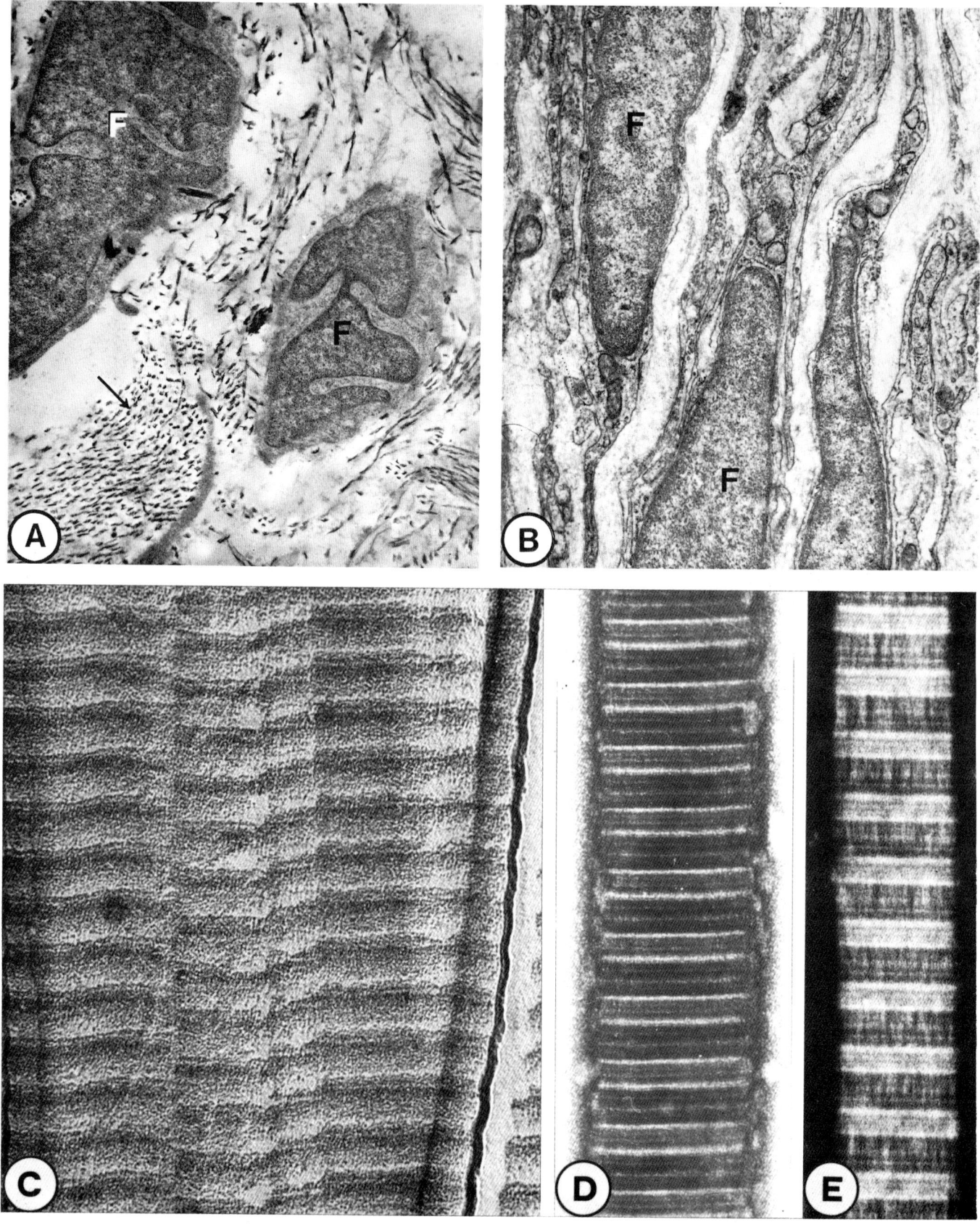

A   **Fibrocytes and collagen fibers from human connective tissue (EM, x8.000). F** = highly differentiated fibrocytes with deeply folded nuclei and cytoplasm containing few organelles. (→) = collagen fibers.

B   **Fibroblasts in connective tissue from rabbit ovary stroma (EM, x8,000). F** = fibrocytes less differentiated than those in preceding plate. Between the cells are layers of ground substance with few fibers.

C   **D,E Collagen fibers in tendon of rat tail (EM, x60,000, x170,000, x170,000).** With negative staining (uranyl acetate, PTA), one sees the typical banding pattern of collagen fibers. The stains show the typical spacing of bands (60-70 nm) on the collagen fibers. By courtesy of A. Ruggeri

Plate 3.5   77

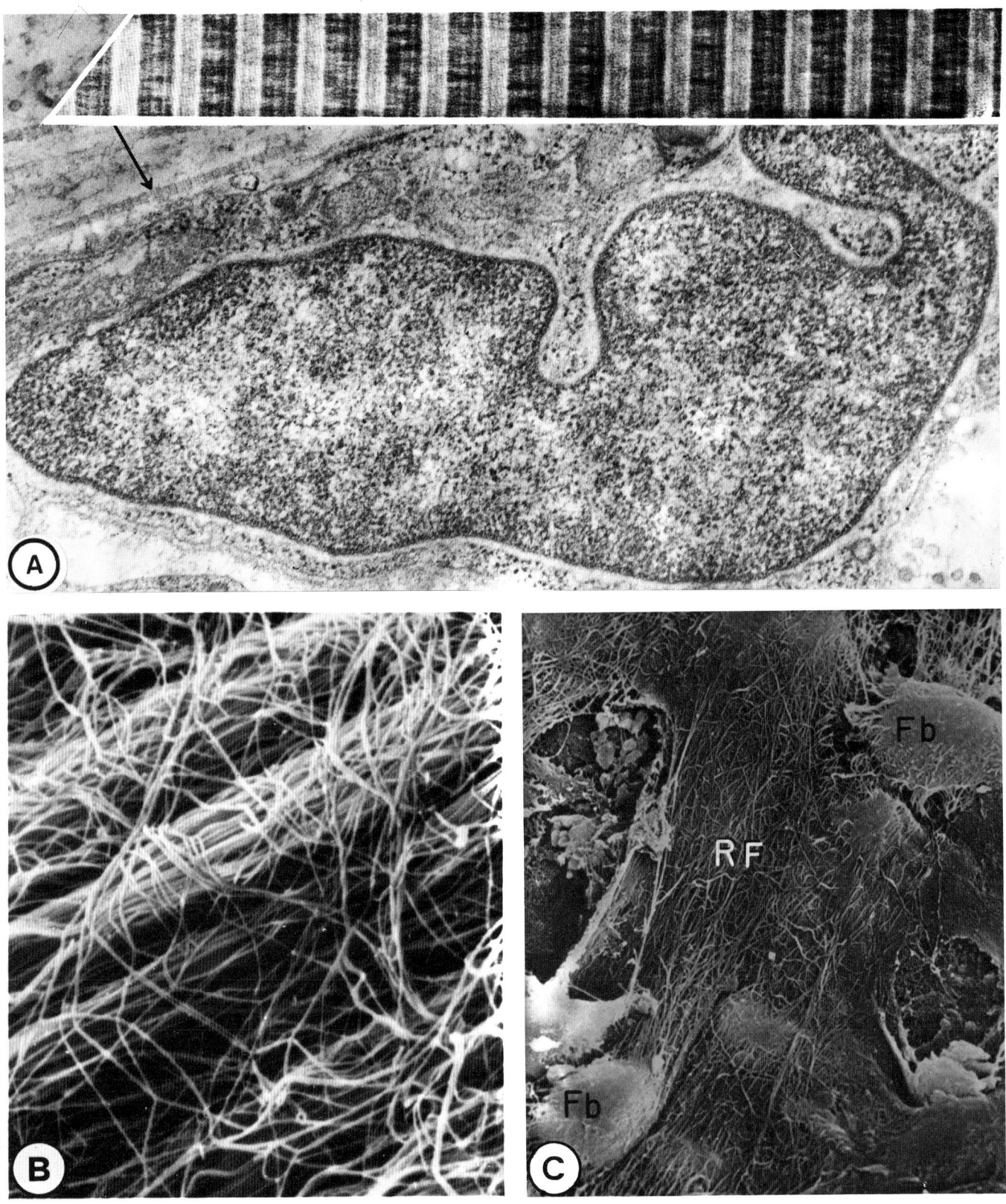

A **Fibrocyte of human connective tissue and (inset) negatively-stained collagen fiber (EM, x20,000).** The elongated cells have sparse cytoplasm containing few organelles and a markedly indented nuclear envelope. An extracelluar collagen fiber is seen in longitudinal section (→). **Inset: high magnification of a collagen fiber (x180,000),** showing typical repeating pattern of 60-70 nm.

B **Bundles of collagen fibers from human knee ligament (scanning EM, x8,500).** By courtesy of G. Marinozzi.

C **Collagen fibers and fibroblasts from rat ovary stroma (scanning EM, x800). Fb** = fibroblasts interacting with and connecting to thin reticular fibers (RF). From J. Van Blerkom and P.M. Motta. Cell Tiss. Res. 189:131, 1978.

Plate 3.6

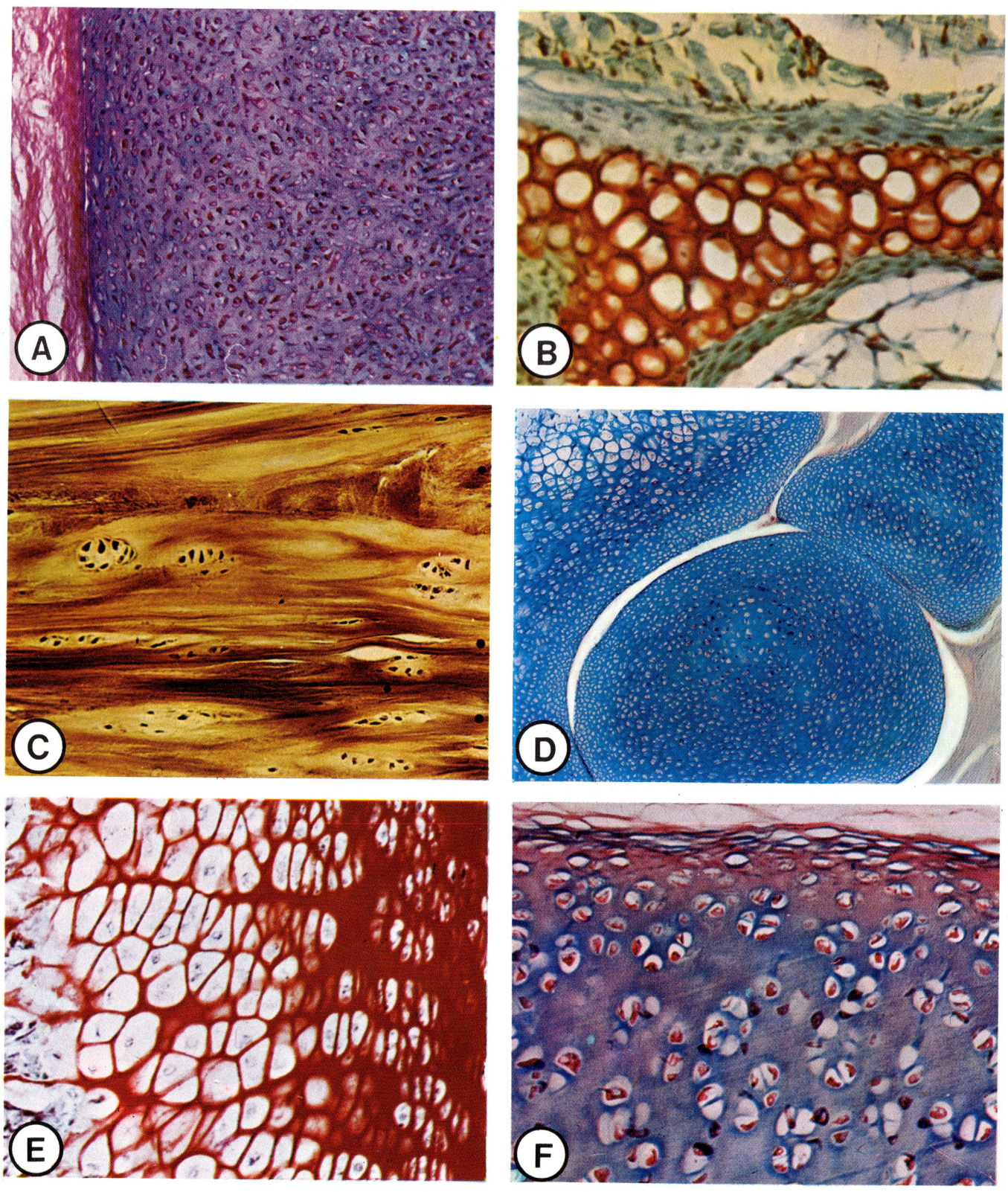

A   **Rib cartilage from human fetus (Alcian blue & PAS, x40).** Left: the perichondrium (red), right: the cartilage with abundant cells and ground substance.

B   **Elastic cartilage from rat ear (Safranine orange & Weigert's fast-green/hematoxylin, x1,200).**

C   **Fibrous cartilage from human symphysis pubis (bromphenol blue, x20).**

D   **Hyaline cartilage from epiphysis of newborn rat (Safranine orange, Weigert's fast-green/hematoxylin, x120).** The columnar arrangement of cartilage cells can be seen at upper left.

E   **Hyaline cartilage from metaphysis of rat (Safranine orange, Weigert's fast-green/hematoxylin, x120).** The columnar arrangement of cartilage cells can be seen, particularly at right.

F   **Hyaline cartilage from rabbit trachea (Alcian blue & PAS, x120).** Above: (red) the perichondrium, below: capsules containing chondrocytes in the ground substance. By courtesy of G. Quintarelli.

Plate 3.7   79

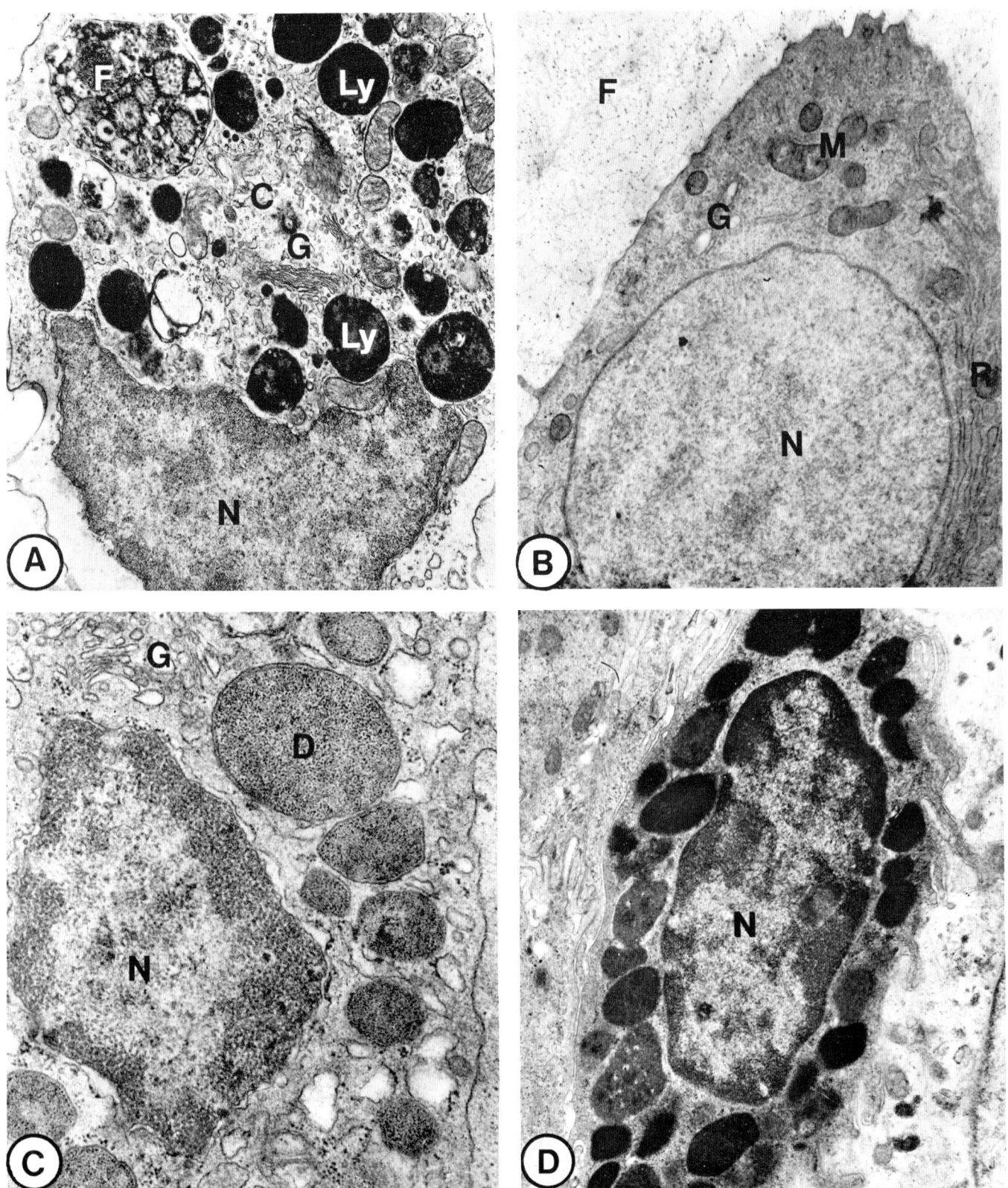

A   **Macrophage of rat lymph node (EM, x11,000). N** = nucleus. **G** = Golgi complex in proximity to a centriole **(C)**, surrounded by numerous dense bodies, the lysosomes **(Ly)**. Top left: a phagosome **(F)** containing partially digested material.

B   **Cartilage cell from tibia of chick embryo (EM, x13,500). N** = round nucleus with uniformly dispersed chromatin. In the cytoplasm, which is basophilic due to the presence of rough endoplasmic reticulum **(R)** and free ribosomes, are the Golgi complex **(G)** and a number of mitochondria **(M)**. In the intercellular space are collagen fibers **(F)**.

C   **Granulocyte from the peripheral circulation of rabbit (EM, x13,000). N** = irregularly shaped nucleus. Large opaque basophilic granules **(D)** in the cyotplasm are in proximity to the Golgi complex **(G)**.

D   **Mast cell of loose connective tissue from rat (EM, x11,500).** The elongated nucleus **(N)** contains chromatin that has aggregated at the periphery. The cytoplasm has a number of dense, large granules. Mast cell granules usually contain heparin and histamine.

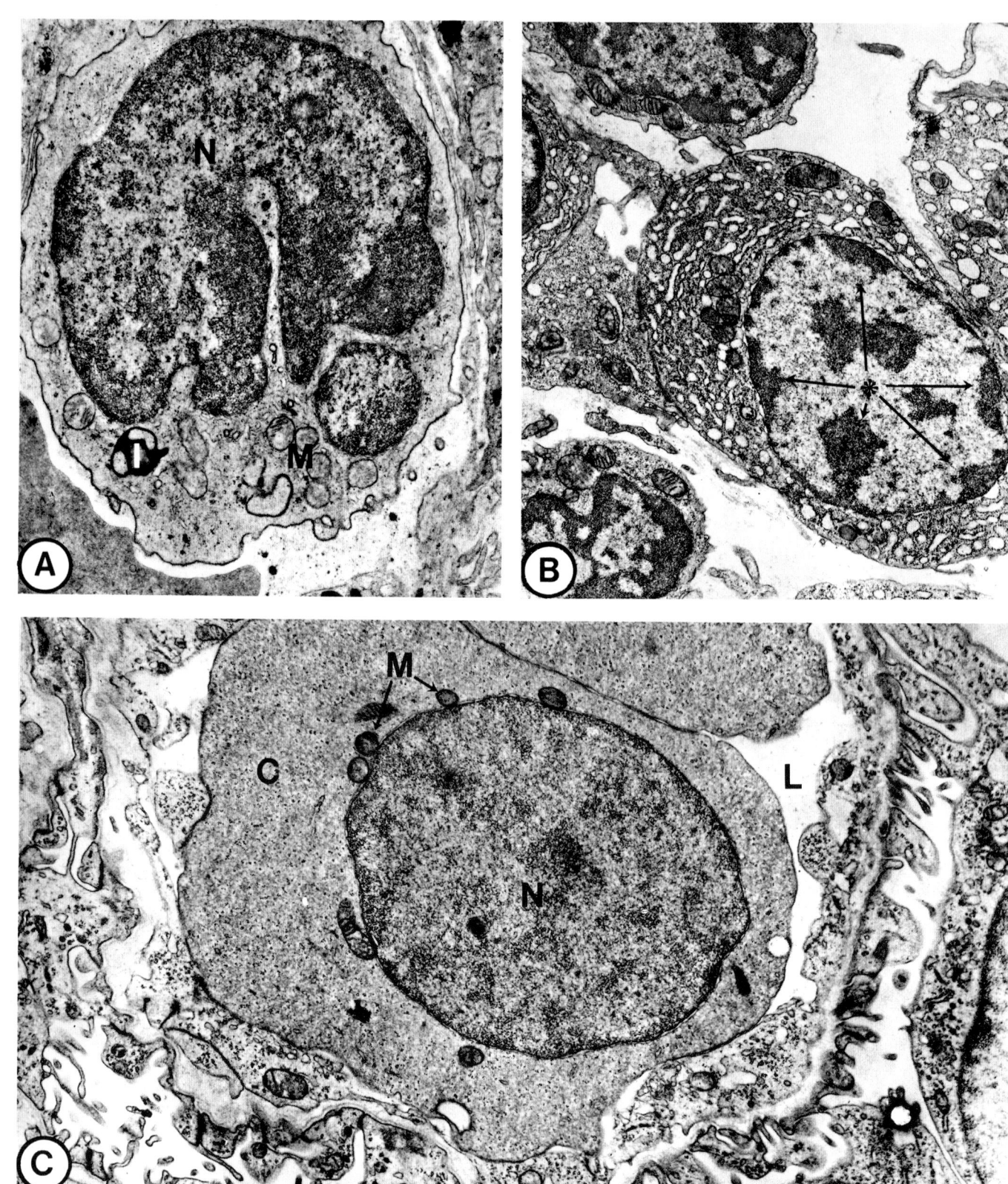

A   **Monocyte from peripheral circulation of rabbit (EM, x11,500). N** = kidney-shaped nucleus. **M** = mitochondria. **I** = cytoplasmic inclusions.

B   **Plasma cell from submandibular lymph node of bat (EM, x68,000).** The chromatin in the nucleus of this cell is organized into clumps at the periphery (*→) to form a cartwheel pattern. The cytoplasm abounds with rough endoplasmic reticulum and is therefore highly basophilic. The main role of plasma cells is antibody production. By courtesy of G. Azzali.

C   **Polychromatophilic erythroblast from human mesonephros (EM, x22,000).** Hemoglobin begins to appear in the cytoplasm (**C**) among the polysomes. A few mitochondria are present (**M→**). In the mature erythrocyte the nucleus (**N**) will have been extruded, and the cytoplasm will be filled almost entirely by hemoglobin. **L** = lumen of blood capillary. By courtesy of C. De Martino.

Plate 3.9   81

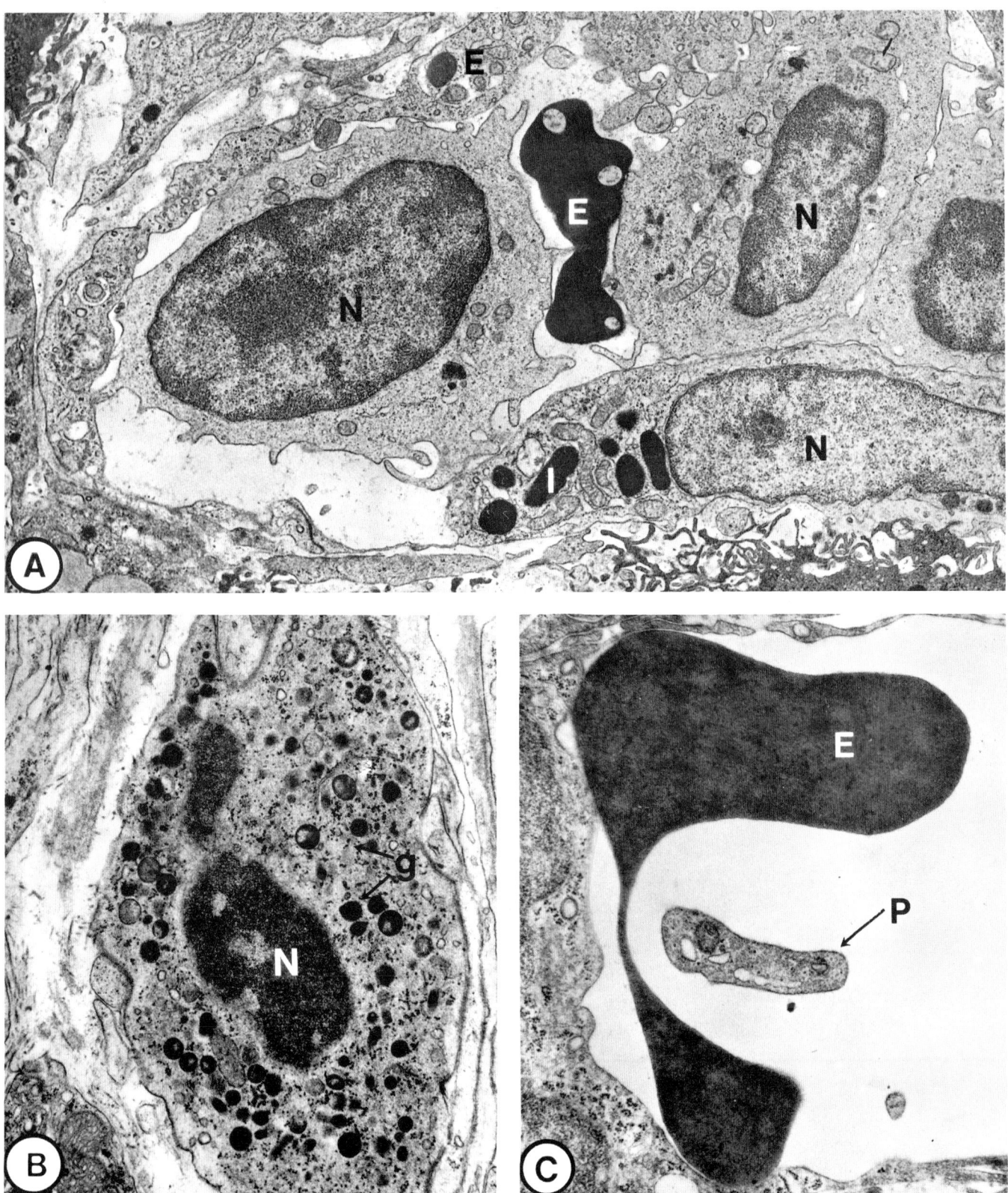

A   **Lymphocytes and red corpuscles in human liver sinusoid (EM, x8,500).** The capillary wall is made up of squamous endothelium (dark **E**). In the lumen of the sinusoid two lymphocytes can be seen, each having a cytoplasm rich in ribosomes and an ovoid nucleus (**N**) containing dense chromatin. Between the two lymphocytes an erythrocyte is visible (white **E**). Below is a reticuloendothelial cell (macrophage) with cytoplasmic inclusions (**I**). Original by C. Inferrera.

B   **Neutrophilic granulocyte in guinea-pig connective tissue (EM, x14,000).** The section shows only a small part of the polylobular nature of the nucleus (**N**). Neutrophil granules (**g**→) (lysosomes) can be seen in the cytoplasm.

C   **Erythrocyte and platelet in rat liver capillary (EM, x22,000).** E = erythrocyte. The cytoplasm appears homogenous due to the presence of hemoglobin. (**P**→) = platelet.

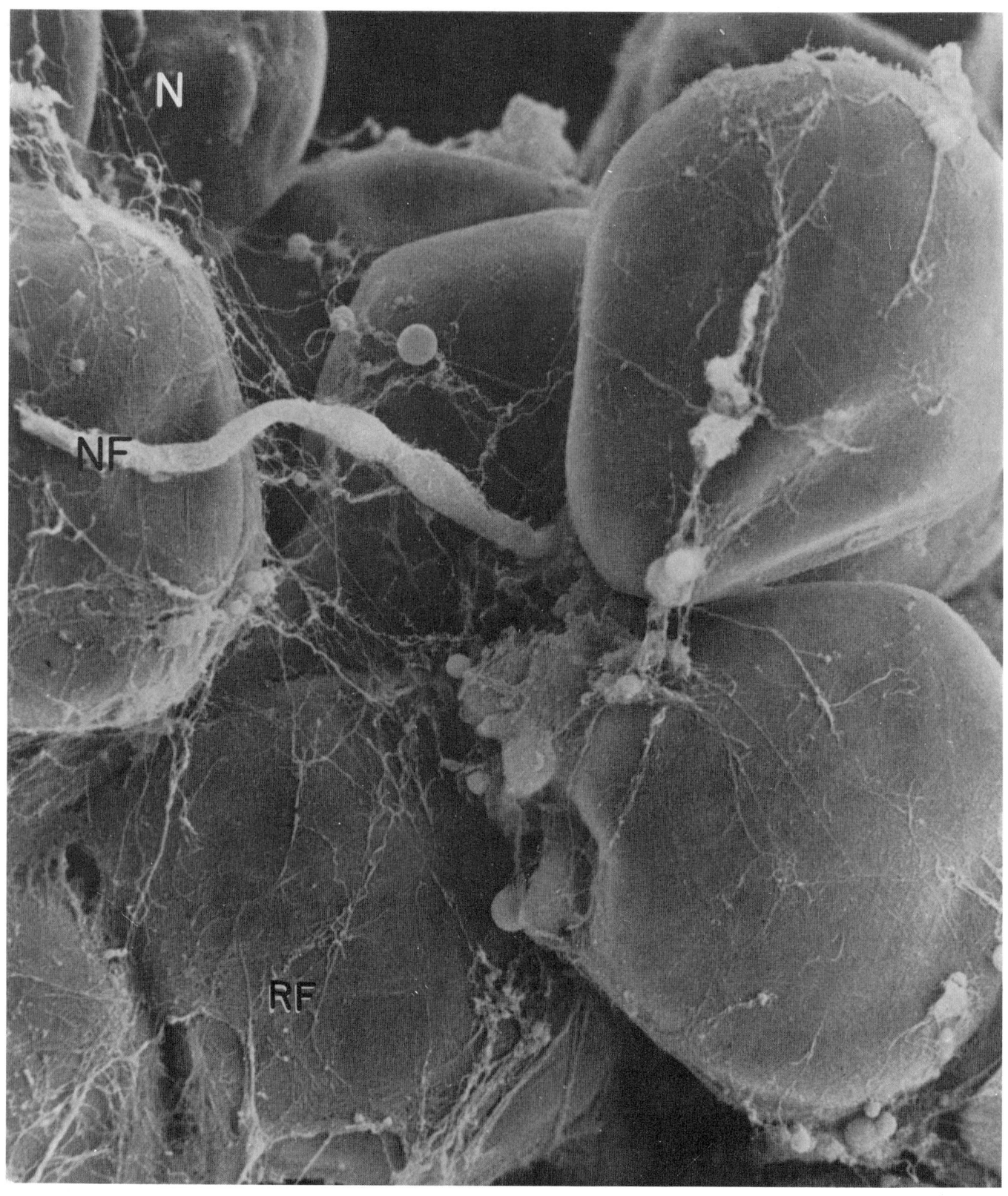

Rat adipose tissue (scanning EM, x1,500). Adipose tissue consists of large round cells wrapped in a fine web of reticular fibrils **(RF). NF** = nerve fiber. **N** = nucleus bulging from under the plasmalemma of an adipose cell. From P.M. Motta. J. Microscopic Biol. Cell. 22:15, 1975.

Plate 3.11   83

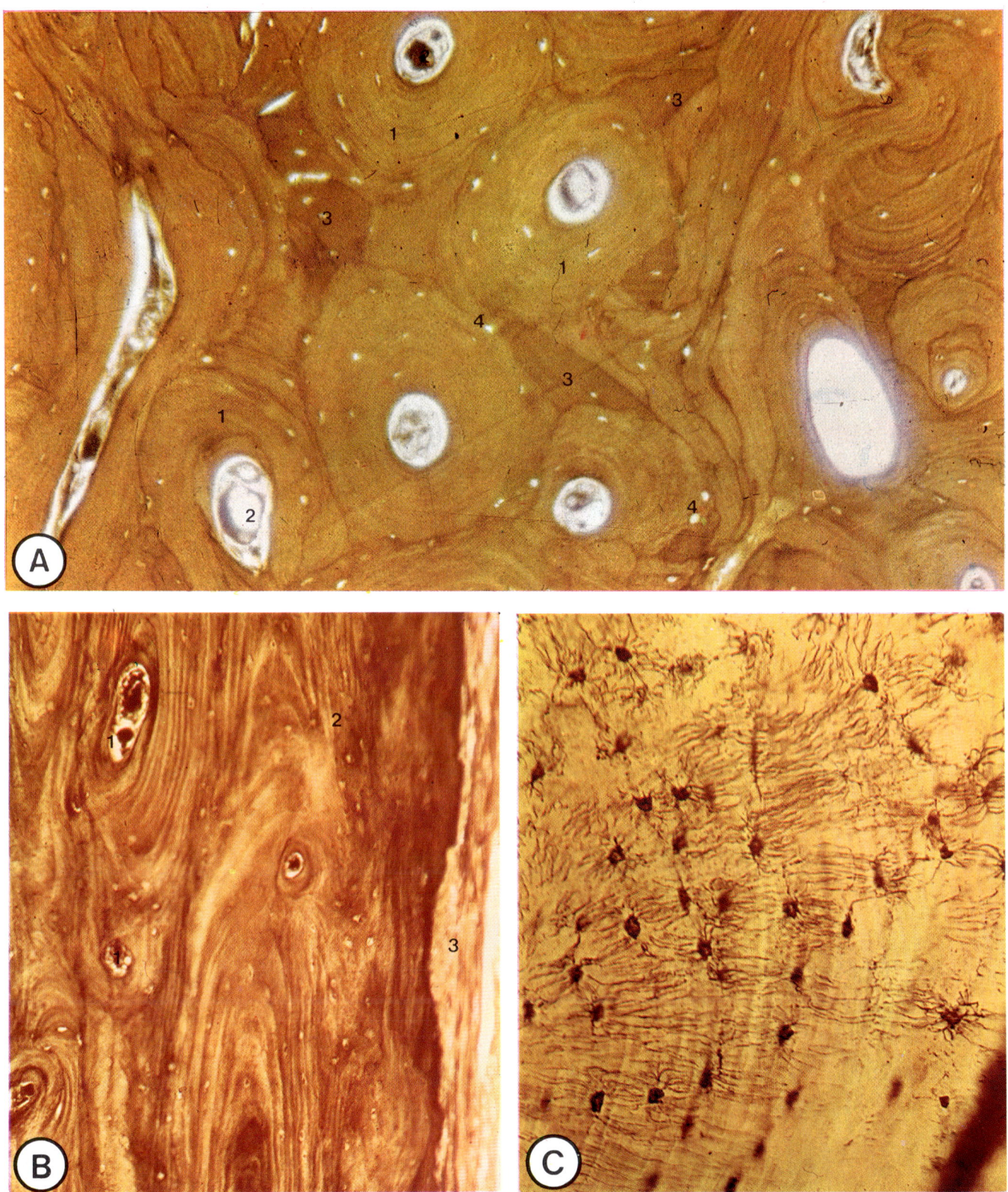

A   **Bone tissue from head of human femur in cross section (Delafield's hematoxylin and eosin, x142). 1** = osteons with Haversian canals containing blood vessels **(2). 3** = interstitial lamellae. **4** = unstained lacunae containing osteocytes.

B   **Bone tissue from head of human femur in longitudinal section (Delafield's hematoxylin and eosin, x180). 1** = Haversian canals with blood vessels. **2** = lamellae of the osteon in tangential section. **3** = periosteum.

C   **Osteocytes in decalcified human femur (silver impregnation, x420).**

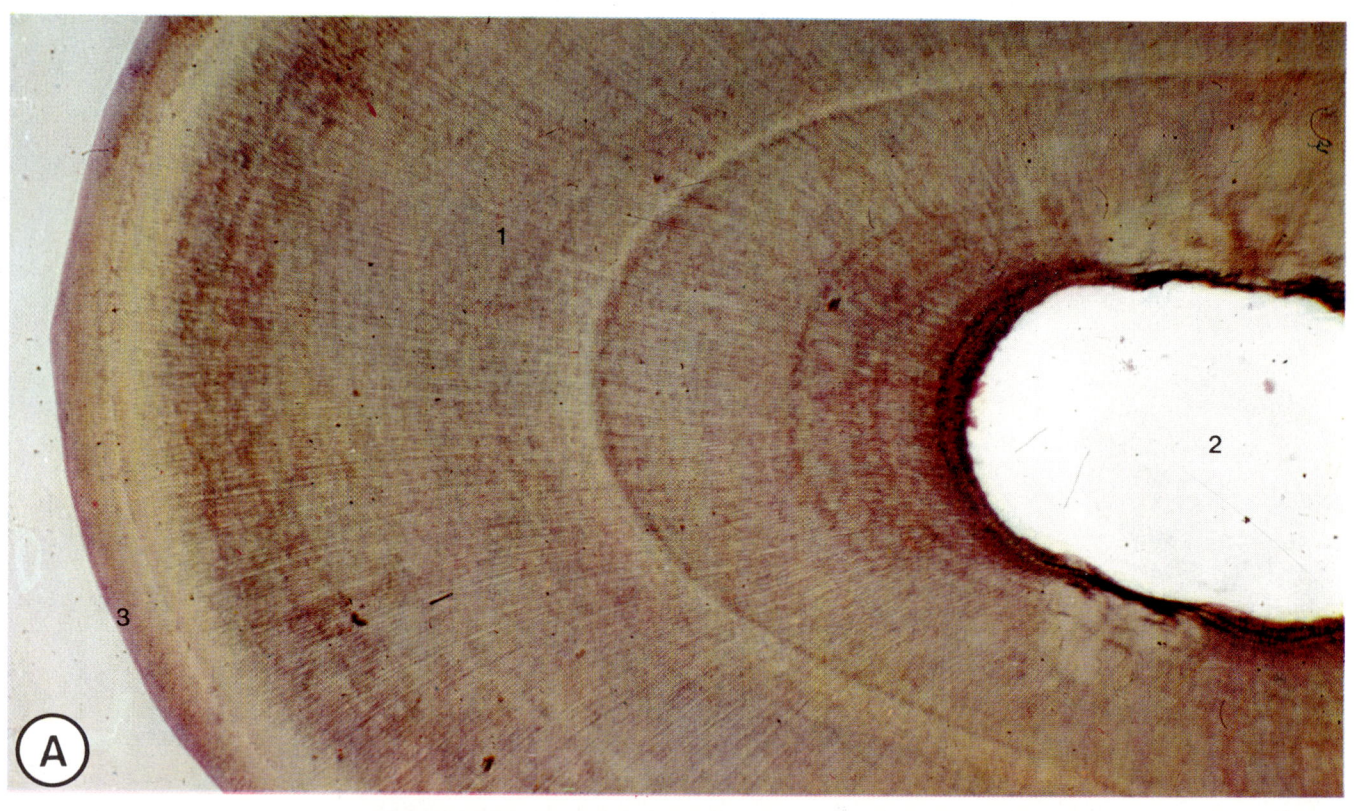

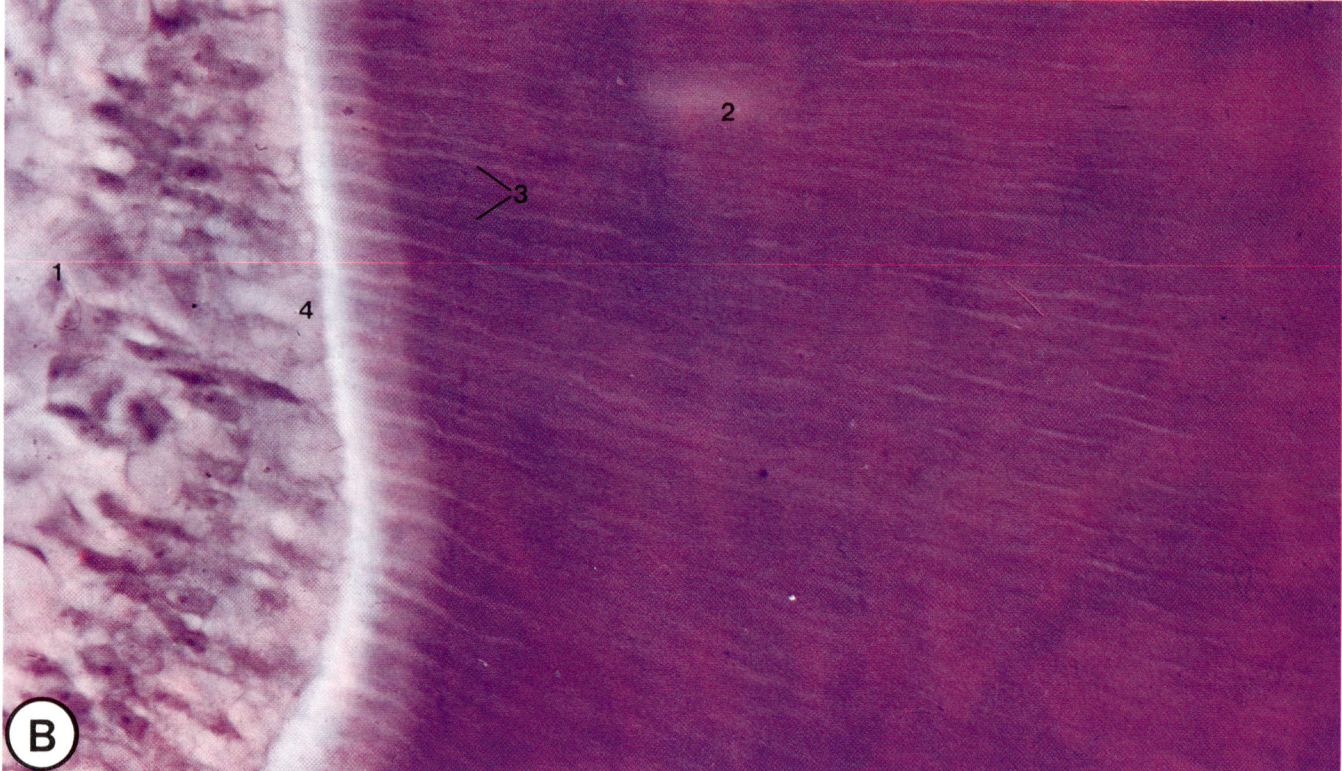

A **Dentin from human tooth at lower crown in cross section (Delafield's hematoxylin and eosin, x70). 1** = dentin. The radiating striations indicate the canaliculi, and the concentric pattern reflects the successive laying down of layers in the dentin. **2** = dental cavity that contained live pulp. **3** = thin layer of enamel.

B **Dental pulp and dentin from mouse tooth in cross section (H & E, x320).** The pulp **(1)** is made up of a mature mucous connective tissue rich in blood vessels and nerves. The dentin is crossed radially by canaliculi **(2)** containing the cytoplasmic processes **(3)** of the odontoblasts. The boundary between pulp and dentin is marked by a line of odontoblasts **(4)** beyond which is a recently deposited layer of dentin that is incompletely calcified.

Plate 3.13 85

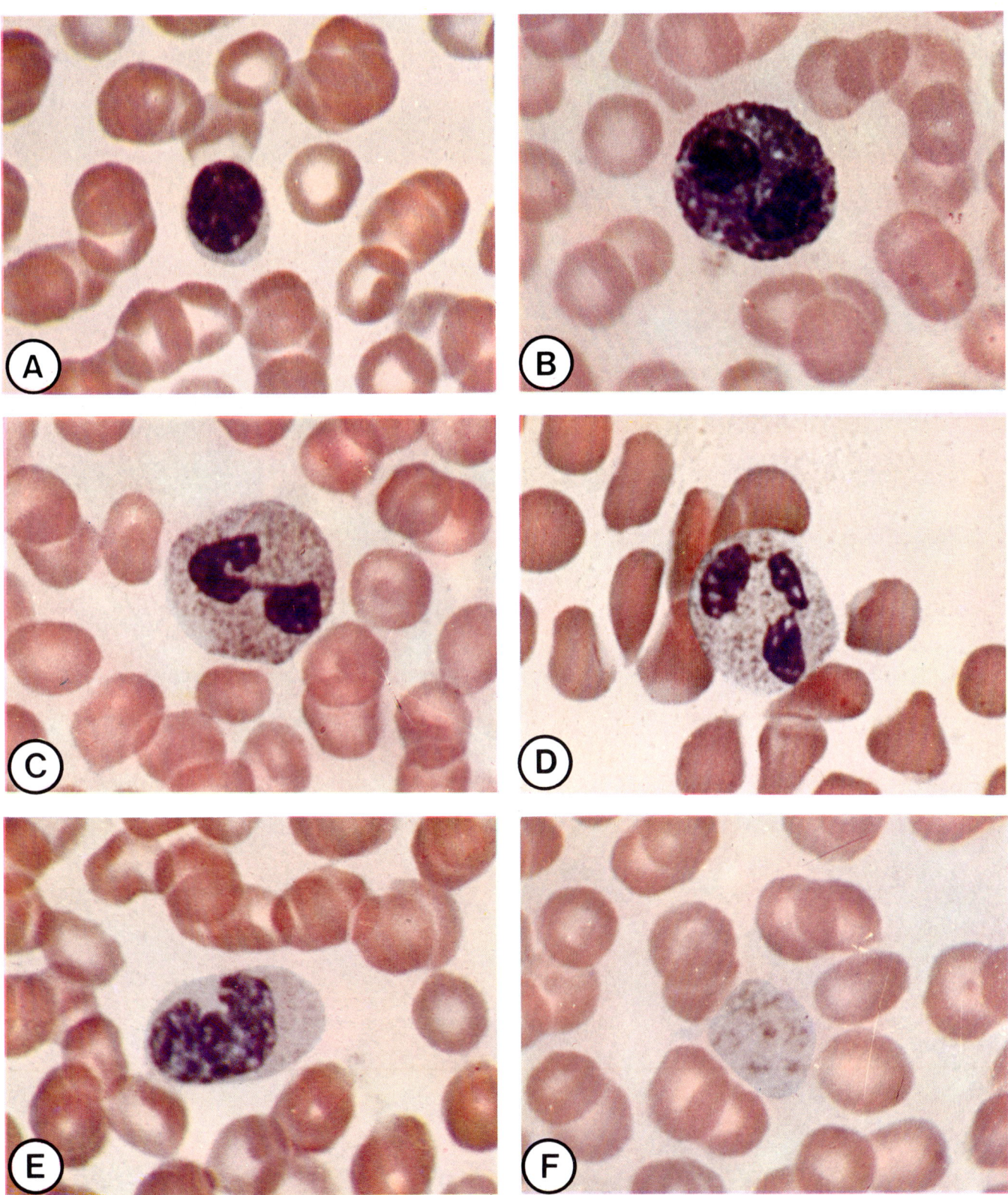

Human blood smears (May-Grunwald-Giemsa, x1,500).
A   **Small lymphocyte with round nucleus and sparse basophilic cytoplasm.** The cell is surrounded by a number of biconcave erythrocytes with a thin, light-staining center and a thicker, dark-staining periphery.
B   **Basophilic granulocyte with bilobed nucleus, acidophilic cytoplasm and large basophilic granules.**
C   **Neutrophilic granulocyte with multilobular nucleus, small neutrophilic granules and acidophilic cytoplasm.**
D   **Eosinophilic granulocyte at center with multilobular nucleus.**
E   **Monocyte with basophilic cytoplasm and kidney-shaped nucleus.**
F   **An aggregate of platelets.**

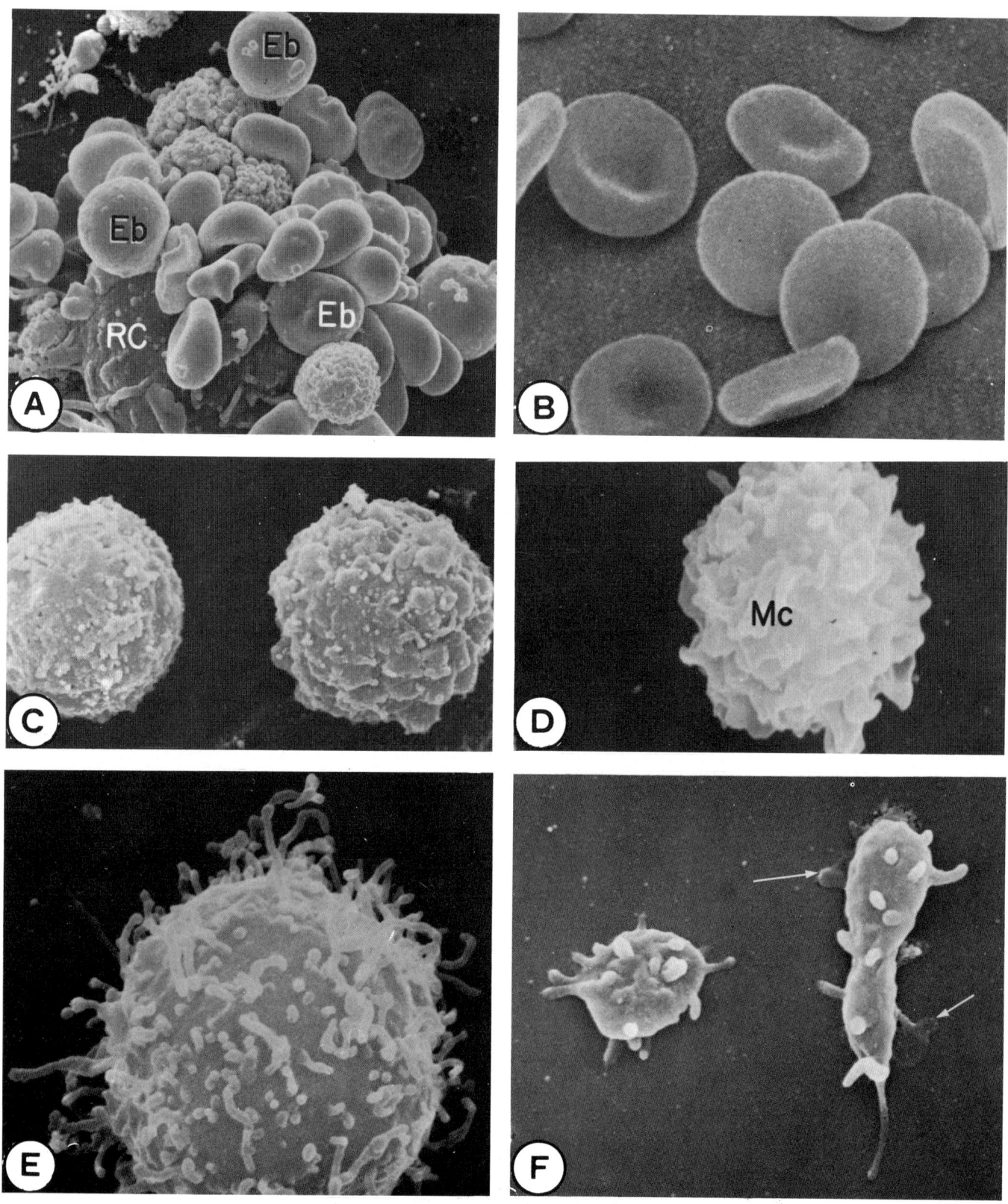

Scanning EM of human blood cells.

A   **Bone marrow cells in culture (x3,000).** Islets of erythroblasts **(Eb)** are gathered around a reticular cell **(RC)**.

B   **Erythrocytes (x5,000).**

C   **Neutrophilic granulocytes (x6,500).** From a patient with acute granulocytic leukemia.

D   **Monocyte (x6,500).** Lamellipodia (Mc) abound on the cell surface.

E   **B Lymphocyte (x9,000).** Microvilli abound on the cell surface.

F   **Platelets (x8,000).** The platelets adhere to a substratum by short filopodia (→). By courtesy of H.R. Toben and P.M. Andrews.

MUSCLE TISSUE

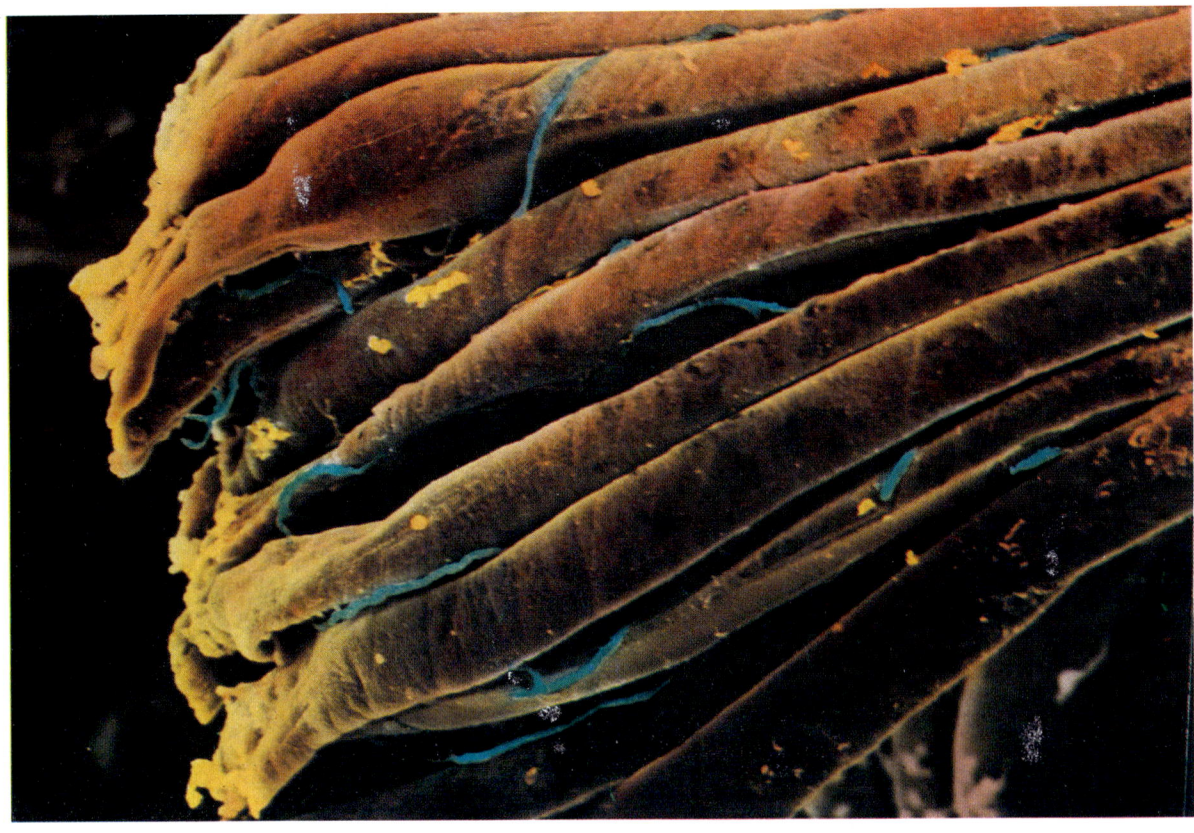

Isolated striated fibers of rat skeletal muscle. (Colored SEM; 820 x).

Muscle is composed of cells (*myocytes*) that are multinucleate and elongated. Muscle cells are referred to as fibers (*muscle fibers*). The cytoplasm of *striated muscle* cells contains a special contractile apparatus, the *myofibrils*. Myofibrils are present in large numbers and are made up of units called *sarcomeres* which are aligned in register with adjacent fibrils and which give rise to the cross bands (striations) that are characteristic of skeletal muscle. Although almost all types of cells are capable of some degree of contraction, only in skeletal muscle and cardiac muscle is the contractile apparatus so highly organized.

In addition to striated skeletal muscle, which moves the skeleton and parts of the skin, there are two other types of muscle, *cardiac*, which is striated and found only in the heart, and *smooth* (involuntary) muscle, which is found in the viscera and the wall of many blood vessels. In smooth muscle the contractile apparatus displays no cross-banded pattern.

There are also specific cells with a contractile function, but the myofilaments that make up the contractile apparatus are not organized into a band pattern. *Pericytes* (perivascular cells whose contraction is thought to cause narrowing of the capillary) are of this type, as well as *basket cells* (in the secretory units of certain exocrine glands) and *myoepithelial cells* (with characteristics both of epithelium and muscle cells), found in some exocrine glands (Plate 4.2 A,C).

Smooth muscle

Smooth muscle tissue is made up of spindle or ribbon-shaped myocytes whose length varies from 30-200 um but whose diameter is constant (5-10 um). These cells may occur singly in interstitial connective tissue, or as simple or stratified layers with connective tissue between them. Single or small bundles of cells adhere to the connective tissue surrounding them. Each bundle of myocytes is enclosed by a connective tissue covering in which the cells may run lengthwise or circumferentially around it (Plates 4.1, 4.2 B, 4.3

A).

The cytoplasm of smooth muscle cells is largely filled with filaments running lengthwise. It is only near the nucleus that the centrioles, the Golgi complex, mitochondria, endoplasmic reticulum and glycogen granules can be seen. The single, rod-shaped nucleus is parallel to the long axis of the cell (Plates 4.2 B, 4.3).

Smooth muscle fibers, like those of striated muscle, are highly differentiated and rarely undergo mitosis. The cells are, however, capable of hypertrophy in certain conditions. The smooth muscle cells of the uterus, for example, are capable of considerable enlargement during pregnancy.

The thin myofilaments of smooth muscle tissue are gathered into nonstriated bundles. The bundles are attached to a framework of dense plates which may be found within the cell and on the inner surface of the plasmalemma. These plates resemble the plates of desmosomes in epithelium, the Z line in skeletal muscle and the intercalated disks of myocardial cells. The cell membrane (or *sarcolemma*) of each smooth muscle cell is covered with a glycocalyx to which numbers of reticular fibers are attached. The glycocalyx is interrupted in some areas where contiguous cells form junctions. These are communicating or gap junctions, providing for the transmission of stimuli from one cell to another. Myofilaments of myosin and actin have been shown to be present in smooth muscle, and the contractile mechanism is thought to be similar to that of striated muscle.

Striated muscle

The cells making up striated muscle are cylindrical. In humans their length can vary from a few millimeters to several centimeters. Their average diameter is from 10-100 um (Plates 4.4, 4.5). The myofibrils can extend the length of the muscle they constitute. Each fiber, as in smooth muscle, is limited by a sarcolemma that consists of three layers, an inner, plasma membrane, a middle layer of glycocalyx 8-12 nm thick, and a third outermost layer composed of a fine web of reticular fibers. The reticular layer is a continuation of the surrounding connective tissue (*endomysium*). The *perimysium* is the connective tissue layer that binds groups of muscle fibers together. The *epimysium* is a connective tissue sheath enclosing the entire muscle, and is in some places continuous with the tendon.

In the cytoplasm of striated muscle fibers, besides the abundant myofibrils, there are mitochondria and endoplasmic reticulum (Plates 4.6, 4.7). The endoplasmic (or *sarcoplasmic*) reticulum is a complex network of smooth-surfaced membranes and cisternae arranged in a characteristic fashion around the myofibrils. At certain points the reticulum is functionally related to infoldings of the plasmalemma (T system). The sarcoplasmic reticulum transports and concentrates calcium ions. Depolarization of the sarcolemma and the T system causes release of calcium ions from the sarcoplasmic reticulum. Following contraction the calcium ions are resequestered into the sarcoplasmic reticulum. The sarcolemma depolarizes as a result of nervous stimulation of the myoneural junction (Plate 4.6).

The cross-banded *myofibrils* have a diameter of 1-2 um. They run parallel to the main axis of the muscle fiber and extend the length of the muscle fiber (Plates 4.6, 4.7). Myofibrils are in turn composed of segments of sarcomeres. Sarcomeres are made up of thin actin and myosin filaments. When seen in the light microscope, the sarcomere has dark *A bands* (birefringent anisotropic) separated by light staining *I bands* (isotropic). The I bands are in turn bisected by the *Z lines*. Adjacent myofibrils are arranged so that their bands are in register. The sarcomere is considered to extend from Z line to Z line.

In the middle of the A band is a less dense region called the *H* or *Hensen band*, which is identified by the particular arrangement of the filaments within the sarcomere. The H band is in turn divided into two parts by a darker and thinner line in the middle (*M line*). On both sides of the M line are two slightly paler sections.

In the I band of each sarcomere there are only thin myofilaments with a diameter of 5.5 nm, and in the A band there are both thin and thick (14 nm) myofilaments. The two arrays of filaments slide past each other during contraction. In the middle part of the H band there are only thick myofilaments. The two arrays of myofilaments are connected by bridges which project from the myosin filaments at regular intervals.

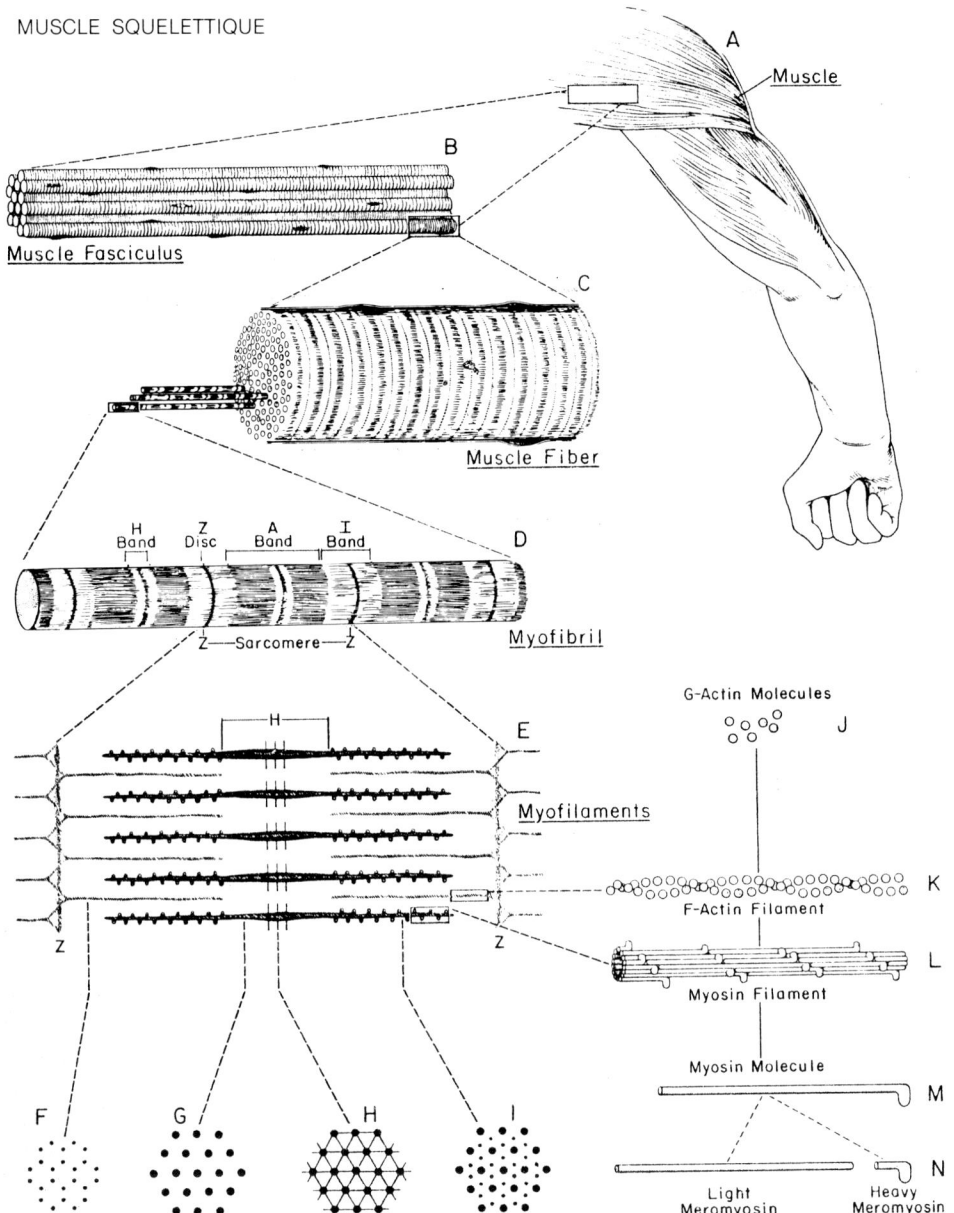

MUSCLE SQUELETTIQUE

Diagram illustrating the structure of skeletal muscle from the macroscopic to the molecular level. Letters F,G,H and I show the cross sections of a myofibril at the points indicated by the dotted lines. Illustration by S.C. Keene, by courtesy of D.W. Fawcett. In: W. Bloom and D.W. Fawcett. A textbook of Histology. 10th ed. W.B. Saunders Co. Philadelphia, Toronto and London, 1975.

Research on the biochemical composition of myofibrils has revealed that they are composed mainly of special contractile proteins. Actin, troponin and tropomyosin constitute the thin myofilaments, and the thicker filaments contain myosin. Alpha-actinin is found in the Z lines.

During contraction the length of the sarconere can decrease by as much as 35%. The shortening is thought to be caused by the thin myofilaments sliding along the myosin filaments towards the M line. This sliding decreases the distance between the Z lines, while the I band and H band disappear.

Heart muscle

Myocardial tissue is made up of elongated cells gathered into bundles that branch to form a network. There are two types of heart muscle, common and specialized.

Common heart muscle

The atrial and ventricular walls are composed largely of common heart muscle tissue. This tissue is innervated by fibers of the autonomic nervous system. One or two nuclei can be found in the cells of heart muscle. The myofibrils of cardiac tissue take up less of the volume of the fiber than those of skeletal muscle fibers. Cardiac muscle has a striated appearance, and thus is similar to skeletal muscle. The myofibrils of this tissue have the same characteristics as those of striated skeletal muscle. Between the bundles of myofibrils are numerous mitochondria. Lipid droplets occasionally can be seen.

Myocardial cells are sheathed in a sarcolemma. The nuclei are usually centrally located in the cytoplasm (Plate 4.3). Heart muscle fibers are bound together by step-like *intercalated disks,* which in the light microscope appear as fine wavy lines at right angles to the main axes of adjacent cells. The disks interlock the plasma membranes of cardiac muscle cells. They consist of two types

of regions. One resembles the desmosome or adhering junction; others comprise gap junctions or communicating junctions (Plates 4.9, 4.10).

Specialized heart muscle

Specialized heart muscle tissue consists of thin, branched cells that conduct the stimulus for contraction. Conduction fibers have fewer myofibrils than common heart muscle fibers. Within the connective tissue of the heart they form a network that spreads throughout the myocardium and branches to make functional contact with the contractile fibers. These specialized fibers have few nuclei irregularly distributed in the sarcoplasm, but have many mitochondria and glycogen granules.

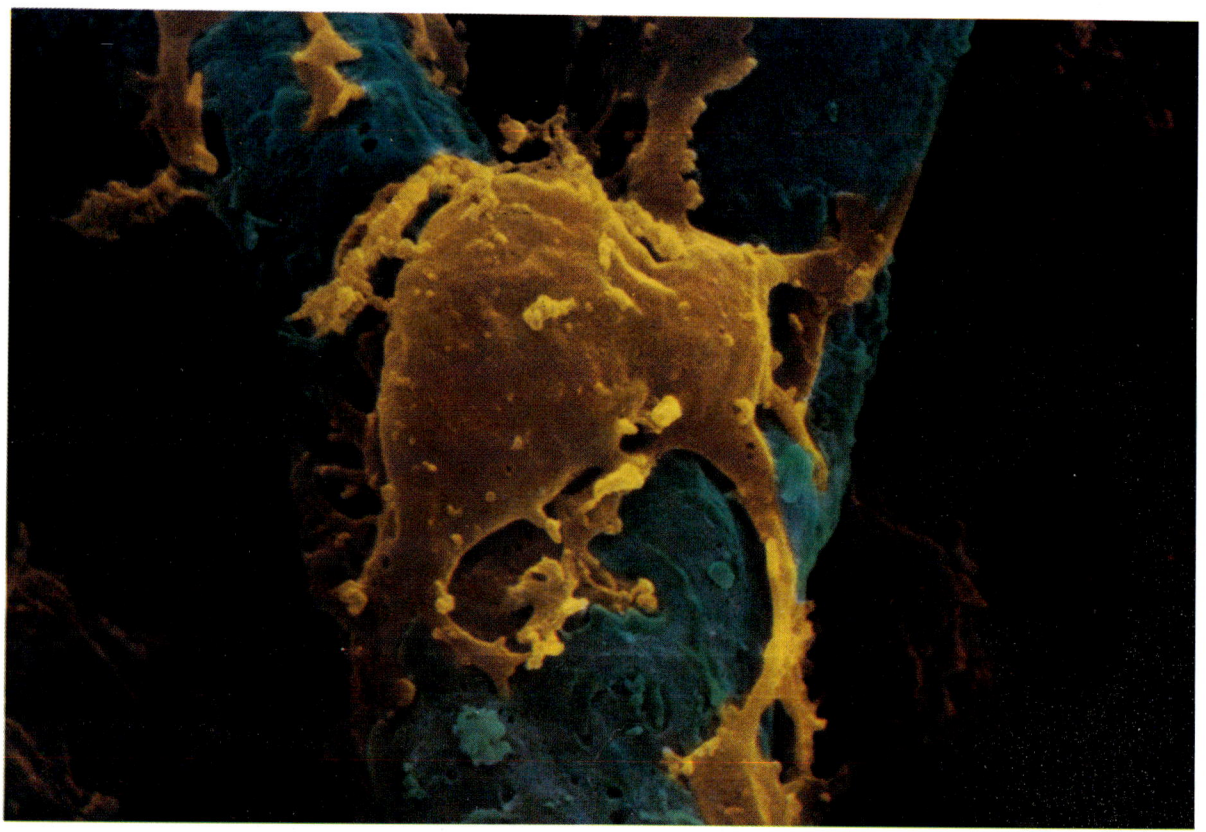

Pericyte branching over a blood capillary wall of rabbit. (Colored SEM; 6,200 x; by courtesy of M. Murakami).

Plate 4.1   91

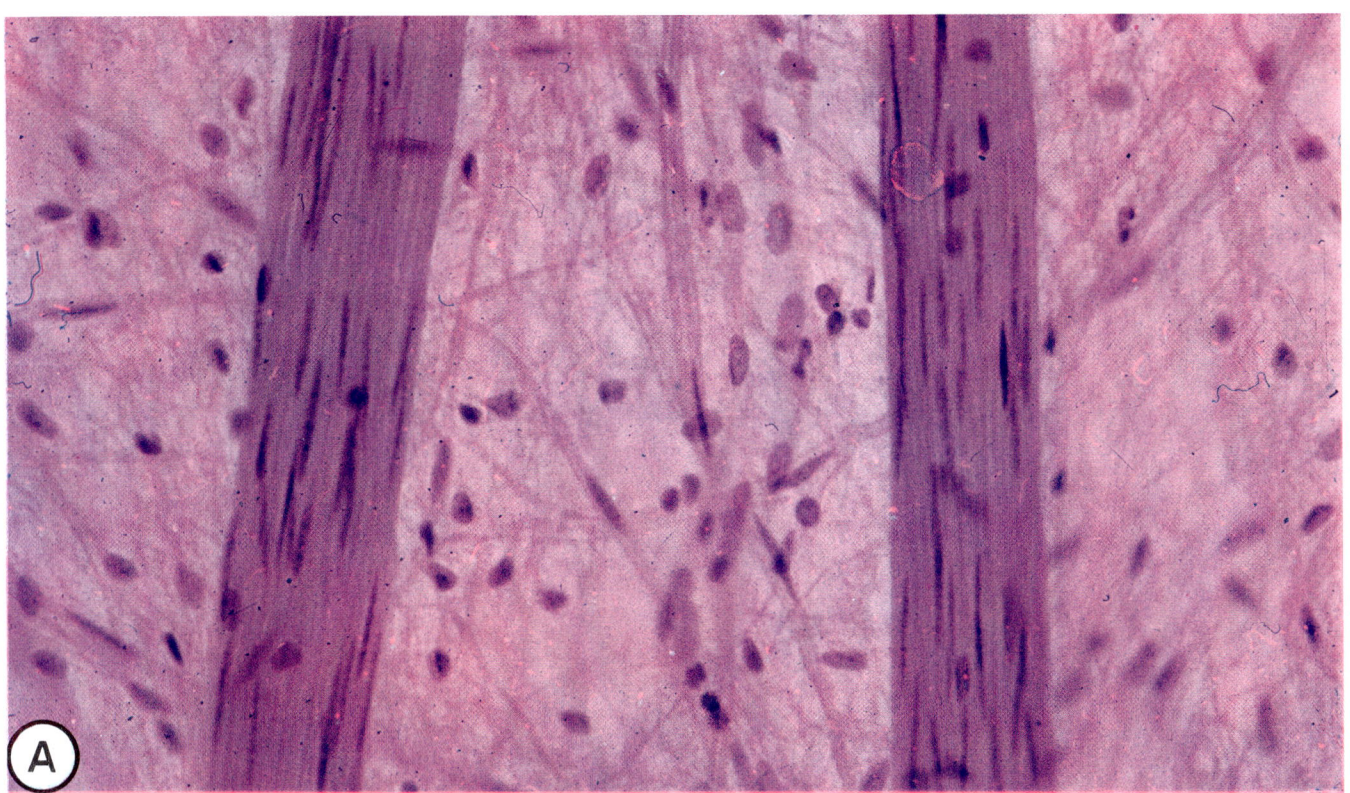

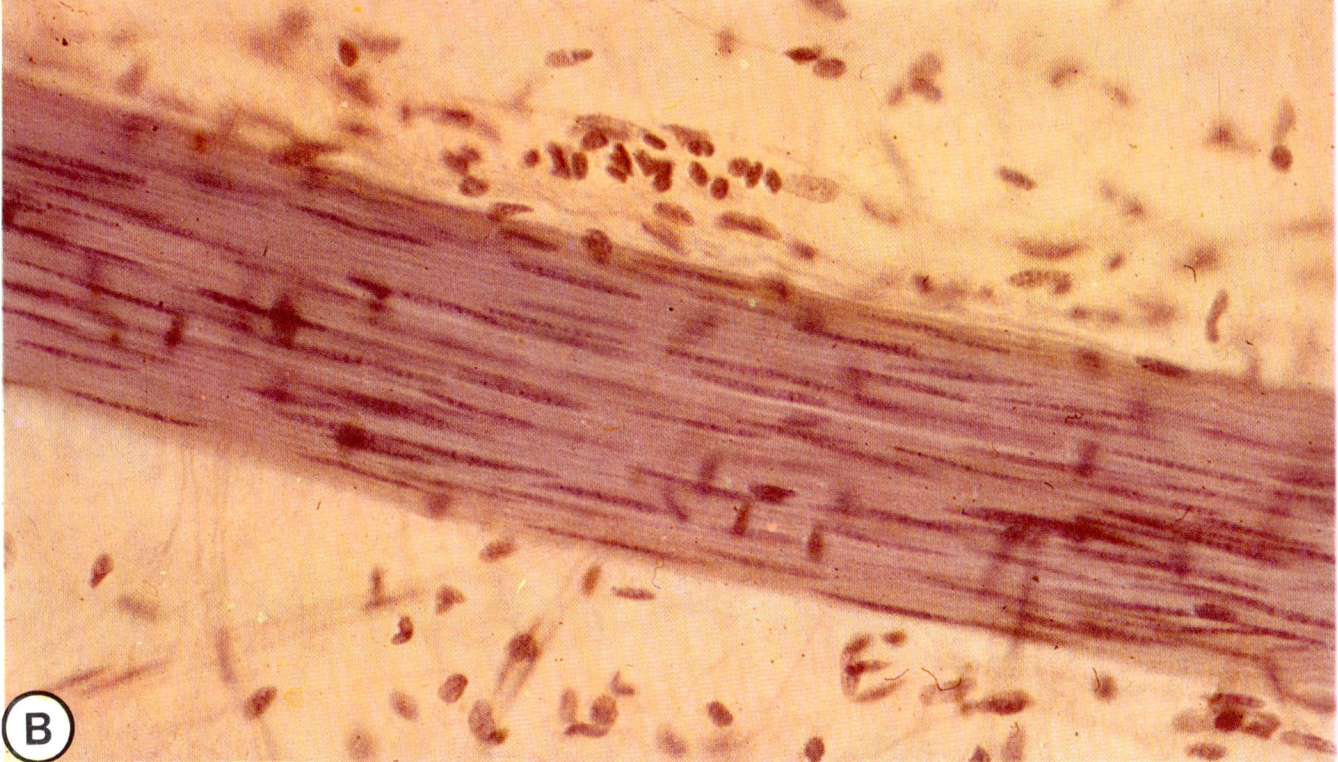

A **Longitudinal section of bundles of smooth muscle fibers from frog bladder (H & E, x850).** In the translucent matrix between the small bundles of smooth muscle can be seen elements of connective tissue.

B **Details of a small bundle of smooth muscle cells (H & E, x1,200).**

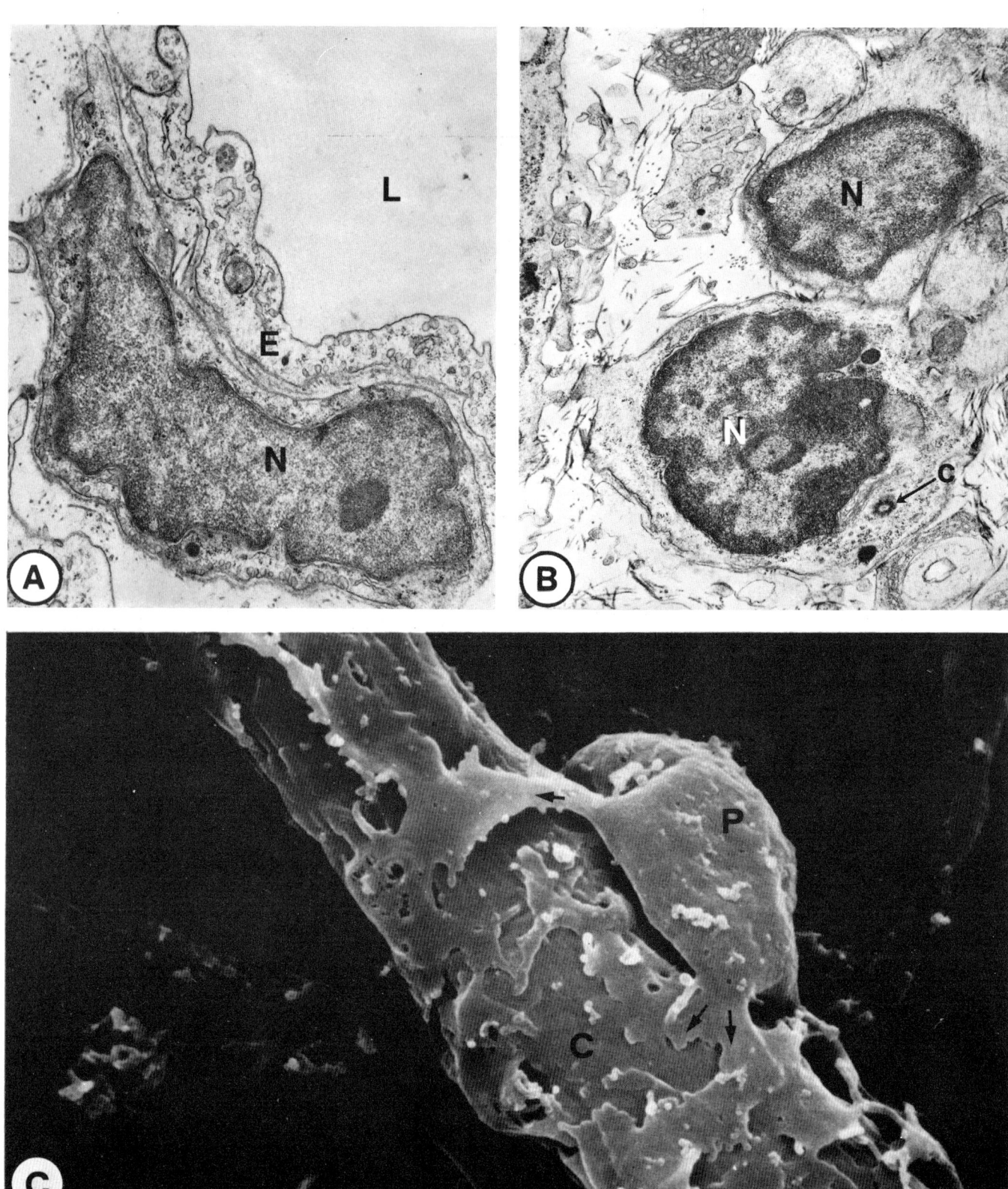

A   **Pericyte of capillary from rabbit pancreas (EM, x26,000).** A pericyte with a large irregular nucleus **(N)** is in close proximity to the surface of a capillary endothelial cell **(E)**. **L** = lumen of the capillary. Pericytes are thought to be contractile cells.

B   **Cross section of smooth muscle cells of mouse ovary (EM, x23,500).** In the plane of section are two nuclei **(N)**. The cytoplasm contains many myofilaments. A centriole **(C→)** in cross section is in the cytoplasm, near the nucleus. From Z. Fumagalli, P. Motta and S. Calvieri. Experientia 27:1250, 1971.

C   **Pericyte of capillary from rabbit retina (scanning EM, x12,300).** Long processes (→) from the body of the pericyte cells **(P)** clasp the wall of the capillary **(C)**. By courtesy of M. Murakami.

Plate 4.3   93

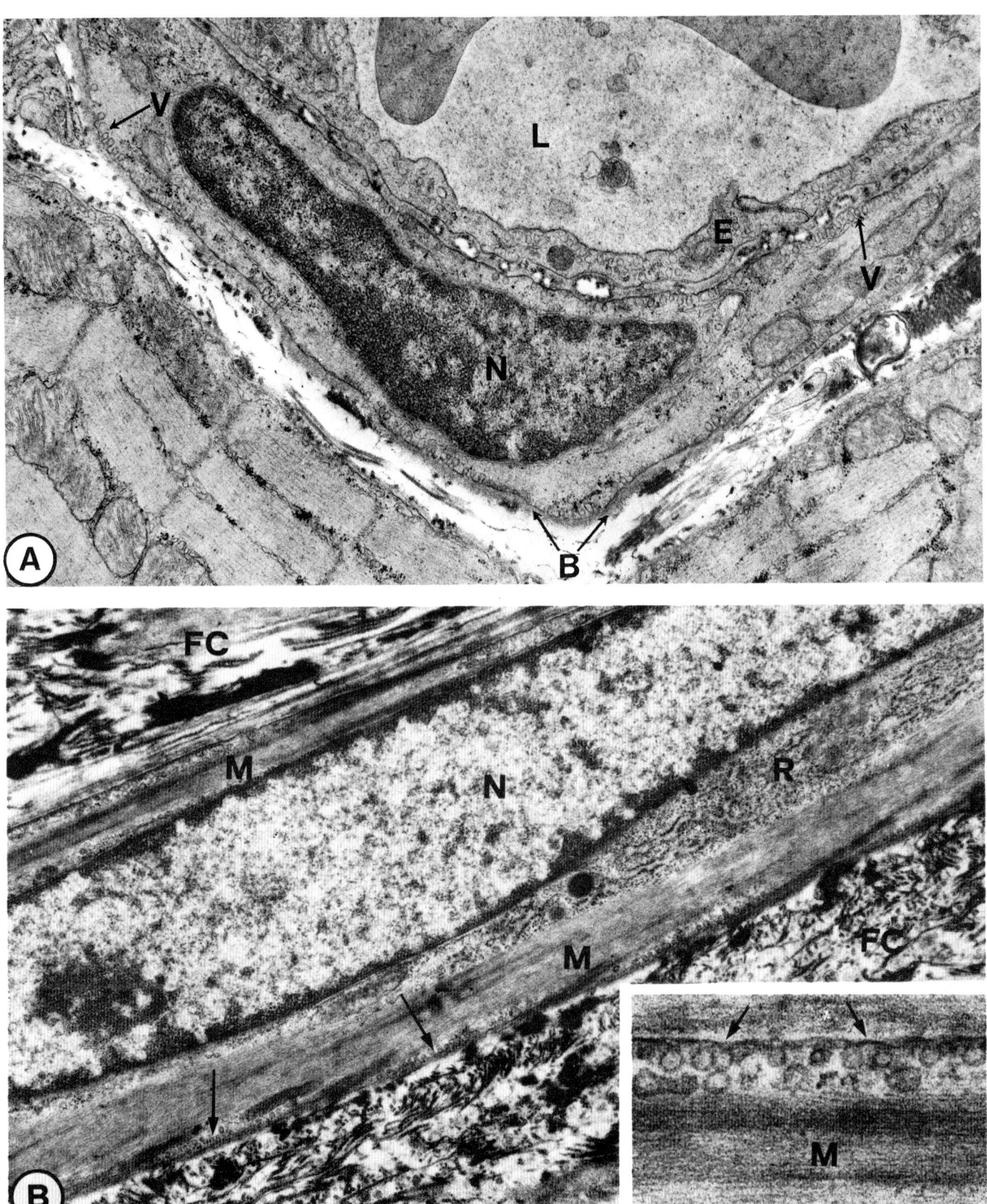

A   **Longitudinal section of smooth muscle cell from arteriole wall of a rat (EM, x22,000). N** = elongated nucleus with dense
chromatin. **(V→)** = pinocytotic vesicles along the outline of the cell membrane. **(B→)** = basal lamina consisting of a dense
layer entwined with reticular fibers. **E** = endothelial cell of vessel. **L** = lumen of vessel with erythrocyte. Below: striated
muscle fibers.

B   **Smooth muscle cell from wall of rat femoral artery (EM, x49,000).** The longitudinal section of the muscle cell shows an
elongated nucleus **(N)** surrounded by endoplasmic reticulum **(R)** and a number of microfilament bundles **(M).** The
indentations of the plasmalemma (→) are pinocytotic vesicles. In the intercellular spaces are collagen fibers **(FC). Inset: high
magnification of pinocytotic vesicles along the plasmalemma (→) and subcortical microfilaments (EM, x110,000).** Original by
G. Macchiarelli and F.G. Magliocca.

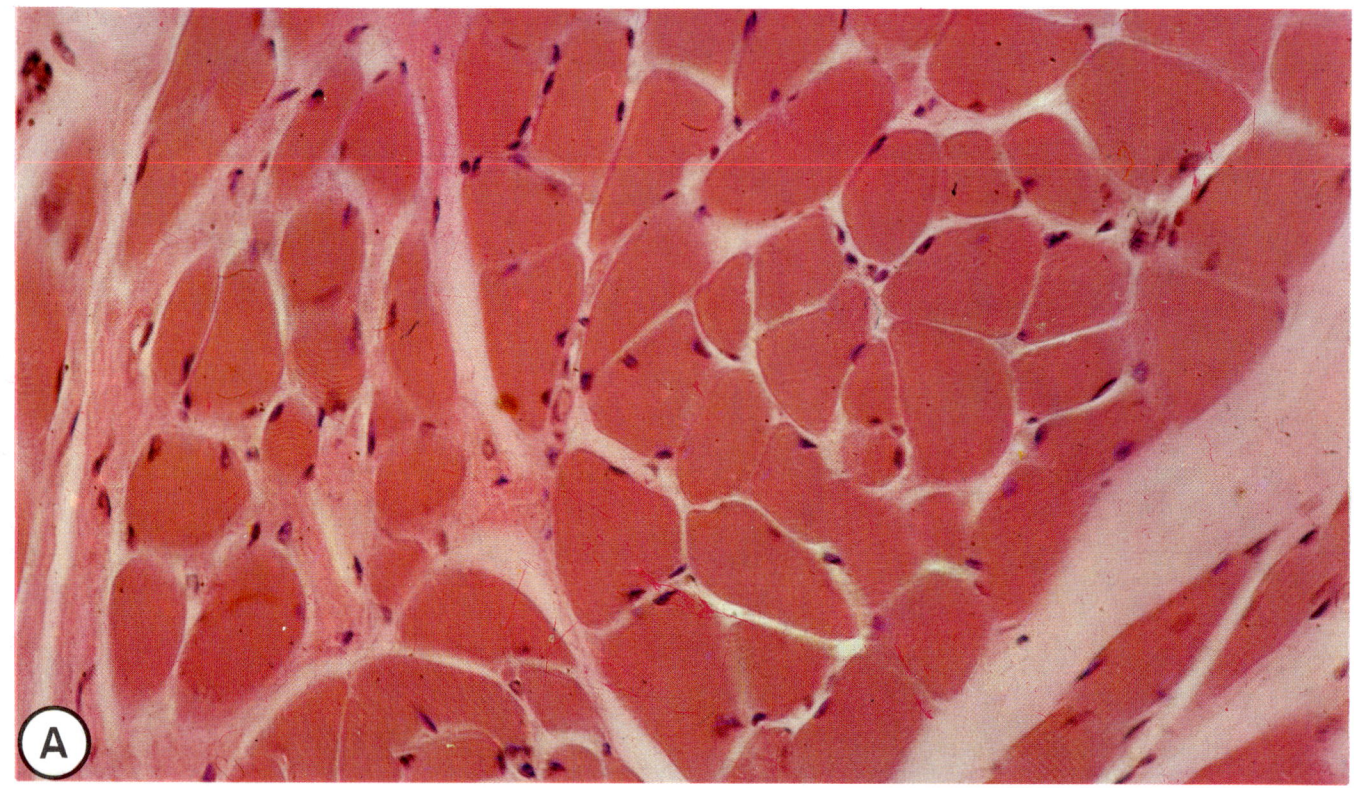

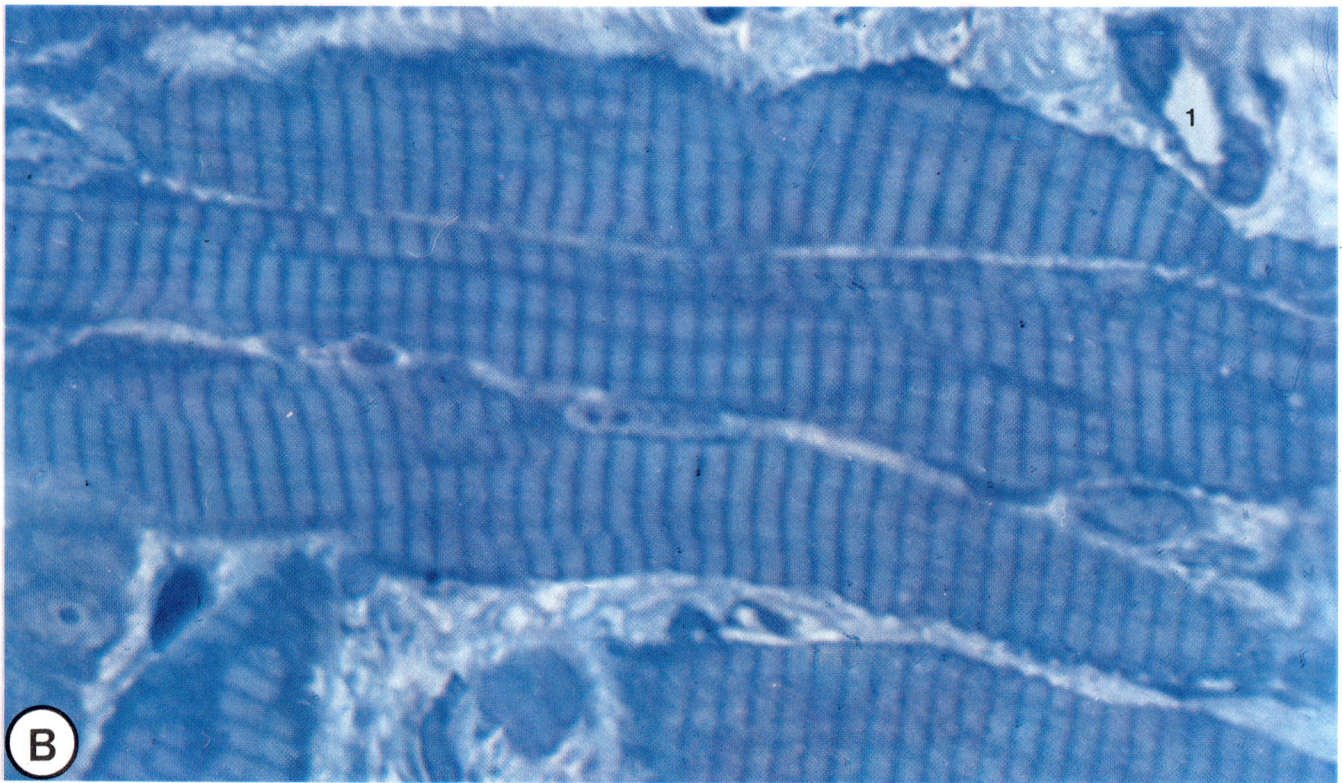

A   **Cross section of striated muscle fibers of mouse tongue (H & E, x340).** Against the sarcolemma are the darkly staining nuclei, with more than one nucleus per fiber. Sparse connective tissue (endomysium) separates each fiber from its neighbor.

B   **Semithin longitudinal section of striated muscle fibers from mouse tongue (methylene blue, x580).** The dark and light bands of the muscle fiber can be distinguished. The nuclei are positioned peripherally near the sarcolemma. **1** = small blood vessel in cross section.

Plate 4.5   **95**

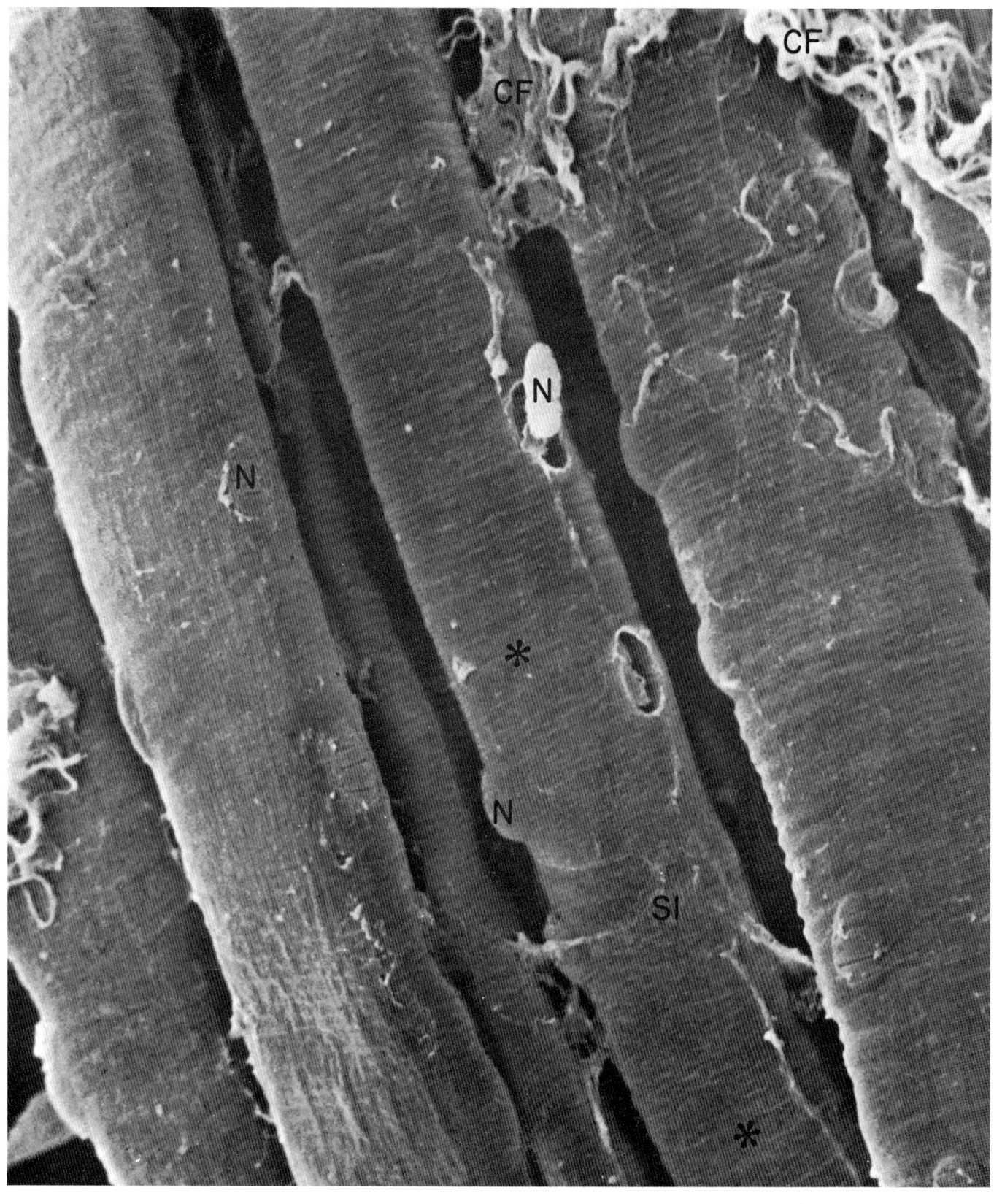

Skeletal muscle fibers from a rat (scanning EM, x1,200). In the cylindrical fibers (*) the nuclei (N) are under the sarcolemma. The nucleus in the upper center of the micrograph has apparently been everted from the fiber. The banding of the fibers can be discerned through the sarcolemma (SI). Above: collagen fibers can be seen (CF) attaching to the sarcolemma. Original by J. Vial. In: P.M Motta, P.M. Andrews and K.R. Porter. *Microanatomy of Cell and Tissue Surfaces. An Atlas of Scanning Electron Microscopy.* Lea & Febiger, Philadelphia, 1977.

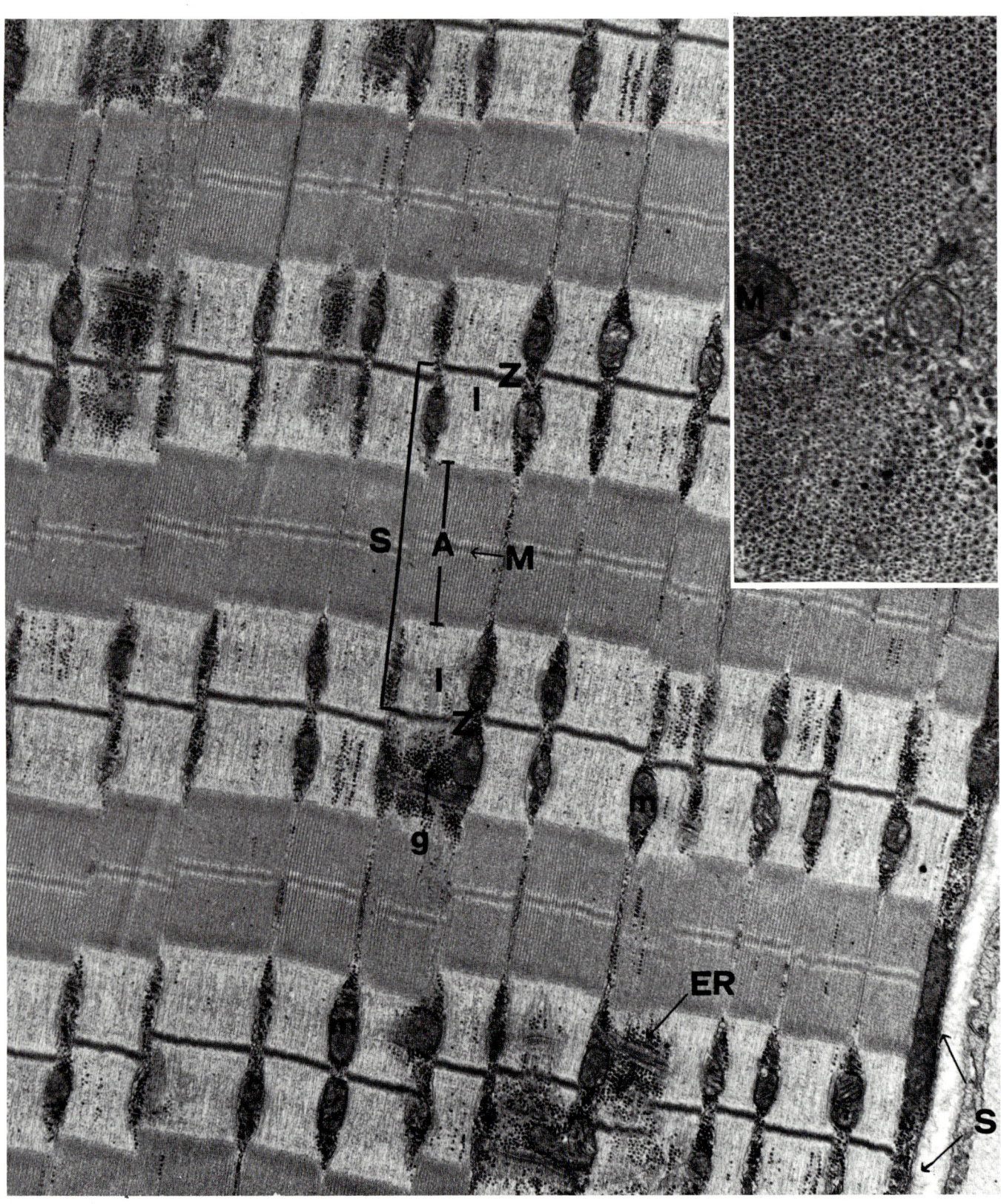

Striated skeletal muscle from a rat (EM, x25,000). Note regular occurrence of sarcomeres (**S**) limited by Z lines (**Z**). **M** = M line (in the middle of the H band). **A** = anisotrope band. Between the myofibrils are mitochondria, sarcoplasmic reticulum (**ER→**) and glycogen granules (**g→**). **The sarcolemma (S→)** delimits the muscle fiber. **Inset: Rat striated muscle fiber in cross section (EM, x60,000).** Cross section showing details of myofilaments in myofibrils. In the cytoplasm between the myofibrils glycogen granules and mitochondria (**M**) can be seen. Within the myofibrils the thinner "pin points" are actin myofilaments in cross section, and the coarser dots are myosin filaments. By courtesy of F. Caramia.

Plate 4.7   97

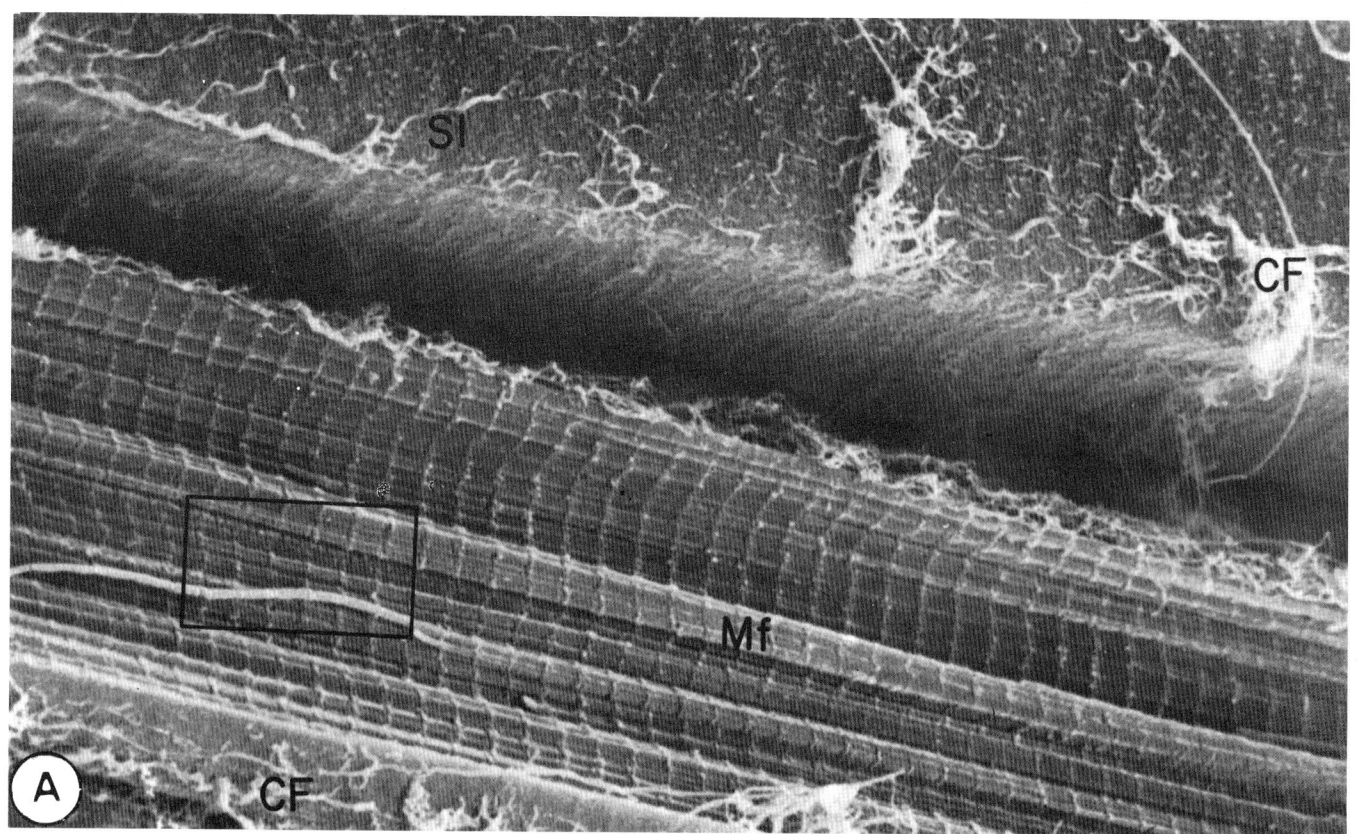

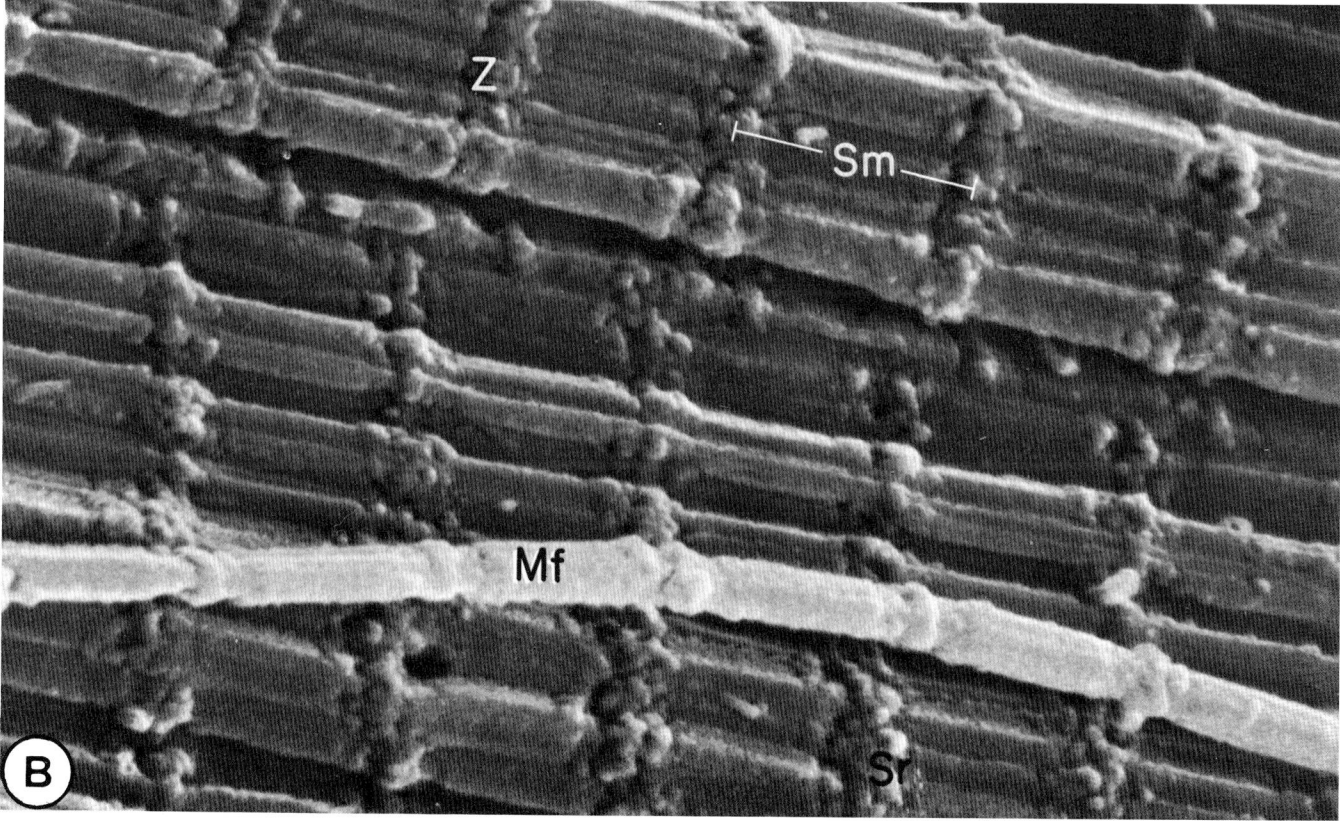

A   **Striated muscle fibers from a rat (scanning EM, x5,000).** Above and below the fiber the sarcolemma is intact. Numerous reticular and collagen fibers **(CF)** adhere to the sarcolemma. Center: the striated myofibrils **(Mf)** are arranged in register and show the typical striations.

B   **Striated myofibrils from a rat (scanning EM, x17,000).** Enlargement of the area outlined in A above. Here one can see the sarcomeres **(Sm)**, myofilaments **(Mf)**, and regions where the sarcoplasmic reticulum **(Sr)** is associated with the Z lines **(Z)**. From P.M. Motta, P.M Andrews and K.R. Porter. In: *Microanatomy of Cell and Tissue Surfaces. An Atlas of Scanning Electron Microscopy.* Lea & Febiger, Philadelphia, 1977.

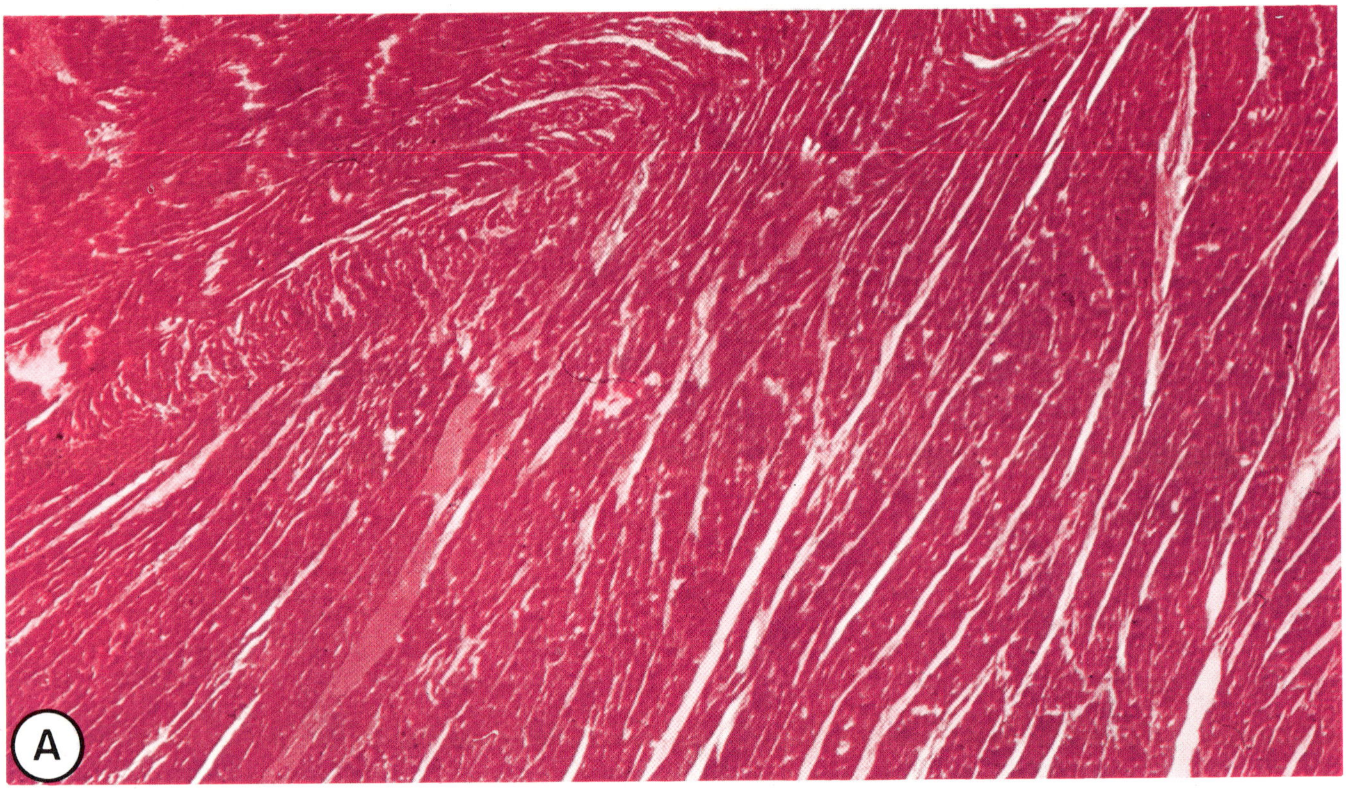

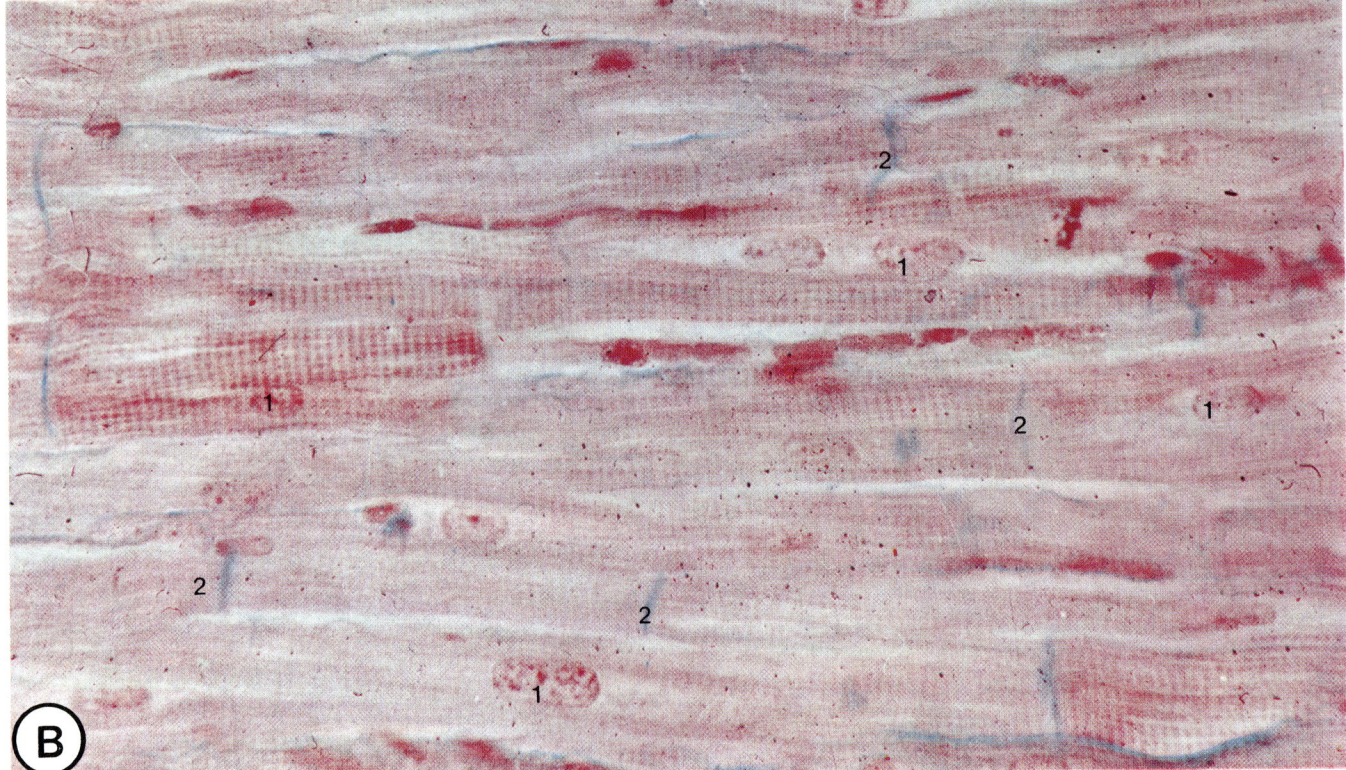

A   **Longitudinal section of papillary muscle from human heart (H & E, x120).** The bundles of muscle fibers are in a typical branched array and are interspersed with connective tissue.

B   **Human cardiac muscle fibers (azan-Mallory, x380).** Cardiac muscle fibers have striations similar to those of skeletal muscle. The nuclei are centrally located in the muscle fibers **(1).** The small vertical lines are intercalated disks **(2).**

Plate 4.9   **99**

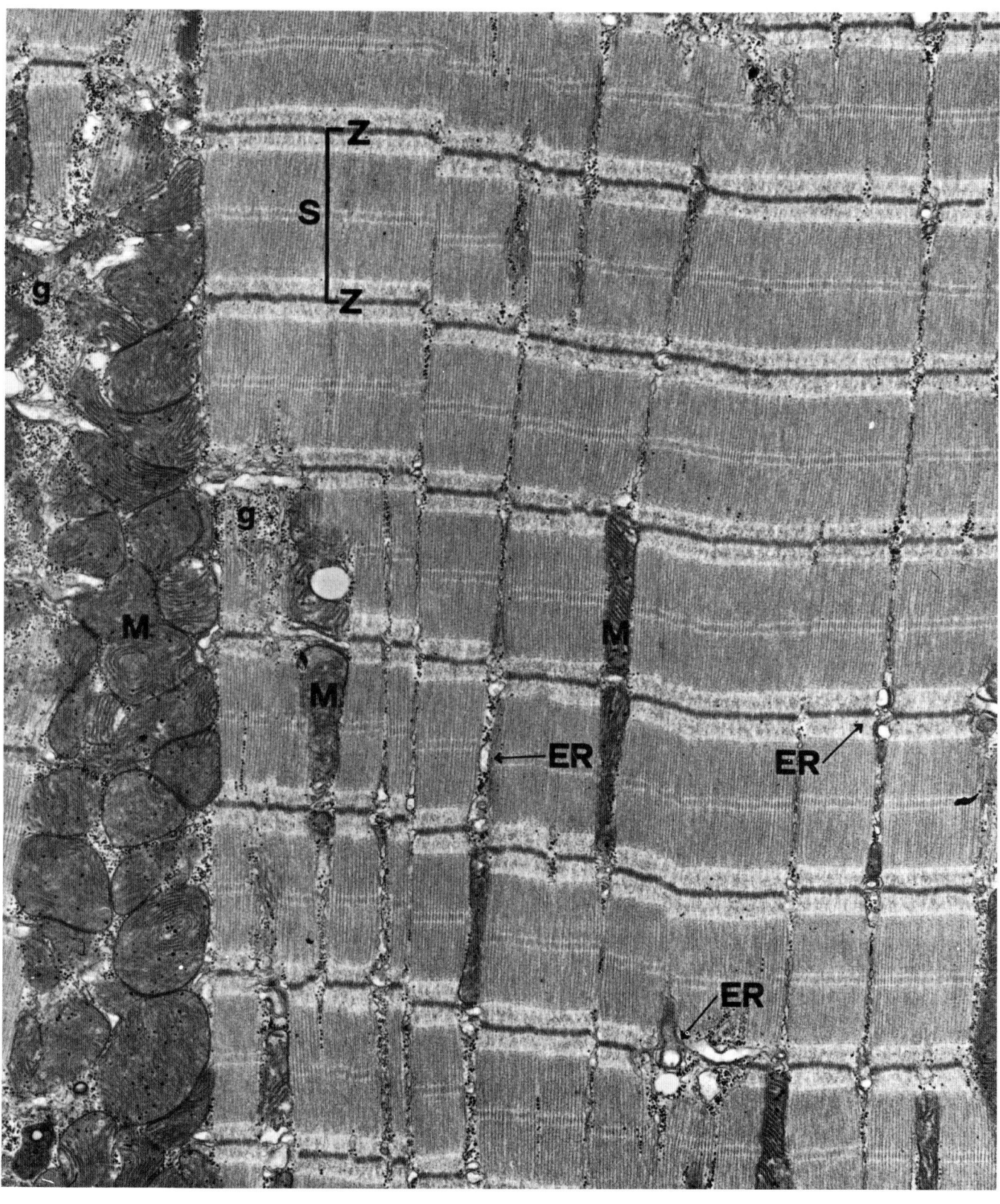

Rat cardiac muscle (EM, x18,000). Cardiac muscle fibers are smaller and contain fewer nuclei than skeletal muscle fibers. The primary difference between the two types of tissue is the presence of intercalated disks. Between bundles of myofilaments sectioned lengthwise are endoplasmic reticulum (**ER**→) and mitochondria (**M**) with glycogen granules (**g**). The Z lines (**Z**) clearly establish the limits of the sarcomeres (**S**). Original micrograph by F. Caramia.

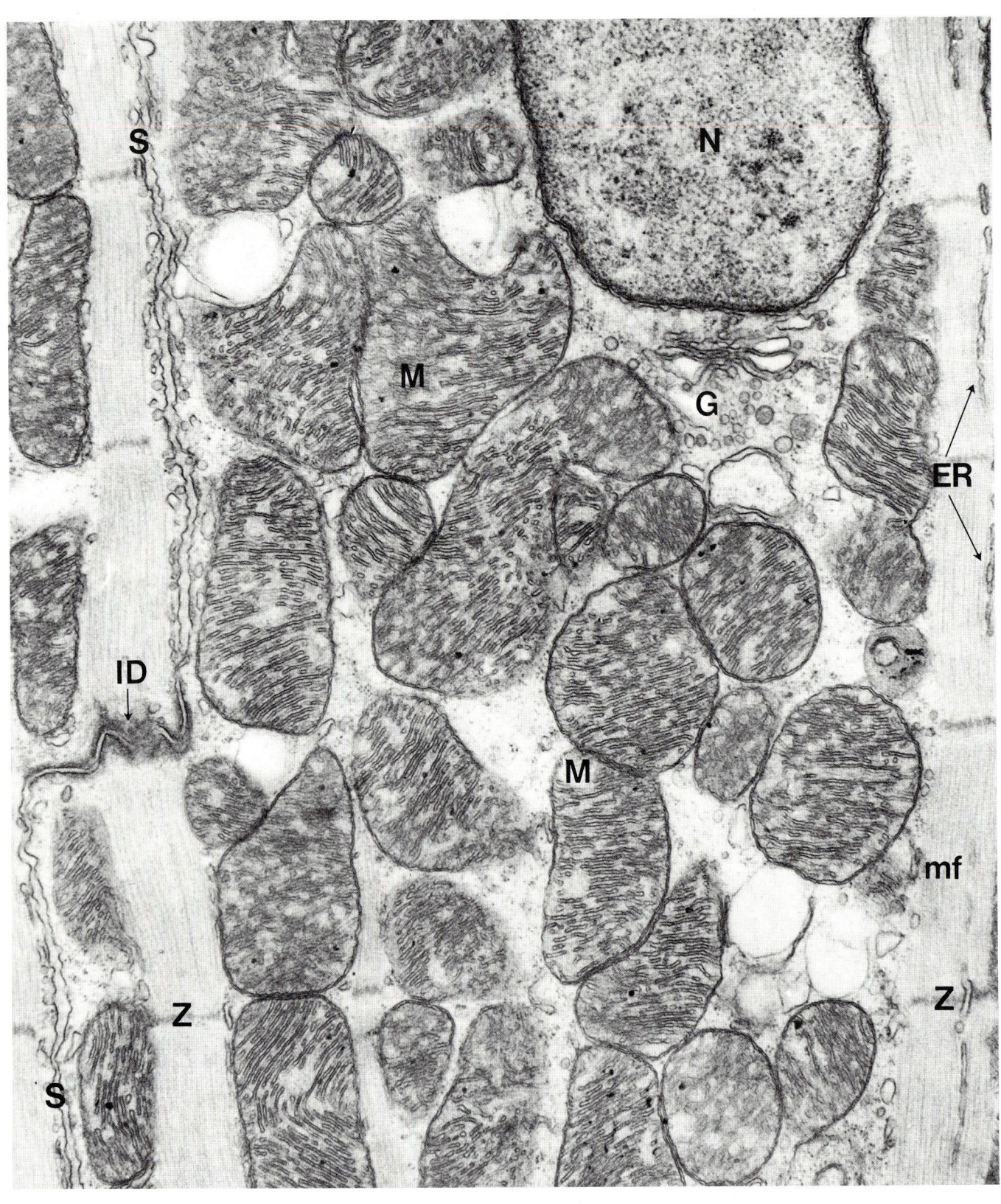

Ventricular myocardial tissue from a hummingbird (EM, x50,000). N = nucleus. **G** = Golgi complex. **ER** = endoplasmic (sarcoplasmic) reticulum. **M** = mitochondria with abundant cristae. **mf** = myofilaments. **Z** = Z lines. **(ID→)** = part of an intercalated disk. The intercalated disks form, as the picture shows, at the plane corresponding to the Z lines. The plasma membranes **(S)** of the two adjacent cells lie close to each other. By courtesy of L.J.A. DiDio. Anat. Rec. 159:335, 1967.

NERVOUS TISSUE

Nervous tissue is composed of cells that are specialized for conducting and transmitting impulses. The nerve cells (*neurons*) are directly associated with satellite cells (*neuroglia* and accessory peripheral cells) that support and maintain the neurons. Neurons and satellite cells originate from the ectoderm of the embryo.

Neurons

The neuron is a highly differentiated cell, incapable of division when mature (Plate 5.1). It is composed of the cell body (*perikaryon*) containing the nucleus and one or more processes. The axon occurs singly; the *dendrites* are branched and numerous.

The perikaryon contains a large, round nucleus with a conspicuous nucleolus. In the cytoplasm (*neuroplasm*) are found the organelles common to all cells, plus *pigment granules* and neurofibrils made up of *neurofilaments,* and *neurotubules* (microtubules). The mitochondria are small and round with mainly transverse cristae. They are especially abundant in the perikaryon but can be found in the neural processes, both the dendrites and the axon. The Golgi complex is highly developed, especially in large neurons. Centrioles are seen more rarely.

Two types of pigment are found in nerve cells: melanin and yellow pigment. *Melanin* is a brownish pigment present as granules in the perikaryon of certain neurons (Sommering's black substance, red and dentate nucleus of the cerebellum). *Yellow pigment (lipochrome)* is a lipofuchsin produced by cell catabolism. Lipochrome is not eliminated and therefore increases in quantity with aging (*age pigment*).

Neurofibrils are made up of thin filaments which can be enhanced by silver-staining techniques. They are present in the perikaryon and in the dendrites and axon. In the neuroplasm and dendrites the neurofibrils are arranged in bundles that branch to form a network, whereas in the axon the neurofibrils run parallel. Neurofibrils are stable structures that have a supporting function. They are formed of an aggregate of elementary filaments which are 10-15 nm in diameter.

The neuroplasm contains rough endoplasmic reticulum enclosing a network of interconnecting cavities. The rough endoplasmic reticulum and attendant polysomes constitute a chromatophilic substance (*Nissl's bodies*). These basophilic regions are distributed throughout the perikaryon except at the periphery of the cell and immediately adjacent to the nucleus. In pathological states Nissl's bodies may disappear (*chromatolysis*).

Protein synthesis in the cell takes place in the neuroplasm. The proteins are quickly transported to the axon and the dendrites. Many of these proteins are involved in producing other substances that act as neurosecretions or chemical mediators. *Neurosecretory products* such as oxytocin and vasopressin (antidiuretic hormone) are produced in the perikaryons of certain neurons of the supraoptic and paraventricular nuclei of the hypothalamus and are gradually transported as granules through the axons to their endings in the neurohypophysis. There the material accumulates before it is secreted and passed into the blood vessels. These neurons thus behave as endocrine cells and their products (neurosecretions) are true hormones.

Many other neurons of the hypothalamus and the central nervous system produce peptide substances with a hormonal function (e.g., factors inhibiting or stimulating the hypothalamus, substance P, somatostatin, enkephalins, endorphins) while maintaining the characteristics of neurons. Hence, neurosecretion should be considered a phenomenon common to many nerve cells (Plate 5.6). The *chemical mediators* (acetylcholine, biogenic amines such as norepinephrine, dopamine, serotonin, and amino acids such as gamma-aminobutyric acid) produced in neurons are substances that have an important role in promoting or inhibiting the transmission of the impulse through the synapse (see below).

Dendrites are thin cytoplasmic processes that branch out from the perikaryon into tree-like formations. Each type of neuron has its own particular and intricate arrangement of dendrites. The nerve impulse in dendrites is directed towards the center (centripetally).

The *axon* usually originates from the perikaryon in the form of an axon hillock and then immediately tapers. It may remain unbranched or have only a few collateral branches. It is limited by a plasma membrane (*axolemma*) that is a continuation of the membrane of the perikaryon. Axons have a neuroplasm rich in mitochondria and neurofibrils arranged parallel to the axis of the axon. In axons the nerve impulse is directed outward from the center (centrifugally).

A classification of neurons based on function includes 1) *afferent neurons* or *receptors* such as those that receive stimuli from outside the body, so that they are located peripherally or have nerve processes that extend to peripheral receptors (Plates 5.3, 5.4, 5.5 A,B), 2) *Efferent* or *motor neurons* that transmit impulses that excite or inhibit effector organs (glands or muscles) (Plates 5.1 B,C,D; 5.5 C), and 3) *Interneurons* that connect the other two types (Plates 5.1 A, 5.4 A,B).

The impulse conducted through the axon is transmitted to another neuron by means of a contact area called a *synapse.* Two categories of synapses are distinguished, one in which the synapse transmits the impulse from one nerve cell to another, and another in which the synapse transmits the excitation from the axon of a neu-

ron to another type of cell (e.g., muscle cell or secretory epithelium). In the first category the impulse passes from one nerve cell to another without alteration, while in the second it is transformed into another activity (primarily contraction or secretion). Synapses of the first type (true synapse) can be 1) *axo-somatic,* in which the synapse is between the axon of a neuron and the perikaryon (or soma) of another neuron, 2) *axo-dendritic,* in which the synapse is between an axon and a dendrite, and 3) *axo-axonic,* in which the contact is between one axon and another.

The synapses between nerve processes and cells of a different type are commonly called *cytoneural junctions* if the contact is between axons and epithelial cells, and *myoneural junctions* if the contact is between axons and muscle cells.

The synapse is an area of the cytoplasm specialized morphologically and functionally to promote or inhibit the transmission of impulses. It is usually the extremity of an axon swelling into a knob shape (bouton) that forms the synapse fitting the membrane of another neuron. The membrane at the terminus of the cell is called the *presynaptic membrane,* that of the adjacent neuron the *postsynaptic membrane,* and the space in between being the *synaptic gap.* The pre- and postsynaptic membranes are each about 6 nm thick. The synaptic gap is 10-20 nm wide. Inside the synaptic bouton are numerous mitochondria and *synaptic vesicles* whose cavities accumulate chemical mediators. These vesicles aggregate near specialized areas near the presynaptic membrane (*active points*) and then open to discharge the chemical mediator into the synaptic gap (exocytosis). This causes the postsynaptic membrane to depolarize or hyperpolarize (Plate 5.4).

Neuroglia

The nonconducting accessory cells that are in the central nervous system in order to support and control their environment belong to a large class called neuroglia or *gliocytes.* Some of these cells are also found in the peripheral nervous system and form the *Schwann cells* and *satellite cells* of the nerve ganglia. The common characteristic of these cells is the presence of processes varying in length, number and shape by means of which they are related to the neurons. In the central nervous system the glial cells form a network that supports and binds the neurons, thus maintaining their stability for both neural transmission and for exchange of nutrients. Some glial cells (*ependymal cells*) line the neural canal of the spinal cord and the cavities of the brain. Some of these cells are involved in a filtering system that forms and reabsorbs the cerebrospinal fluid. Other cells derived from the mesenchyme and classified as connective cells exist in the nervous system with neuroglia and neurons. As a group these cells constitute the *microglia*, which have a phagocytic function like that exercised by the macrophages in connective tissue.

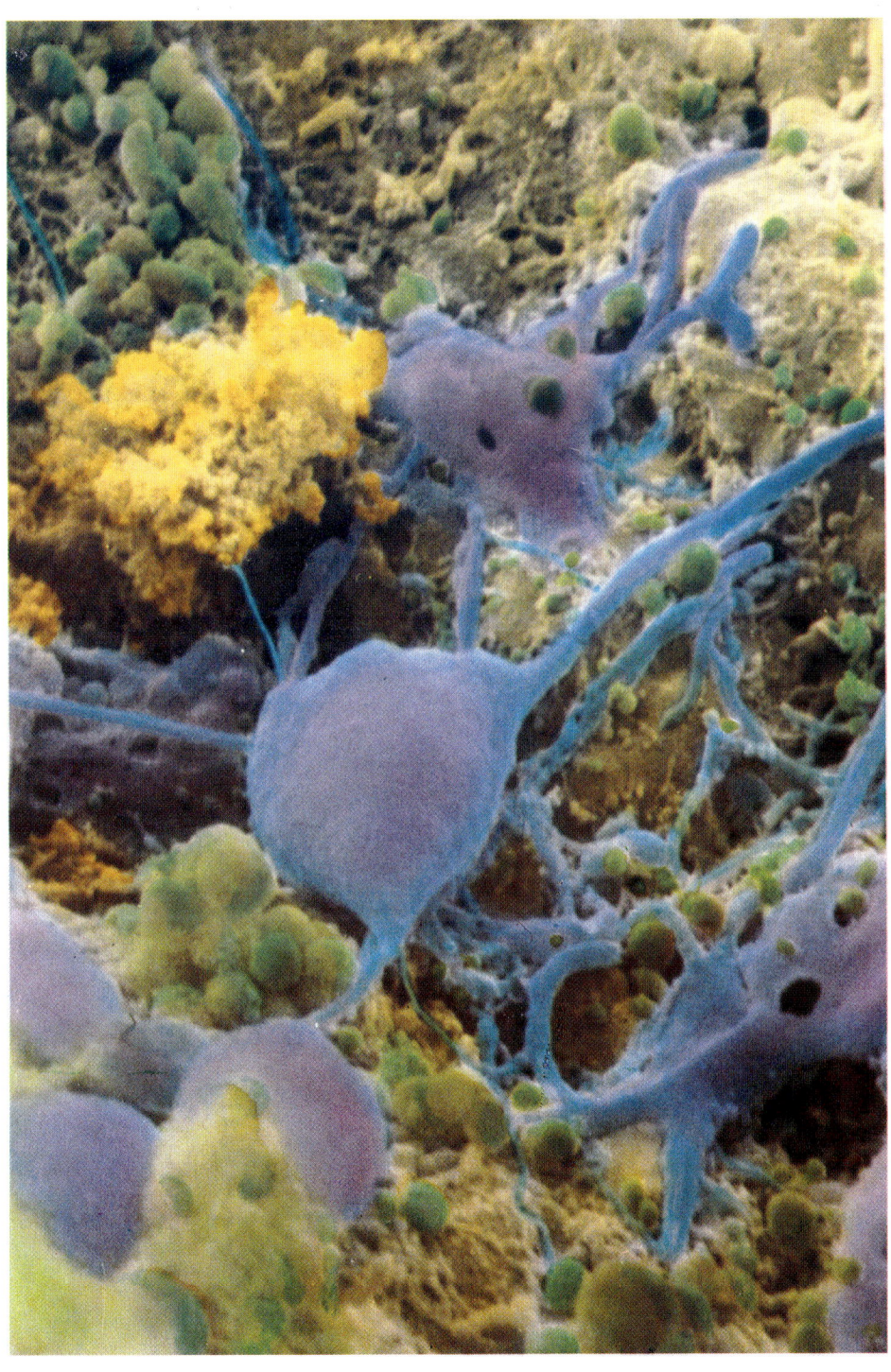

Fine dendrites and neurites of a rat neurons form a delicate network. (Colored SEM; 4,250 x).

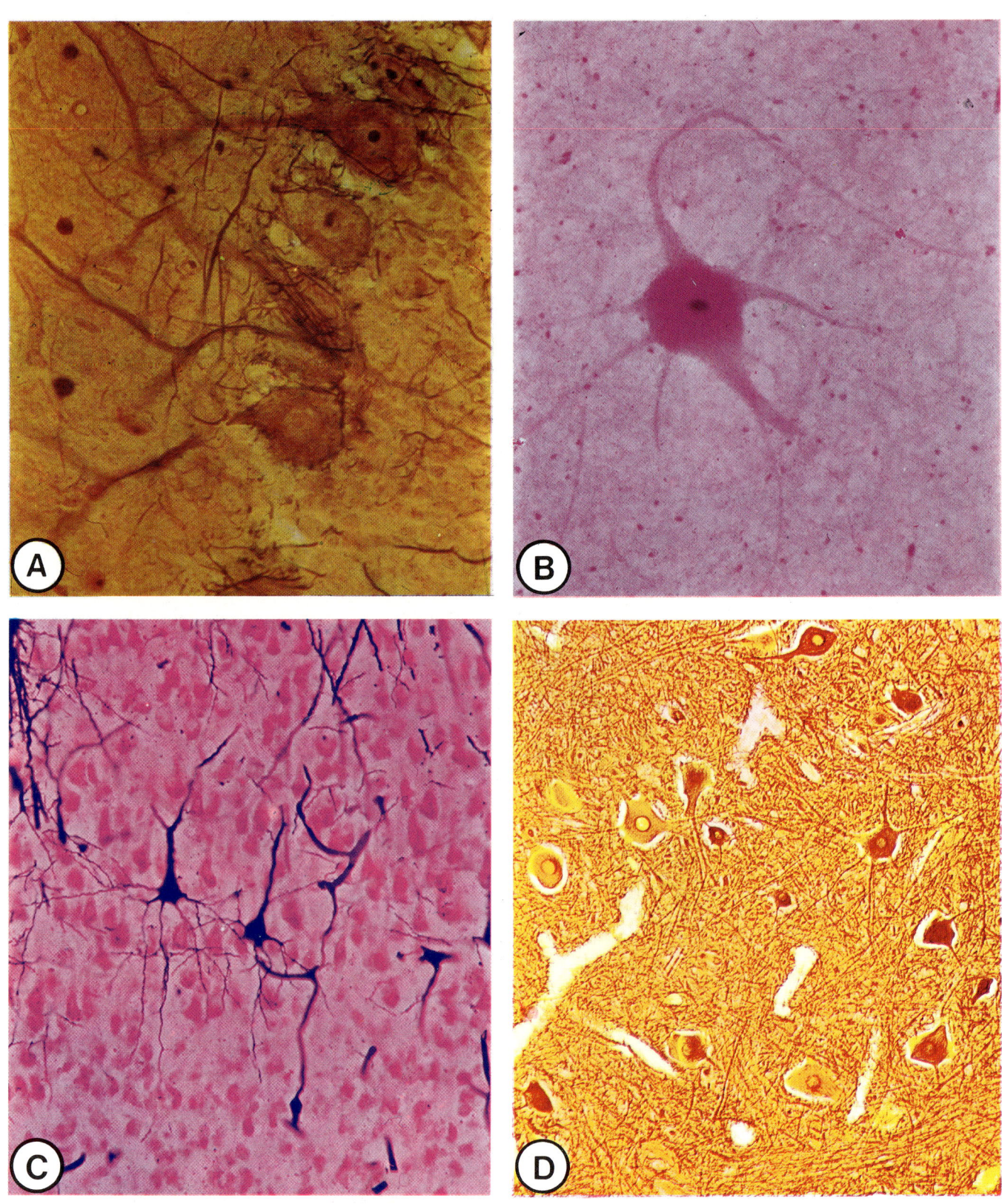

A   Purkinje cells from the cerebellar cortex of a cat (silver impregnation, x450).
B   Single ganglion cell of bovine autonomic nervous system (carmine-alum, x425).
C   Pyramidal cells from cat cerebral cortex (silver impregnation, x180).
D   Motor nerve cells from anterior horn of human spinal cord (Cajal method, x200).

Plate 5.2 105

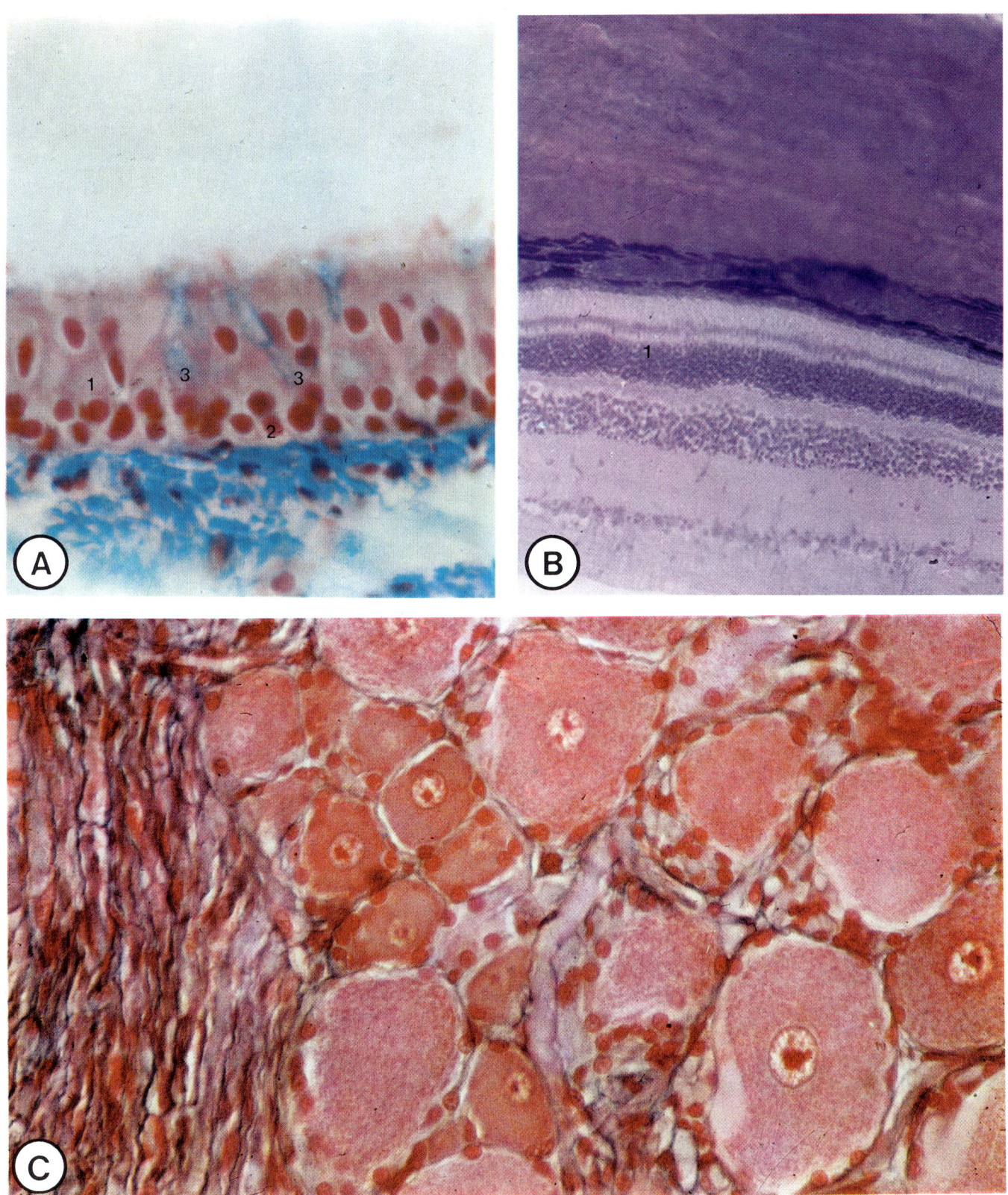

A **Epithelium from human olfactory mucosa (azan-Mallory, x780).** Between the supporting cells **(1)** and the basal cells **(2)** the olfactory cells (neuron receptors) **(3)** are intercalated.

B **Pig retina cells (H & E, x120).** The rod and cone cells **(1)** are classified as receptor (or afferent) neurons.

C **Sensory neurons from cat spinal ganglion (azan-Mallory, x620).** The cell bodies of sensory neurons are large and surrounded by satellite cells (glial type). Left: nerve fiber bundles.

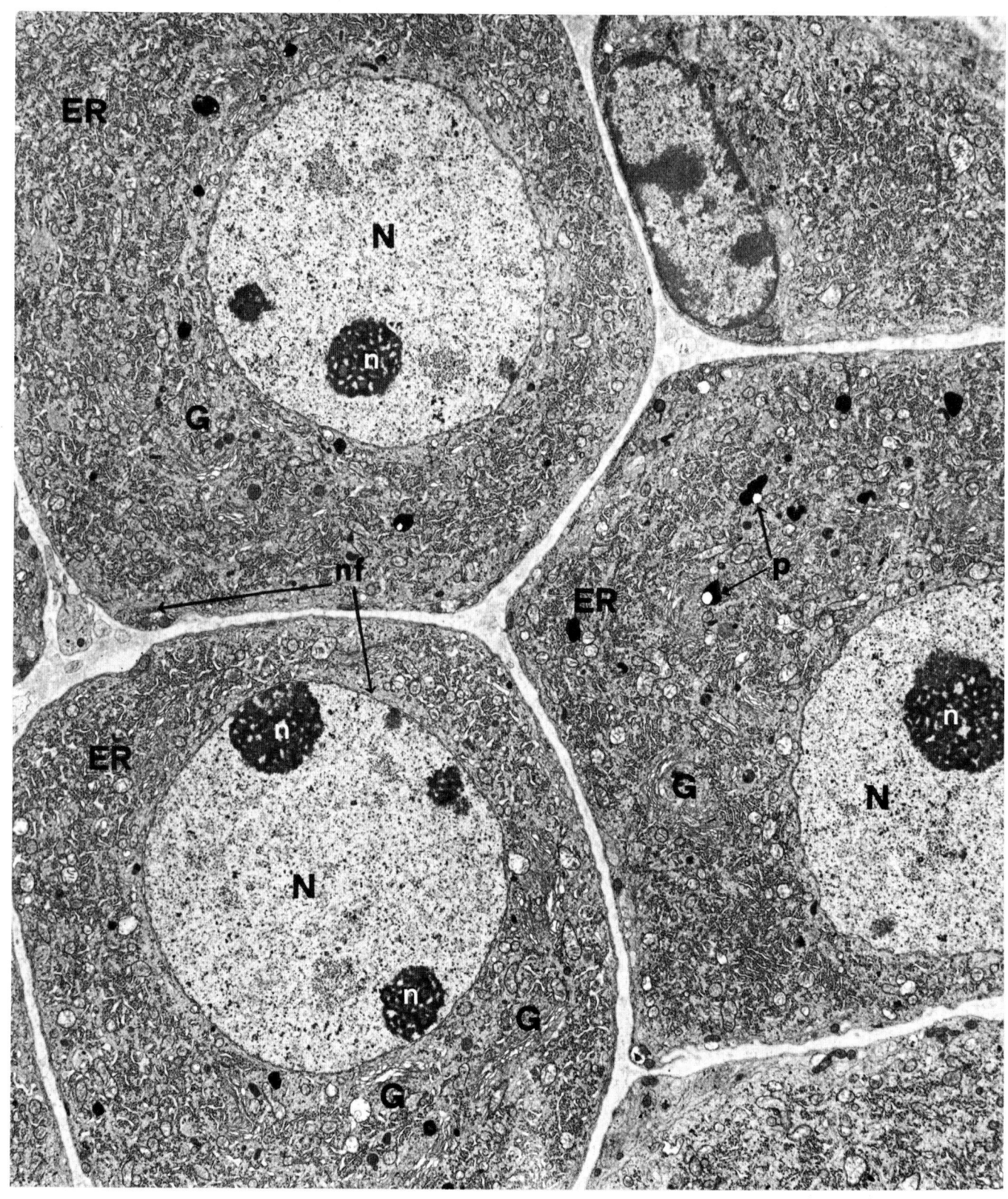

Neurons of mouse spinal ganglion (EM, x8,500). The perikarya of these neurons contain a vesicular nucleus (**N**) with one or more nucleoli (**n**) and a cytoplasm rich in ribosomes and rough endoplasmic reticulum (Nissl's chromophilic areas). Golgi complexes (**G**), pigment granules (**p→**), neurofilaments (**nf→**) and small mitochondria are scattered throughout the cytoplasm. By courtesy of F. Caramia.

Plate 5.4 107

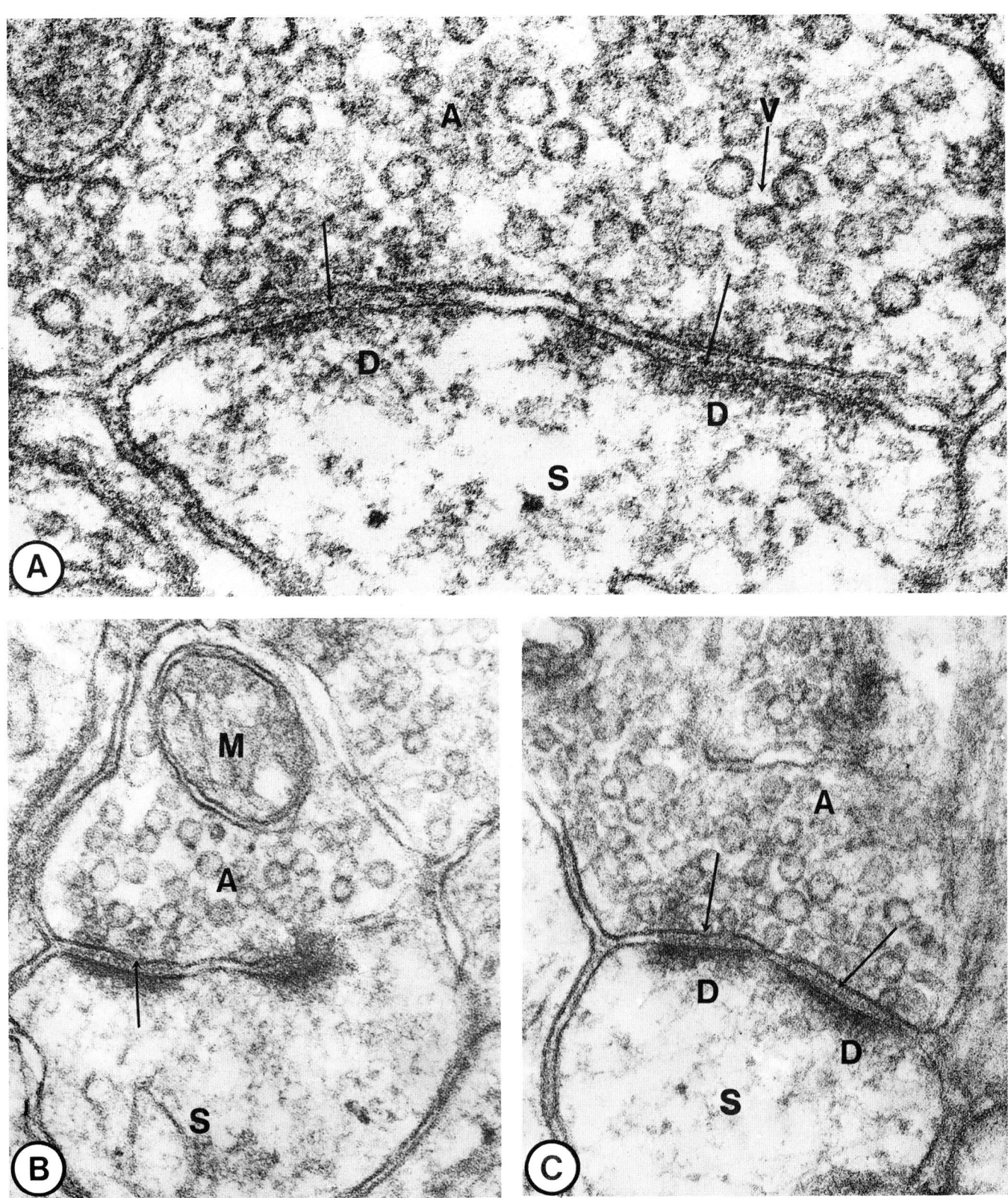

A   **Axo-dendritic synapse in rat cerebral cortex (EM, x180,000).** The synapse is between an axon ending (**A**) containing many synaptic vesicles (**V→**) and a dendritic spine (**S**). The synaptic junction has two dense postsynaptic areas (**D**) and in the synaptic gap dense material can be seen (**→**).

B   **C Axo-dendritic synapses of rat cerebral cortex (EM, x120,000). A** = axon ending. **S** = dendritic spine. The pre- and postsynaptic membranes are separated by the synaptic gap, which contains dense material (**→**). On the cytoplasmic surface of the postsynaptic membrane are denser areas (**D**) (active points). In the axon endings are many synaptic vesicles and some mitochondria (**M**). By courtesy of A. Peters. Z. Zellforsch. 100:487, 1969.

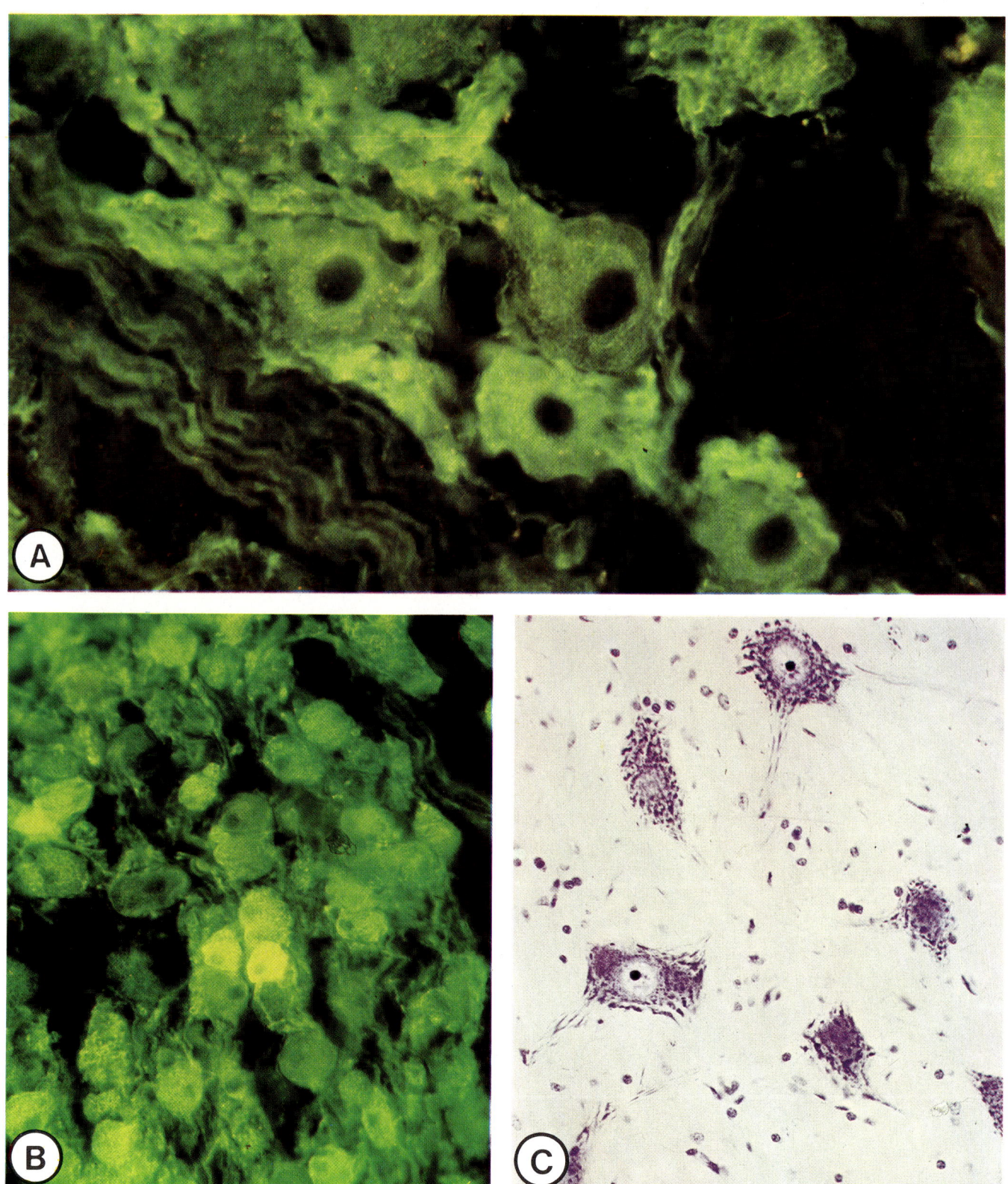

A   **Neurons of sympathetic ganglion from a dog (Falk and Hillarp fluorescence method, x425).** Catecholamine is shown to be present by the yellow-green fluorescence in the cytoplasm and the axons. The nerve cell nucleus is seen as a dark vesicle. By courtesy of V. Tessitore.

B   **Bundle of ganglion neurons (fluorescence method, x220).** The neurons are markedly fluorescent.

C   **Somatomotor neurons from anterior horn of human spinal cord (Nissl method, x340).** The perikaryon abounds in tigroid substance (violet granules). They have a vesicular nucleus and a dense nucleolus. Between the neurons are a number of glial cells.

Plate 5.6   **109**

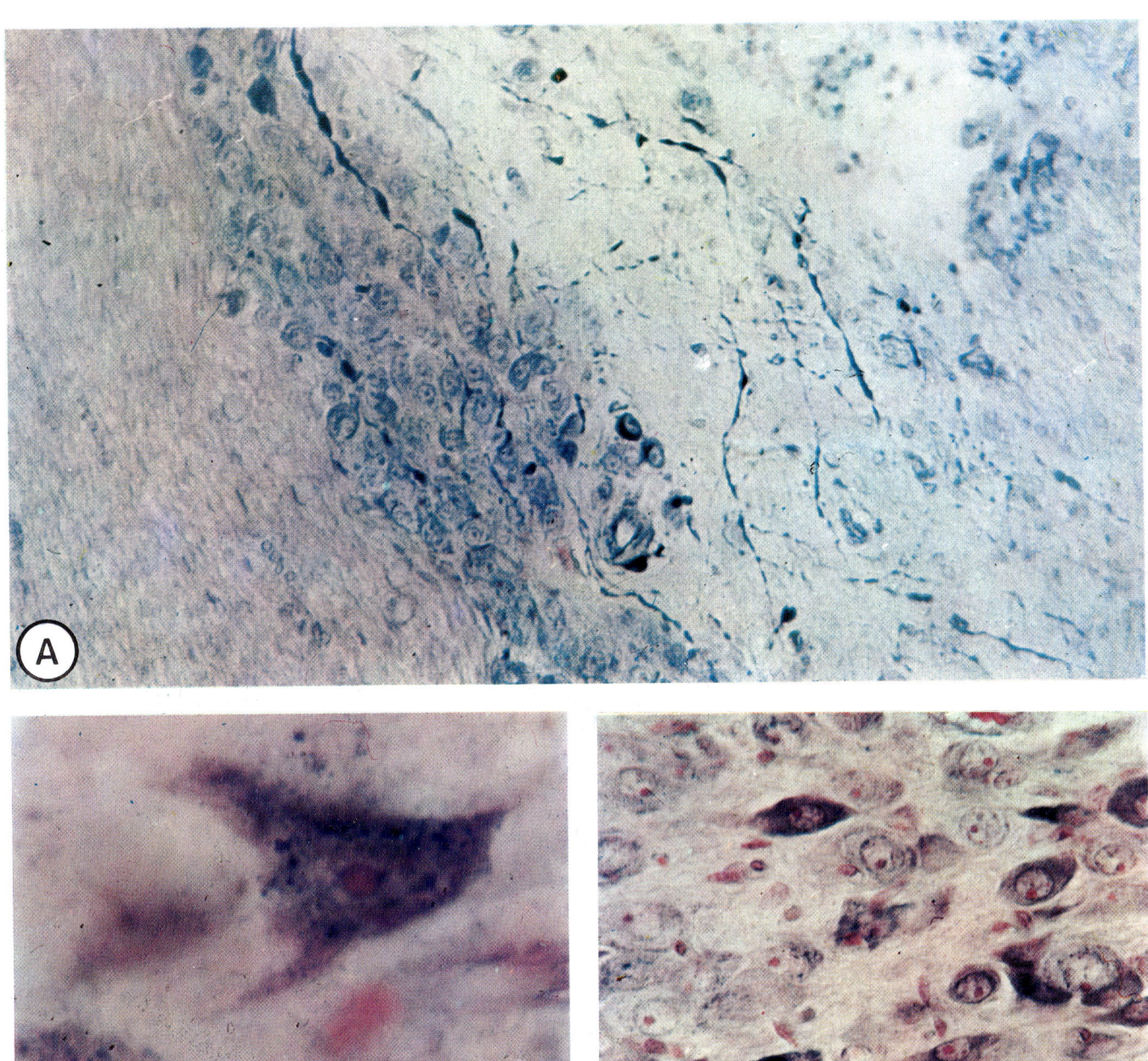

A **Supraoptic nucleus from a rat (chrome-hematoxylin-phloxin, x200).** Around the nucleus are fibers filled with neurosecretory products (Herring bodies).

B **Perikarya from neurons of rat supraoptic nucleus (chrome-hematoxylin-phloxin, x380).** The cytoplasm of the neurons contains many neurosecretory granules.

C **Supraoptic nucleus from a rat (chrome-hematoxylin-phloxin, x220).** Note many neurons with neurosecretory material stained blue-violet. By courtesy of A. Pasqualino.

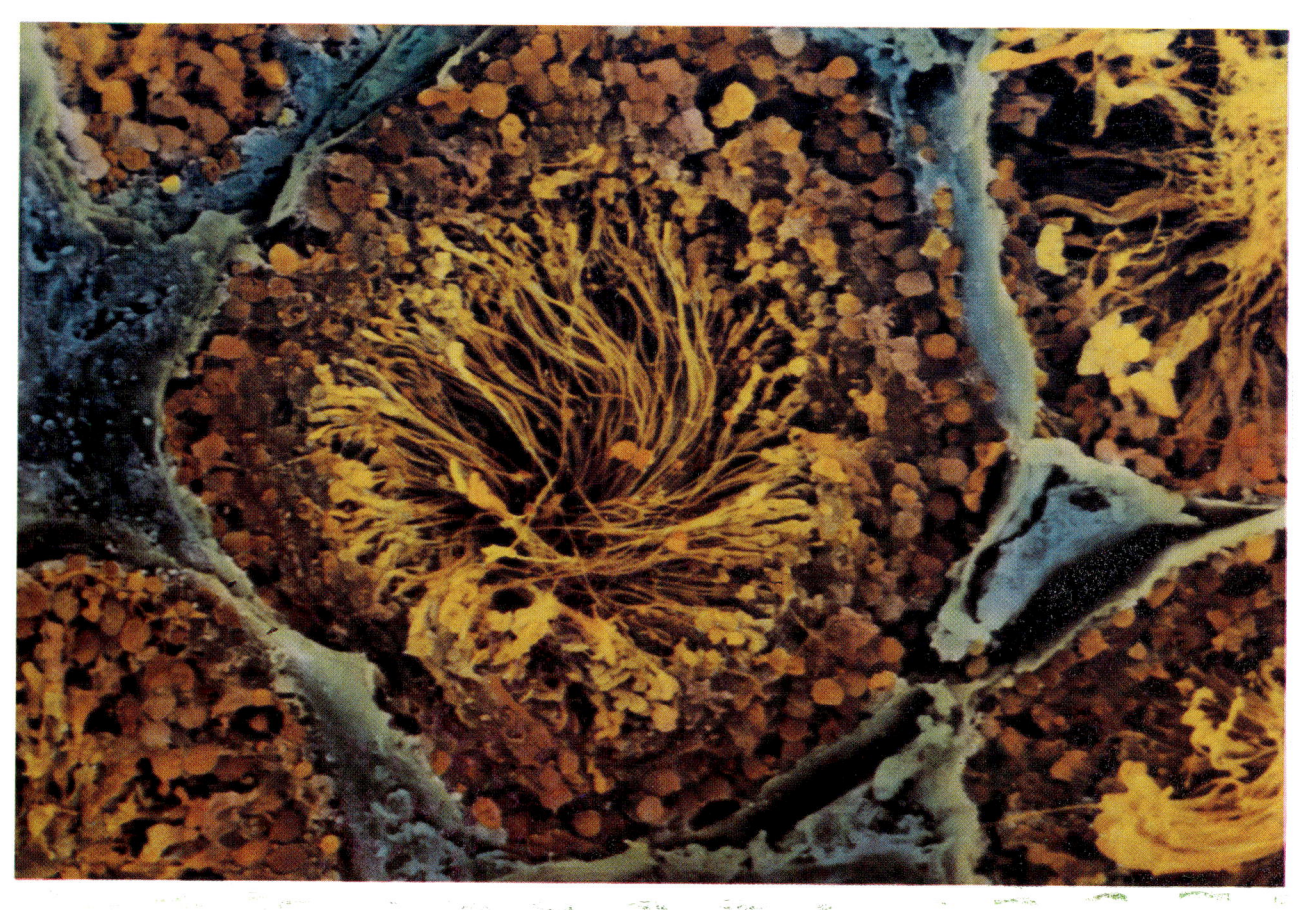

Testis. A rat seminiferous tubule. (Colored SEM; 630 x).

GERMINAL TISSUE

The myriad variety of cells that make up the adult organism is derived from the union of two cells, the *oocyte (egg)* and the *spermatazoon.* The tissues that are formed of cells specialized both morphologically and functionally for reproduction are called *germinal tissues.* Oocytes and spermatozoa develop as a result of a complex maturing process (*gametogenesis*), which can be divided into specific stages.

The primordial germ cells (*gonocytes*), from which the oocytes and spermatozoa are derived, originate in the developing human embryo with the appearance of the yolk sac about three weeks after fertilization. The germ cells migrate to the caudal portion of the digestive tract by moving along its mesentery. After about a week they reach the gonadal ridge of the gonad. Primordial germ cells have a relative abundance of cytoplasm and are capable of ameboid movement by which they migrate to their definitive sites in the gonads. The primordial germ cells can also reach the gonads via the blood stream, which is typical of birds, and perhaps also occurs in humans and other mammals. Once the primordial germ cells have reached their destinations they enter into a stable relationship with other types of cells (nutrient or satellite cells). Together these cells form complex units (ovarian follicles and seminiferous tubules).

The female gametes (oocytes) mature in the ovary through a process called *oogenesis,* and the spermatozoa mature in the testis through a process called *spermatogenesis.* Oogenesis and spermatogenesis are comparable events, and take place in three main phases: 1) *proliferation,* 2) *growth,* 3) *maturation.*

The primary consequence of oogenesis and spermatogenesis is the formation of gametes whose nucleus has the haploid number of chromosomes. Gametes are differentiated morphologically so that their union during fertilization re-establishes the diploid number of chromosomes characteristic of the species (Plates 6.11, 6.12, 6.13).

Oogenesis

The primordial germ cells have the diploid number of chromosomes. These cells undergo frequent mitoses in the gonad, greatly increasing in number (proliferation phase). A number of these cells then increase in volume (growth phase), and in their cytoplasm there is an accumulation of ribosomes for protein synthesis as well as lipid and glycogen. The growth phase in the ovary is dependent on the presence of other cells (*satellite cells* or *follicle cells*) which surround the growing ovum. The follicle cells and the oocyte together are called the *follicle* (Plates 6.1, 6.4).

The oocyte, in the course of its growth and maturation, is in contact with the follicle cells by means of gap junctions. These areas of continuity are essential for maturation of the oocyte and provide for a symbiotic relationship between the germ cell and follicle cells (Plates 6.2, 6.3, 6.5).

The chromosomal complement of the oocyte becomes haploid only in the maturation phase, through meiosis, which produces cells with the haploid number of chromosomes.

The oocyte is usually a large cell with ample cytoplasm containing rough endoplasmic reticulum, free ribosomes, a Golgi complex and large numbers of mitochondria. The nucleus is large and has a conspicuous, characteristic nucleolus (Plates 6.2, 6.3, 6.4).

Spermatogenesis

Spermatogenesis takes place in the testis and is similar to oogenesis in all its basic stages. The primordial cells (spermatogonia) originate outside the mesenchymal structure that will become the gonad, and once they have migrated into the gonad they proliferate by mitosis. The growth phase of these cells, especially in terms of the accumulation of reserve material, is much less marked than in oocytes. The growth and maturation of male gametes depend on the presence in the testis of large supporting cells (*Sertoli cells*), which are equivalent to the follicle cells surrounding the oocyte. The male germ cells are arranged in several layers (*seminiferous epithelium*). The Sertoli cells and the gametes together constitute the wall of the seminiferous tubule (Plates 6.6, 6.7, 6.8, 6.9).

The spermatozoon is made up of three parts, the *head, middle piece* and *tail*. The head contains the nucleus, in which the chromatin is a condensed and homogeneous mass, and in which the chromosomes cannot be individually observed. At the tip of the nucleus is a membranous cap containing lytic enzymes (*acrosome*) (Plates 6.8, 6.9, 6.10). At the base of the nucleus can be seen a pair of centrioles from which the middle piece projects and continues as the tail. The tail of the spermatozoon has a structure similar to that of a cilium or flagellum, being formed from a central pair of microtubules (the *axoneme*) surrounded by a ring of nine pairs of peripheral microtubules. The axoneme originates at the base of the sperm head and extends to the tip of the tail. Around the middle piece of the tail there is a sheath composed of mitochondria, and around the principal piece of the tail there exists a fibrous sheath.

Genetically speaking, the head of the spermatozoon is the most significant portion of the sperm, because it contains the chromosomes. The middle piece, rich in mitochondria, provides energy for motion of the flagellum. The flagellum as a whole propels the sperm.

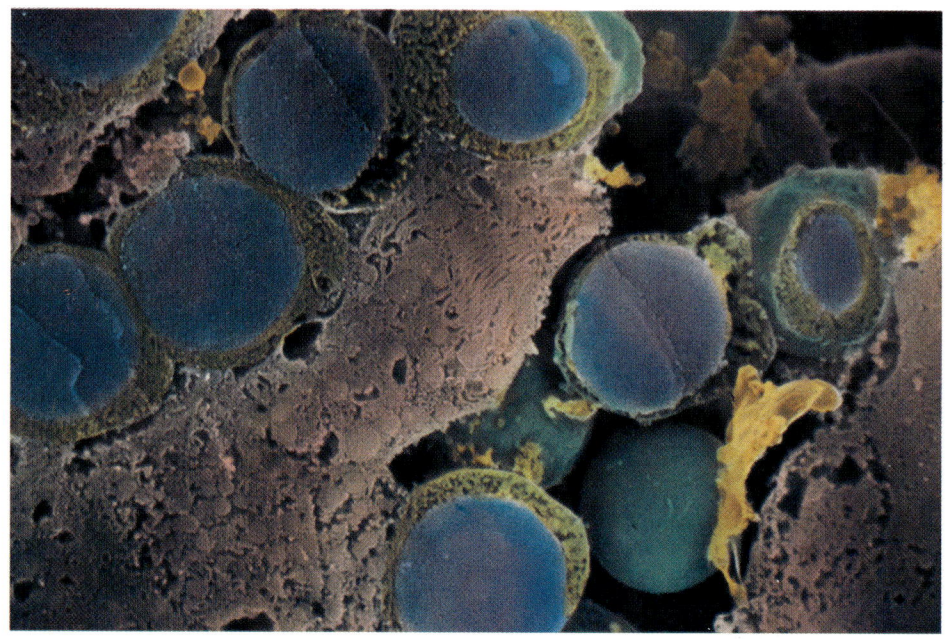

Oocytes proliferating and emerging from the cortical areas of a human fetal ovary. (Colored SEM; 2,100 x).

Plate 6.1   113

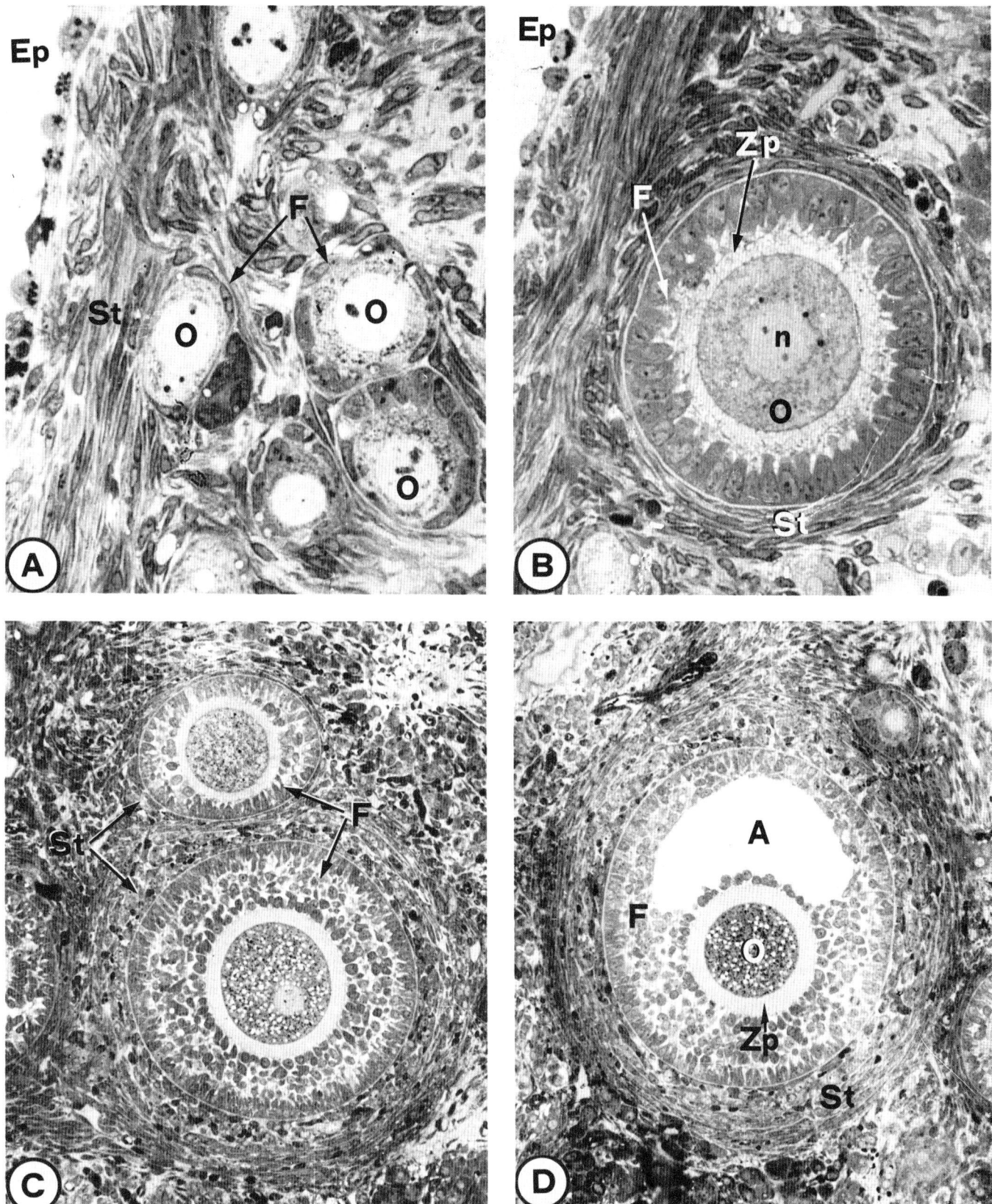

A   **Semithin section of primordial follicles from the cortex of mouse ovary (methylene blue, x710).** Oocytes (**O**) and satellite follicle cells (**F→**) are present in the stroma (**St**) under the superficial epithelium (**Ep**) of the ovary.

B   **Growth phase of primary follicle in mouse ovary (semithin section, basic fuchsin, x980).** The oocyte (**O**) is surrounded by the zona pellucida (**Zp→**) and a layer of cylindrical follicle cells (**F**). **St** = perifollicular stroma. **Ep** = superficial epithelium of ovary. **n** = nucleus of oocyte.

C   **Maturation of follicles in mouse ovary (Semithin section, methylene blue, x580).** Two oocytes can be seen wrapped in several layers of follicle cells (**F→**) and in a perifollicular stroma of spindle-shaped cells (**St→**) from which the theca interna and theca externa derive.

D   **Semithin section of secondary follicle of mouse ovary (methylene blue, x650).** The oocyte (**O**), surrounded by the zona pellucida (**Zp→**) and by follicle cells (**F**), is contained in cumulus cells facing the antrum (**A**), where the liquor folliculi accumulates. The perifollicular stroma (**St**) is abundant and already differentiated into an internal layer (theca interna) and an external layer (theca externa).

Plate 6.2

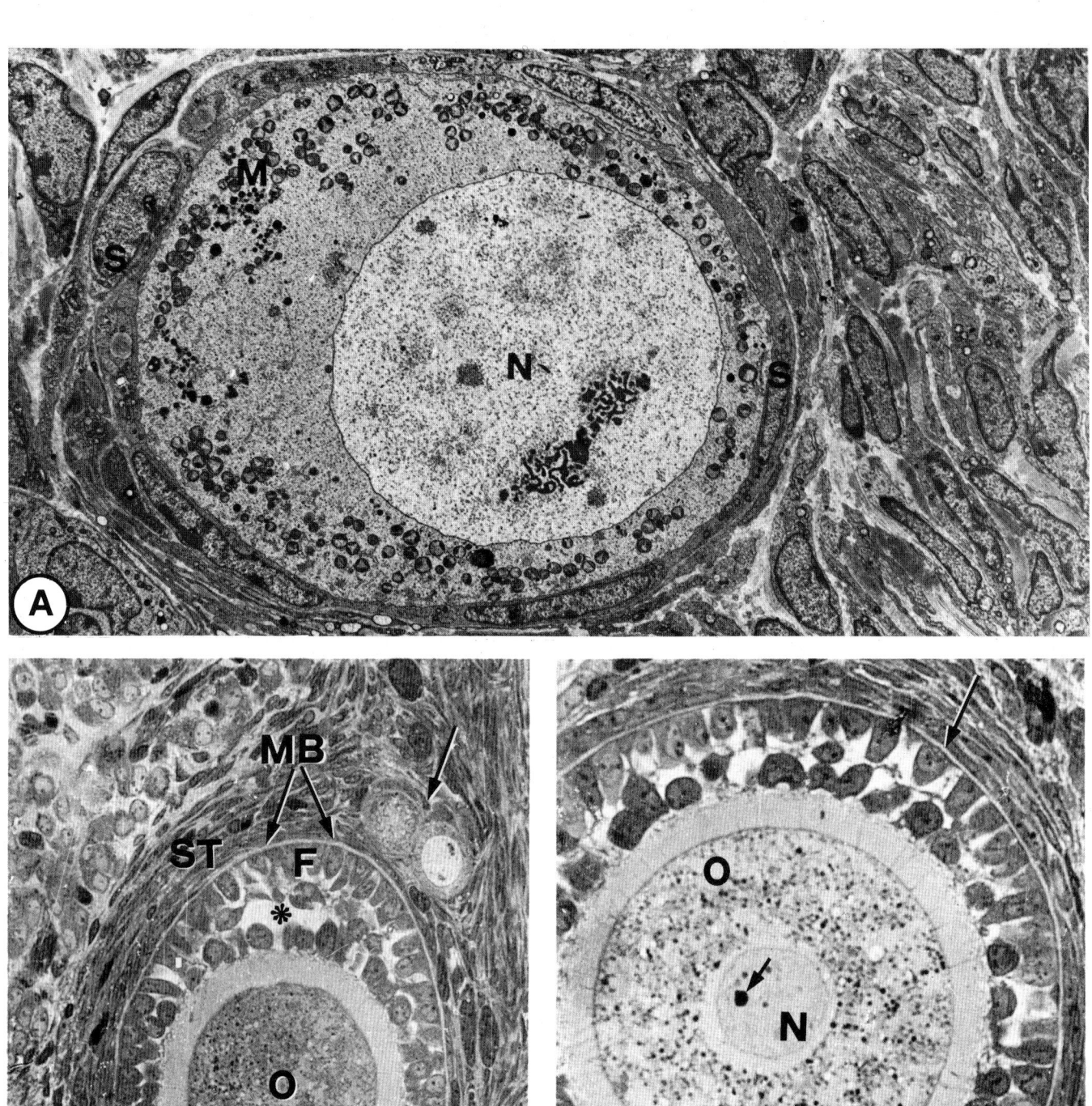

A **Rabbit oocyte (EM, x6,200).** The primordial follicle consists of an oocyte surrounded by follicle cells **(S)**. The oocyte has a large spherical nucleus **(N)** and numerous mitochondria **(M)** in the peripheral cytoplasm.

B **Semithin section of a secondary follicle from mouse ovary (methylene blue, x950).** The oocyte **(O)** is covered by a thick zona pellucida **(Zp)** and surrounded by two layers of follicle cells **(F)**. * = liquor folliculi. **MB→** = basal lamina of the follicle. The unlabeled arrow shows two small primordial follicles in the perifollicular stroma **(ST)**.

C **Growth phase of follicle (semithin section, methylene blue, x1,250).** The cytoplasm of the oocyte **(O)** contains numerous mitochondria, a nucleus **(N)** and nucleolus (→). The zona pellucida **(Zp)** contains thin microvilli extending between the oocyte and the follicle cells **(F)**. A thick basal lamina (→) clearly separates the follicle from the perifollicular stroma **(St)**.

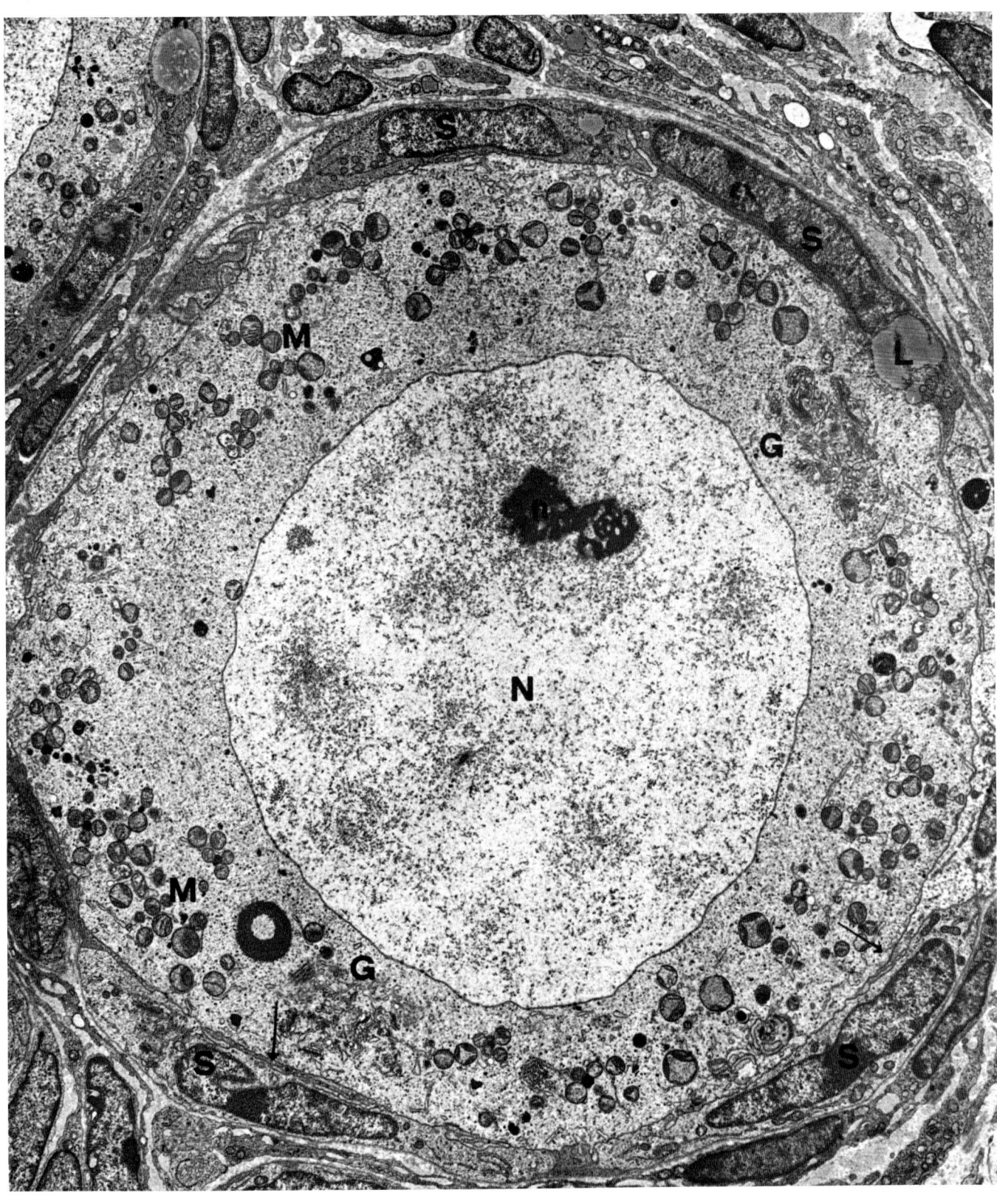

Plate 6.3   **115**

Rabbit oocyte and follicle cells (EM, x16,300). The oocyte is surrounded by follicle cells **(S)**. A narrow intercellular space (→) separates the follicle cells from the oocyte. The cytoplasm of the oocyte contains a number of scattered mitochondria **(M)**, ribosomes and Golgi complexes **(G)**. A large nucleolus is present in the spherical nucleus **(N)**. There are lipid droplets **(L)** in the cytoplasm of the follicle cells.

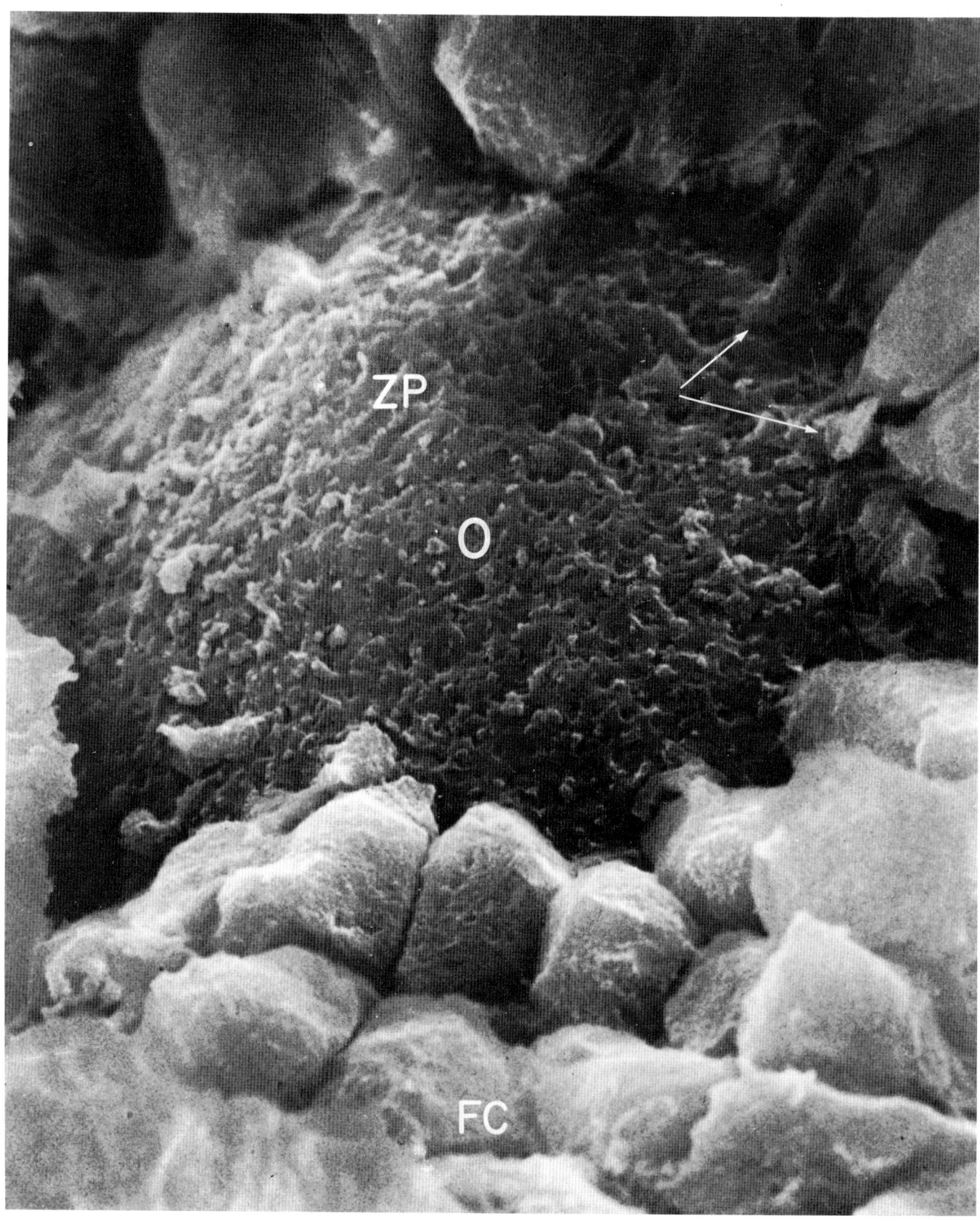

Oocyte and follicle cells in a rabbit secondary follicle (scanning EM, x6,200). A number of the cells of the cumulus oophorus (**FC**) have been artificially removed in order to render more visible the surface of the zona pellucida (**ZP**), which covers the oocyte (**O**). The zona pellucida has a porous appearance and in it are embedded the cytoplasmic processes of the follicle cells (→). From P.M. Motta and J. Van Blerkom. J. Submicr. Cytol. 6:297, 1974.

Plate 6.5   **117**

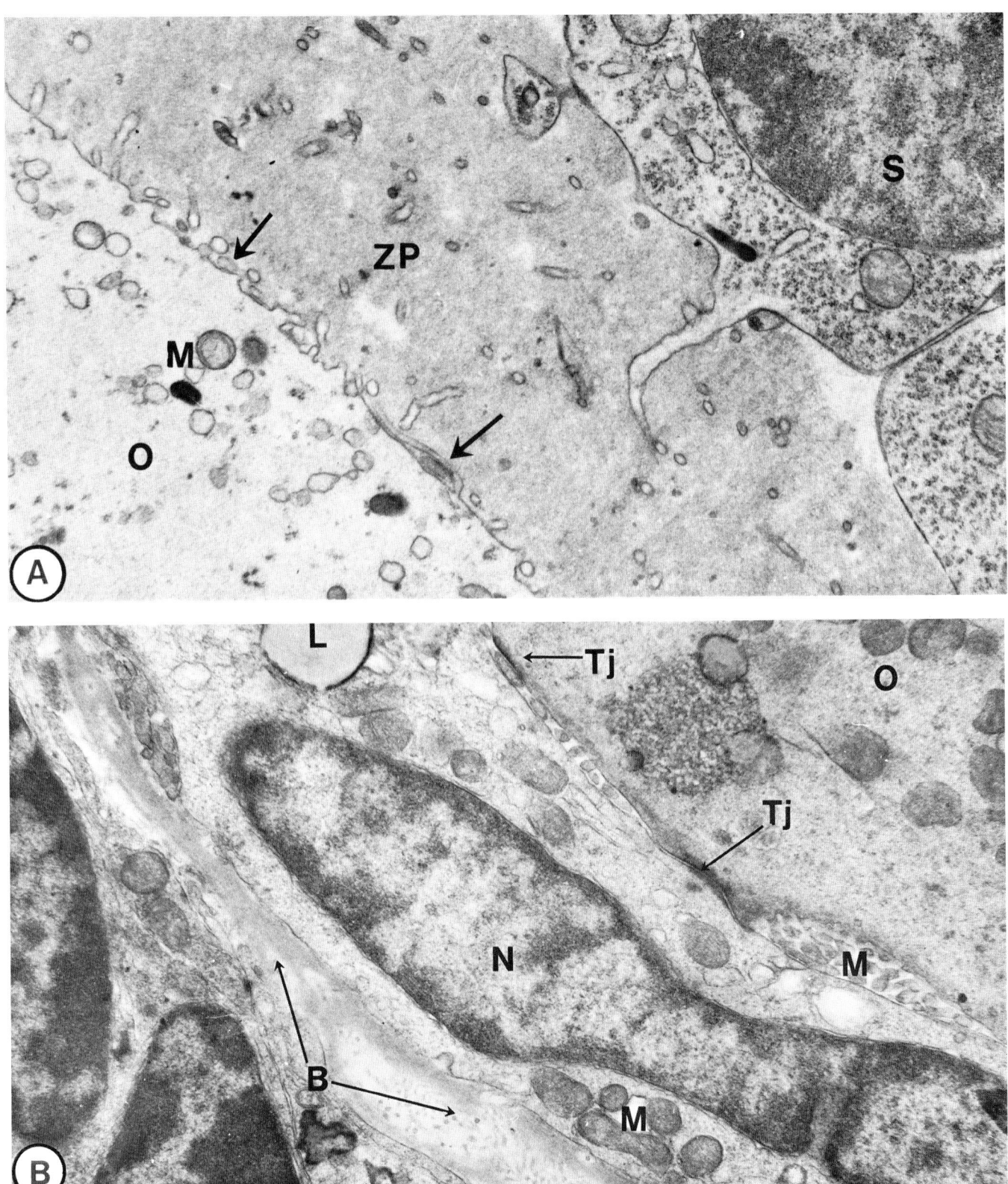

A   **Oocyte and follicle cells of mouse ovary (EM, x31,000).** The cytoplasm of the oocyte **(O)** contains mitochondria **(M)** and endoplasmic reticulum. The follicle cells **(S)** are in communication with the oocyte by means of finger-like extensions of the plasmalemma (→). The zona pellucida **(ZP)** has formed between the oocyte and the follicle cells.

B   **Oocyte and follicle cells of a cat ovary (EM, x28,500).** Detail of connections between the oocyte **(O)** and follicle cells in a primordial ovarian follicle. The cell membranes of the oocyte and of an underlying follicle cell form microvilli **(M)** in some areas. In other areas tight junctions **(Tj)** are present. The follicle cell shows an elongated nucleus **(N)**, lipid droplets **(L)** and mitochondria **(M).** It is separated from the surrounding connective tissue by a basal lamina **(B→).** From P.M. Motta, Z. Takeva and E. Nesci. Acta Anat. 80:537, 1971.

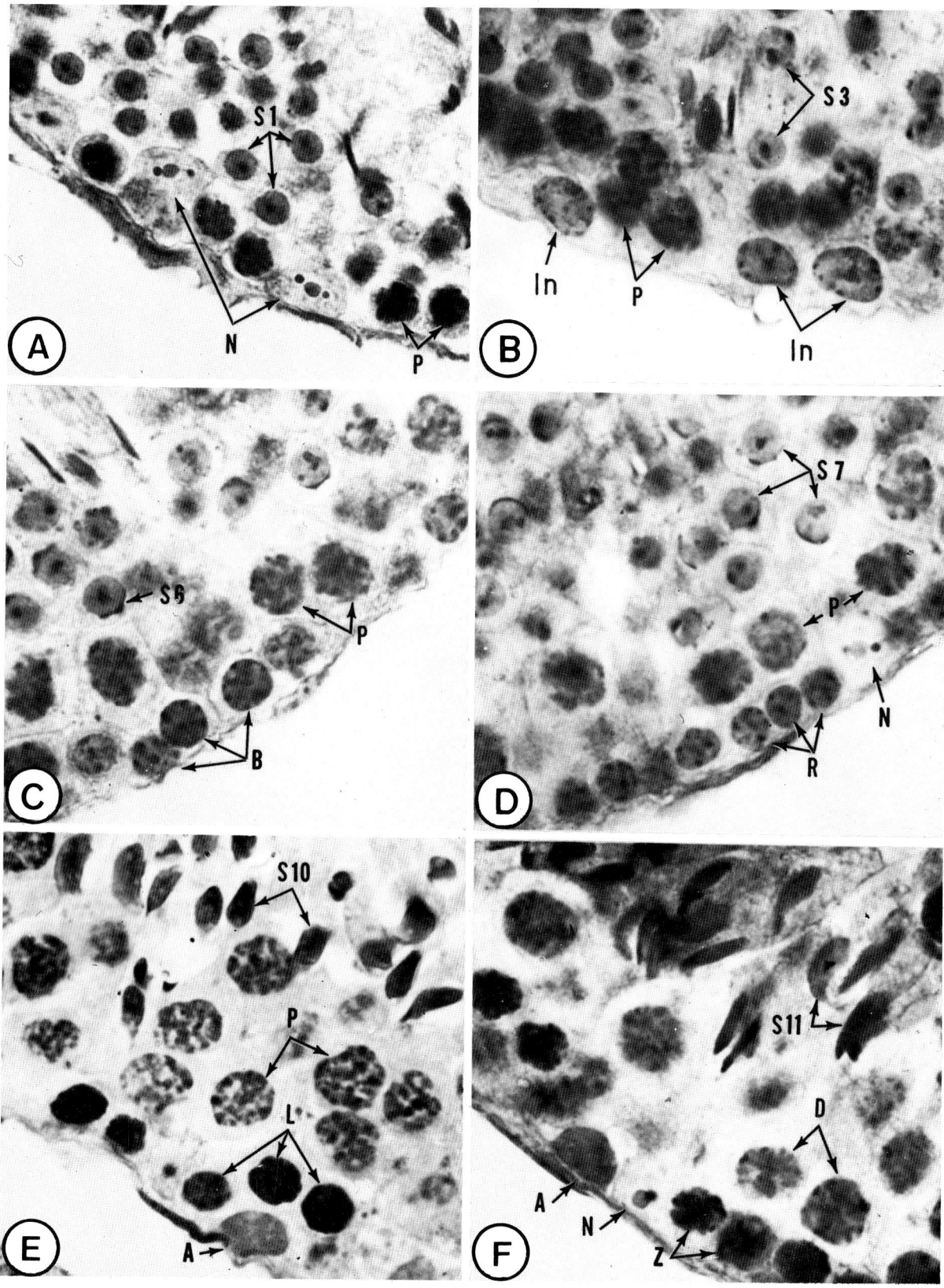

Spermatogenesis in the mouse (PAS & hematoxylin, x1,000). Cross sections of seminiferous tubules showing various phases of spermatogenesis **(A-F)**. The order of spermatogenesis is the following: Type A spermatogonia, lying at the base of the epithelium; **(A→)**, Type B spermatogonia, with a spherical nucleus containing condensed chromatin **(B→)**; and intermediate type spermatogonia **(In→)**. Primary spermatocytes in the various stages of prophase of the first meiotic division can be seen: leptotene **(L→)**, zygotene **(Z→)**, pachytene **(P→)** and diakinesis **(D→)**. **S1, S3, S6, S7, S10, S11** = spermatids in various stages of spermiogenesis. Next to the germ cells are Sertoli cells **(N→)**. By courtesy of V. Monesi. Riv. Istoch. Norm. Pat. 13:15, 1967.

Plate 6.7   **119**

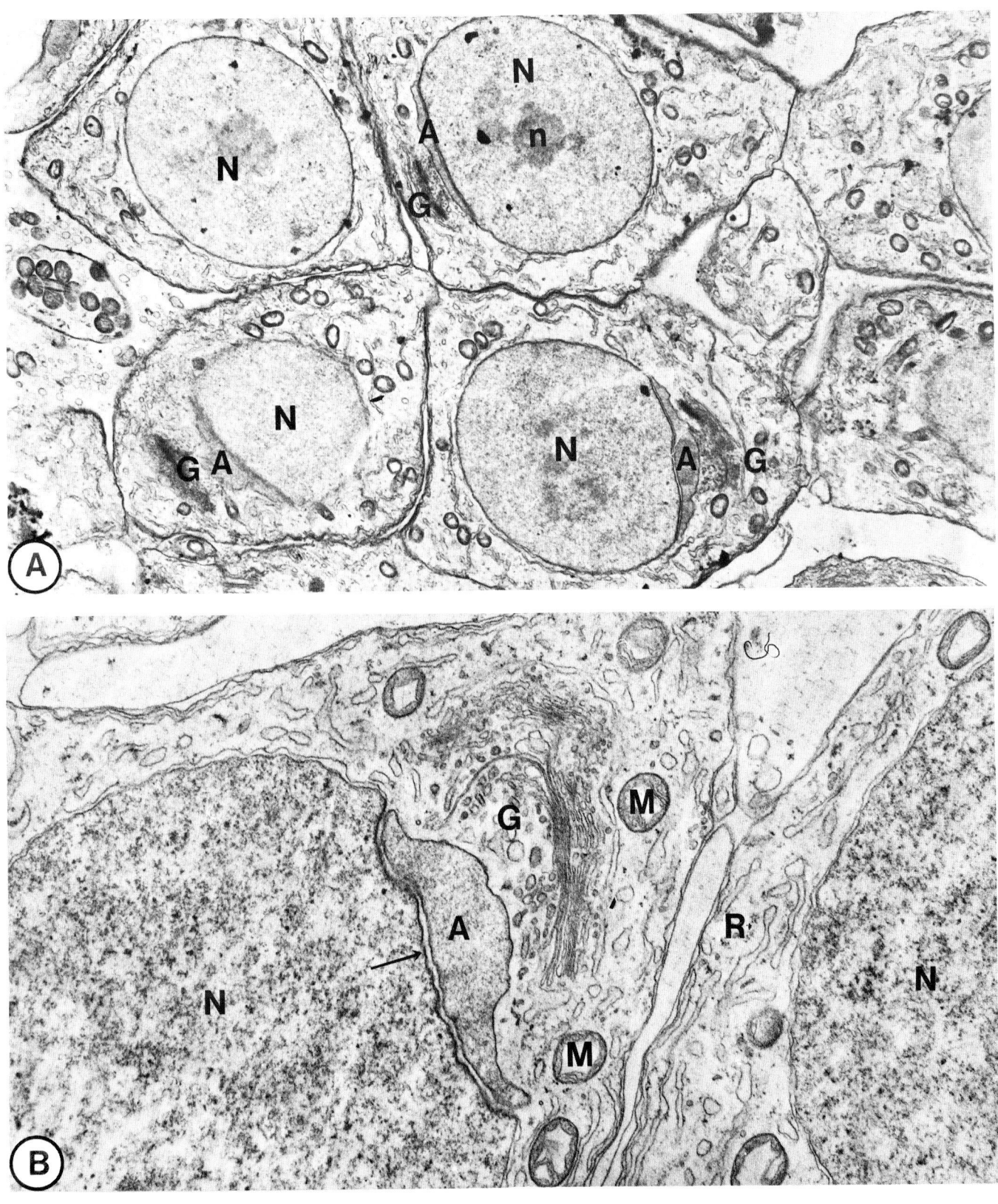

A   **Spermiogenesis in the mouse (EM, x4,500).** A convoluted seminiferous tubule shows within its wall a number of germinal cells (spermatids) which are closely related to one another. **N** = nucleus. **n** = nucleolus. **G** = Golgi complex in the process of giving rise to the acrosomal vesicle that is forming **(A)**.

B   **Spermiogenesis in the mouse: Golgi complex and acrosome (EM, x18,000).** In the nucleus of the spermatid **(N)** chromatin is dispersed. The Golgi complex **(G)** is forming the acrosomal vesicle **(A)**, which is beginning to associate with the future anterior head of the nucleus. The mitochondria **(M)**, now scattered about the cytoplasm, will congregate at the posterior pole of the nucleus to form a typical mitochondrial sheath. Right: detail of a secondary spermatid with abundant elements of the endoplasmic reticulum membranes **(R)**.

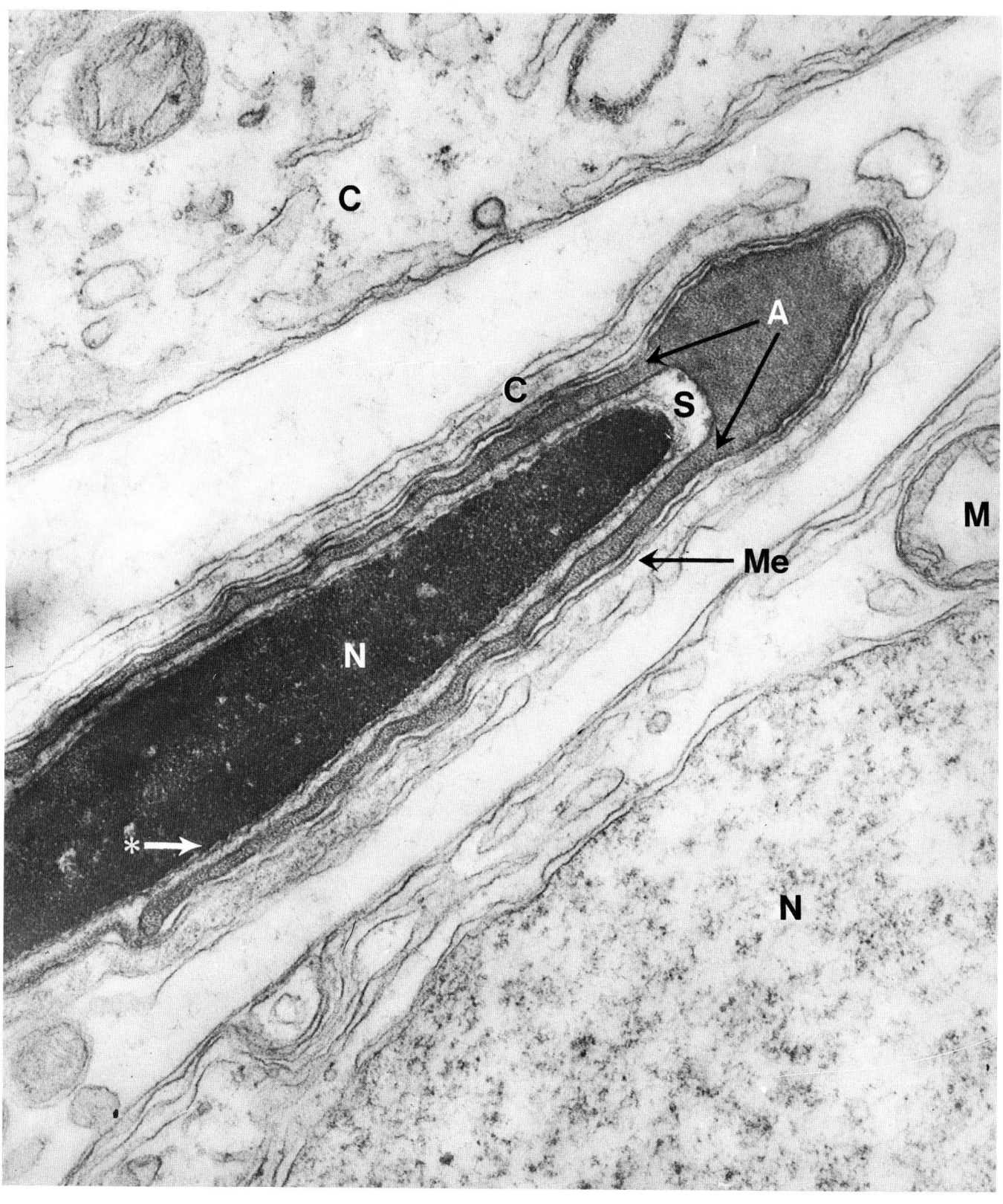

Spermiogenesis in the mouse: acrosome and nucleus (EM, x48,000). A spermatozoon now almost differentiated is seen in close association with a Sertoli cell. The head of the sperm is composed of a nucleus (white **N**) having highly condensed chromatin and a typical nuclear envelope (*→). The anterior region of the nucleus is covered with an acrosomal vesicle that contains dense material and envelops the tip (**S**) and much of the lateral nuclear surface (**A**→) like a cap. The plasma membrane of the sperm lies immediately outside the outer acrosomal membrane. The plasma membrane (**Me**→) lies next to the limiting membrane of the sperm. Areas of cytoplasm (**C**) from the Sertoli cells can be seen. Lower right: the nucleus (black **N**) and highly modified mitochondrion (**M**) of a spermatid.

Plate 6.9 121

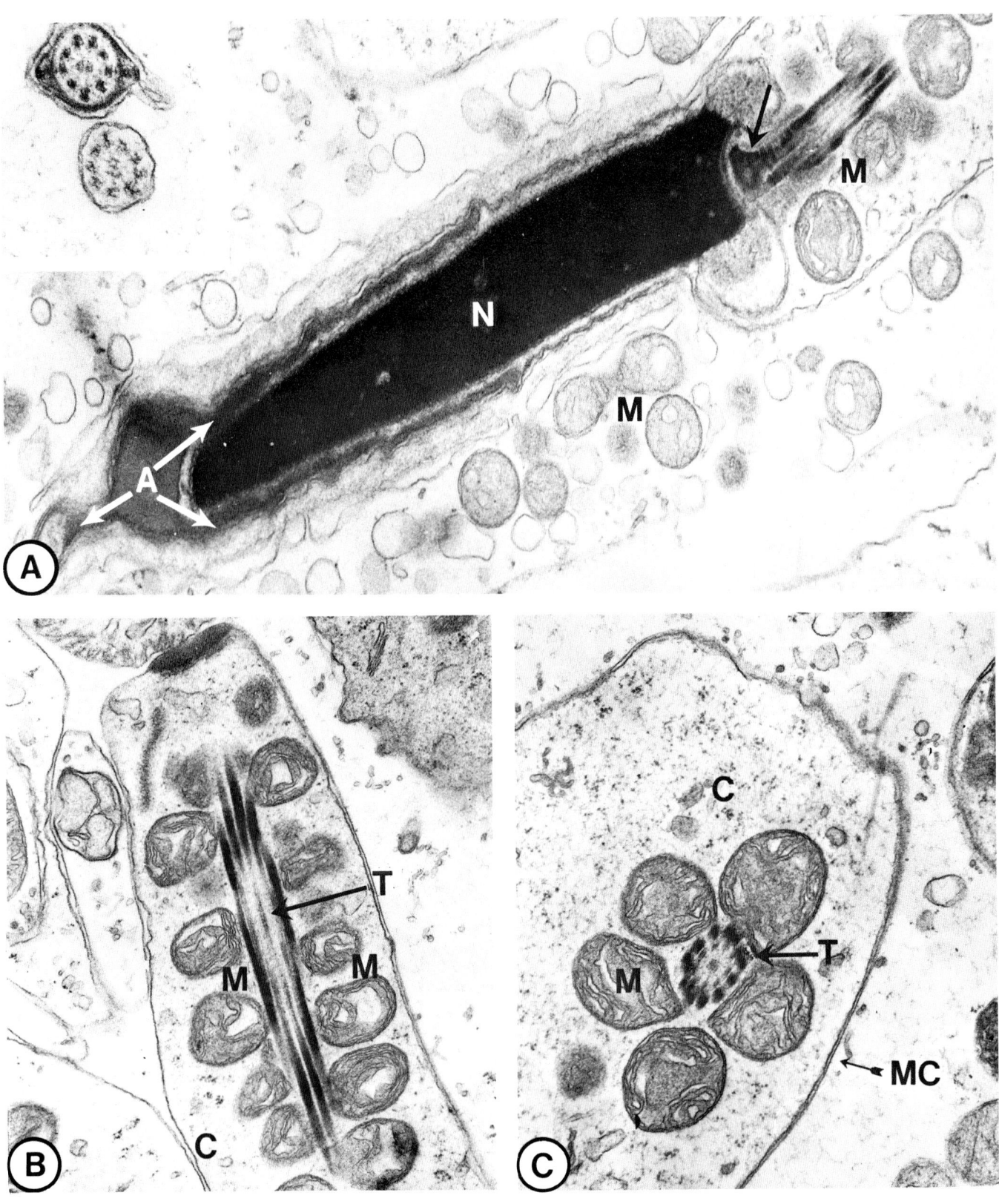

A **Mouse spermatid (EM, x40,000).** An almost completely mature spermatid (spermatozoon) surrounded by a Sertoli cell in which numerous mitochondria **(M)** can be seen. The head of the sperm is composed of the nucleus **(N)** covered with an acrosomal cap **(A→).** At the base of the head lies the connecting piece (→), where the axoneme is joined to one of the two centrioles. The flagellar structure is wrapped by a mitochondrial sheath **(M). Inset: two tails of spermatozoa in cross section.** The section is through the principle piece in one sperm (above), where the tail has a fibrous sheath, and through the end piece in the other sperm.

B **Longitudinal section of the middle piece of the flagellum of a mouse sperm (EM, x32,000).** The middle piece is visible. The axoneme, sectioned tangentially **(T→),** is covered with a sheath of mitochondria **(M)** and surrounded by a thin layer of cytoplasm **(C).**

C **Cross section of middle piece of flagellum of mouse sperm (EM, x38,000). (T→)** = axoneme. **M** = mitochondrial sheath. **C** = *cytoplasm.* **(MC)** = cell membrane.

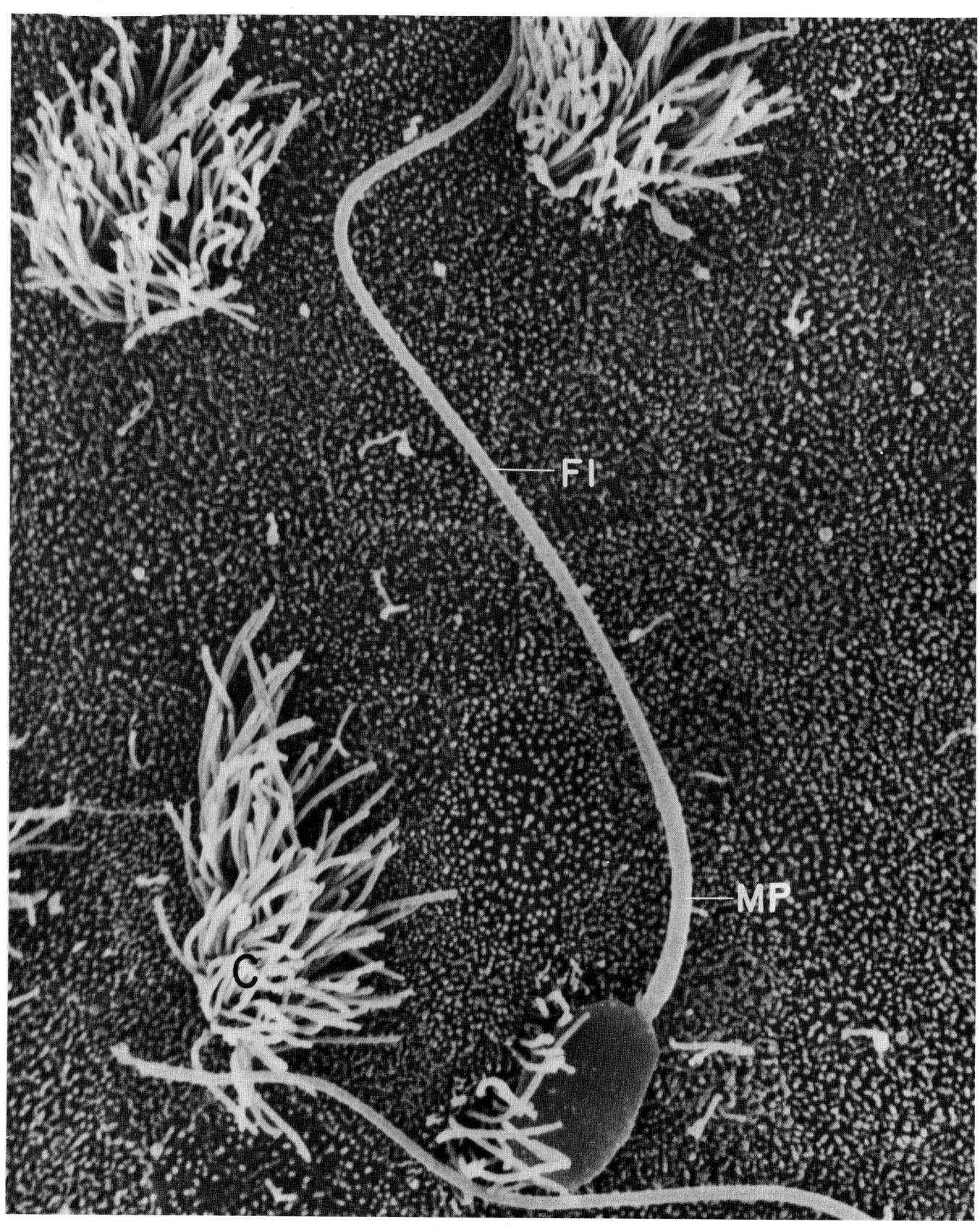

Rabbit spermatozoon (scanning EM, x4,500). The sperm is on the surface of the uterine mucosa, and its head is in contact with the cilia **(C)**. The proximal portion of the tail **(MP)** is thicker than the terminal portion because it contains a mitochondrial sheath. **Fl** = flagellum. From P.M. Motta and J. Van Blerkom. Cell Tiss. Res. 163:29, 1975.

Plate 6.11   **123**

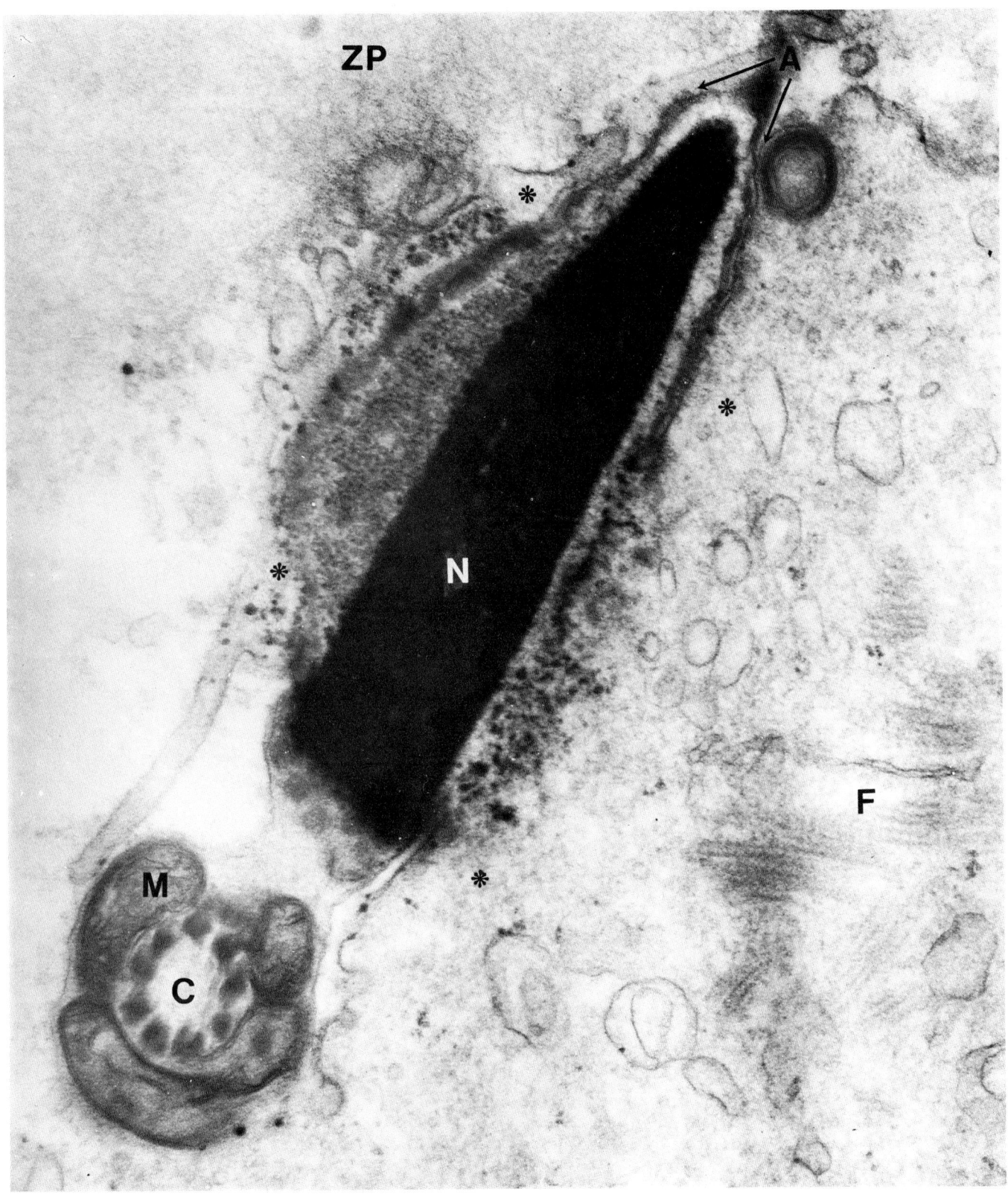

Penetration of spermatozoon into a mouse oocyte (EM, x44,500). The section has been taken tangentially, behind the acrosome of the sperm head at the moment of fertilization. The membranes of the two gametes are dissolving at the lateral surfaces of the sperm head (*). (A→) = acrosomal cap. **N** = nucleus of spermatozoon. **C** = axoneme. **M** = mitochondria of sperm flagellum. **F** = spindle fibers in the cytoplasm of the egg. **ZP** = fragment of zona pellucida. By courtesy of M. Stefanini, C. Oura and L. Zamboni. J. Submicr. Cytol. 1:1, 1969.

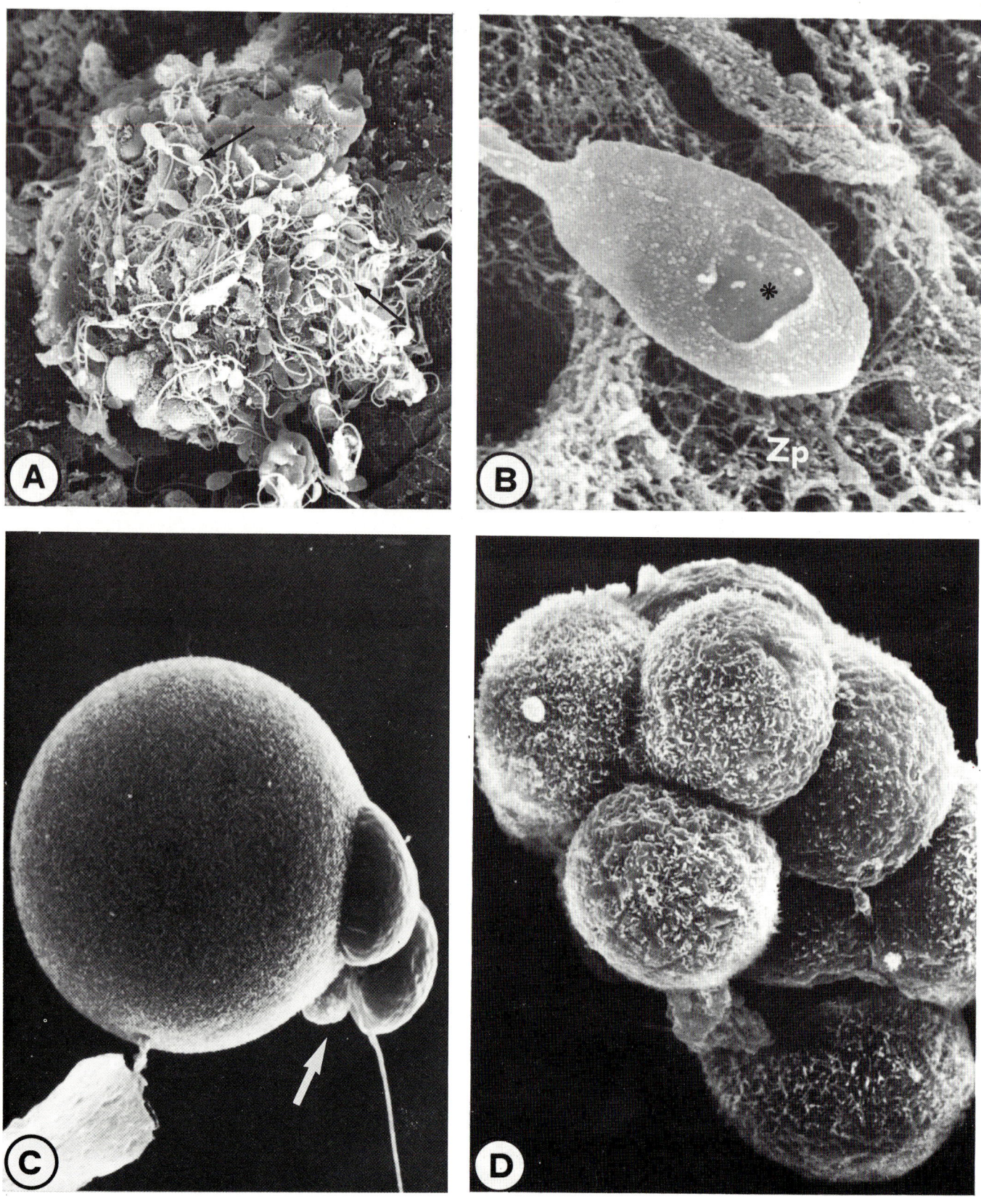

A **Fertilization of an oocyte in the oviduct of a rabbit (scanning EM, x1,800).** The mass visible in the picture contains an ovum still surrounded by the zona pellucida and by follicle cells of the corona radiata with which numerous spermatozoa (→) are associated. From P.M. Motta and J. Van Blerkom. *Amer. J. Anat.* 143:241, 1975.

B **Rabbit sperm in contact with the zona pellucida during fertilization (scanning EM, x10,200).** The head of the sperm (*) can be seen. The underlying amorphous material is partially digested zona pellucida **(Zp)**.

C **Fertilized egg of mouse embryo (scanning EM, x2,000).** The zona pellucida has been removed by enzymatic digestion in order to reveal the surface of the egg, which is covered by small microvilli covering the surface of the blastomeres. The three polar bodies and the tail of the sperm can be seen (arrow). By courtesy of G. Siracusa and M. De Felici.

D **Morula of a mouse (scanning EM, x3,100).** The blastomeres are still covered with numerous microvilli except for the areas of contact between the cells. From J. Van Blerkom and P.M. Motta. *The Cellular Basis of Mammalian Reproduction.* Urban & Schwarzenberg, Munich/Baltimore, 1979.

Plate 6.13   125

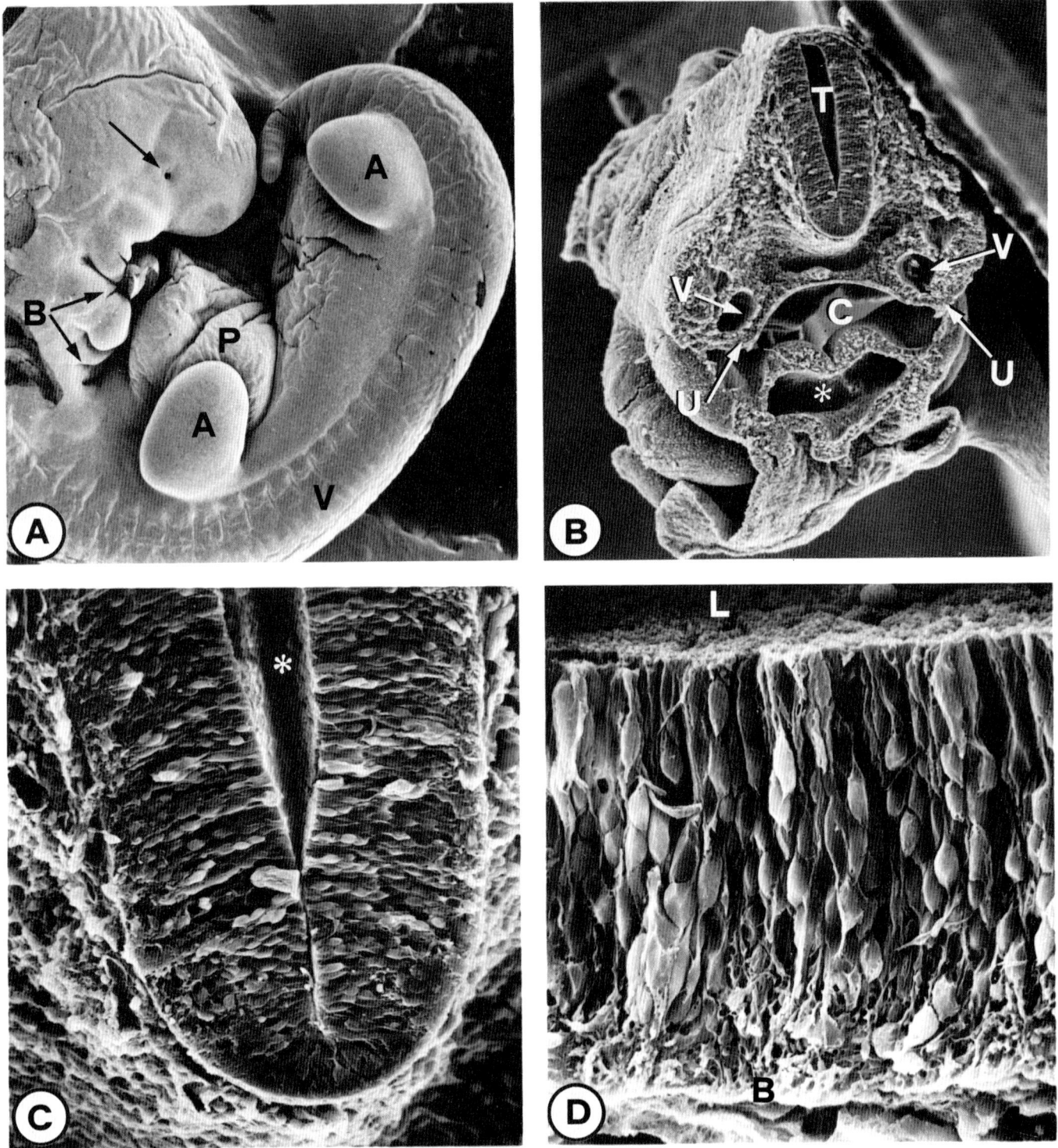

A **Human embryo at five weeks of gestation (scanning EM, x150).** At this stage are visible the buds of the upper and lower limbs (**A**), the somites (**V**), the pericardium (**P**). The head with the optic vesicle (→) and the branchial arches (**B**→) are prominent.

B **Human embryo at the end of the fifth week of gestation (scanning EM, x190).** Cross section through the developing heart. The neural tube (**T**), the cardinal veins (**V**), the urogenital ridge (**U**) and the midgut united to the yolk sac (*) can be seen.

C **Neural tube of a human embryo at five weeks of gestation (scanning EM, x380).** Several layers of proliferating neuroblasts, which line the wall of the canal (*), can be seen.

D **Wall of the neural tube of human embryo at five weeks of gestation (scanning EM, x720).** From the base (**B**) towards the lumen of the canal (**L**) the neuroblasts arranged in layers are proliferating and differentiating. The cells nearest to the lumen will become ependymal cells. By courtesy of S. Makabe.

PART THREE

MULTI-TISSUE STRUCTURES AND THE ORGANS

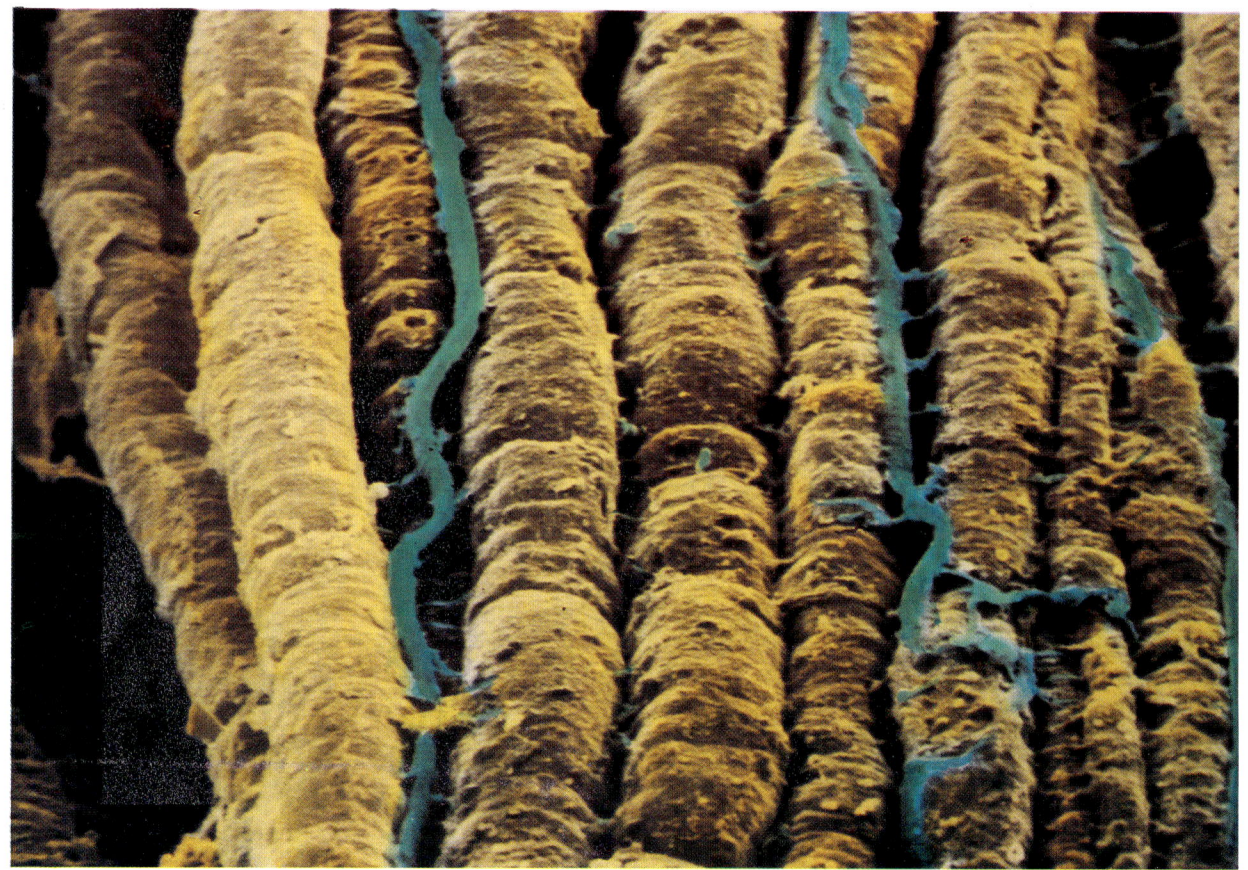

Bundle of nerve fibers with associated blood vessels (blue) running parallel. (Rat. Colored SEM; 1,630 x).

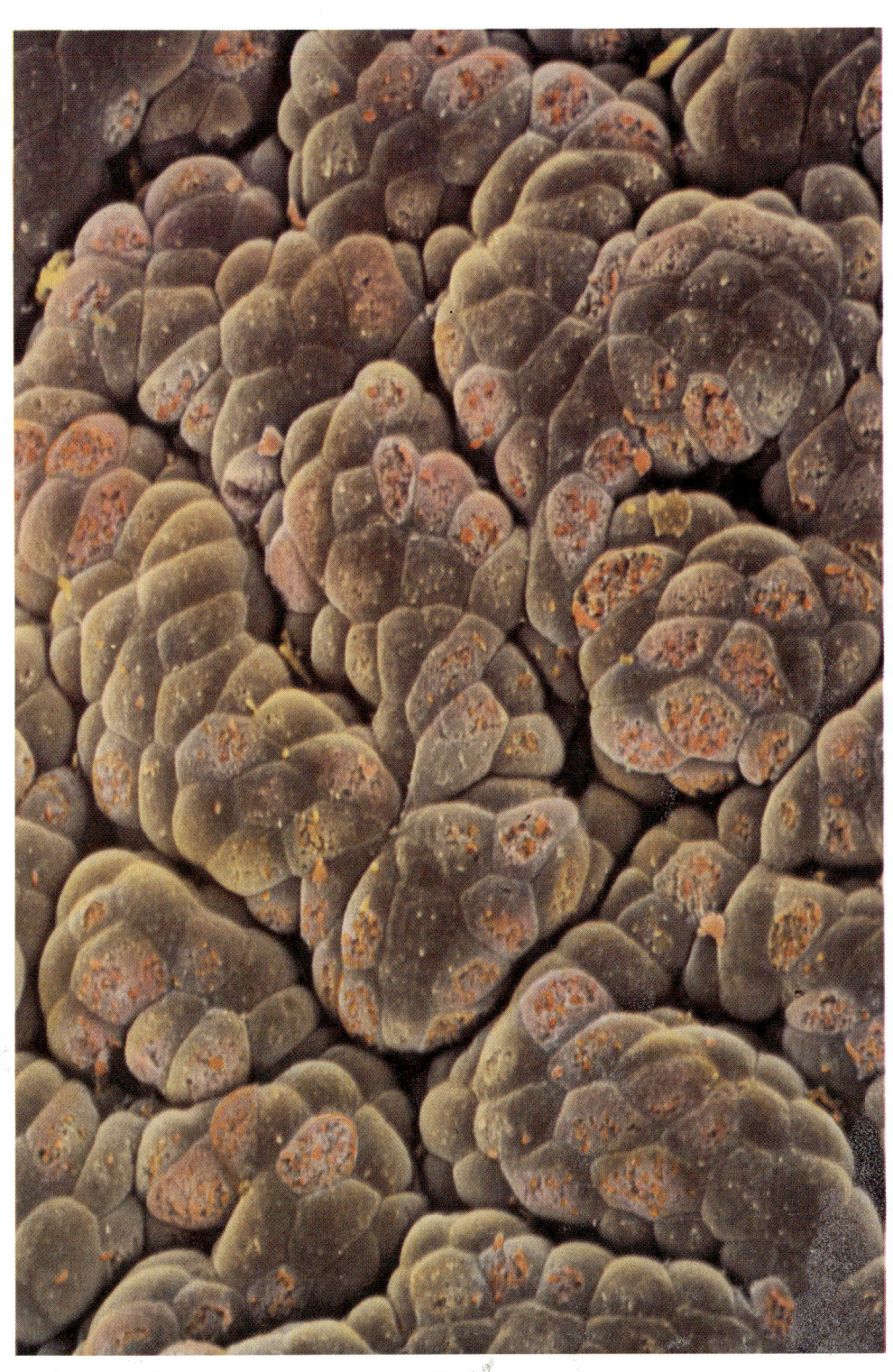

Pancreas: an overview of glandular acini in a rat. (Colored SEM; 1,100 x).

MULTI-TISSUE STRUCTURES

The term "multi-tissue structure" is defined as the association of two or more tissues in which one of the tissues generally predominates both quantitatively and functionally over the other(s) and is responsible for the specific activity that characterizes the structure (Fumagalli). The associated tissue(s) aids the primary tissue by contributing in some specific way to the primary function.

Skin, mucosa and serosa

Multi-tissue structures whose primary function is to provide a covering epithelium are the *skin,* which covers the outside surface of the body, *mucous membranes,* which cover the internal surfaces of hollow organs that communicate with the exterior, and *serous membranes,* which cover the internal surfaces of the walls of body cavities that do not communicate with the outside. The latter cover the outer surface of the organs residing in these cavities.

Skin and hair

The skin (see diagram) covers the entire body surface externally and merges into the mucosa in natural orifices. The skin is divided into two superimposed layers of which one, the *epidermis,* is epithelium and that under it, the *dermis,* is connective tissue. The two layers are separated by a basal lamina. Below the dermis lies the hypodermis (Plates 7.1 A, 7.4 A).

The epidermis is a covering epithelium of the stratified squamous keratinized type in which, according to the location of the skin, various layers can be distinguished. Among these layers are the basal layer (*stratum germinativum*) and a superficial layer (*stratum corneum*). The latter is formed of flattened cells that are completely keratinized and lacking a nucleus. These scalelike cells slough off (*stratum disjunctum of the epidermis*). In certain areas of the skin that are subject to abrasion there is, below the stratum corneum, the *stratum lucidum.* The next deeper layer is the *stratum granulosum.* Overlying the cuboidal cells that make up the stratum germinativum (or *stratum basale*) lie several layers of cells firmly attached to one another by numerous desmosomes (*stratum spinosum*) (Plates 7.2 A, 7.4 A,B).

The dermis is a layer formed of fibrous connective tissue with a thickness varying from 0.2 to 0.3 mm. It is made up of a subepithelial layer having projecting ridges (*dermal papillae*) in the boundary zone with the epithelium, as well as a deeper layer. Below the dermis is the hypodermis of connective tissue that connects the dermis to the muscle fascia and periosteum. Its construction varies according to the location of the skin. Usually it contains groups of adipose or fat cells (Plate 7.4 A,B).

Special skin appendages are derived from the epidermis. Examples are hairs, nails and various glands (sebaceous, sweat and mammary glands).

Hair is composed of a portion that projects from the skin surface (*hair shaft*) and another region embedded obliquely in the skin (*hair root*) and wrapped in a *hair follicle.* The part beneath the skin surface is contained in a deep goblet-shaped invagination of the epidermis that extends into the hypodermis. In cross section the hair shaft is circular or oval. The root, which is implanted in the follicle, swells at the end into a cup-shaped bulb. The bulb contains material derived from the connective tissue sheath of the follicle, the *papilla* (Plates 7.1, 7.2 B, 7.4 A,C). Sebaceous glands and small smooth muscle cells (*erector pili*) are appendages of the follicle.

The cells of the hair proper are modified epidermal epithelium. In cross section the constituent epithelium of the hair is present in three layers. The inner layer, not always present, is the *medulla;* the middle, principal layer is the *cortex;* the surface layer, which is the thinnest, is the *cuticle.* In the hair root these layers are less distinct. The hair is covered also with a sheath of epithelium in three layers, which are (from the inside) the *root sheath cuticle, Huxley's layer* and

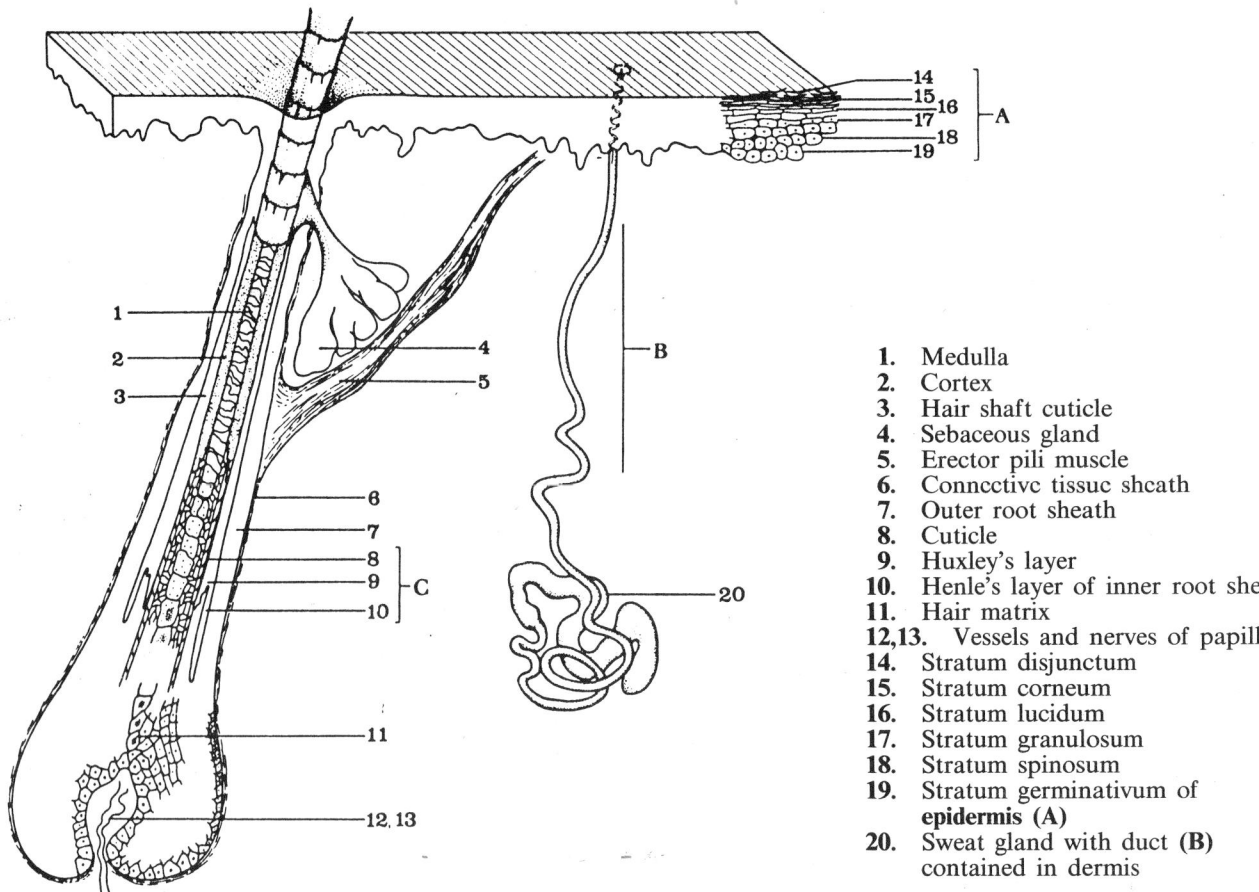

1.   Medulla
2.   Cortex
3.   Hair shaft cuticle
4.   Sebaceous gland
5.   Erector pili muscle
6.   Connective tissue sheath
7.   Outer root sheath
8.   Cuticle
9.   Huxley's layer
10. Henle's layer of inner root sheath
11. Hair matrix
12,13. Vessels and nerves of papilla
14. Stratum disjunctum
15. Stratum corneum
16. Stratum lucidum
17. Stratum granulosum
18. Stratum spinosum
19. Stratum germinativum of **epidermis (A)**
20. Sweat gland with duct **(B)** contained in dermis

Diagram of skin and hair follicle

Henle's layer. The outer root sheath of the follicle is in turn wrapped by a basal lamina (*glassy membrane*) to which is attached a sheath of connective tissue, the surface of which has the erector pili muscle deeply embedded in it (Plates 7.1, 7.3 B). Around the bulb the epithelial cells are undifferentiated and proliferate continually in order to ensure hair growth.

The *sebaceous glands* are always associated with a hair follicle. The lining of these glands is derived from the epidermis, which grows down around the hair follicle as the outer root sheath (Plate 7.3 B). The secretion of these glands is described as holocrine and results from the periodic shedding of certain gland cells whose cytoplasm is filled with fatty secretion droplets. The glandular epithelum rests on a basal lamina wrapped in connective tissue.

The *sweat glands* are appendages that are distributed almost throughout the skin. They are coiled tubular glands classified according to their mode of secretion into *apocrine sweat glands* and *eccrine sweat glands* (Plates 7.3 A, 7.5 C). The secretory part of these glands is located at the junction of the dermis and hypodermis. It is a series of convolutions, with a coiled secretory part and a straight duct passing up through the dermis into the epidermis. The orifice by which these glands open onto the outside of the skin surface is called a sweat pore. The secretory portion of the gland is made up of cuboidal stratified epithelium.

The *mammary glands* are formed from 12-20 distinct gland structures, each having a secretory duct. These are glands of the alveolar type, having an apocrine secretion mechanism (Plates 7.3 C,D; 7.5 A,B). Each gland opens at the tip of the nipple by means of a lactiferous duct leading from a saclike dilation (*sinus lactiferous*). At the nipple the lactiferous ducts are supported by elastic connective tissue reinforced by smooth muscle cells. Near its opening the duct is lined by a non-keratinized stratified squamous epithelium. In the lactiferous sinus it is lined by a stratified cuboidal epithelium, which becomes a single layer of columnar or cuboidal cells throughout the remainder of the duct system.

During pregnancy the parenchyma of the

glands increases, and the lactiferous ducts take the form of numerous solid epithelial buds which originate by proliferating from the lateral branches of the ducts. The solid buds then become alveoli lined by cuboidal epithelium and having a stratum basale of myoepithelial basket cells. Preparation for the secretory process begun in pregnancy reaches its peak during lactation (Plates 7.3 D, 7.5 A,B).

Mucous membranes

Three superimposed laminae form the mucous membranes. These vary in thickness according to location and consist of *epithelium, basal lamina* and *lamina propria.* Beneath the basal lamina is a connective tissue layer reinforced by reticular fibers. The lamina propria is a connective tissue layer with a plexiform pattern of interwoven fibers. Lymphoid cells can aggregate in this layer to form *lymphoid nodules.* Various types of glands also occur in this layer, as well as thin networks of nerves, blood vessels and lymph vessels (Plate 7.7 A,C). Some mucosae have a thin layer of smooth muscle cells (*muscularis mucosae*) at the junction with the submucosa layer (see also chapter 8).

Serous membranes

The serous membranes are composed of simple squamous epithelium resting on a basal lamina. Beneath the basal lamina is the tunica serosa, which generally is thin and is made up of laminar connective tissue (Plate 7.7 B). Serous membranes include the *peritoneum,* the *pleura* and the *pericardium.*

GLANDS

Glands are multi-tissue structures whose primary function is performed by secretory epithelium. Glands contain a lining epithelium, connective tissue, vessels and nerves (Plate 7.6). Certain glands secrete products to the skin or to the surface of the mucosae via ducts (*exocrine glands*). Glands can also be ductless and secrete their products (*hormones*) directly into the lumen of the blood vessels (*endocrine glands*). Specific glands are described in Chapter 8.

Exocrine glands

Exocrine glands originate in the epithelium covering the skin or mucosa and are always connected to the surface by a secretory duct. Exocrine glands can be classified according to their position relative to the internal part of the body, whether *intraparietal (intraepithelial, intrachorial* and *submucosal)* or *extraparietal.* These glands can also be classified according to the number of cells that make up the gland, and thus can be either *unicellular (goblet cells)* or *multicellular glands.* The shape of the secretory unit also can be used as a criterion for classification, in which the gland is considered *alveolar* if the cavity of the adenomere is spherical, *tubular* if the outer shape and the cavity are cylindrical, or *acinar* if the adenomere is spherical and its cavity cylindrical. Exocrine glands also can be grouped according to the type and degree of branching of the duct, in which case the glands are *simple, compound or ramified* exocrine glands. A final type of classification is based on the nature of the secretory product. *Serous, mucous* or *mixed* exocrine glands are those in which the product contains an enzyme, a mucopolysaccharide, or both, respectively.

Endocrine glands

Endocrine glands produce hormones and, being without ducts, discharge the hormone into the vascular system. These glands can exist separately (e.g., pituitary, pineal, thyroid, parathyroid, adrenal glands) or can be found in association with other organs (e.g., islets of Langerhans in the pancreas, interstitial cells in the testis or ovary, corpus luteum, endocrine cells in the digestive tract). These glands have an abundance of blood vessels and capillaries which are often sinusoidal and are associated directly with the secretory cells. Based on the distribution of cells in the glands, endocrine glands can be divided into four groups: 1) *follicular endocrine glands* (e.g., the thyroid gland), 2) *endocrine glands with cords* (e.g., the adrenal gland), 3) *interstitial endocrine glands* (e.g., Leydig cells in the testis), and 4) *unicellular endocrine glands* (e.g., scattered endocrine cells in the alimentary canal).

Bone

Bones making up the skeleton are multi-tissue structures whose primary function is performed by specialized connective tissue, the bone (Plate 7.8). These bones consist of 1) bone tissue,

2) periosteum (and in long bones endosteum), 3) articular cartilage, 4) epiphyseal cartilage, found in developing long bones, 5) loose connective tissue, which pervades the bone cavities and contains nerves and blood vessels, and 6) bone marrow contained in the cavities of bone.

Bone tissue (see chapter 3).

Periosteum and endosteum are membranous fibrous connective tissue covering all bones and lining marrow spaces. They contain an abundant supply of blood vessels, nerves and nerve endings. They act as the connective substratum from which bone tissue originates. After a fracture the periosteum and endosteum form the bone callus, the periosteum making the outer and the endosteum the inner callus. Lymph vessels terminate at the periosteum and do not penetrate the bone tissue.

Articular cartilage is a hyaline cartilage found on the surfaces of bones making up the area of the joint that functions in articulation. This cartilage is characterized by mechanical resistance, elasticity and a smooth surface, features that are necessary for the contact areas of the joint to slide smoothly against each other.

Epiphyseal cartilage is a platelike region between the epiphysis and the diaphysis of long bones and some short bones. It is found only in bones that are developing. When the bone has reached its full length and growth ceases, the plate disappears. The epiphysis increases in width as a result of the proliferation of the cartilage cells (*chondroblasts*), which face the marrow cavity. These cells continually produce intercellular matrix and differentiate into *chondrocytes.*

Four areas can be distinguished in the epiphyseal plate. These correspond to the different stages of development of the cartilage cells. They are (progressing from the epiphysis toward the marrow cavity) A) *germinal cartilage,* with a structure similar to the hyaline cartilage already described. It lies at the place where the epiphysis merges into the epiphyseal plate. B) *proliferating cartilage,* in which the flattened cells are arranged in columns and are stacked parallel to the long axis of the bone. These cells frequently divide. C) The *area of hypertrophied cartilage,* where glycogen and lipid droplets appear in the cytoplasm. Between the cells the matrix becomes partially calcified and forms trabeculae between the columns of cells. These intercellular networks are

mainly longitudinal but have transverse connections. D) The *area of calcified cartilage matrix and associated spicules of bone,* or *metaphysis.* The penetration of the cartilage by blood vessels leads to the disappearance of the chondroblasts. The spicules of matrix remain and calcify. In the part of the metaphysis near the ossified diaphysis the cartilage matrix begins to disappear, but parts remain for a time to form a scaffolding over which bone is laid down.

Bone is continually renewed by means of a coordinated process of destruction and reconstruction (bone remodeling). The resorption of bone is caused by special multinuclear cells with an osteolytic function (*osteoclasts*), which are contained in relatively large cuplike depressions (*Howship's lacunae*). The appearance of new bone tissue depends on the osteogenic action of the endosteum and periosteum. This continual process of osteolysis and osteogenesis has the further effect of liberating calcium ions. These ions can then move freely from bone to blood, where their concentration is maintained at constant levels.

Blood vessels and *nerves* are widespread within the bone. Nerve endings are especially abundant in the periosteum. Nutrition of long bones is ensured by a nutritive vessel which enters the bone at right angles through the nutritive aperture and branches into a rich capillary network. Branches of the vessel passes through the Haversian canals and the bone marrow.

Bone marrow is a soft connective tissue rich in blood vessels. It is contained in certain bone cavities (in the diaphysis of long bones and spaces in spongy bone) where its function is the production of blood cells (hemopoiesis). In the marrow are found the precursors of all the circulating blood cells and the platelets. In young bones, where hemopoiesis is intense and red blood cells abound, the marrow has a bright red color (*red marrow*). With age the blood-forming activity diminishes and many adipose cells develop, so that the marrow becomes yellowish in color and gelatinous in consistency (*yellow marrow*).

Nerve

The anatomical nerve is a multi-tissue structure whose primary function is performed by nerve tissue. A nerve is made up of a bundle of nerve fibers ensheathed in connective tissue which contains arterial, venous and lymphatic vessels (*vasa nervorum*) and nerve endings (*nerva nervorum*).

The *nerve fibers* or *nerve processes* are wrapped by a special sheath (*axon sheath or myelin sheath*) formed of membranes of *Schwann cells*. The large nerve fibers (also called the neurite) contain a highly viscous cytoplasm rich in mitochondria and neurofibrils. The myelin sheath is composed of cell membranes of Schwann cells wrapped concentrically around the nerve process and in direct contact with it. Schwann cells and the myelin sheath together surround large nerve fibers except at their distal ends (Plates 7.9, 7.10, 7.12, 7.14 A).

The myelin sheath is interrupted at regular intervals by characteristic constrictions (*nodes of Ranvier*). A Schwann cell and its myelin sheath wrap each internode region, and in the internodal region where there is no myelin sheath the layers of peripheral Schwann cell cytoplasm interdigitate. The number of nodes along the length of a determined fiber is constant. Sometimes in the region of nerve fiber between two nodes of Ranvier the Schwann cell cytoplasm remains between the two membranes of the sheath, apparently breaking the continuity of the sheath (the *Schmidt-Lanterman clefts*).

In the case of nerves of small diameter the Schwann cell envelops many nerve processes. Here the nerve fibers do not have a true myelin sheath, and so are called unmyelinated nerve fibers (Plates 7.9 C, 7.14 A).

The outer surface of the Schwann cell is covered by a basal lamina into which are anchored reticular fibers (*neurilemma*).

Within the nerve each fiber is separated from the other by a supporting connecting tissue (*endoneurium*). Small bundles (fascicles) of several fibers, together with their surrounding endoneurium, are in turn bound together by a connective sheath called the *perineurium;* these bundles are in turn wrapped in an outer sheath of connective tissue called the *epineurium.*

In motor nerve fibers the endoneurium (here shown as the *sheath of Key & Retzius,* or *Plenk's subsidiary sheath)* is very thin. In sensory fibers the endoneurium thickens considerably and is known as *Ruffini's subsidiary sheath.* By analogy the perineurium of fibers that reach their target organ individually can form a rather thick covering (*Henle's perineural sheath*).

Every nerve fiber, just before reaching the point where it makes functional contact with a gland or a muscle, loses its myelin sheath and immediately subdivides, branching into a large number of dilated, bulbous endings. The endings of nerves in the central nervous system are in functional contact with other neurons at the synapse (see Nerve Tissue, Chapter 5).

The endings of nerve fibers differ according to the cells with which the nerve ending comes into contact. At the periphery the specialized endings may be sensory or motor (Plates 7.ll, 7.13, 7.14, 7.15).

Afferent nerve endings

Afferent nerve endings include naked nerve endings within epithelium and connective tissue. These endings have a variety of morphological characteristics and may have accessory cells associated with them. Specialized sensory endings include the *taste buds* of the tongue (nerve endings and taste cells), the *cristae of the membranous labyrinth* (ampulla sensory cells and nerve fibers), *static maculae of the membranous labyrinth* (sense cells of the utricle and saccule relating to nerve fibers), *spiral organ of Corti* (acoustic sense cells and nerve fibers (Plates 2.6, 2.7).

Complex accessory nerve endings also occur in connective tissue. Here the nerve endings usually are wrapped in connective lamina resembling a capsule. There exist several different types of these so-called corpuscles in connective tissue, and each has a specialized function. Among these are the *Vater-Pacini (Pacinian) corpuscles,* with a straight nerve fiber at its center and an envelope of connective tissue (Plates 7.11, 7.13). *End bulbs of Krause* are smaller than Pacinian corpuscles, with a spheroidal morphology. Structures intermediate between the end bulb of Krause and the Pacinian corpuscle are the *Golgi-Mazzoni corpuscles, genital nerve corpuscles* and *Herbst's corpuscles* (Plates 7.11, 7.13). Meissner's corpuscles have an oval capsule containing flattened Schwann cells and an internerve fiber that ramifies and forms a series of spirals. The terminal arborization of the nerve fiber within the corpuscle extends from the end of the spiral (Plate 7.ll). Dogiel's and *Grandi's corpuscles* resemble Meissner's corpuscles. The *Ruffinian corpuscle* is spindle-shaped and has a supporting capsule of connective tissue rich in elastic fibers. A reticulate

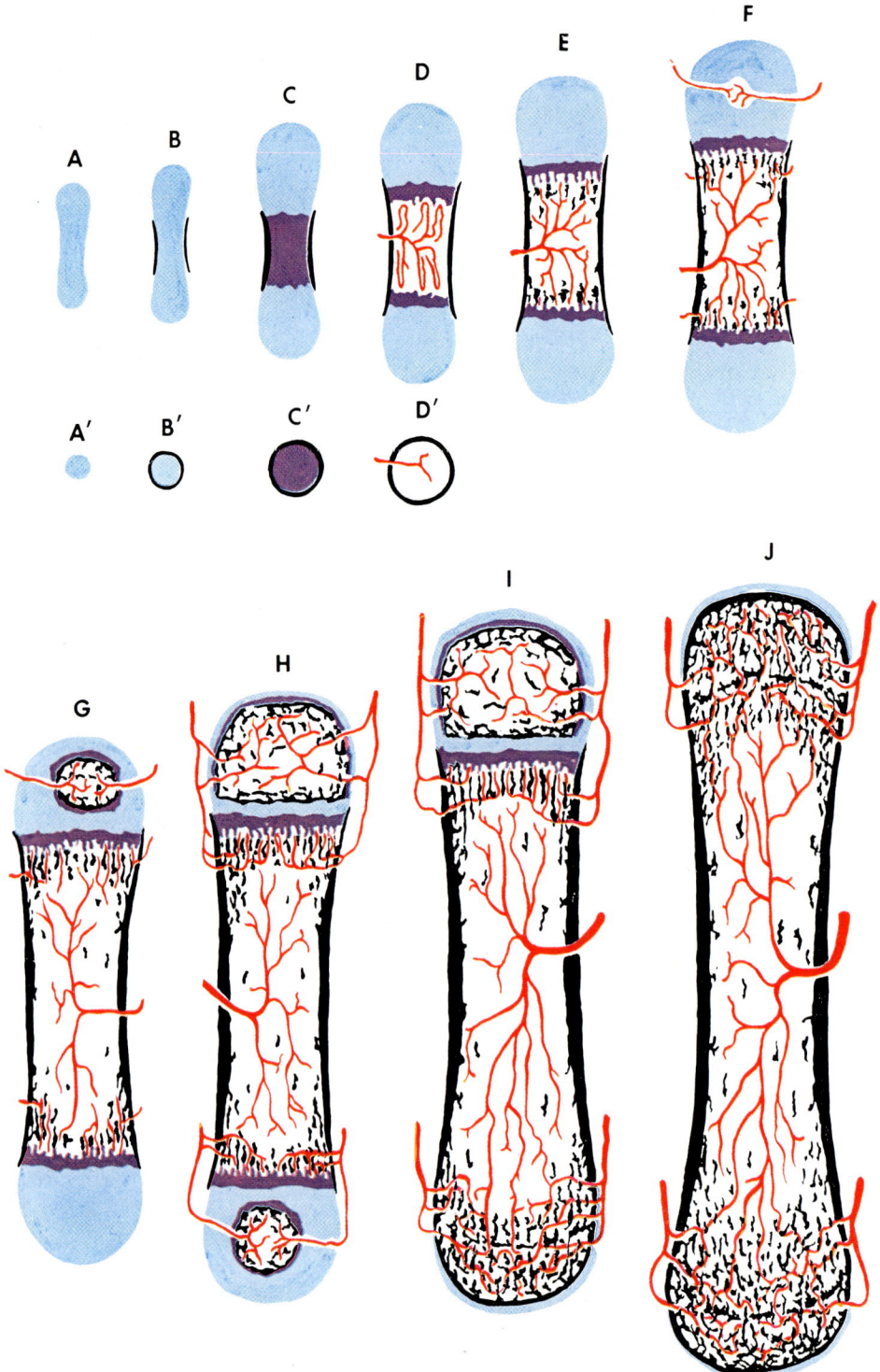

Diagram of the development of long bone. *A-J* are longitudinal sections; *A',B',C',D'* are cross sections of *A,B,C,D* taken at mid-diaphysis. Light blue = cartilage. Violet = calcified cartilage. Black = bone. Red = arteries. *A,* cartilage model; *B,* formation of the periosteal bone collar before calcification of the cartilage; *C,* early calcification of cartilage; *D,* penetration of vascular mesenchyme into the matrix of calcified cartilage, dividing it into two zones of ossification *(E); F,* penetration of blood vessels and mesenchyme into the epiphyseal cartilage (upper portion of figure) where the epiphyseal ossification center develops *(G); H,* a similar ossification center developing in the lower epiphyseal cartilage; *I,* disappearance of the lower epiphyseal disk when the bone ceases to grow in length, followed by disappearance of the upper epiphyseal disk *(J).* The marrow cavity then extends throughout the length of the bone, and the blood vessels of the diaphysis, metaphysis and epiphysis unite. By courtesy of D.W. Fawcett. In: W. Bloom and D.W. Fawcett. A Textbook of Histology. 10th ed. W.B. Saunders Co. Philadelphia, Toronto and London, 1975.

nerve ending is contained within the spindle.

Corpuscular nerve endings can also be found within muscle tissue. Muscle spindles are of this type. They are elongated structures enclosed by a capsule that has within it groups of specialized striated muscle fibers and abundant nerve endings.

Golgi's musculo-tendinous organs are spindle-shaped corpuscles parallel to the long axis of the muscle with one end fixed to the muscle fiber and the other to the tendon.

Efferent nerve endings

Efferent nerve endings include the nerve endings of secretory cells in glands (*cytoneural junctions*), smooth muscle (*myoneural junctions*) and striated muscle fibers (*motor end plates*) (Plates 7.14 A, 7.15).

Blood and lymph vessels

Blood and lymph vessels are a multi-tissue structure whose primary function is performed by connective tissue. Blood vessels are composed of arteries, veins, capillaries and sinusoids.

Arteries

Arteries are tubes in which the blood flows from the heart towards a capillary network. These vessels have two basic properties, elasticity and contractility. Both of these properties are found in various degrees in the different types of artery. There are always three layers in arterial vessels, regardless of diameter. These are the internal layer or *tunica intima,* the middle layer or *tunica media, and the external layer* or *tunica adventitia.* It is the diameter of the vessel that determines variation in the structure of these layers (Plate 7.16).

Large arteries (elastic type) have a diameter exceeding 7 mm. The tunica intima comprises an endothelial layer and a subendothelial layer made of thin elastic and collagen fibers. The tunica media is rich in smooth muscle cells, between which can be seen many layers of elastic connective tissue. The tunica adventitia consists of spirally arranged layers of collagenous connective tissue. Between the tunica intima and the tunica media is an *internal elastic membrane* made up of a web of elastic fibers oriented both longitudinally and circumferentially. The tunica media is

demarcated from the tunica adventitia by an *external elastic membrane,* which is also a layer of elastic fibers.

Medium-sized arteries (muscular type) are vessels with a diameter of 3-7 mm. Their tunica intima comprises an endothelial layer and a thin subendothelium rich in elastic and reticular fibers. The tunica media is composed of layers of smooth muscle cells separated by layers of elastic fibers. The tunica adventitia is more prominent than in large arteries. There is an internal elastic membrane between the tunica intima and the tunica media, with an external elastic membrane between the tunica media and tunica adventitia.

Small arteries (muscular type) are vessels with a diameter of less than 3 mm. They have a tunica intima consisting of the endothelium only and rest on an internal elastic lamina which is so folded that the endothelial cells seem almost to project into the lumen of the vessel. The tunica media is constituted wholly of smooth muscle cells. The tunica adventitia is composed primarily of collagen fibers and elastic fiber bundles running longitudinally (Plates 7.17 A, 7.18 A,B).

The adventitia of large and medium-sized arteries has a blood vessel network (*vasa vasorum*) and a nerve network. These vessels give rise to the capillaries found in the tunica media.

Veins

Veins are vessels in which blood flows from the capillary network back to the heart. Their walls are thinner than those of arteries. When empty the veins collapse, being fully tubular only when full of blood. Venous pathways are more abundant than arterial pathways, so that for every artery in a given region of the body, expecially if the artery is medium-sized or small, two or more veins may be encountered. Veins resemble arteries structurally, but the three layers are not always easily observable. Veins can be divided into two groups according to the development of the tunica media: those that act as reservoirs, and those that act directly in aiding the flow of blood. In the former the tunica media is poorly supplied with smooth muscle cells, and the veins function as true reservoirs (e.g., the large veins of the neck and mediastinum). In the second type the tunica media is highly developed and rich in smooth muscle cells which, by contracting, aid the flow of blood against gravity (e.g., the popliteal vein, femoral vein, etc.). Veins of this type often have valves.

As with arteries, large veins also have a network of vessels (vasa vasorum) in the adventitia, which reaches as far as the tunica intima (Plate 7.16).

Blood capillaries

Capillaries are very thin vessels with a diameter of 5-30 um and originate from the finer ramifications of the arteries. They are composed of a layer of endothelial cells resting on a thin basal lamina wrapped in a fine network of reticular fibers (reticular adventitia of the capillary). Pericytes and adventitial cells may be associated with the capillary. Certain capillaries have numerous pores in their endothelium (e.g., kidneys, endocrine glands). Those whose course is tortuous are classified as sinusoidal capillaries. There are also specialized capillaries in blood-producing organs and the liver that are characterized by having numerous perforations interrupting their wall (fenestrations), by having a tortuous course, and by having phagocytic cells in their lining (Plates 7.16 E; 7.17 B,C; 7.18 C and 7.19).

Lymph vessels

The lymphatic system is a set of vessels with a structure similar to that of veins and capillaries. This system is composed of *lymph vessels and lymph capillaries.* Lymph flows into these vessels from the periphery towards the heart. Lymph capillaries drain the tissue fluids and transport the lymph into the larger lymphatic vessels. Lymph is derived from two sources: from fluid expressed from the blood capillaries and from fluid that moves out of the tissue cells during normal function. Lymph capillaries resemble blood capillaries in having an endothelial lining. They originate as cul-de-sac vessels with a diameter varying from 5 to 100 um, and they form an anastomosing network that is associated with that of the blood capillaries.

Like veins, the larger lymph vessels have valves, and their wall is made up of an endothelial lining resting on a connective tissue layer. In the larger vessels this wall has elastic fibers and often bundles of smooth muscle cells. Only in the lymph vessels of considerable size are the three tunics similar to those in blood vessels.

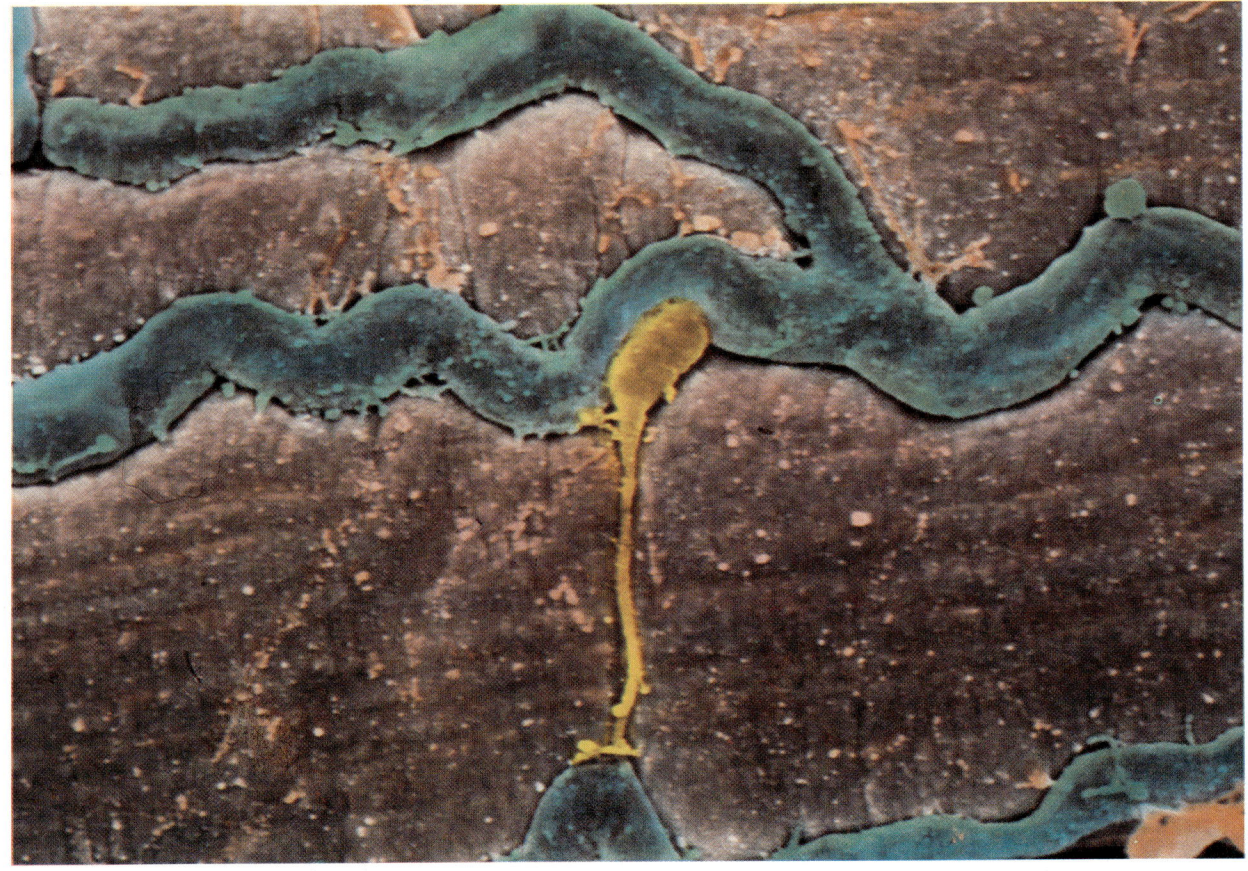

Capillaries running over the surfaces of rat skeletal muscle fibers. A thin pericyte (yellow) is associated with the vessels. (Colored SEM; 2,300 x).

Plate 7.1 137

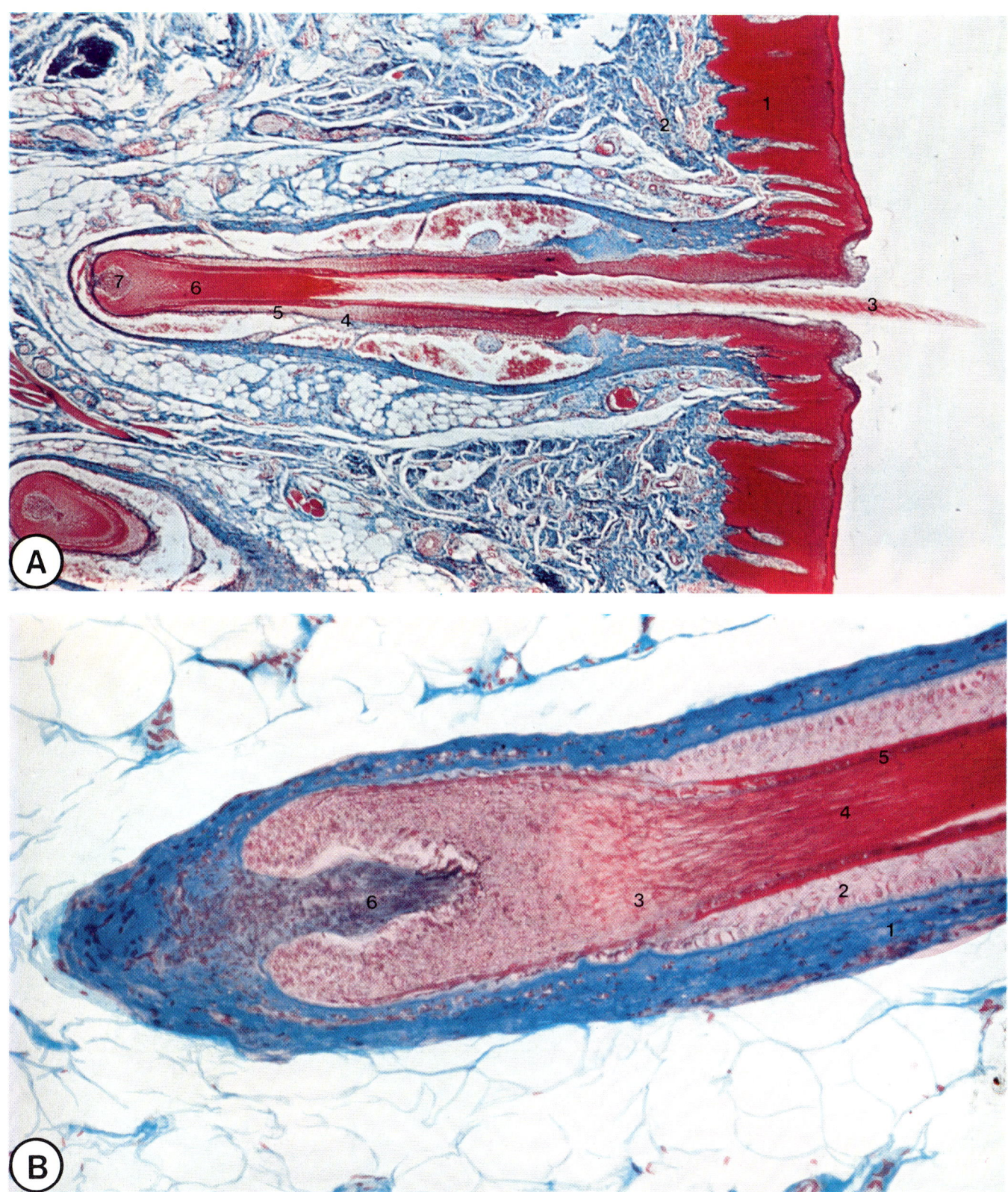

A **Longitudinal section of hair from human scalp (azan-Mallory, x30). 1** = epidermis with superficial stratum corneum. **2** = dermis with papillae. **3** = hair shaft. **4** = epidermis of follicle. **5** = root sheath epithelium. **6** = root of hair. **7** = papilla of hair follicle.

B **Longitudinal section of human hair follicle (azan-Mallory, x210). 1** = connective tissue sheath of follicle. **2** = root sheath epithelium. **3** = area of differentiation. **4** = medulla. **5** = cortex. **6** = papilla of follicle.

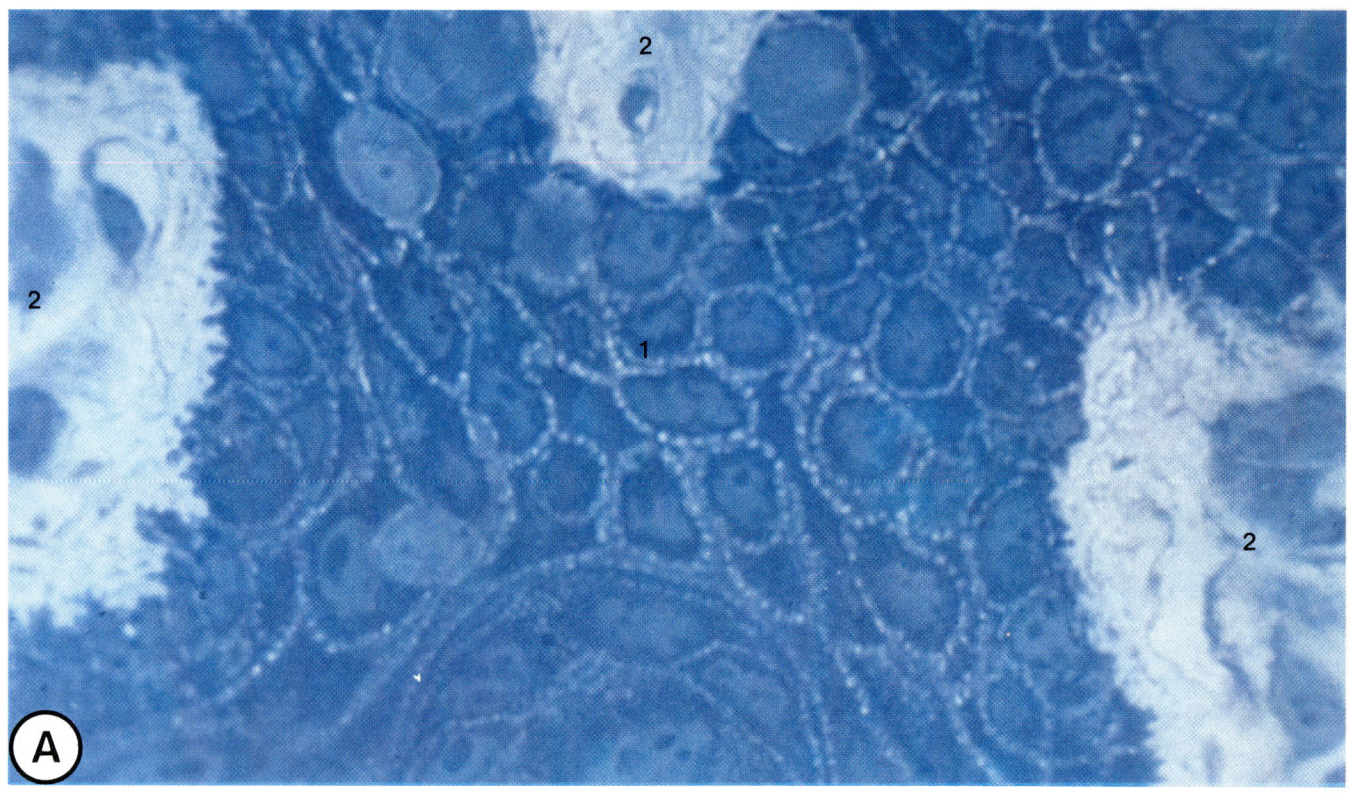

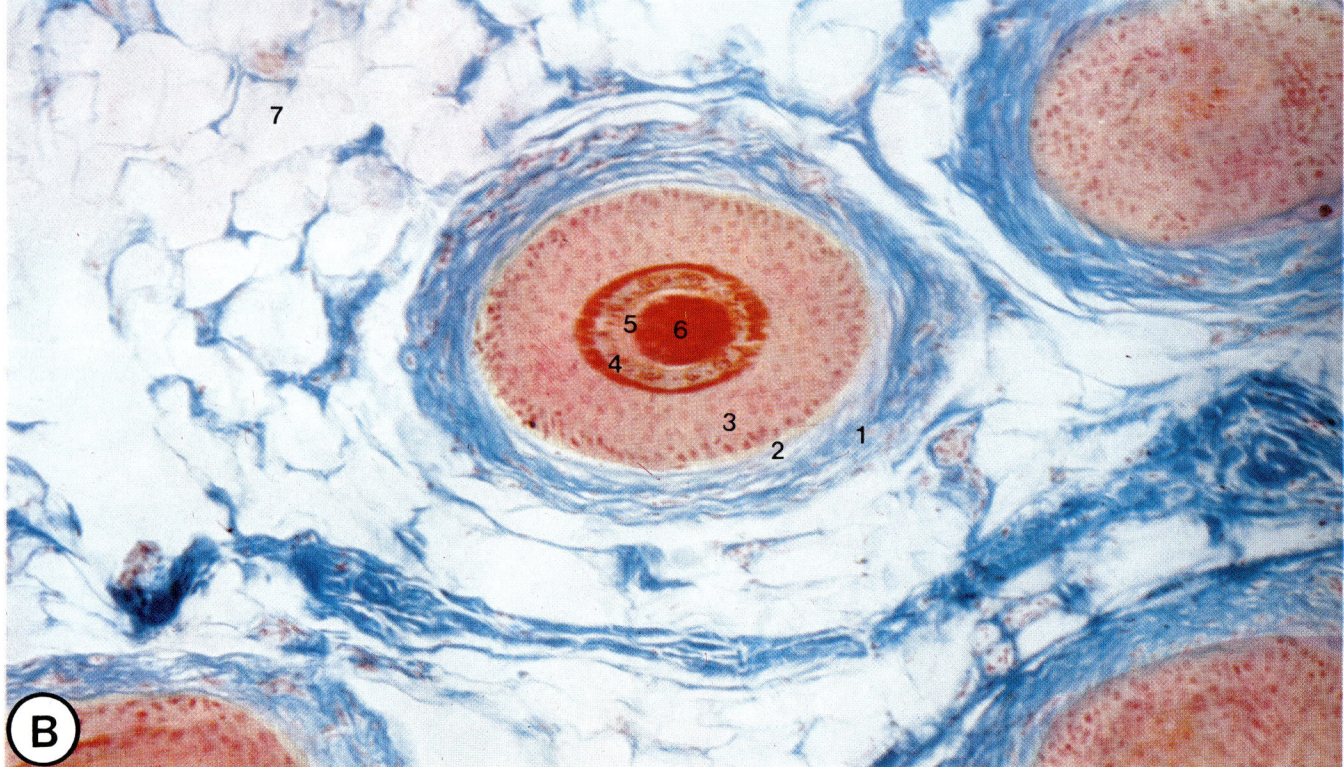

A **Stratum spinosum of human epidermis (methylene blue, x800). 1** = tangential section of stratum spinosum showing many cells with the thin cytoplasmic processes (spines) marking the attachment of adjacent cells by desomosomes. The spaces between the spines are clearly visible. **2** = cross section of dermal papillae.

B **Cross section of the root of a human hair follicle from the scalp (azan-Mallory, x160). 1** = connective sheath of follicle. **2** = glassy membrane. **3** = epidermis of follicle. **4** = root sheath with (outer) Henle's layer and (inner) Huxley's layer. **5** = cortex. **6** = medulla. **7** = adipose cells of hypodermis.

Plate 7.3   **139**

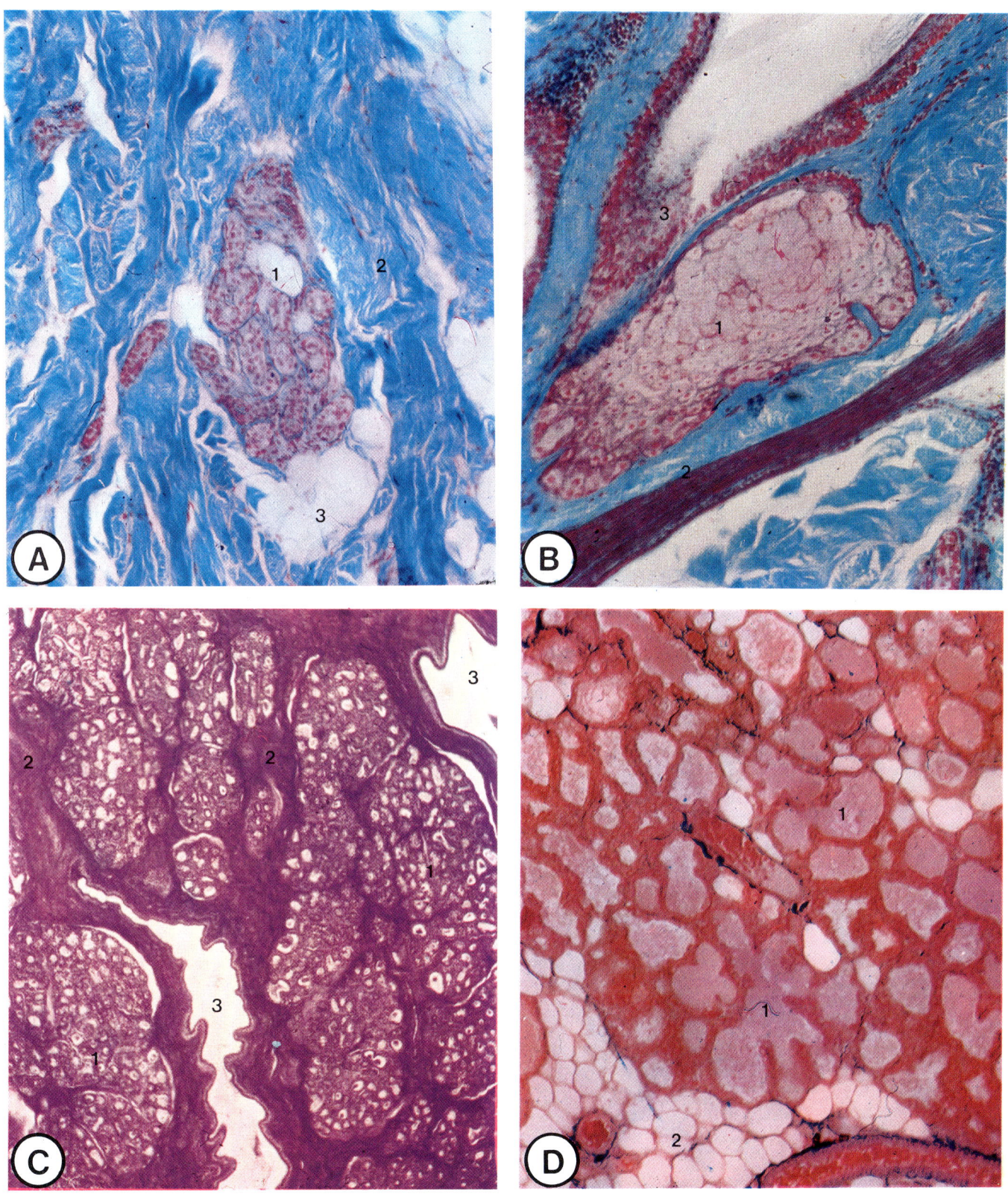

A   **Eccrine sweat gland from skin of human lip (azan-Mallory, x220). 1** = secretory units of the sweat gland. **2** = connective tissue of dermis. **3** = adipose cells.

B   **Sebaceous gland from human scalp (azan-Mallory, x220). 1** = secretory cells of the sebaceous gland. **2** = erector pili muscle. **3** = tangential section of gland duct. Sebaceous glands are found only in association with hairs.

C   **Human mammary gland (H & E, x80). 1** = gland lobules with secretory ducts in various degrees of dilatation. **2** = interlobular connective tissue septa. **3** = large lactiferous ducts.

D   **Mammary gland of lactating rat (H & E, x350). 1** = Alveoli of the gland fully dilated by the secretion. **2** = adipose tissue of the gland.

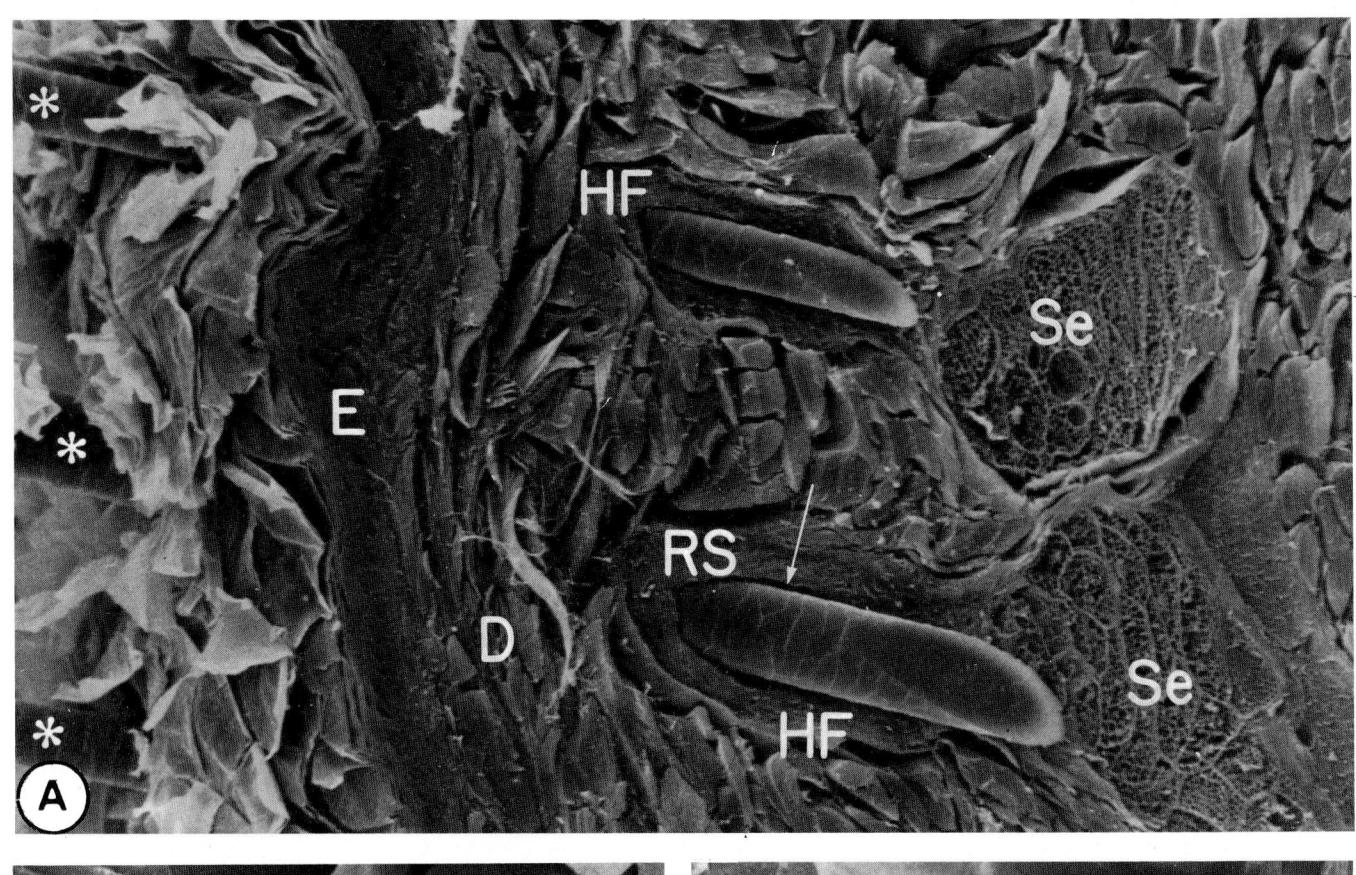

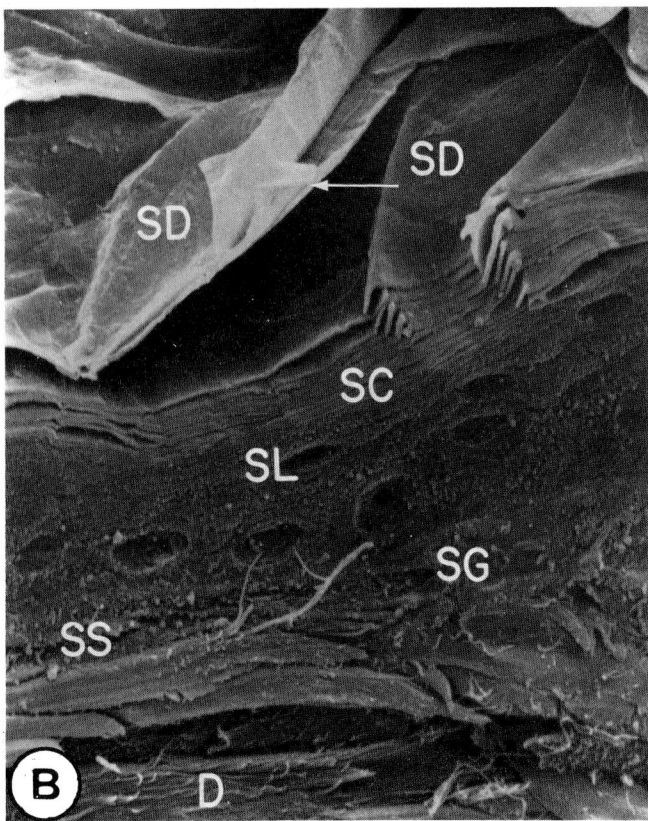

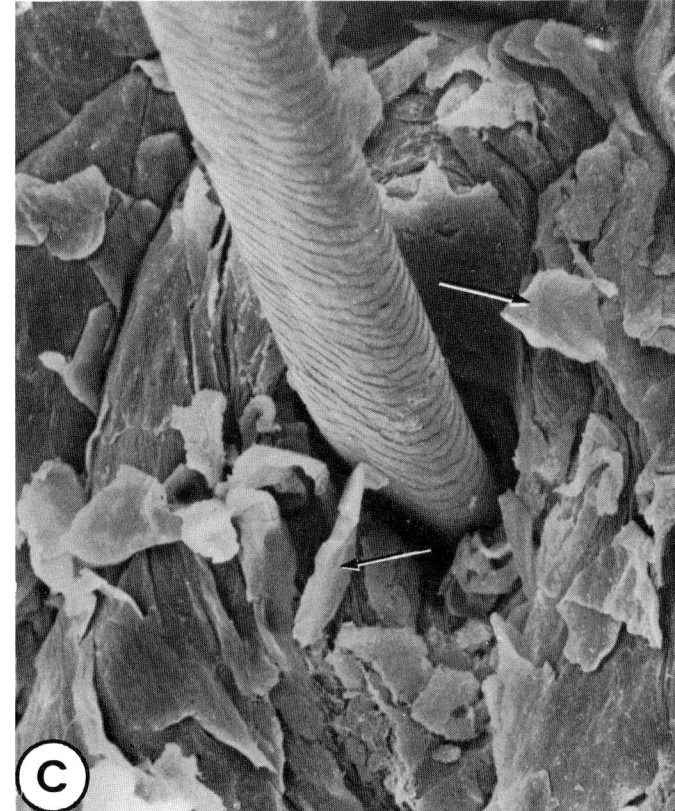

A   **Oblique section of monkey scalp (scanning EM, x450).** Hairs from deep within the hair follicle **(HF)** are visible, emerging obliquely through the skin surface (*). **RS** = outer root sheath. **E** = epidermis. **D** = dermis. **Se** = secretory cells of a sebaceous gland whose product is secreted into the cleft between the hair and the follicle (→).

B   **Cross section of monkey scalp (scanning EM, x1,400).** From bottom to top: dermis **(D)** rich in collagen fibers. In the epidermis can be seen the stratum spinosum **(SS)**, stratum granulosum **(SG)**, stratum lucidum **(SL)**, stratum corneum **(SC)** and stratum disjunctum **(SD)**, which is sloughing off at the surface (→).

C   **Human hair from the leg (scanning EM, x3,500).** A flattened hair is seen on the surface where it emerges from its follicle. Around the orifice the epidermis is sloughing off (→). From P.M. Motta, P.M. Andrews and K.R. Porter. In: *Microscopic Anatomy of Cell and Tissue Surfaces. An Atlas of Scanning Electron Microscopy.* Lea & Febiger, Philadelphia, 1977.

Plate 7.5   141

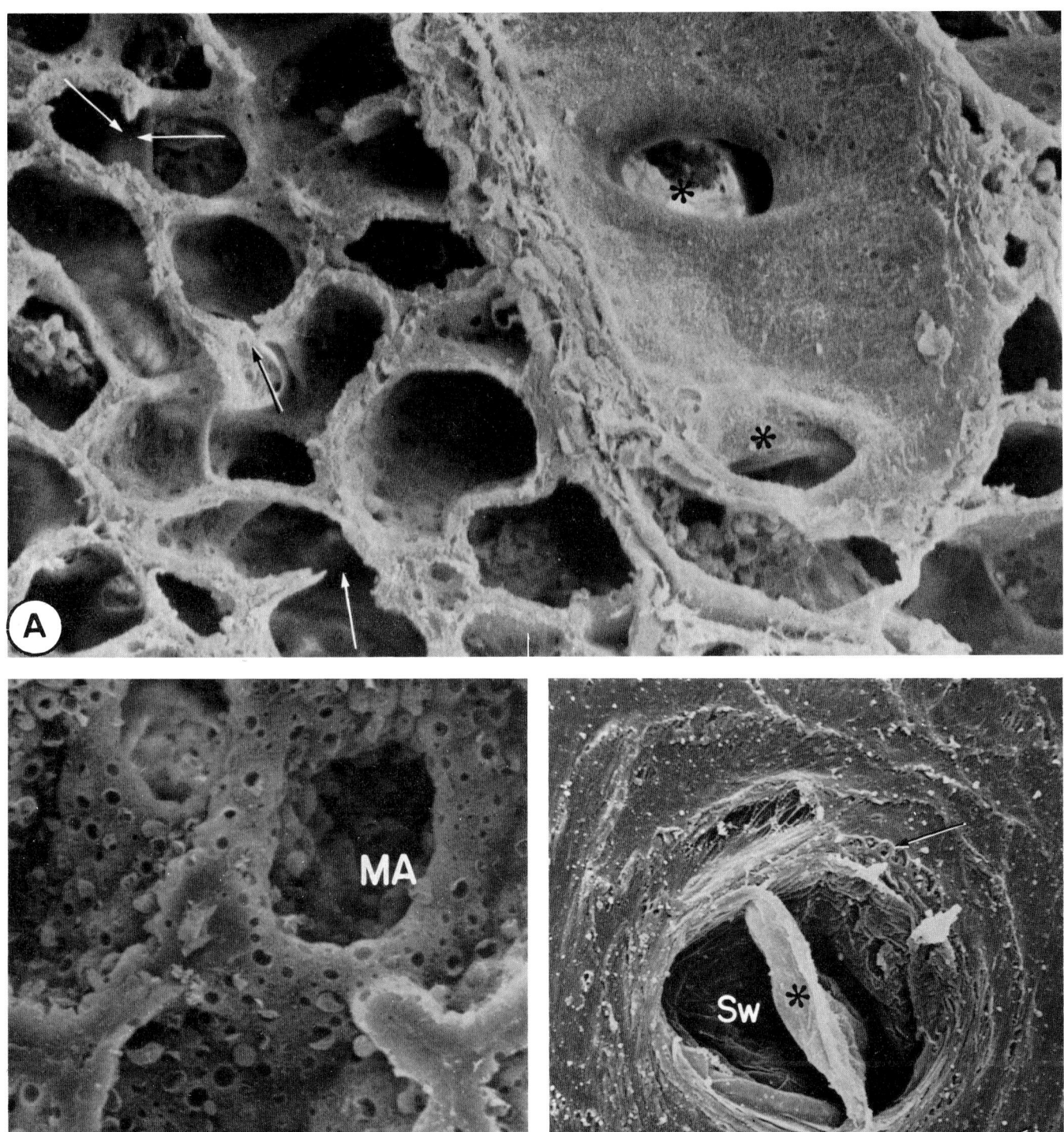

A **Mammary gland of lactating mouse (scanning EM, x600).** Along the wall of a large lactiferous duct are the openings of two secondary ductules (*). Around the duct are many dilated alveolar ducts which may communicate with each other (→). Original micrograph by K.M. Nemanic and D.R. Pitelka.

B **Alveolar sac of mouse mammary gland during lactation (scanning EM, x600).** Along the inner surface of the two alveoli (MA) are small vacuoles and secretion droplets.

C **Human sweat gland (scanning EM, x2,700).** The epidermal cells lining the spiralling gland duct (**Sw**) are firmly joined to each other (→). At the orifice of the gland is a cell being sloughed off (*).

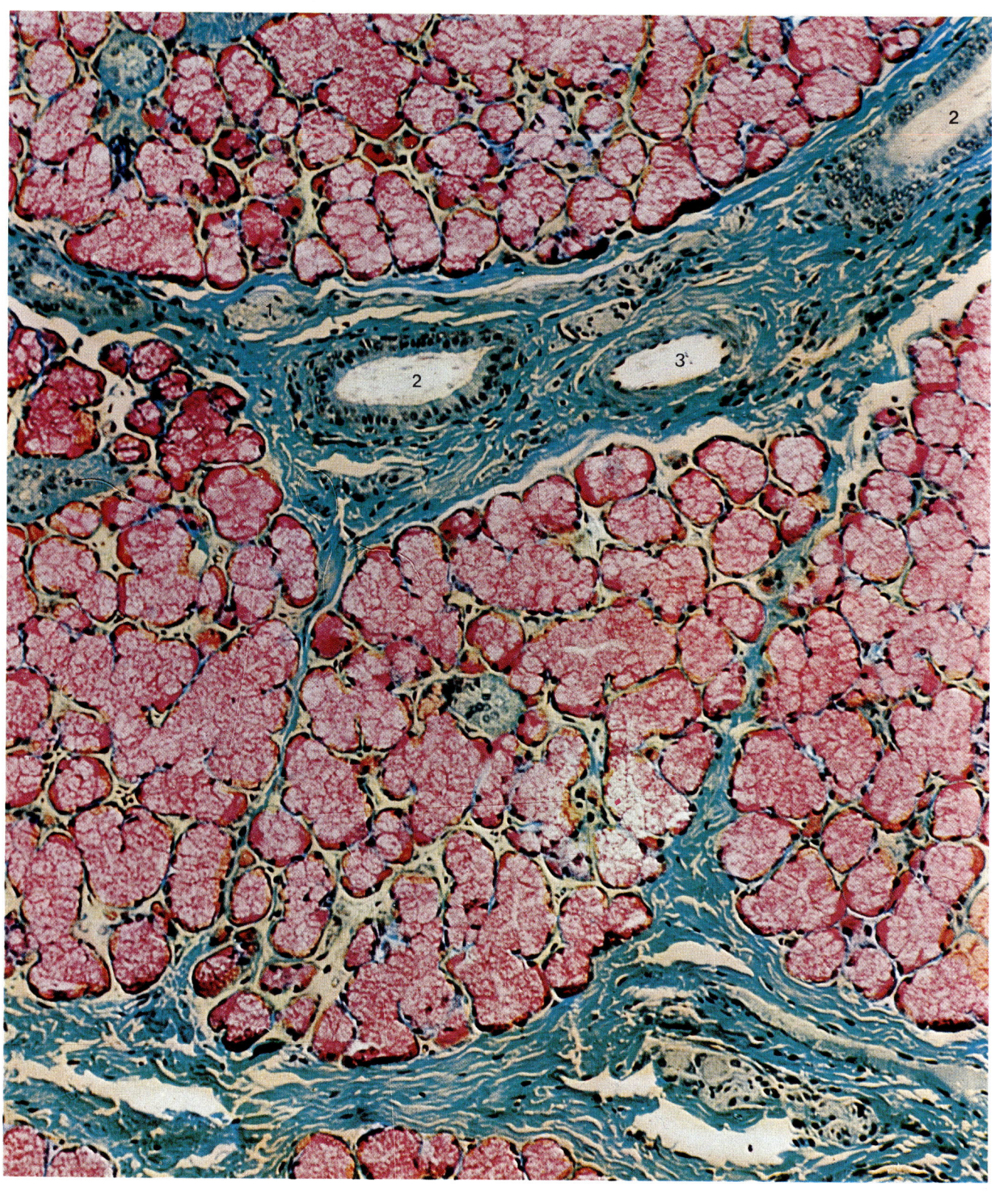

Canine submandibular gland (safranine orange, Weigert's fast-green/hematoxylin, x260). In the interlobular connective tissue are nerve bundles **(1)**, excretory ducts **(2)** and an arteriole **(3)**. Mixed secretory units can be seen with characteristic demilunes. By courtesy of G. Quintarelli.

Plate 7.7 143

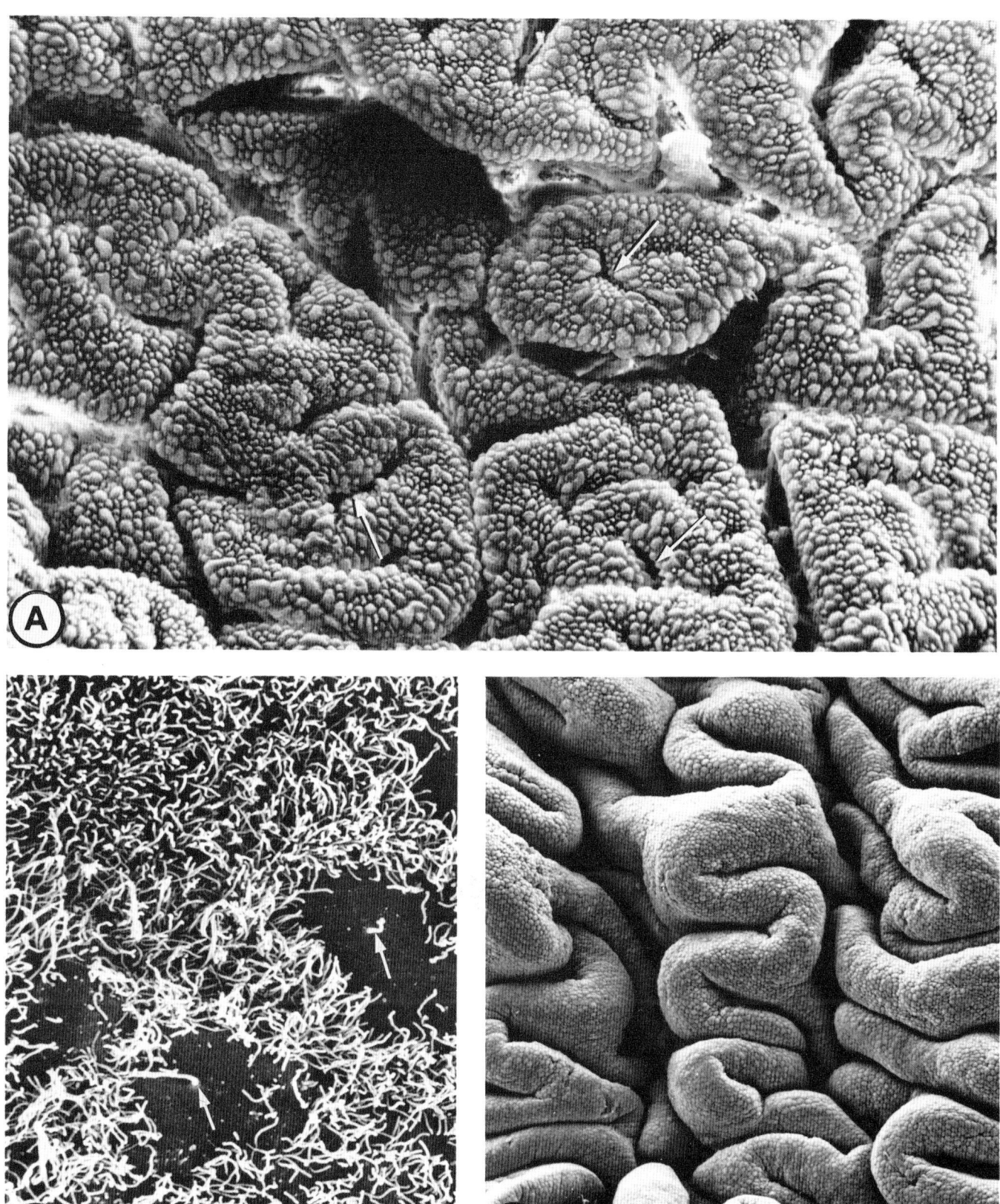

A **Rabbit uterine mucosa (scanning EM, x850).** In the secretory (luteal) phase the mucosa has large folds. Between the folds are deep furrows. The small fissures are glandular crypts (→). From F. Barberini, S. Sartori, J. Van Blerkom and P.M. Motta. Cell Tiss. Res. 190:207, 1978.

B **Peritoneal surface of rat liver (scanning EM, x7,500).** The serosal cells are coated with numerous microvilli and in some cases have thin, single cilia (→). From P.M. Motta, T. Fujita and M. Nishi. In: *Basic and Clinical Hepatology,* P.M. Motta and L.J.A. DiDio, eds. M. Nijhoff Publishers. The Hague/Boston/London, 1982.

C **Folds from the mucosa of cat gallbladder (scanning EM, x3,200).** The depth of the folds is partly caused by the contraction of the muscular wall of the gallbladder. The invaginations increase the surface area of the mucosa for water reabsorption. By courtesy of M. Castellucci and A. Caggiati.

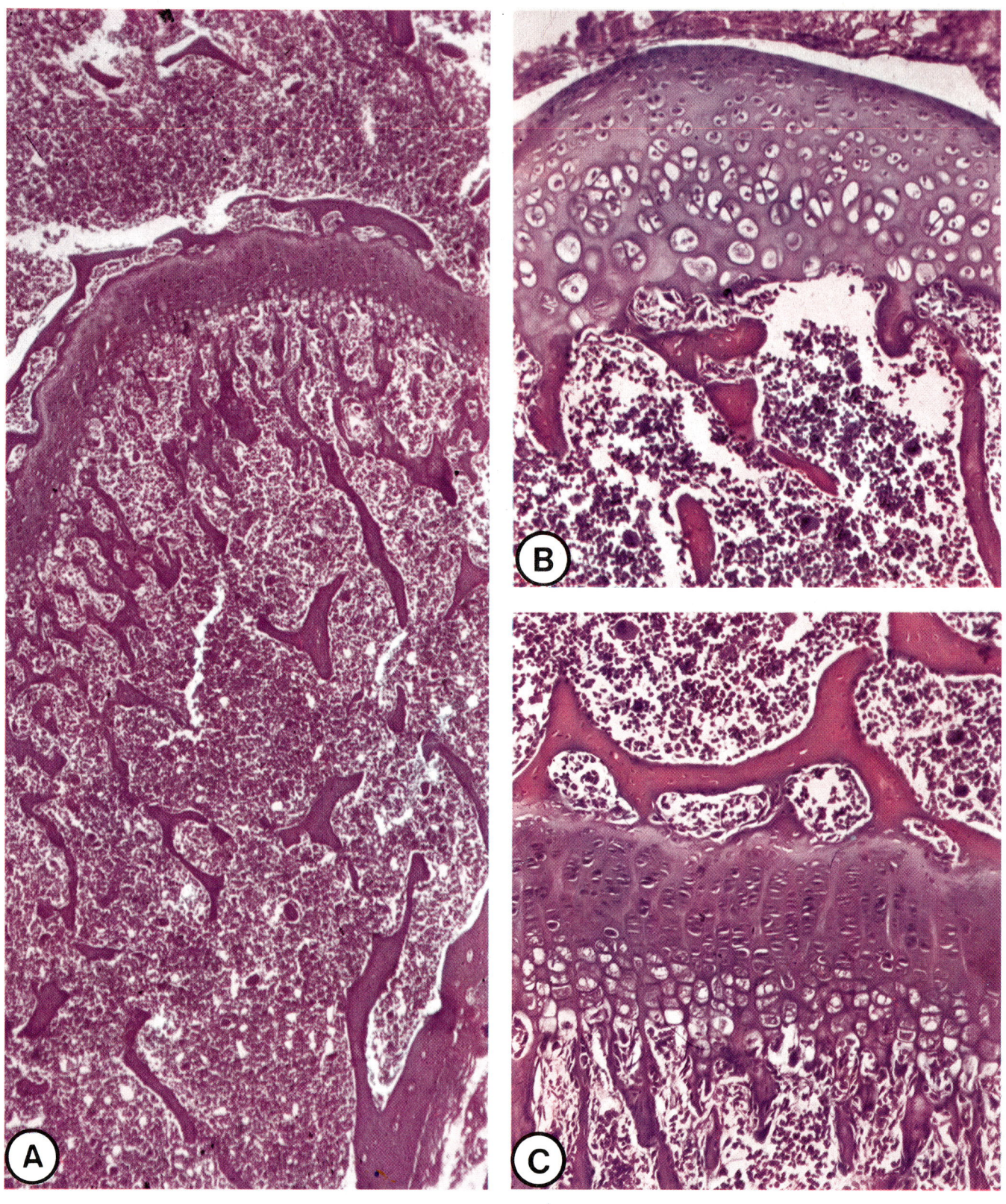

A Ossification in the tibia of fetal rat (H & E, x60). The longitudinal section of the bone shows part of the epiphysis (above) and part of the diaphysis (below). Networks of calcified cartilage are distributed irregularly throughout the section.

B Epiphyseal cartilage in the tibia of fetal rat (H & E, x175). The cartilage cells are dividing and beginning to hypertrophy while the intercellular substance is forming.

C Epiphyseal plate from a rat (H & E, x175). The cartilage cells are arranged in columns. Below: the ossification zone can be seen with networks of calcified cartilage.

Plate 7.9   145

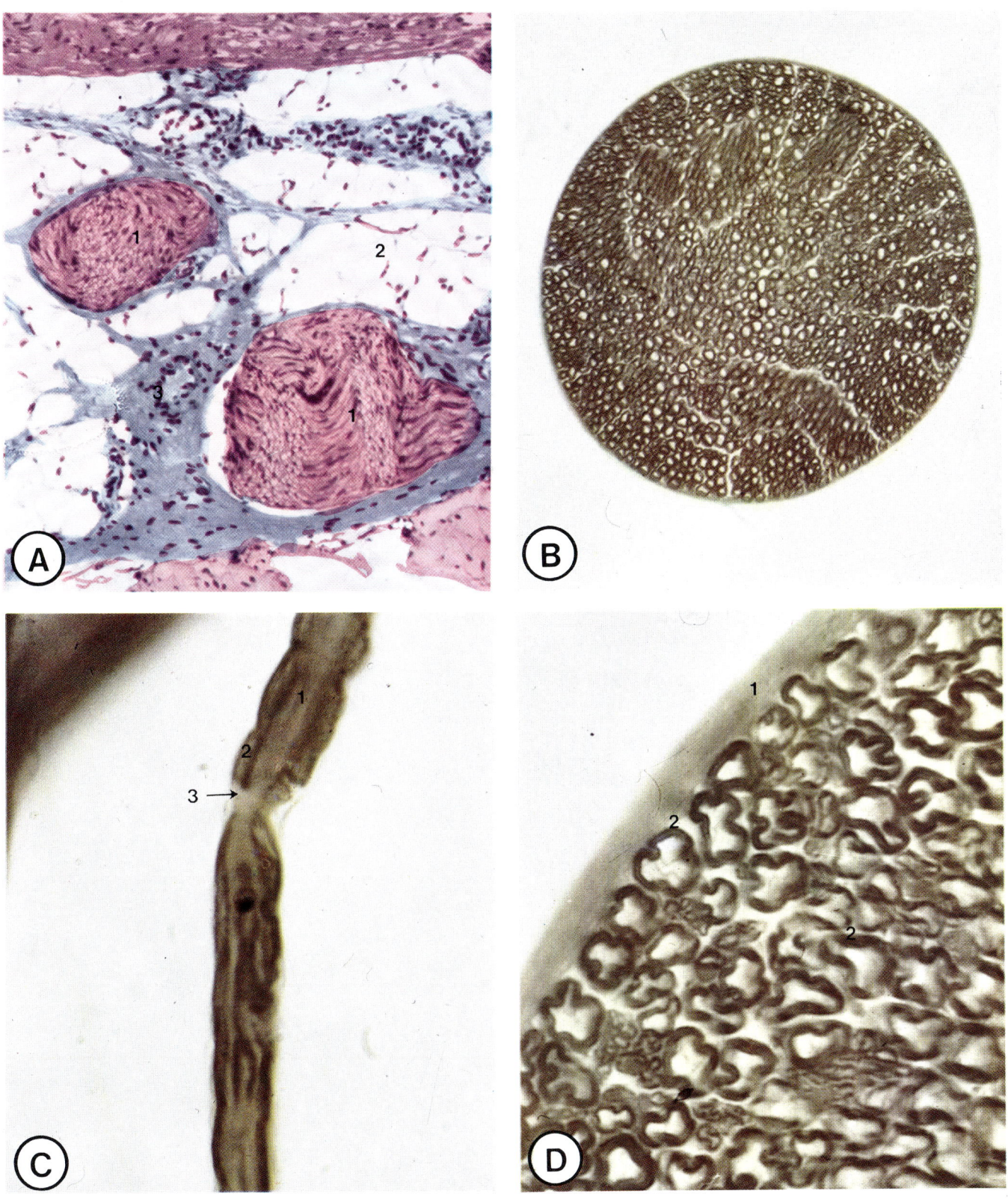

A   **Nerve fibers in tracheal adipose tissue (Mallory, x220). 1** = nerve fibers in oblique section. **2** = adipose tissue. **3** = blood vessel.

B   **Cross section of a bundle of myelinated nerve fibers from the ischial nerve of a frog (osmium tetroxide, x100).**

C   **Longitudinal section of a nerve fiber with node of Ranvier (constriction) (osmium tetroxide, x480). 1** = axon. **2** = myelin sheath. **3** = node of Ranvier.

D   **Detail of myelinated nerve fibers from a frog (osmium tetroxide, x380). 1** = epineurium. **2** = myelin sheath.

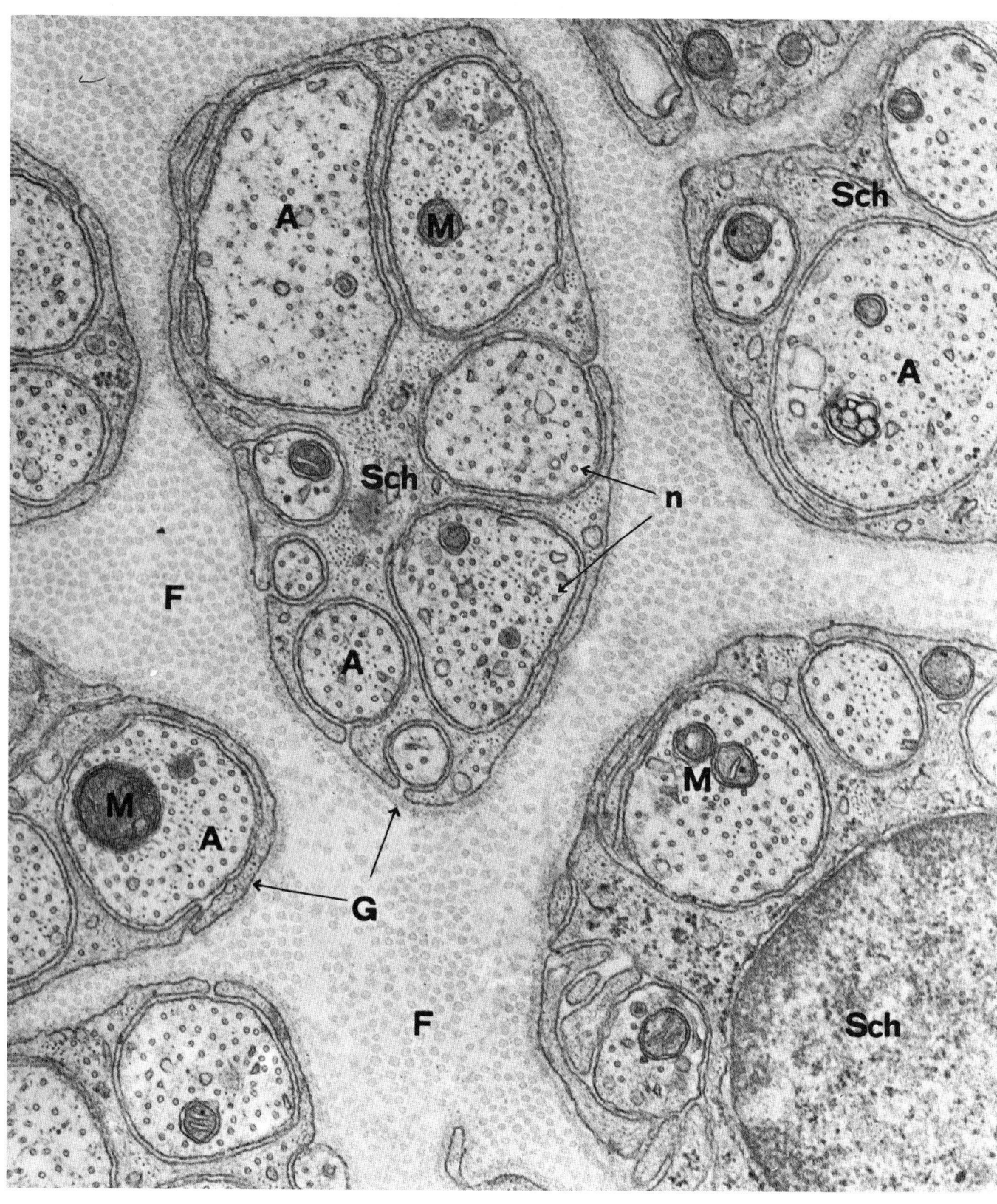

Cross section of unmyelinated nerve fibers (EM, x42,000). A number of axons **(A)** are contained in the cytoplasm of a single Schwann cell **(Sch).** Neurotubules (microtubules) **(n→)** and mitochondria **(M)** are in the axoplasm. The plasma membrane of the Schwann cells is covered with a thin glycocalyx **(G→)** with which numerous collagen fibers **(F)** are associated. The fibers are also distributed in the intervening spaces (endoneurium). Original micrograph by F. Caramia.

Plate 7.11   147

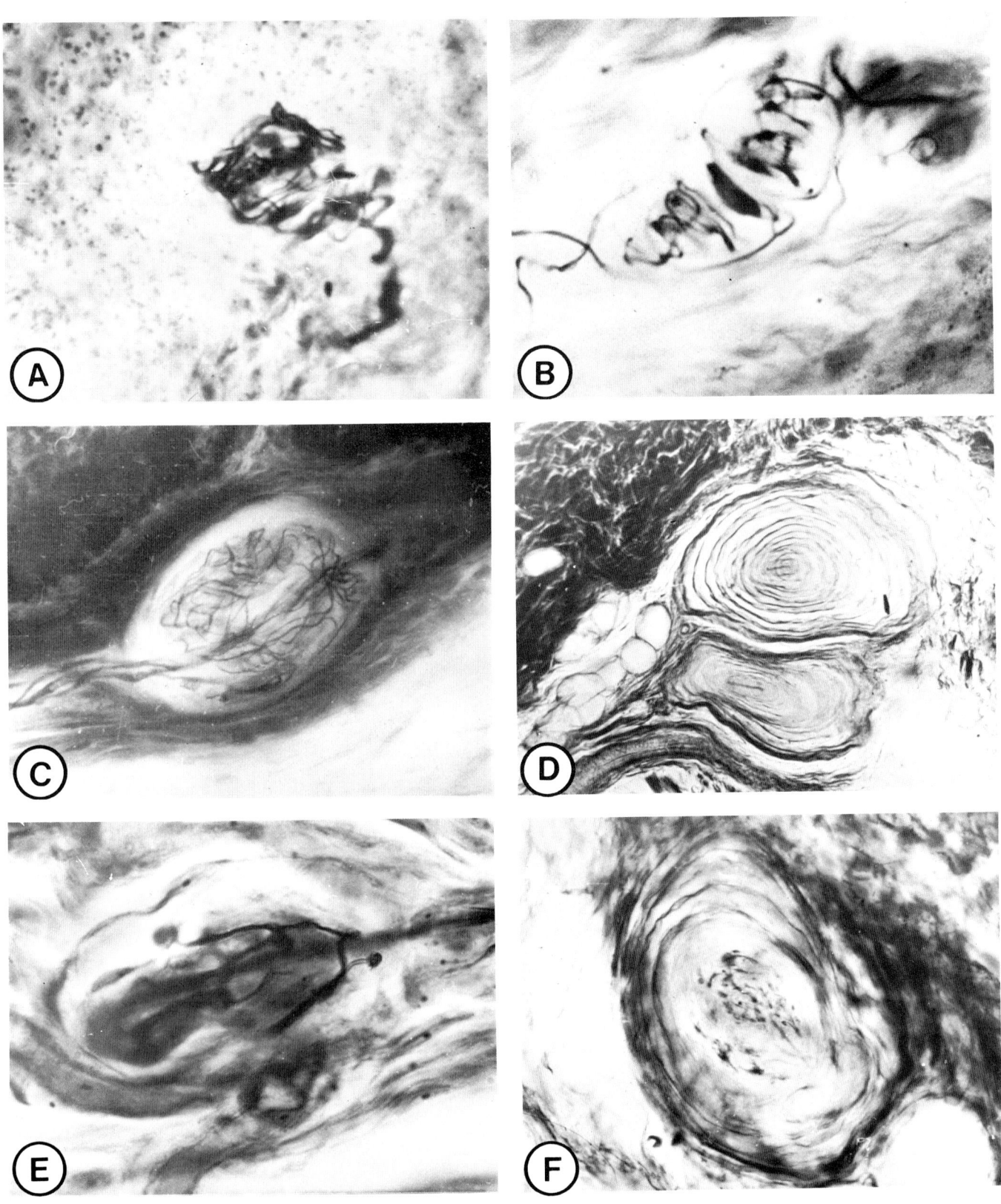

A   Human tongue nerve ending (bundle) (silver impregnation, x400).
B   Meissner's corpuscle in skin from sole of monkey foot (silver impregnation, x120).
C   Sensory end bulb of Krause (silver impregnation, x220).
D   Vater-Pacini corpuscles in skin from palm of monkey hand (silver impregnation, x400).
E   Golgi-Mazzoni small corpuscle from skin of human nail bed (silver impregnation, x1,000).
F   Golgi-Mazzoni corpuscle from skin of human toe (silver impregnation, x400). By courtesy of D. Kadanoff.

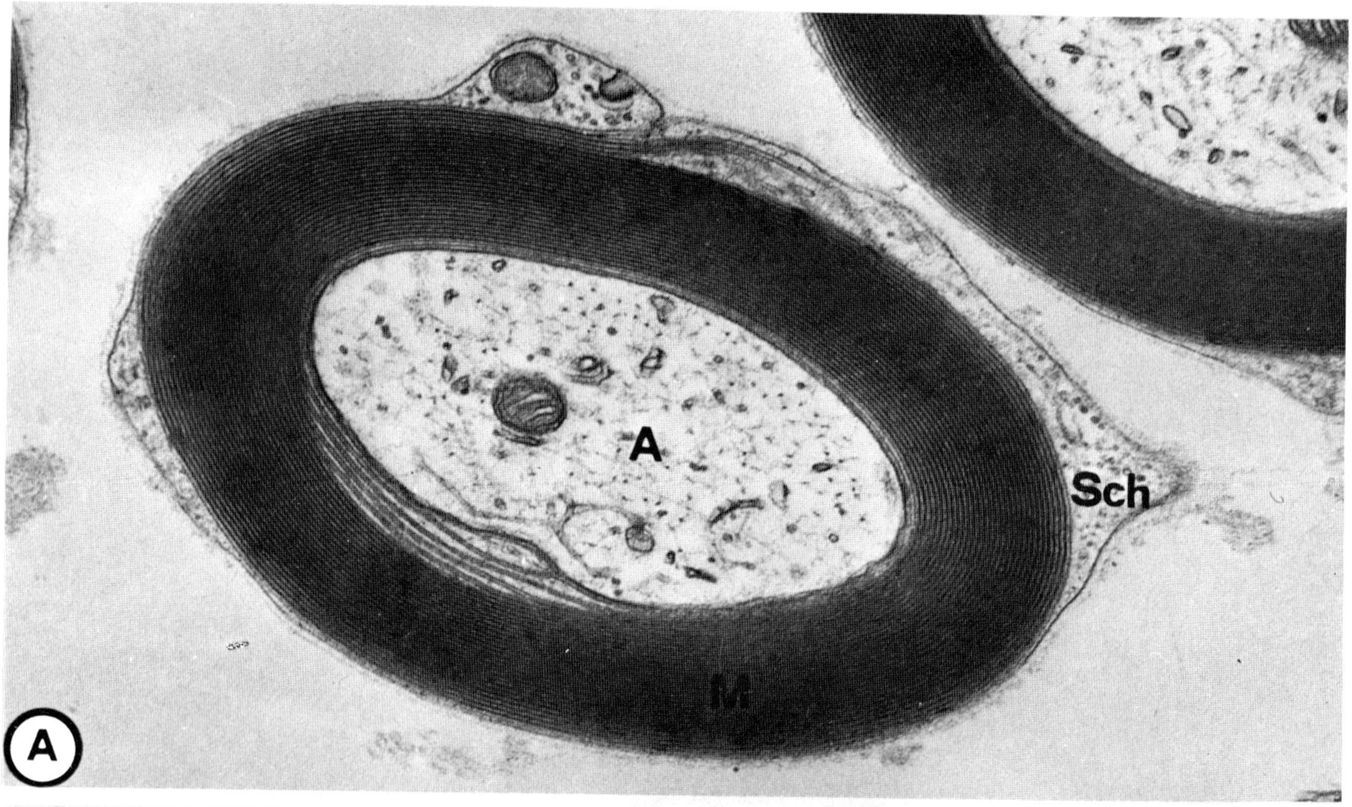

Plate 7.12

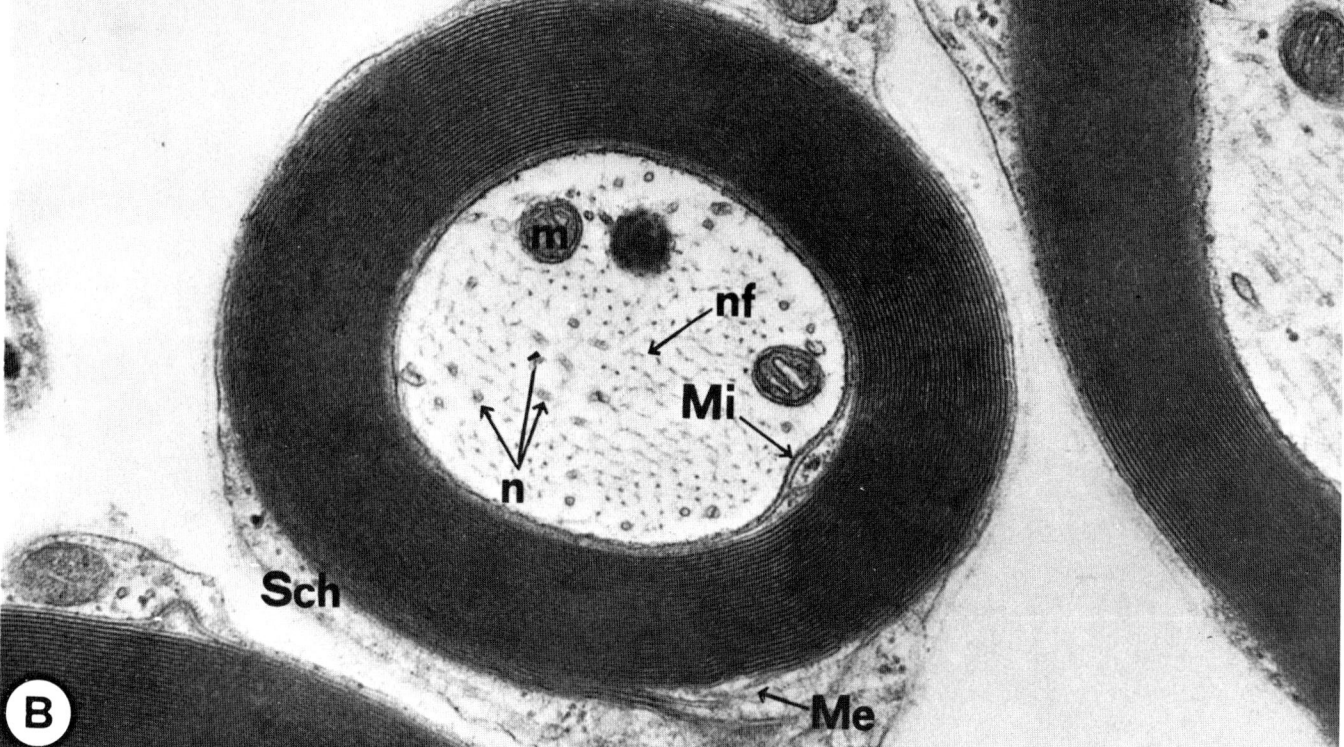

A Oblique section of myelinated nerve fiber (EM, x62,000). **M** = myelin sheath of concentrically wrapped plasma membranes of Schwann cells **(Sch)**. **A** = axon with axoplasm having neurotubules, neurofilaments and mitochondria.

B Cross section of myelinated nerve fiber (EM, x62,000). **Mi** = internal mesaxon. **Me** = external mesaxon formed of cytoplasm from Schwann cell **(Sch)**. Mitochondria **(m)**, neurotubules **(n)** and neurofilaments **(nf)** are contained in the axon. By courtesy of F. Caramia.

Plate 7.13

149

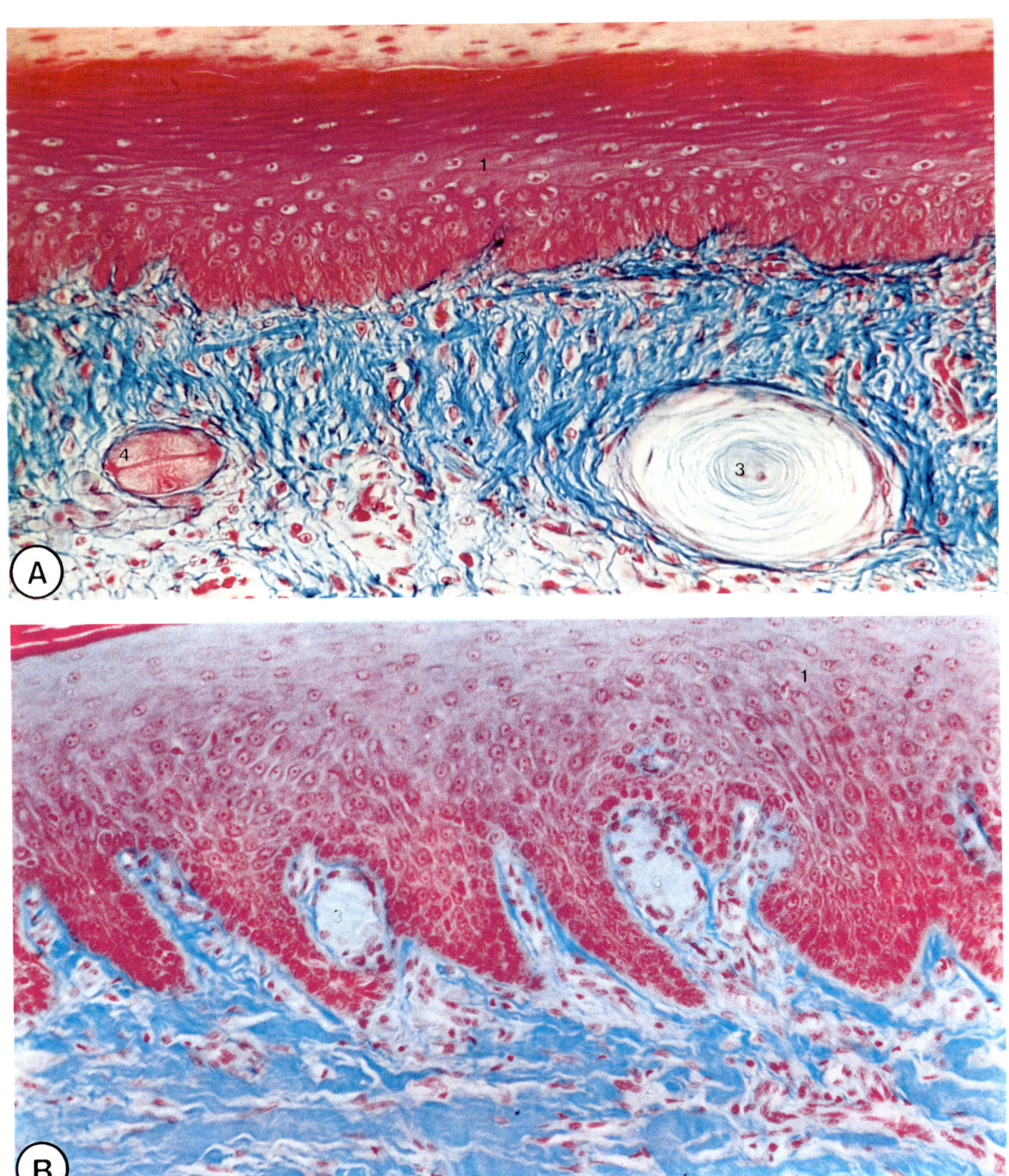

A **Sensory corpuscles in skin from duck beak (azan-Mallory,x180). 1** = epidermis. **2** = dermis. **3** = Vater-Pacini corpuscle. **4** = Herbst's corpuscle.

B **Meissner's corpuscles in the dermal papillae of human finger (azan-Mallory, x180). 1** = epidermis. **2** = dermis with numerous Meissner's corpuscles **(3)** in the corium papillae.

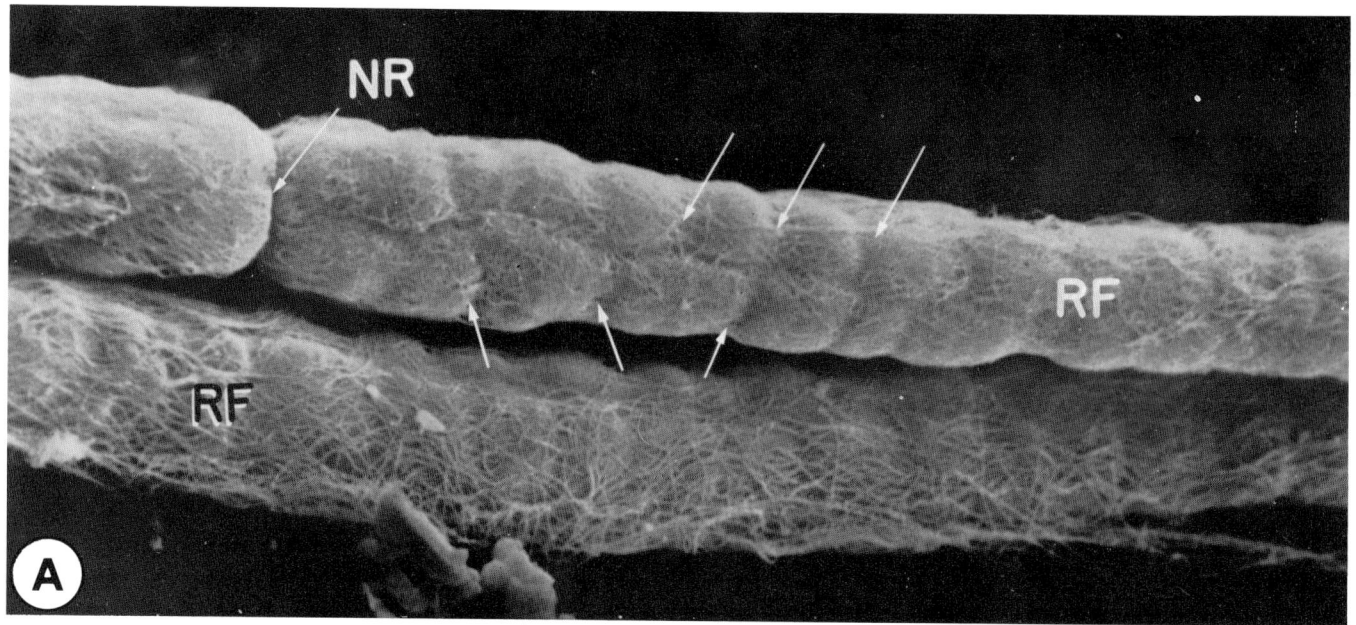

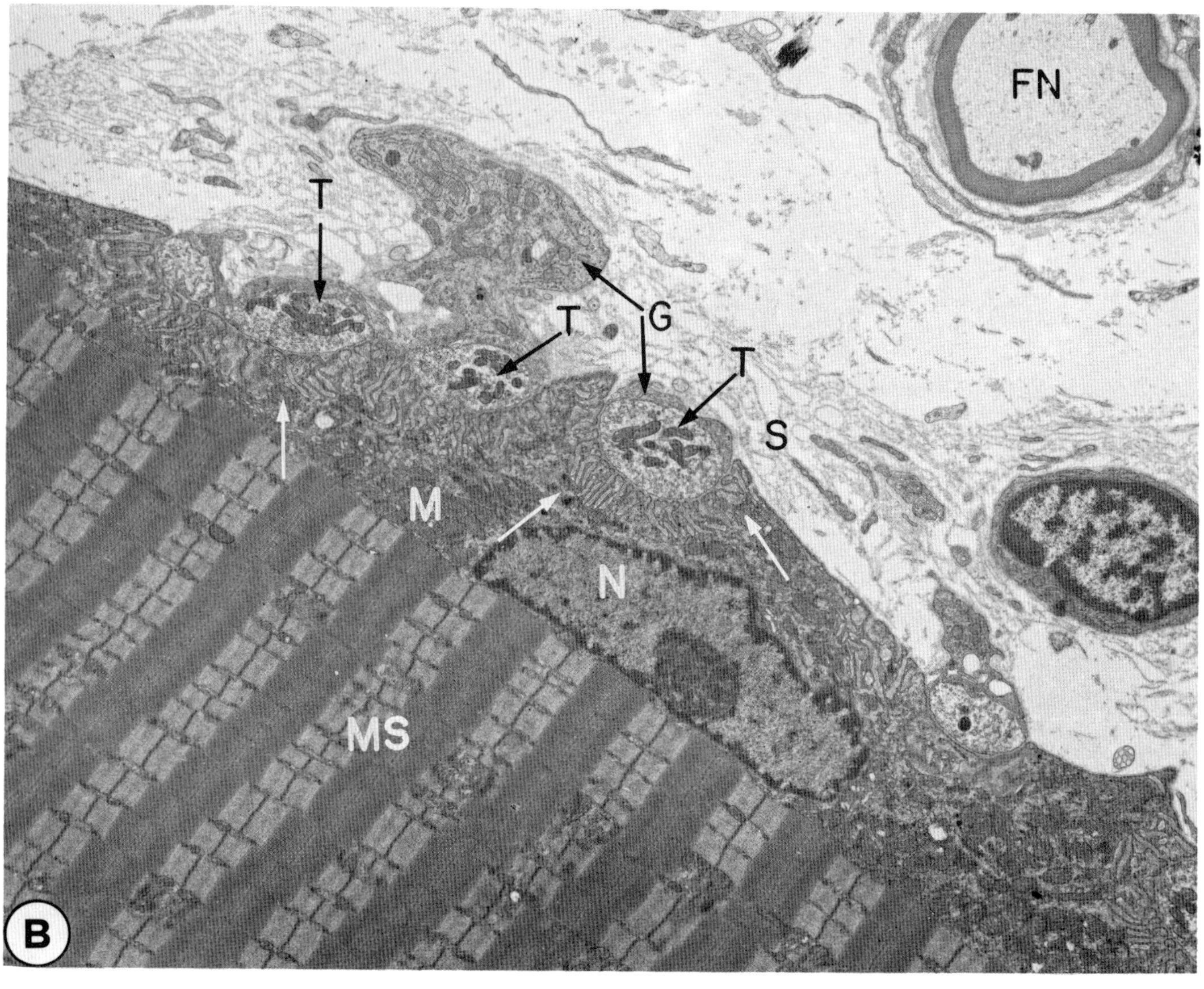

A **Isolated myelinated fibers from the sciatic nerve of a rat (scanning EM, x2,200).** A web of delicate reticular fibrils **(RF)** forms a sheath around each nerve fiber. A node of Ranvier **(NR)** is visible in one fiber. The smaller furrows along the fiber (→) mark the site of the clefts of Schmidt-Lanterman. Original micrograph by J. Vial.

B **Motor end plates from rat muscle (EM, x12,500).** Abundant vesicles and mitochondria are in the terminal axons **(T),** which are partly covered by glial cells **(G)** and are in close relation to a striated muscle fiber **(MS).** The plasma membrane of the muscle fiber forms numerous folds (→) lined by an amorphous extracellular substance continuous with the dense outer coating of the sarcolemma **(S).** The nucleus **(N)** and the mitochondria **(M)** of the muscle fiber **(MS)** are at the periphery of the cell. Above right **(FN):** a myelinated nerve fiber in cross section. The terminal branches of the axons of the motor end plate terminate here. By courtesy of J.E. Rash and M.H. Ellisman.

Plate 7.15   **151**

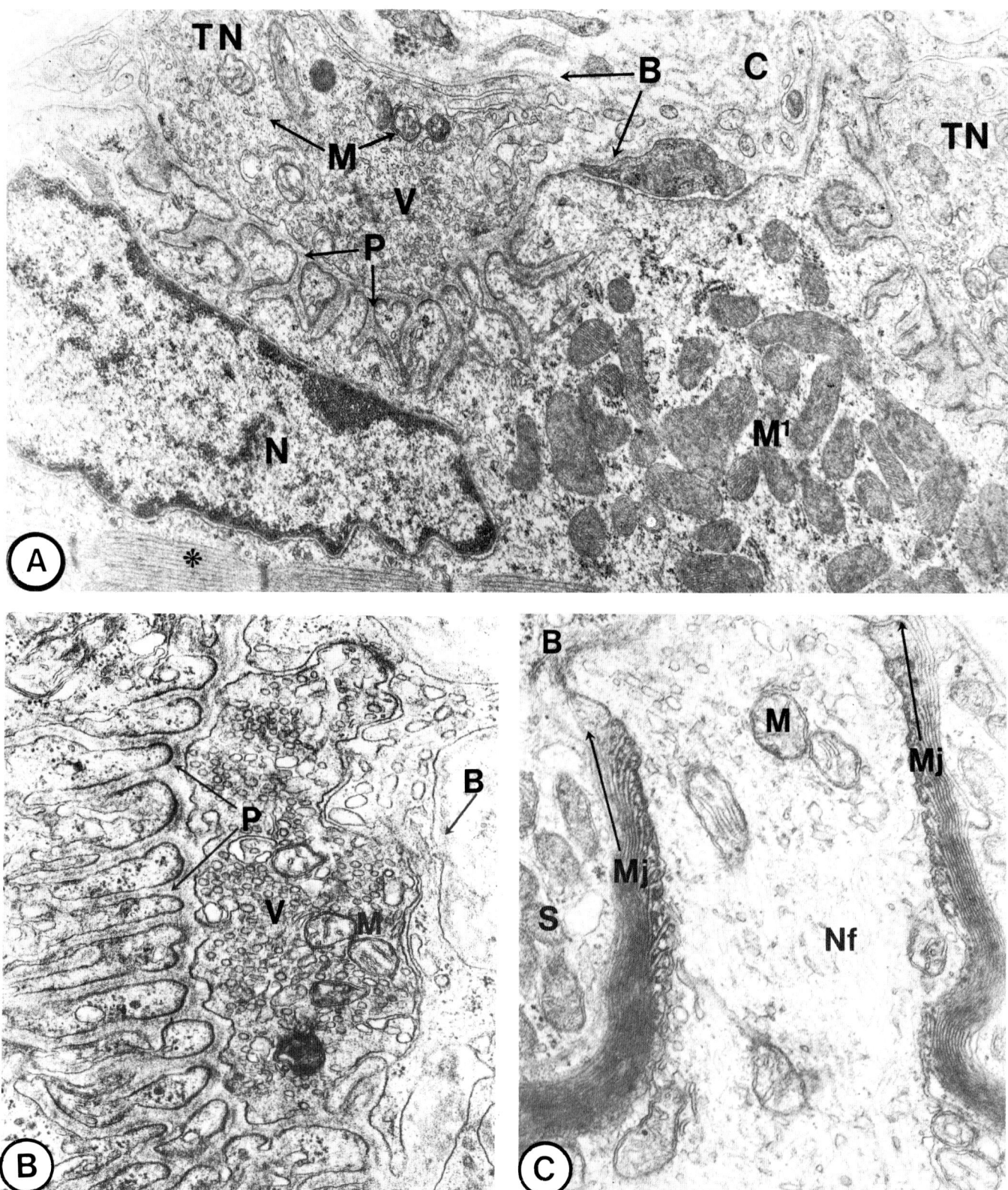

A **Motor end plate from the diaphragm muscle of a rat (EM, x18,000).** The terminal parts of the axon **(TN)**, lacking a myelin sheath and containing many synaptic vesicles **(V)** and mitochondria **(M)**, are in contact with a grooved surface of the striated muscle fiber in a region rich in mitochondria **(M1)**. The membrane of the muscle fiber is invaginated with numerous folds **(P)** containing amorphous material associated with the sarcolemma. The same material is visible on the surface of the muscle fiber where it forms a dense layer covering the sarcolemma **(B→)** to which fibrils of the connective tissue adhere **(C)**. Below left: the nucleus **(N)** and the myofibrils **(*)** of the striated muscle fiber.

B **Detail of motor end plate from a rat (EM, x31,000).** The figure shows a nerve ending containing synaptic vesicles **(V)** and mitochondria **(M). (P)** = folds of the sarcolemma. The terminal part of the axon is covered with a neurilemma composed of an outer layer **(B→)** and connective tissue fibrils.

C **Termination of a myelinated nerve fiber (EM, x34,000).** Where the myelin sheath **(Mj)** approaches the ramification at the nerve ending it tapers and finally terminates **(→)**. The axon contains neurofilaments **(Nf)** and mitochondria **(M). S** = cytoplasm of a Schwann cell. **B** = external coating of the neurilemma. The myelin sheath displays the same morphology at the point where a node of Ranvier occurs. By courtesy of S. Manolov.

Plate 7.16

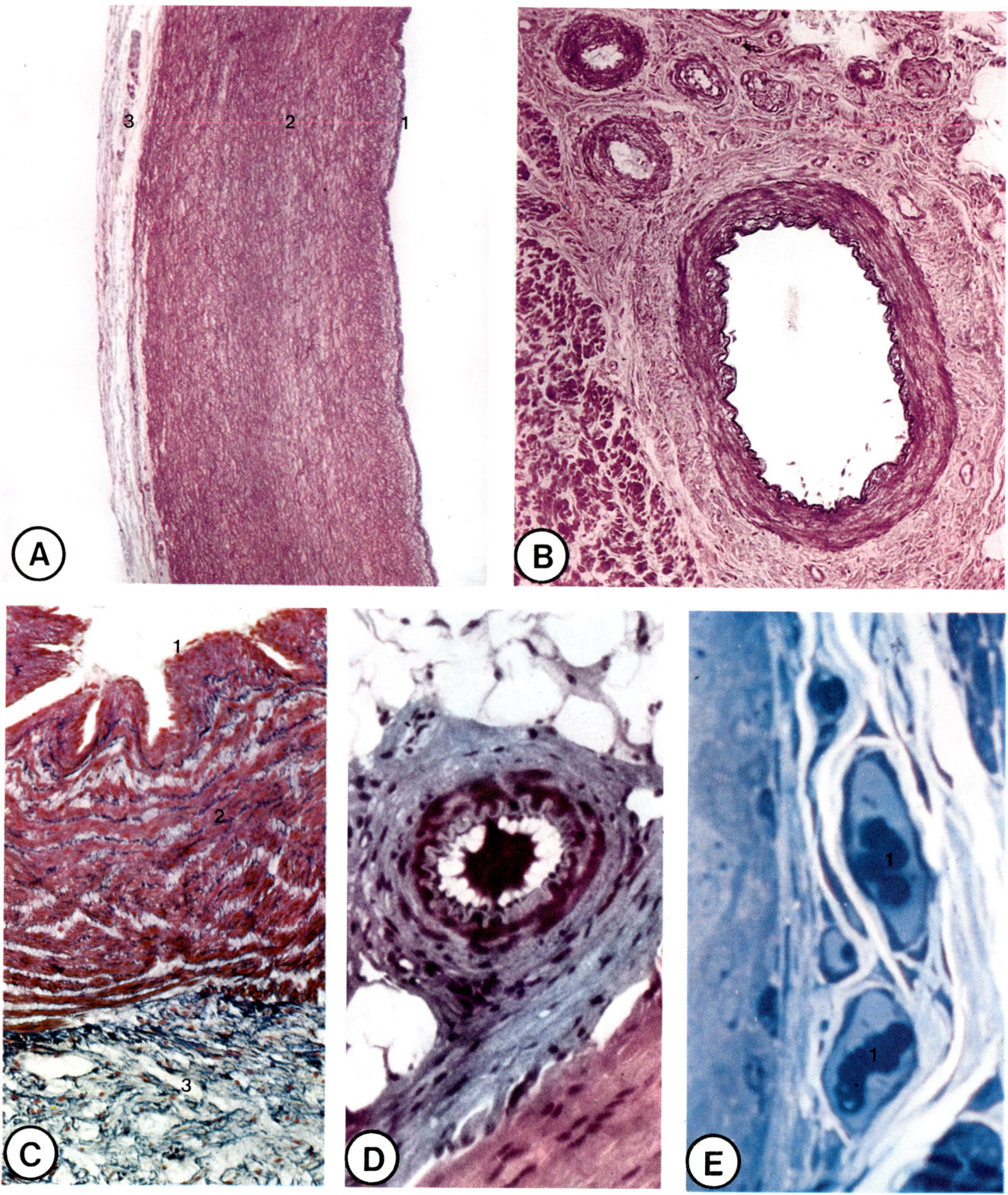

A   Section of the wall of the aorta from a monkey (H & E, x50). 1 = tunica intima. 2 = tunica media. 3 = tunica adventitia with vasa vasorum.

B   Muscular artery from human pampiniform plexus (resorcin & fuchsin, x85). The internal elastic lamina is visible as a black line circling the lumen. The tunica media comprises smooth muscle cells and elastic fibers. Above left: small vessels.

C   Artery of human umbilical cord (azan-Mallory, x120). 1 = endothelium of tunica intima. 2 = tunica media composed of elastic fibers (blue) and smooth muscle cells (red). 3 = tunica adventitia merging with Wharton's jelly. The internal elastic lamina can be seen.

D   Tunica adventitia in artery of esophagus (azan-Mallory, x85).

E   Blood capillaries in the lamina propria of bladder mucosa from a rat (methylene blue, x820). The capillary walls are composed of endothelial cells. Red blood cells (1) can be seen in the lumen.

Plate 7.17   153

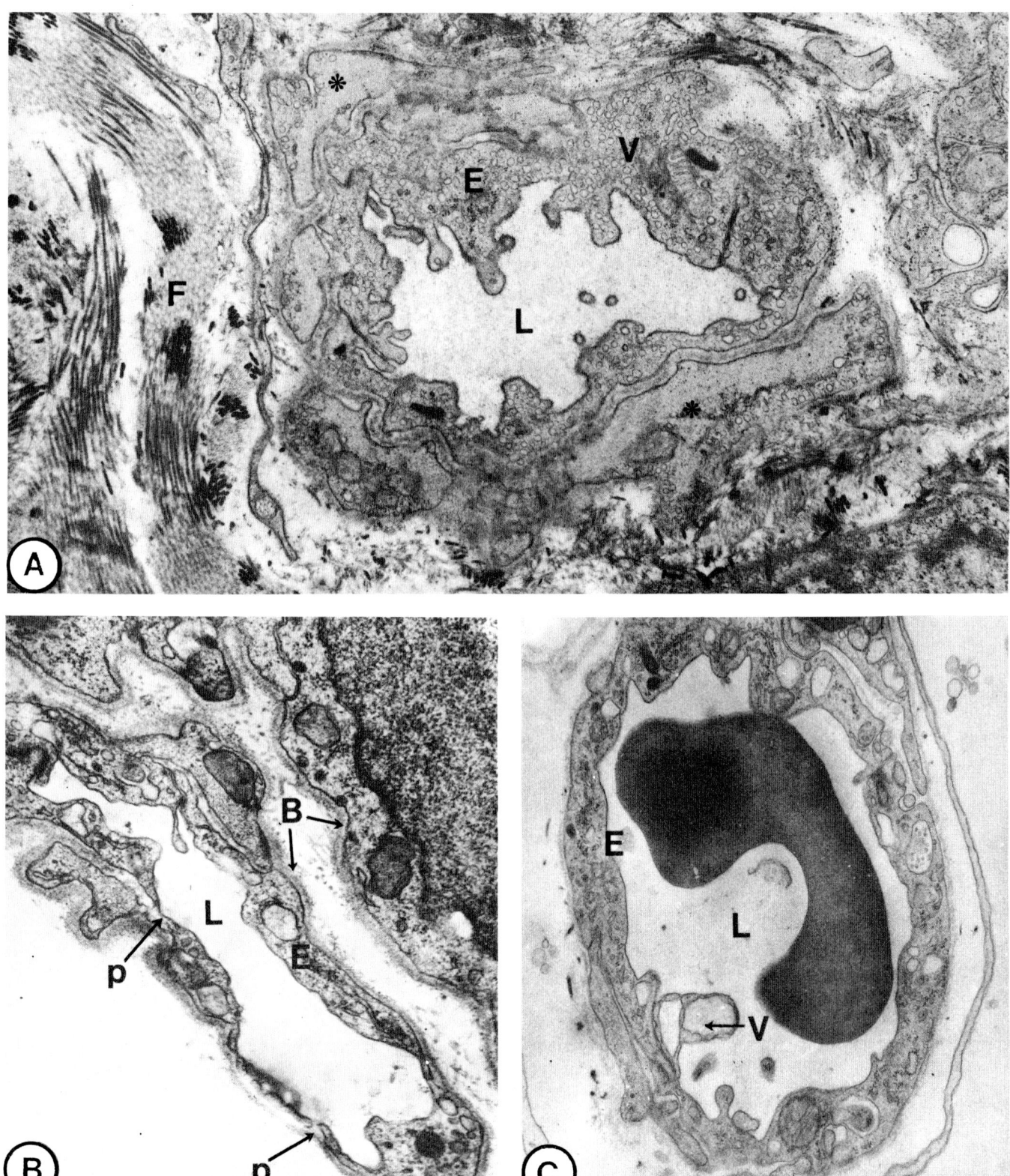

A   **Arteriole from a mouse (EM, x11,500). L** = lumen of vessel. **E** = endothelial cell with cytoplasm abounding in pinocytotic vesicles **(V)**. The endothelium is covered by smooth muscle fibers **(*)**. **F** = collagen fiber bundles in the surrounding connective tissue.

B   **Oblique section through a fenestrated blood capillary from rat hypophysis (EM, x26,000). L** = lumen of capillary. **E** = endothelial cell with pores **(p→)**. **B** = basal lamina of the capillary and of a surrounding cell. By courtesy of A. Santoro.

C   **Cross section through a blood capillary (non-fenestrated) from a mouse (EM, x12,000).** An erythrocyte can be seen in the lumen **(L)** of the capillary. The endothelial cells **(E)** extend into the lumen to form vacuoles **(V→)**.

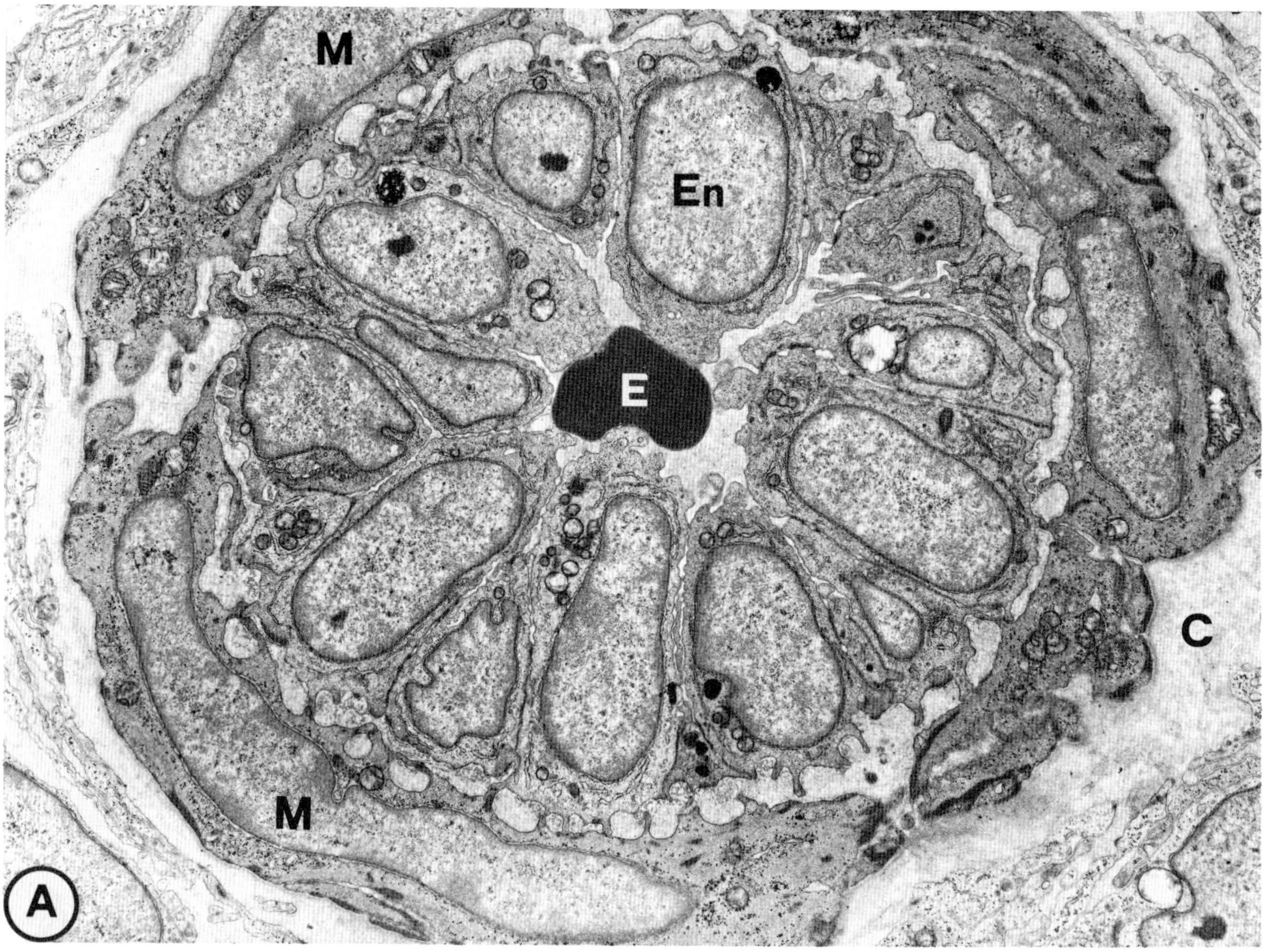

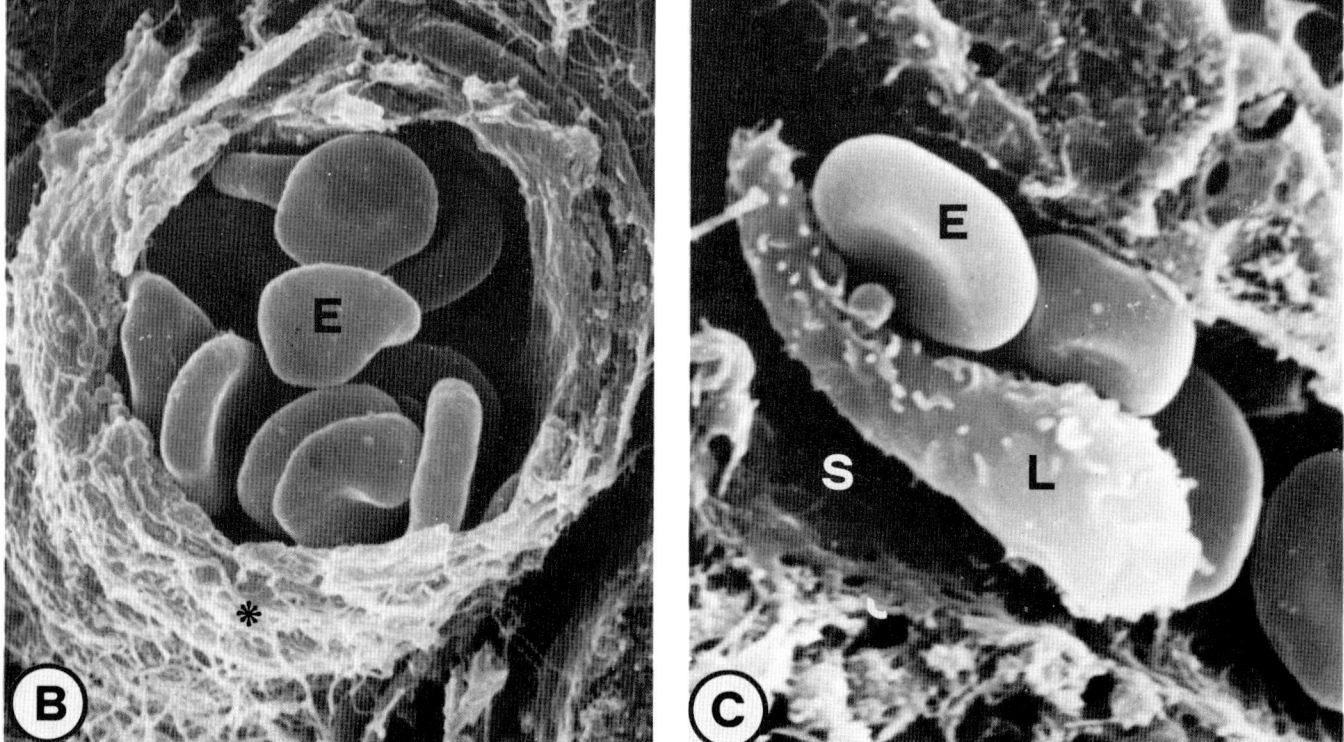

A **Arteriole from rabbit ovary (EM, x16,400).** The vessel has greatly contracted and its lumen, in cross section, is reduced to a star-shaped fissure containing a partly deformed erythrocyte (**E**). **En** = endothelium. **M** = smooth muscle cells of the arteriole wall. **C** = connective tissue.

B **Arteriole from rat hypophysis (scanning EM, x8,100).** The wall of the vessel is slightly contracted and contains in its lumen a mass of erythrocytes (**E**). The vessel is wrapped in a thin web of collagen fibers (*****). Original micrograph by S. Correr.

C **Sinusoidal capillary from rat liver (scanning EM, x14,200).** The erythrocytes (**E**) and a leukocyte (**L**), deformed perhaps by the narrowness of the capillary lumen (**S**), can be seen. Original by F. Barberini.

Plate 7.19   155

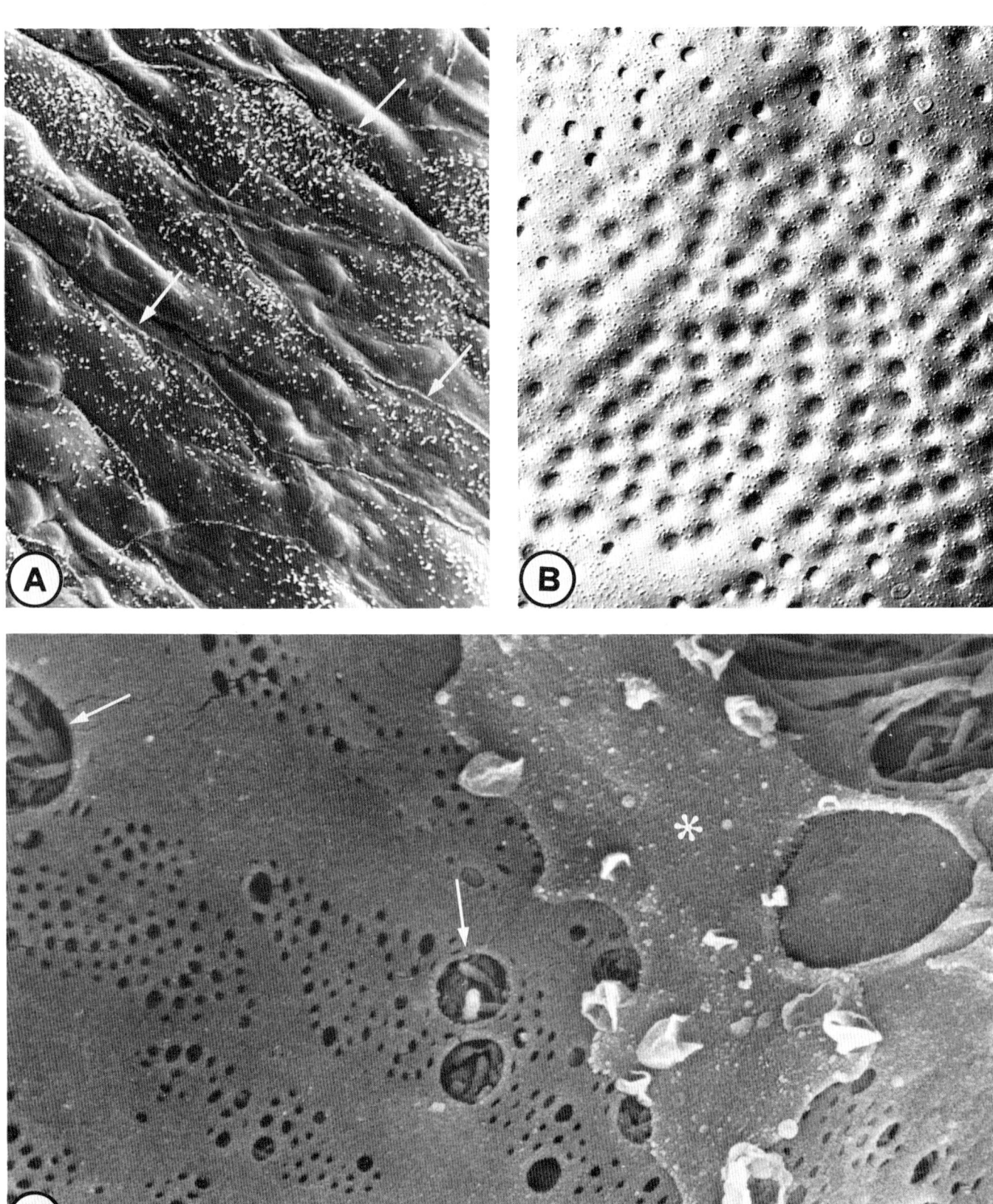

A   **Endocardium from a rat (scanning EM, x1,700).** The flattened endothelial cells form a continuous wall. The microvilli are arrayed on the central part of the cells, whose raised edges are clearly visible (→).

B   **Fenestrated endothelium from a thyroid capillary (EM, freeze-fracture, x42,000).** The endothelial wall of the vessel has many characteristic small pores. The capillaries of many internal secretion glands have this appearance. By courtesy of K. Ishimura and H. Fujita.

C   **Fenestrated endothelium from sinusoidal capillary in the liver (scanning EM, x14,200).** The very thin endothelium has large and small pores (fenestrations) (→). The wall of the sinusoid has a macrophage whose cytoplasm spreads to cover the inner surface of the endothelial lumen (Kupffer cell). From P.M. Motta. In: *Progress in Liver Diseases, Vol VII.* H. Popper and P. Schaffner (eds). Grune & Stratton Inc., New York, 1982.

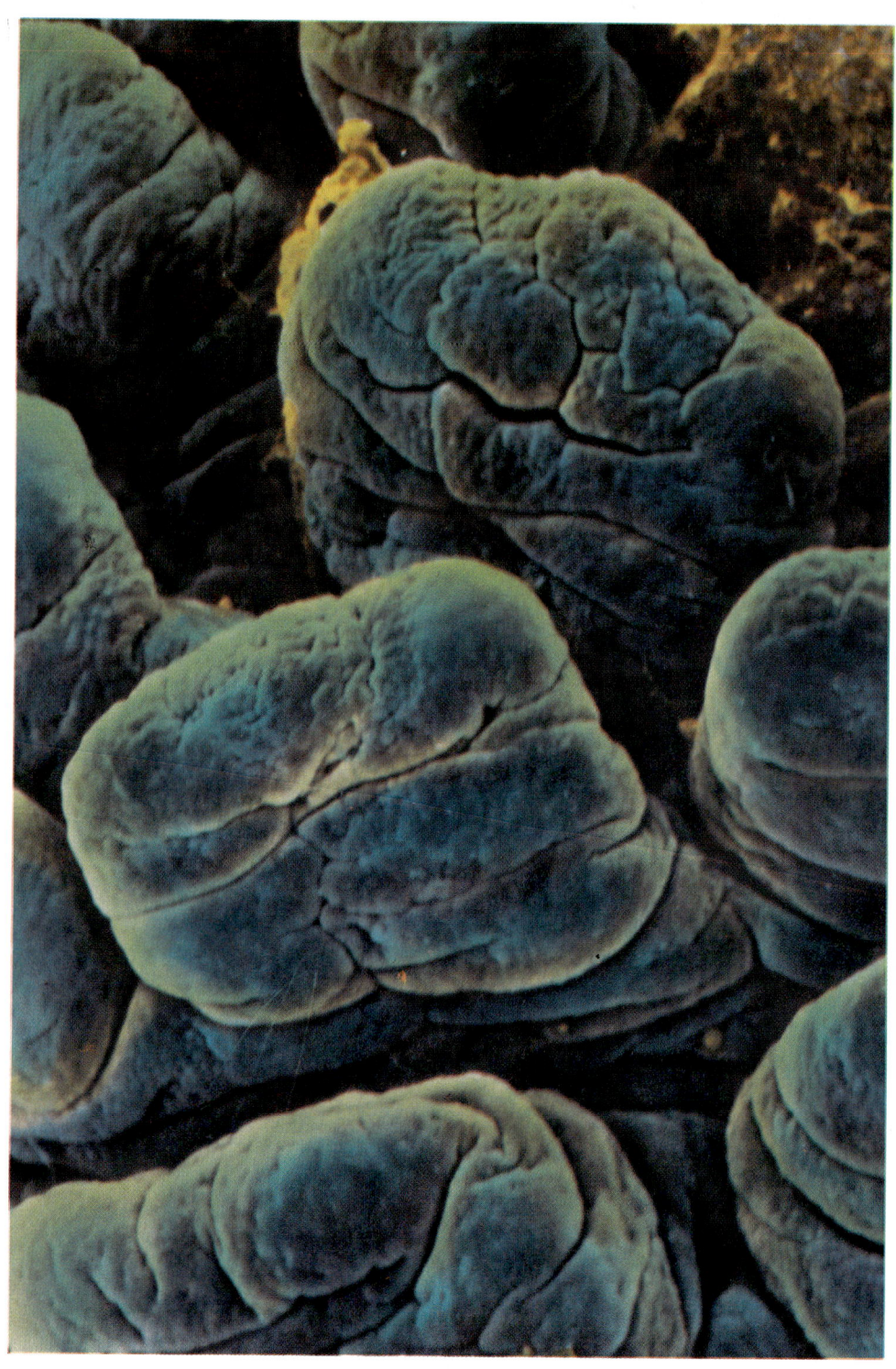

Surface view of intestinal villi of rat duodenum. (Colored SEM; 290 x).

ORGANS OF THE ORAL CAVITY

Teeth

The teeth are very hard structures attached within the sockets of the alveolar bone of the jaws. They function in mastication.

The *fully grown tooth* (Plates 3.12, 8.1 C).

Every tooth has a *crown,* a *neck,* and one or more *roots.* The crown projects from the gingiva. The neck is the constricted portion between the crown and the root. The root is implanted firmly into the cavity of the jaw-bone, the alveolus. At the tip of the root is an aperture (*apical foramen*) leading into a canal that extends the length of the root and expands at the level of the crown (*dental cavity*). Inside this cavity is the *dental pulp,* consisting of connective tissue with an abundant network of vessels and nerves. A special connective tissue (dentin) is the principal tissue of the teeth (see Chapter 3). Covering the crown is a layer of *enamel* which is a *cuticle* derived from epithelium. Enamel is formed of apatite crystals arranged in thin *prisms* which are bound together by a calcified material. Adhering to the dentin around the root and much of the neck is a layer of bone tissue (*cementum*) containing fibers (*Sharpey's fibers*) of the periodontium that fix the tooth in the alveolus. In the cavity containing the dental pulp the *odontoblasts* are arranged on the surface that faces the dentin. The hard tissues of the tooth (dentin, enamel and cementum) lack blood vessels.

Tooth buds (Plate 8.1 A,B). At the beginning of the second month after birth the epithelium thickens along the edge of the future upper and lower jaws to form the *dental ridges* of the oral cavity. The thickening forms a layer that lies over the underlying mesenchyme. At the sites of the future teeth the epithelium grows down into the mesenchyme to form the tooth germs. Each germ hollows out to form an inverted cup while the surrounding mesenchyme condenses to form a

thin layer (*dental sac*) on the outside of the tooth germ, and the *dental papilla* that will form the pulp of the tooth. The more superficial layers of the tooth germ are transformed into the *enamel organ* in the following manner. The cells that line the dental papilla lengthen into cylinders and become a uniform layer (the *adamantine membrane*). The cells in the outermost layer of the tooth germ flatten to become the external enamel epithelium, while the innermost layer becomes the internal enamel epithelium. Between these two layers the cells become stellate and form the enamel pulp. The cells of the dental papilla adjacent to the internal enamel epithelium differentiate into odontoblasts, which begin to produce dentin in one direction only, that is, on the surface facing the adamantine membrane. While the odontoblasts produce dentin the enamel organ forms a covering of enamel. The dental papilla transforms into the dental pulp. Thus the hard and soft structures of the tooth are created.

The roots form relatively late in tooth development, and in this instance the epithelial tooth germ does not form a layer of enamel; rather, the mesenchyme of the dental papilla forms odontoblasts, which in turn form dentin. Cementum forms around the dentin of the root where the disappearance of the enamel organ allows the root to come into direct contact with the connective tissue of the dental sac.

Tongue

The tongue can be described as a flattened cone. It is mobile and composed of a web of striated muscle covered by the mucosa of the oral cavity. Anatomically, the tongue is divided into the *root,* the *corpus* and the *tip.*

The mucosa that covers the upper (dorsal) surface of the tongue, especially the corpus and the tip, looks velvety to the naked eye. This appearance is due to the presence of many small elevations, the *papillae.* There are four types of

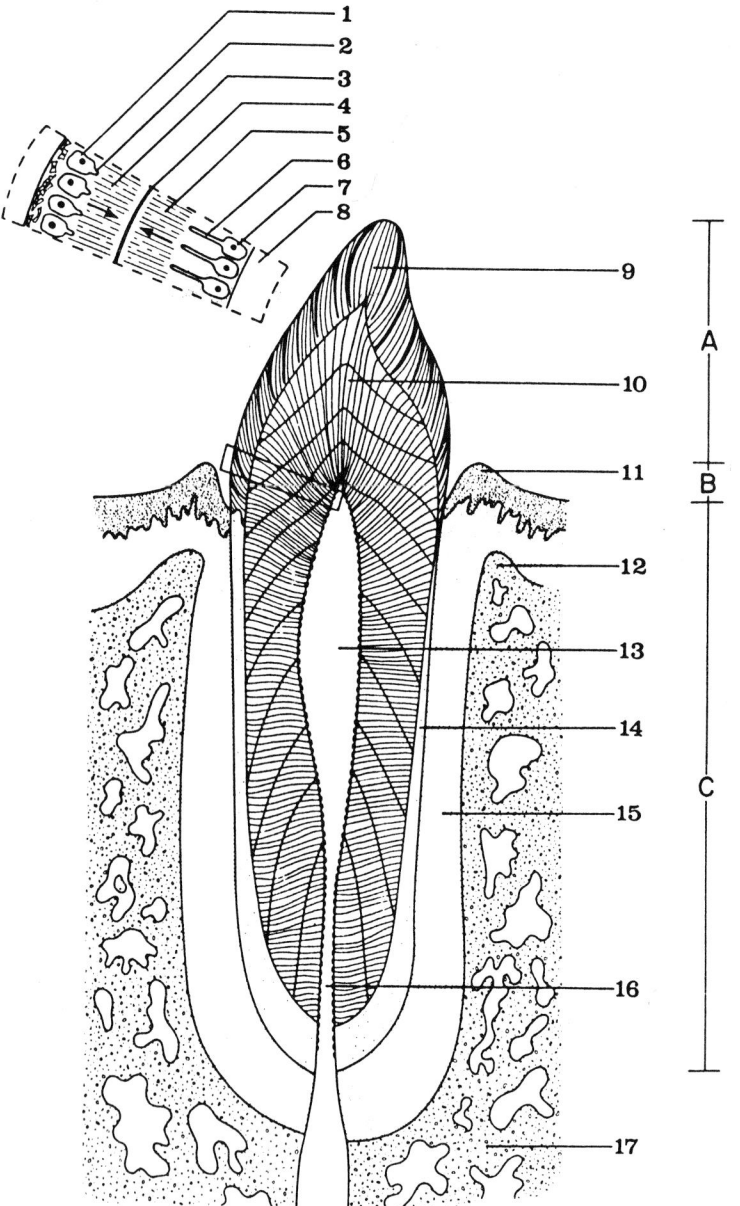

Longitudinal section of a tooth

The inset (above left) shows a small area of the tooth during the development of enamel and dentin. The arrows indicate the direction in which both enamel and dentin are deposited.

  1 Ameloblasts
  2 Tomes' processes of ameloblasts
  3 Enamel
  4 Enamel-dentin junction
  5 Dentin
  6 Tomes' fibers of odontoblasts
  7 Odontoblasts
  8 Connective tissue of pulp cavity
  9 Enamel (mature tooth)
 10 Dentin (mature tooth)
 11 Gingiva
 12 Rim of alveolus
 13 Pulp cavity
 14 Cementum
 15 Periodontal membrane
 16 Apical foramen
 17 Bone
  A Crown of tooth
  B Neck
  C Root

From P.M. Motta, P.M. Andrews and K.R. Porter. *Microanatomy of Cell and Tissue Surfaces. An Atlas of Scanning Electron Microscopy.* Lea & Febiger, Philadelphia, 1977.

papillae in the mucosa of the human tongue (Plates 8.2, 8.3 A,B). *Filiform papillae* are the most numerous. They have an elongated conical shape and are arranged in rows that run obliquely from the median sulcus to the margins. *Foliate papillae* are rudimentary in humans but highly developed in other mammals. Occurring on the back margins of the corpus they comprise 4-8 fine transverse ridges with furrows between the ridges. *Fungiform papillae* are larger and covered with non-keratinizing stratified squamous epithelium. *Circumvallate papillae* lie in a V-shaped array in front of a depression called the sulcus terminalis. Each of these papillae is composed of a cylindrical elevation surrounded by a deep furrow and bounded by a rim (vallum). They are well sup-

plied with taste buds (see Chapter 2 and Plate 2.6 A). In the furrow of the vallum are the openings of *von Ebner glands.*

The lamina propria of the tongue mucosa (Plate 8.3 A,B) is a connective tissue composed of dense fibrils adhering to the muscle layer underlying the upper side and margins of the tongue. On the ventral side of the tongue the lamina propria adheres loosely because of an intervening submucosal layer. Masses of lymphocytes occur in the root and form lymphatic nodules that are part of the palatine and lingual tonsils. On the tip and dorsal surface of the corpus the elevations that reflect the underlying connective tissue framework of the papillae can be seen. On the papillae themselves are secondary elevations which enclose a core of connective tissue beneath the papilla under the stratified epithelium.

Glands of the oral cavity

Salivary glands are located either within the lamina propria of the mucosa lining the oral cavity or within the tongue muscle itself (*lingual glands*). Salivary glands can also occur in the submucosa of the palate. In addition, there are 3 pairs of large glands which constitute the salivary glands proper. They are the parotid, the submandibular and the sublingual glands. All salivary glands are composite glands, each classified according to the type of secretion they produce. The glands may be serous (parotid and taste, or von Ebner's glands), mucous (glands of the palate and tongue root), or mixed (containing serous and mucous secretion units), all the remaining glands.

The main excretory duct of salivary glands has secondary branches which subdivide as far as the so-called *intercalated ducts* that lead to the secretory units.

Parotid gland (Plate 8.6 C). In the parotid gland each lobule is made up of secretory units with intercalated (*preterminal*) ducts joining each of them to a branch of the excretory duct. The lobules are separated by septa of connective tissue usually rich in adipose cells. The epithelium in the excretory ducts is double-layered. The main excretory duct branches into ducts classified as interlobular, sublobular and intralobular. Between the interlobular ducts and the secretory units are the intercalated ducts, which are particularly long in this gland and are lined by a flattened epithelium. In some cases a group of secretory units can be seen grouped around the intercalated duct. In histological sections each unit has the appearance of a large acinus whose lumen merges with the intercalated duct. In such instances the cells of the intercalated duct resemble the centroacinar cells typical of the pancreas. In both interlobular and sublobular ducts the double-layered epithelium has at the basal region of the cells perpendicular striations that result from the alignment of the mitochondria. For this reason ductal areas with this appearance are called *striated ducts (salivary canaliculi)*. Their function is the active resorption of sodium ions.

The epithelium of intercalated ducts passes

abruptly to that of striated ducts. In non-striated sublobular ducts and in interlobular ducts the basal cells are more evident, and the surrounding duct membrane, which is composed of elastic connective tissue, is thicker. In the parotid duct the epithelium is trilaminar up to the intersection of the buccinator muscle and the mucosa of the vestibulum of the mouth. The epithelium then becomes multi-layered and is sheathed in a thick lamina propria of elastic connective tissue.

The secretory units can either be acinar or shaped like branched tubules. These units are lined by secretory cells whose nuclei, in the light microscopic image, appear in a row. The secretory cells are pyramid-shaped and contain granules. The basal part of the cells has abundant rough endoplasmic reticulum. Between the cells are narrow intercellular spaces or canaliculi (*secretory capillaries*). Tight junctions join the cells near their bases so that the canaliculi communicate with the lumen of the gland. The secretory cells have an underlying layer of myoepithelial cells (basket cells) which rest on a basal lamina.

Von Ebner's taste glands (Plate 8.3 A) in humans are associated with the circumvallate and foliate papillae. They are serous glands, although they have tubular branching secretory units. The secretory cells are usually buried within the muscle fibers of the tongue. Typical intercalated and striated ducts are not encountered in their duct systems.

The glands occurring in the palate and tongue root are, as we have seen, pure mucous glands and have a duct system that lacks striated ducts or obvious intercalated ducts. There are two types of cells in their secretory epithelium, so that two kinds of mucus are produced. The two types of cells are mixed at random in the mucous glands of the tongue, whereas in those of the palate there are secretory tubules lined by one cell type only, as well as mixed tubules. Like other salivary glands, the ducts are lined by a double layer of epithelium, and isolated goblet cells are found in the interlobular ducts.

Mixed glands vary greatly in structure.

In the *submandibular glands* (Plates 7.6, 8.6 D, 8.7 A) some of the secretory units are serous and some are mucus-secreting. In shape they are predominantly tubuloacinar, and they may be simple or branched. The mucus-secreting acini not only secrete mucus, but are usually mixed, having serous cells arranged in a sort of cap covering the end of the unit (*demilunes of Giannuzzi*). The serous cells have canaliculi between them, and occasionally they are intercalated individually among the mucous cells. The mucin produced by the latter cells does not stain with aniline dyes. In the intercalated ducts either the mucin does not stain at all or the cells show a simultaneous seromucous reaction. The basal myoepithelial cells are stellate, while the intercalated ducts have variations in shape, branching and length. The intercalated ducts can, as in the pancreas but less so, penetrate the lumen of the serous acini so that the cells of the ducts are said to be centroacinar cells. The interlobular ducts have constrictions and dilations that give the ducts an irregular caliber, and also blind tubular diverticula whose lining cells stain like mucous cells but are not goblet-shaped. The epithelium of the excretory ducts has two layers of cells; the main duct is also lined by a stratified epithelium. The superficial cells in these ducts occasionally have cilia.

The *sublingual glands* (Plate 8.7 B), which open into the sublingual duct, are partly mixed and partly pure mucous glands. The serous cells are rather mucoserous and produce mucin with liquid rather than viscous characteristics. It is the shape of the secretory portions and the cell arrangements that determine the variability of these glands, so that intercalated ducts with mucous cells are found interspersed with ducts that contain no mucus cells. Muciferous and non-muciferous ducts can occur without the presence of striated ducts in the mucus-secreting regions of the glands. As in the duct of the submandibular gland, the interlobular excretory ducts include striated ducts having dilations or constrictions with blind diverticula.

The *small sublingual glands* (excluding the linguo-palatal glands, which are mucous) have in part the characteristics of the submandibular gland and in part those of the major, large sublingual gland. The anterior *labial and buccal salivary glands* are similar in structure to the submandibular gland. The glands situated behind the outlet of the parotid duct have no striated ducts. The intercalated ducts are short and most of the secretion is of the mucous type. The more rostral of the anterior lingual glands are mucoserous,

while the aboral glands are purely mucous. These glands lack striated ducts.

The different glands are clearly distinguishable histologically. In section the submandibular gland shows a uniform distribution of mucous and serous units with the interlobular excretory ducts having a broad lumen. In the sublingual gland, however, translucent secretory regions predominate with few excretory ducts with broad lumens. The secretory cells of the parotid gland are serous only. In the other mixed glands lightly staining cells (mucous) are visible, each having a flattened nucleus at its base. Associated with them are basophil cells having a round central nucleus (serous cells).

DIGESTIVE TRACT

The digestive tract is a long tube extending from the base of the pharynx to the anus. Its constituent parts vary in width, shape and function, and are classified as esophagus, stomach, small intestine and large intestine. The wall of the digestive tract is composed primarily of four layers, the *mucosa, submucosa, muscularis* and *serosa* or *adventitia.*

Esophagus

The esophagus connects the pharynx to the stomach.

The *inner surface of the esophagus* (Plate 8.3 C,D) displays longitudinal folds. The mucosa consists of a layer of stratified non-keratinized squamous epithelium which is a continuation of the epithelium lining the pharynx and extends as far as the gastric epithelium. In certain areas the esophagus contains islets of epithelium similar to that of gastric mucosa. At the esophago-gastric junction there is in the mucosa an abrupt transition from stratified squamous to simple columnar epithelium of the stomach. The lamina propria of the mucosa is composed of a membranous layer of fibrillar connective tissue with sparse and irregularly distributed elastic fibers. In the lamina propria there is a certain area facing the epithelium that is in the form of small crests (with and without papillae) or rows of papillae. These papillae, in the lower part of the esophagus where the folds are less frequent, can push up the epithelium and give it an irregular appearance. The muscularis mucosae is distinct and consists of

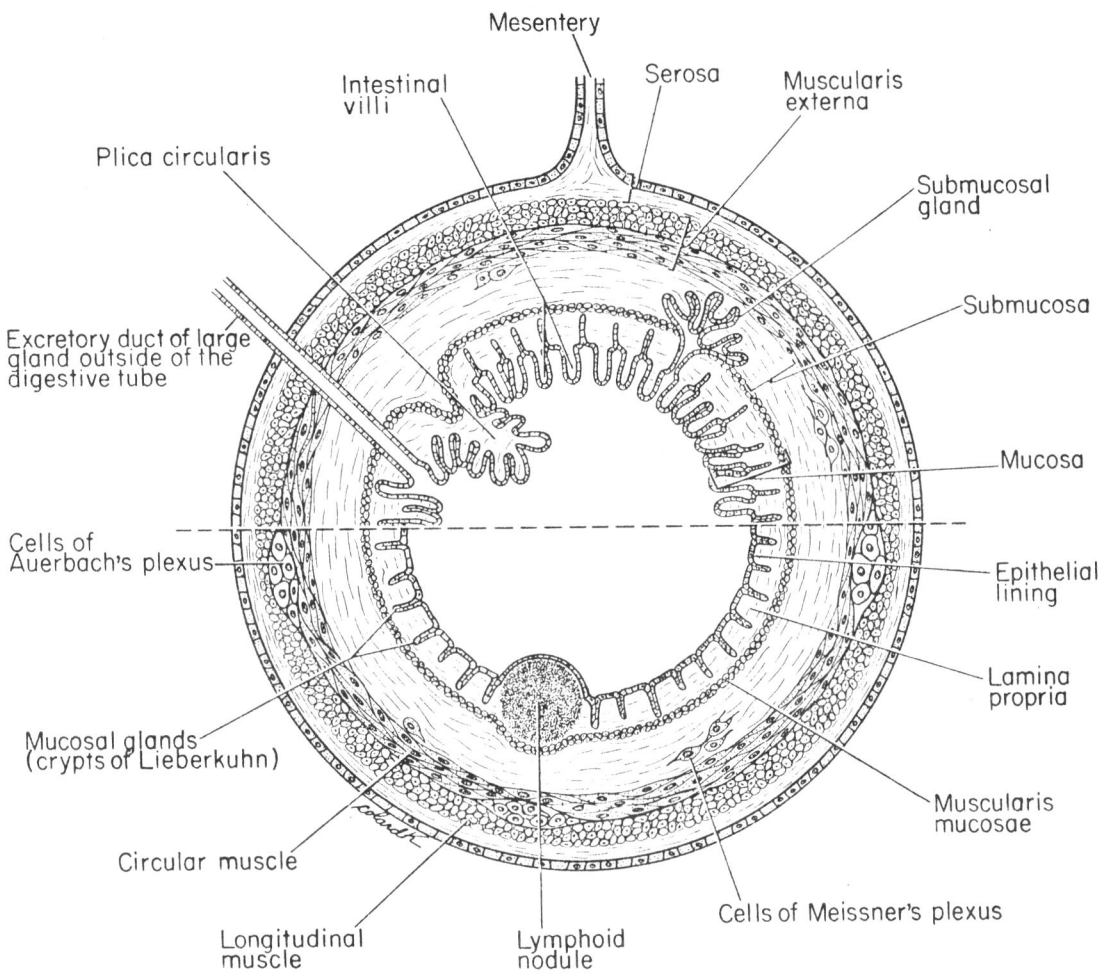

Mesentery

Intestinal villi

Serosa

Muscularis externa

Plica circularis

Submucosal gland

Submucosa

Excretory duct of large gland outside of the digestive tube

Mucosa

Cells of Auerbach's plexus

Epithelial lining

Lamina propria

Mucosal glands (crypts of Lieberkuhn)

Circular muscle

Muscularis mucosae

Longitudinal muscle

Lymphoid nodule

Cells of Meissner's plexus

Diagram of the wall of the digestive tract. The concentric layers, the serosa, muscularis, submucosa and mucosa are present throughout the length of the gut. In the upper half of the figure the mucosa has villi and glands as it does in the small intestine, but in the lower half it has only glands, as in the colon. By courtesy of D.W. Fawcett. In: W. Bloom and D.W. Fawcett, *A Textbook of Histology*. 10th ed. W.B. Saunders Co., Philadelphia/London/Toronto, 1975.

bundles of smooth muscle tissue running longitudinally. The thick submucosa is composed of a layer of loose connective tissue.

The glands of the esophagus are of two types. The *esophageal glands,* having the same structure as mucous salivary glands, are in the submucosa. The *cardiac glands* are in the lamina propria. These glands are classified as superior cardiac glands when in association with the islets of gastric mucosa in the esophagus and inferior cardiac glands when found in the transition zone between esophageal mucosa and gastric mucosa. The latter glands have a structure typical of cardiac glands in the stomach. Histologically they are branched tubular glands with numerous mucoid cells.

The muscularis includes one internal circular layer and an external longitudinal layer of muscle. Its fibers are mainly striated in the upper third,

smooth in the lower third and mixed in various proportions in the middle third. The adventitia is composed of loose connective tissue that is rich in elastic and collagen fibers with several lobules of adipose tissue. This layer appears to be joined to the connective tissue that forms a sheath around the neighboring organs. In the abdominal part of the esophagus the tunica adventitia becomes the tunica serosa.

Stomach

The stomach is the dilated segment of the digestive tract between the esophagus and the small intestine. Its function is to receive and mix food while initiating digestion. The inner surface of the stomach is subdivided into small *gastric areas* which are further subdivided by small grooves and perforated at regular intervals by invaginations, the *gastric pits (foveolae gastricae),* which lead into the gastric glands of the fundus of the stomach.

Wall of the stomach (Plate 8.4 A,B,C). The lining epithelium of the gastric mucosa consists of simple columnar mucous cells. In the gastric pits the epithelium is thinner and the cells are often in mitosis. The lamina propria is composed of fibrillar connective tissue that surrounds the many glands. This tissue varies in structure and shape according to its location in the stomach. The well-differentiated muscularis mucosae comprises two or three layers of muscle cells oriented in different planes of space.

The glands of the stomach, which can be simple or branched, lie in the mucosal layer. There are four types of stomach glands: *cardiac glands, gastric glands proper, pyloric glands* and *intestinal glands* (Plate 8.8 C). The cardiac glands are tubular, highly branched glands with cyst-like dilations. They are composed primarily of mucous cells with occasional parietal cells, and resemble pyloric glands.

The gastric glands proper occupy the body and the fundus of the stomach. They are simple tubular glands opening into the gastric pits. The gland is composed of a bulbous basal part, the *fundus,* the *corpus,* and a tapering apex, the *isthmus,* which is a transitional area leading to the gastric pit. The secretory cells of the fundic part of the gland are principally of two types: *zymogenic* or *chief cells,* filled with pepsinogen granules which may stain only lightly, and *parietal cells,* which are large, stain readily and contain intracellular secretory canaliculi which are the sites of hydrochloric acid secretion. In addition, these glands are composed of mucous, argentaffin and APUD cells. These two latter types are endocrine cells. All these types of cells rest on a basal lamina.

The pyloric glands are tubular or branched, formed mainly of one type of cell that is similar to the chief cells of the gastric glands proper that occur in the fundus of the stomach. Mucous cells are found among the other type of secretory cells in these glands.

The intestinal glands occasionally encountered in the pre-pyloric region and the lesser curvature may be considered tubular crypts of the mucosa.

The lamina propria of the stomach is a supporting framework of fibrillar connective tissue which becomes reticular where it surrounds the glands and directly underlies the epithelium. In its deeper regions are elastic fibers and bundles of smooth muscle extending from the muscularis mucosae. The extensive submucosa is composed of loose connective tissue. Scattered lymphocytes, plasma cells and small groups of eosinophils are encountered in the body of the stomach, while more conspicuous aggregations of lymphocytes occur in the antrum of the pylorus. The muscularis is composed of three layers of muscle fibers. The inner layer is disposed obliquely, the middle layer is circular, and the outer layer is longitudinal. In the pyloric region of the stomach the inner circular layer becomes a strong ring of muscle (*pyloric sphincter*). The serosa is called the peritoneum when it lines the abdominal cavity and forms a sheath around the organs of the visceral cavity.

Small intestine

The small intestine is the longest part of the digestive tract (about 6 meters). It consists of 3 segments having many common characteristics: *duodenum, jejunum* and *ileum.* The function of the small intestine is to complete the digestion of proteins, carbohydrates and lipids, and to absorb selectively the final products of the digestive process. Its inner surface is raised in many circular folds (*plicae circulares*). Each of these folds has an underlying framework of connective tissue (from the submucosa), and is covered by the mucosa, which itself is folded to form the villi of the intestine.

The *wall of the intestine* (Plates 8.4 D, 8.5 A,B,C). The mucosal surface of the intestine is lined by a single layer of columnar epithelial cells (absorptive or intestinal cells) having numerous microvilli on their free surface, forming a striated border (Plate 8.9 A), and muciferous goblet cells scattered among them (Plate 2.4 A, 2.5). Among these two types is found another type of cell which stains brown when treated with chromium or silver salts (*argentaffin* or *enterochromaffin cells*). These cells are most numerous in the epithelial lining of the intestinal glands or crypts, but similar cells are also found among the secretory cells of the gastric glands and the glands or crypts of the large intestine (*enterochromaffin cell system*) (Plates 8.10, 8.11).

The lamina propria of the small intestine is

composed of reticular connective tissue with interspersed accumulations of lymphocytes (*solitary lymph nodules*). In certain areas, such as the ileum, these nodules form *aggregated lymph nodules* or *Peyer's patches,* which can extend into the submucosa. The mucosa is demarcated from the submucosa by the muscularis mucosae, a thin layer of smooth muscle cells.

The villi are elevations of the intestinal mucosa (Plate 8.8 A,B) covered by the intestinal epithelium. The supporting stroma of each villus (core of the villus) is made up of the connective tissue of the lamina propria and smooth muscle of the muscularis mucosae. Arterioles enter the villi and become capillaries, thus forming arteriovenous loops that regulate the flow of blood in the capillaries. In the core of the villus are one or two lacteals (lymph capillaries), nerves and a venule that collects the venous blood. The *intestinal glands* (of Galeazzi) open into furrows (sulci) that exist between each villus. These are tubular glands embedded perpendicularly within the lamina propria of the mucosa. The lining of these glands is composed of epithelial cells (which undergo frequent mitosis and are similar to the absorptive cells of the mucosa) and a variable number of goblet cells. In the fundus of these glands, also called the *crypts of Lieberkuhn,* are granular cells thought to secrete lysozyme and peptidases (*Paneth cells*). The intestinal glands are composite tubulo-acinar glands only in the duodenum. Some extend from the lamina propria into the submucosa. Where their secretory units occur they are called *Brunner's duodenal glands.*

The thin submucosa is composed of loose, fibrillar connective tissue containing vessels and nerves (*Meissner's submucosal plexus*). The muscularis has an inner circular layer and an outer longitudinal layer, both composed of smooth muscle. Between the circular and the longitudinal layers is a lamina that is rich in elastic fibers and contains a fine nerve network, *Auerbach's myenteric plexus.* The serosa forms a sheath around the intestine.

Glands associated with the duodenum

Besides the intestinal glands that are present throughout the intestine there are glands in association with the duodenum, i.e. Brunner's duodenal glands (intraparietal glands), the pancreas and the liver (extraparietal glands).

Brunner's duodenal glands (Plates 8.4 C,D)

The excretory duct of the duodenal glands runs either directly into the cavity of the duodenum or into the crypts of the duodenal glands. This highly branched duct, which is already subdivided at the point of intersection with the lamina propria of the mucosa, continues to branch as far as the submucosa. The glands are arrayed in a continuous layer in the upper and descending portions of the organ, but become rare below the lower duodenal papilla. The secretory units occur in both the lamina propria and the submucosa, so that they have a distinct inner portion within the mucosa and an outer region within the submucosa. They are composite tubulo-acinar glands composed of only a single layer of secretory mucoid cells and a few intercalated parietal cells. Among them are found isolated enterochromaffin cells (Plate 8.10 C,D).

Pancreas

The pancreas is a large extraparietal gland associated with the duodenum. It contains two components whose cells have totally different functions, the exocrine pancreas and the pancreatic islets which make up the endocrine pancreas (see p. 183).

Exocrine pancreas (Plates 8.7 C, 8.12). In its construction the pancreas has much in common with the parotid gland. There are two excretory ducts (the *main* and *accessory* ducts) whose function is to empty the pancreatic enzymes into the duodenum. The intercalated ducts of its very low epithelium branch in a way that characterizes the organ. Unlike the parotid gland, the pancreas has its acini located not at the end of the intercalated ducts but along them. Among the acinar cells which contain abundant rough endoplasmic reticulum are often encountered the so-called *centroacinar cells.* These cells can be either undifferentiated gland cells which closely resemble the cells of intercalated ducts, or true intercalated duct cells in the lumen of the acinus and ensheathed by its secretory cells. The glands have myoepithelial basket cells, but they lack striated ducts. The superficial cells of the excretory ducts are mucoid. In histological section the pancreas is

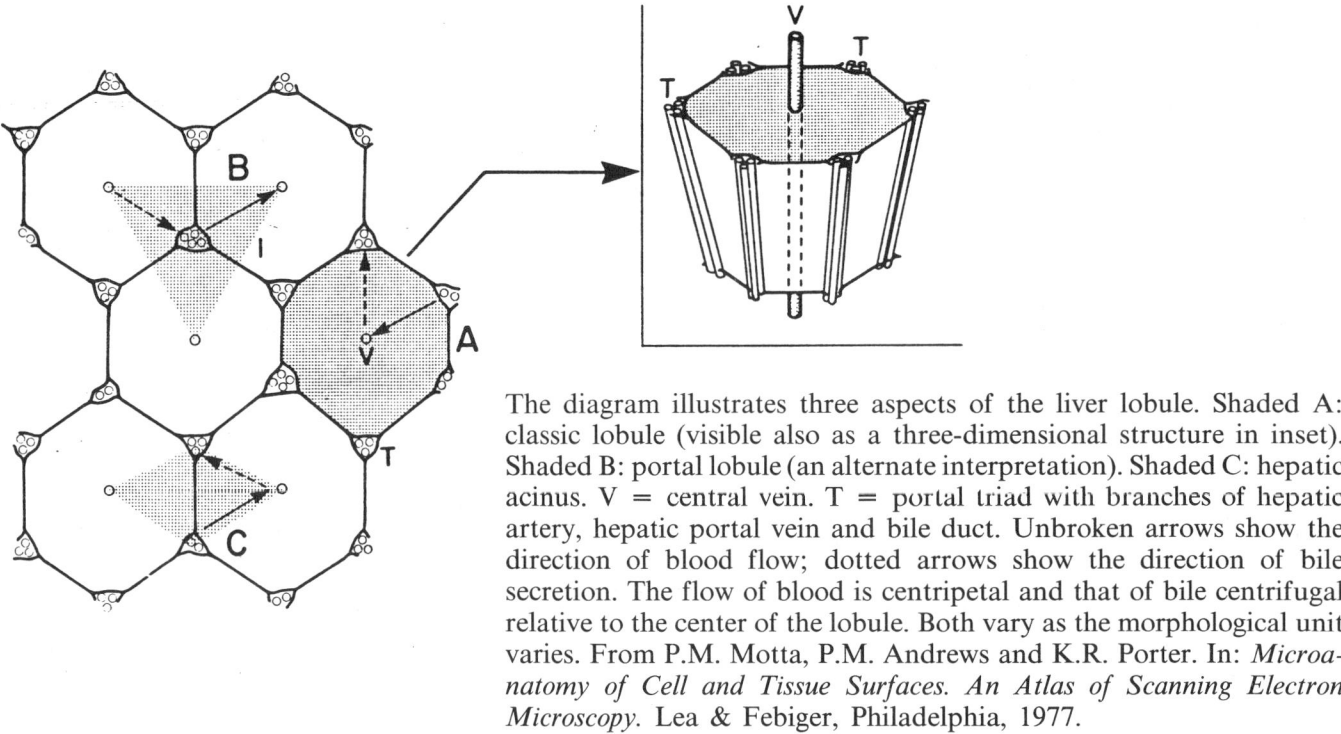

The diagram illustrates three aspects of the liver lobule. Shaded A: classic lobule (visible also as a three-dimensional structure in inset). Shaded B: portal lobule (an alternate interpretation). Shaded C: hepatic acinus. V = central vein. T = portal triad with branches of hepatic artery, hepatic portal vein and bile duct. Unbroken arrows show the direction of blood flow; dotted arrows show the direction of bile secretion. The flow of blood is centripetal and that of bile centrifugal relative to the center of the lobule. Both vary as the morphological unit varies. From P.M. Motta, P.M. Andrews and K.R. Porter. In: *Microanatomy of Cell and Tissue Surfaces. An Atlas of Scanning Electron Microscopy.* Lea & Febiger, Philadelphia, 1977.

distinguishable from the parotid gland (disregarding the pancreatic islands that may be visible), because the system of intralobular excretory ducts, so prominent in the parotid gland, is not visible in the pancreas.

Liver

The liver is a large organ composed of glandular cells and having a complex function. A special network of vessels (portal system) present in this organ brings the blood directly from the digestive tract to the liver. As a glandular organ it produces a secretion, *bile,* which has a role in the digestion of fats. The liver receives through the portal vein blood containing metabolites absorbed from the digestive tract and plays a major role in the metabolism of proteins, carbohydrates and lipids. In the fetus the liver is a blood-producing organ.

Structure of the hepatic lobule (Plates 8.13, 8.17 A). A liver lobule has the shape of a polyhedral prism, often hexagonal in section, and, depending on the species, is more or less demarcated by septa of connective tissue which support the vessels, nerves and bile ducts. Where several lobules abut one sees a thicker layer of connective tissue within which are found a branch of the hepatic artery, hepatic portal vein and bile duct, the so-called portal area. The hepatic portal vein conveys the venous blood, rich in nutrients, as it returns from the gut; the fine

branches of the hepatic artery bring arterial blood to the liver. The bile ducts associated with these vessels collect the bile secreted by the lobule in order to convey it into the common bile duct and thence into the intestine. The branches of the hepatic portal vein and the hepatic artery that pass through the portal areas between the lobules are called the *interlobular branches.* From the portal area the blood vessels enter into the sinusoidal capillaries within the lobule. The blood flows toward the center of the lobule where it is collected into the central vein, the *centrolobular vein,* so called because of its axial position in the center of the lobule. This vein, after passing longitudinally through the lobule, opens at its base into the sublobular vein. The sublobular veins converge to form the hepatic veins, which discharge into the inferior vena cava. The network of sinusoids passes radially through plates of hepatocytes (*hepatic cords*) (Plate 8.18 C).

The liver cell, bile canaliculi and *sinusoids* (Plates 8.13, 8.14, 8.15, 8.16, 8.17, 8.18). The liver cords are composed of at least two adjacent plates of cells which between them form the bile canaliculi. The histological appearance of the hepatocytes varies with the functional phases of the cells. In the hepatocyte cytoplasm can be seen numerous typical mitochondria, as well as rough endoplasmic reticulum, glycogen granules, lipid droplets and often bile pigments and microbodies. The nucleus is large and spheroid (cells with two nuclei occur) and contains one or more nucleoli. The surface of a liver cell forms a small furrow which combines with that of the contiguous cell to enclose a typical bile canaliculus. Within the furrow each of the two cells has numerous microvilli, and they are sealed at the edges of the furrow by tight junctions. Hence, although the sinusoidal network is nearby, the bile cannot leave the canaliculi to enter the intracellular spaces. Because the canaliculi follow the faces of the polyhedral liver cells, in certain preparations they appear as a zig-zag line.

At the periphery of the lobule the bile canaliculi converge into the bile ducts, which are small tubes of cuboid or columnar epithelium resting on a basal lamina and ensheathed by reticular connective tissue, which is continuous with the connective tissue of the portal area. The bile canaliculi are connected to the intrahepatic bile ducts by small ductules, the so-called *cholangioles (Hering ducts)*. At least three faces of every liver cell face a blood capillary. The sinusoid capillaries are lined by a very thin endothelium in which macrophages (*Kupffer's cells*) are present. These stellate cells may derive from monocytes.

The endothelium of sinusoids contains numerous fenestrations and lacks a true basal lamina. Between the liver cells and the endothelium are interwoven thin, scattered reticular fibers.

Between the wall of the sinusoidal endothelium and the hepatocyte is the so-called *space of Disse*, whose size can vary according to the functional state of the gland, and a few star-shaped cells rich in lipid droplets and vitamin A (*Ito's lipocytes* or *fat-storing cells*) can also be found in this space. The subendothelial spaces of Disse lead into the portal spaces in a series of broad prelymphatic lacunae (*Mall spaces*) from which the true lymph vessels found in the portal areas derive.

Extrahepatic ducts

The bile system outside the liver is composed of the *hepatic duct, the cystic duct,* the *gallbladder* and the *common bile duct (ductus choledochus).* The basic composition of these tubes consists of a mucosa covered by simple columnar epithelia possessing glands (*bile glands*) and supported by a layer of fibrillar connective tissue in which are embedded smooth muscle cells. Within the hepat-

ic duct these muscle cells occur in a less organized fashion, but in more compact layers in the gallbladder and common bile duct. In the cytstic duct the muscle fibers are less numerous, their place being taken by abundant elastic fibers. In the distal part of the common bile duct the bundles of muscle fiber cells are in two layers, one circular and the other longitudinal.

Gallbladder

The gallbladder is a pear-shaped sac attached to the visceral surface of the liver. Its function is to store and concentrate bile. Its three parts are the dilated fundus, the body and the neck, which merges with the cystic duct.

Wall of the gallbladder (Plate 2.3 A, 7.7 C, 8.14 C,D).

The epithelium of the mucosa is simple columnar with a striated or brush border. It is capable of secretion, by producing mucus, and absorption of water. The lamina propria is composed of two layers. The inner subendothelium is made up of connective tissue forming irregular folds, which in the fundus and body give a pitted appearance to the inner surface of the mucosa. The folds run circumferentially in the neck. The folds continue as a spiral into the cystic duct (*spiral valve*).

The layer that is peripheral to the lamina propria consists of longitudinal or circular lamellae made up of bundles of smooth muscle fibers with intervening elastic connective tissue. This fibromuscular layer is considered a true muscularis mucosae.

A layer of loose fibrillar tissue (*lamina subserosa*) on the surface separates the above fibromuscular layer from the serosa.

Large intestine

The large intestine is a tube, shorter than the small intestine (about 2 meters) but larger in diameter. It consists of 3 segments having many similar features: *cecum, colon* and *rectum.* Its function is to absorb water and salts and to evacuate the feces. The wall has semilunar folds which project into the cavity (*plicae semilunares*).

Wall of the large intestine (Plate 8.6 A,B). The almost flat surface of the tunica mucosa lacks both circular folds and villi. The mucosa consists of columnar epithelium with a brush border (Plate 2.1 C) and absorptive cells with goblet cells among them (Plate 8.8 D). In the anal region the mucosa forms a series of longitudinal folds (*rectal columns* of Morgagni). Here the crypts become shorter and disappear and the simple columnar epithelium is suddenly replaced by a stratified squamous epithelium. The lamina propria contains simple tubular glands (*crypts*) composed mainly of mucous cells among which can be found some argentaffin cells and occasional Paneth cells. The large intestine has large solitary lymph nodules which project into the epithelium and may extend into the submucosa to disrupt the muscularis mucosae. These nodules occur particularly in the blind-ending evagination of the cecum (the *appendix vermiformis*) where they are closely grouped together to form an almost continuous layer (Plate 8.6 B).

The submucosa is a thin layer and contains occasional lymphocytes. The tunica muscularis is composed of an inner circular layer of fibers and an outer longitudinal layer. Starting at the cecum this outer layer condenses into three thin, long bands, the *teniae coli.*

In the free parts of the colon the serosa separates from the surface of the intestine to form pendulous pockets filled with fat (*appendices epiploicae*).

Endocrine cells of the digestive tract

The endocrine cells responsible for producing the various hormones of the digestive tract are found among the secretory cells of the intraparietal glands of the gut and also in the epithelium of its mucosa. They are seen as small prismatic or spheroid cells always resting on the basal lamina of the mucosal epithelium (Plates 8.10, 8.11). These *gastrointestinal endocrine cells* can only be identified with certainty by using special immunochemical techniques.

The *enterochromaffin (argentaffin) cell system* is composed of cells scattered in the gastric and intestinal glands, and in the epithelium of intestinal villi. They are classified in the category of intestinal endocrine cells and produce a hormone-like substance (serotonin or 5-hydroxytryptamine) capable of stimulating smooth muscle. Other intestinal endocrine cells are responsible for producing hormones such as gastrin, glucagon (in the stomach), secretin, cholecystokinin

(formerly pancreozymin), somatostatin and neurotensin (in the small and large intestine). The endocrine cells of the pancreas (*islets of Langerhans*) could also be considered a part of the intestinal endocrine cell system, because they are contained in a gland which, although extraparietal, is associated with the digestive tract and derives from it embryologically.

RESPIRATORY TRACT

The air passages include the cavities of the nose, pharynx, larynx, trachea, bronchi, alveolar passages and the alveoli.

The pharynx, as well as having a function in respiration (*nasal pharynx*), functions in the digestive system in that the pharynx joins the mouth with the esophagus (*oral pharynx*). The larynx is the voice-producing organ.

The air passages have a mucosal lining that can be categorized into *respiratory mucosa, mucosa of the upper digestive tract and olfactory mucosa.*

Upper digestive tract mucosa is composed of stratified squamous epithelium (Plate 8.3). It is found in the vestibule of the nose as modified skin, on the surface of the tongue, and sometimes on the laryngeal surface of the epiglottis (Plate 8.19 B), on the glosso-epiglottal folds, and frequently in the vestibule of the larynx up to the free margin of the laryngeal folds. The epithelium of the false vocal cords is also stratified squamous. The change from the respiratory type of epithelium to the stratified squamous type of the upper digestive tract can be either gradual or sudden, especially in the supraglottal region of the larynx.

Olfactory mucosa (Plates 5.2 A, 8.20 A,B) is confined to that part of the nasal cavity limited by the lamina cribrosa of the ethmoid bone and by the nasal septum which lies laterally and medially in front of the superior concha. The olfactory mucosa is composed of pseudostratified epithelium in which three types of cells are found: supporting cells (sustentacular), primary sensory cells and basal cells resting on a basal lamina. The lamina propria, which contains collagen fibers and occasional elastic fibers near the surface, is rich in macrophages and other motile cells and contains numerous tubulo-alveolar glands.

Respiratory mucosa (Plates 1.32 A,B, 8.19 A,

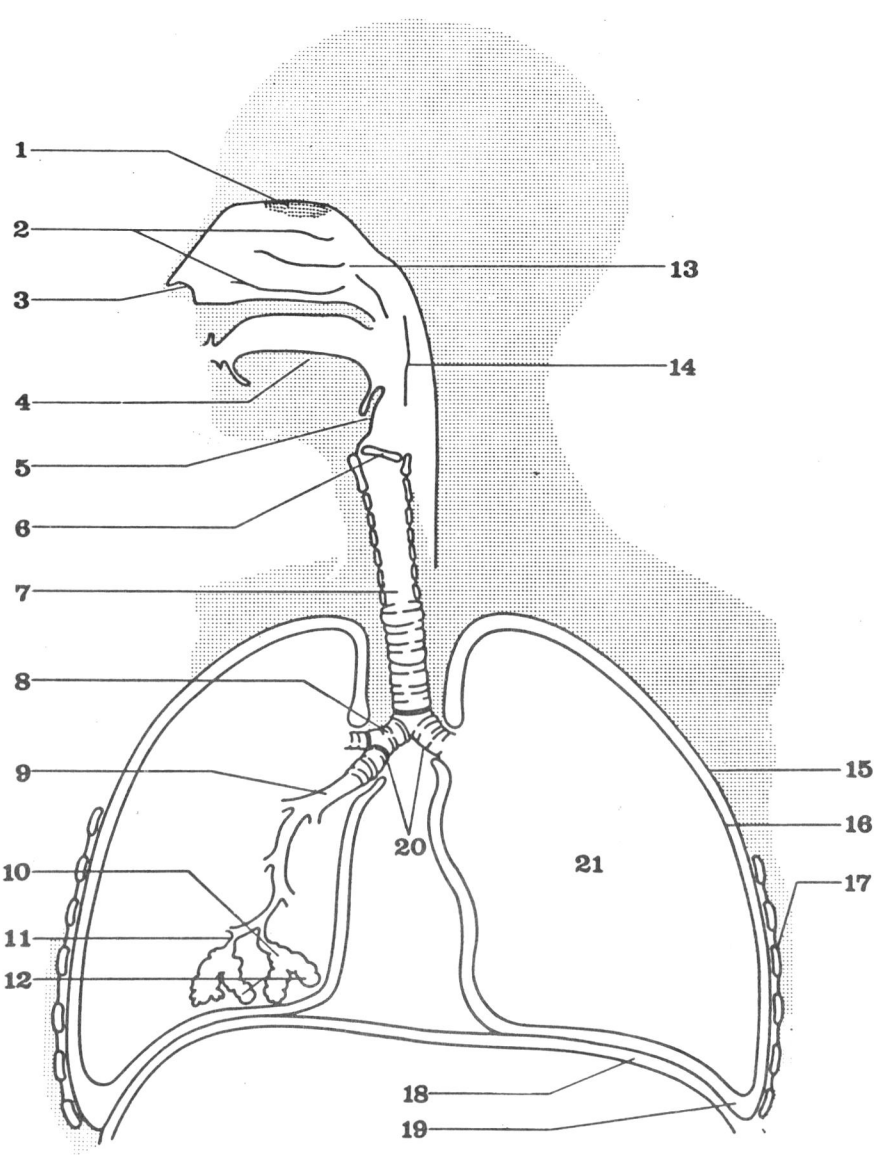

8.20 C) forms the coating of the main and accessory nasal cavities, adhering firmly to the periosteum and perichondrium. The epithelium of this mucosa is columnar with motile cilia. Between the epithelial cells goblet cells may be found either occurring singly or in groups. The thick lamina propria is composed of a subepithelial layer without papillae; this is also called the lymphoid layer because of the scattered or grouped lymphocytes contained there. Sometimes the lymphocytes occupy the subepithelial layer to such a degree that it appears to be a tonsillar glandular tissue. Normally the lymphocytes accumulate as nodules near the mouths of the mucous glands. The lamina propria also contains a middle layer and a deep layer, both of which consist of dense fibrillar connective tissue that is continuous with the periosteum, with no intervening submucosa. Elastic fibers are rare. The middle layer contains the bodies of the glands. The deep layer abounds in blood vessels. In all layers of the lamina propria are found fibrocytes and histiocytes, as well as eosinophilic and basophilic leukocytes, plasma cells and mast cells, and, quite commonly, cells containing a yellow pigment.

The glands are tubular, either composite or branched. The smaller glands remain in the subepithelial layer and the larger ones extend to the vascular layer. Usually they are located in the middle layer. The main excretory ducts are covered by columnar epithelium and have both striated ducts like those of the salivary glands and intercalated ducts composed of undifferentiated cells or mucous cells. The secretory cells of the adenomeres produce a secretion that is serous and mucous. In children and in the hypertrophied mucosa of adults the serous secretion predominates.

The mucosa of the paranasal sinuses is similar to that described above but much thinner. The lamina propria is very thin and inseparable from the periosteum. The reduced vascular layer lacks venous plexes. The epithelium is lower and grades into a single layer of columnar cells with motile cilia. Goblet cells are also present. In the mucosa covering the ethmoid bone the glands are fairly numerous, but they are rare in the maxillary sinus and very rare in the frontal and sphenoidal sinuses.

Trachea

The trachea is a semirigid tube which extends from the opening of the larynx to its division into the two main bronchi.

The *wall of the trachea* (Plates 8.21 A, 8.23 A) has a framework of fibrocartilage. The lamina fibrosa is composed of connective tissue that is rich in elastic fibers. Embedded in the lamina fibrosa are 16-20 C-shaped rings of hyaline cartilage, the open ends of the C being on the dorsal side of the body. The fibroelastic membrane is continuous around the trachea and reinforced by a layer of smooth muscle attached to the inner surface of the C-shaped rings.

The mucosa is typical of the respiratory tract. Beneath it, unlike the case in the nasal cavities, is a submucosa rich in elastic fibers. This connective tissue layer is loose between areas containing cartilage but dense in the region of the cartilaginous rings. Glands are embedded among the muscle fiber bundles.

The connective tissue that forms a sheath around the esophagus thickens around the trachea to form a sort of adventitia.

The trachea bifurcates into the left and right bronchi, which subdivide further into smaller bronchi. The walls of the bronchi have the same structure as that of the trachea. Inside the lungs the bronchi divide to form a finer network of bronchioles, becoming progressively smaller in diameter.

Lungs

It is the countless subdivisions of the bronchi that form the basis of the lungs. The microscopic endings of the tubular system are cul-de-sacs. The terminal parts of the system have numerous diverticula, the *alveoli.* The alveoli have a very thin wall within which is a capillary network fed by the branches of the pulmonary artery and drained by the roots of the pulmonary veins.

The lungs (Plates 8.21 B, 8.23) are divided into equivalent portions, the lobules. The lobules are the functional units of the lungs, being composed of a subdividing complex of *respiratory bronchioles.* Each lobule has roughly the shape of a pyramid. The outer surface of the lungs is covered by the pleura. Deeper inside the lungs each lobule adapts to the shape of its neighbor and so is an irregular polyhedron rather than a pyramid. The individual lobules are separated by interlobular septa of connective tissue. The septa become thicker when surrounding a group of lobules. Macrophages that take up debris from the atmosphere lodge within the large septa and give the surface of the lungs a speckled appearance. From the apex of the pyramid the *alveolar ducts* spread out to the base. They have no longer any trace of bronchial structure. The alveolar ducts can be likened to corridors whose walls are formed by countless pits of alveolar shape. These ducts subdivide further to end in the *alveolar sacs* or *infundibula,* which are dilations with a blind ending having sac-like evaginations arranged side by side to form their walls. The number of sacs in a lobule is about 60, but varies according to the size of each lobule. The walls of the alveoli of the same sac or of adjacent sacs are fused to form the interalveolar septa. The total number of alveoli in a pair of human lungs is about 300 million, with a surface area reaching 80-100 m². Within the lung complex the bronchi and bronchioles can be seen. Their fibrocartilage framework is modified as larger bronchi subdivide into ever smaller ones.

Wall of the bronchi and *bronchioles* (Plates 8.21 B, 8.24). The larger bronchi have the same structure as the trachea, but in smaller bronchi the layer of fibrocartilage has more elastic fibers. In the bronchi of diameter less than 1 mm (bronchioles) the cartilage, which is reduced to more or less irregular plates, finally disappears. The smooth muscle fibers thus tend to form a continuous layer circling the fibrocartilage layer on the inside. The mucosa is composed of simple columnar epithelium with cilia, with many goblet cells. Bronchial glands are numerous in the large bronchi, but their number diminishes as the bronchi subdivide. Bronchioles are characterized by the lack of supporting cartilage and glands. The mucosa of the bronchioles is composed of simple ciliated columnar epithelium without goblet cells and a thin lamina propria of elastic tissue sheathed in a spiral of smooth muscle.

The proximal part of the bronchiole has a ciliated columnar epithelium. In the distal part the epithelium loses its cilia and becomes at first cuboidal and then squamous. The lamina propria is very thin. The bundles of smooth muscle fibers gradually disappear.

Structure of the alveoli (Plates 8.22, 8.23 B,C). Each alveolus has a wall lined with squamous *small alveolar cells (Type I pneumocytes)* and with *large alveolar cells* or *septal cells (Type II pneumocytes)*. The cytoplasm of the latter type is rich in multilamellar osmiophilic bodies (*cytosomes*) and secretes a surface-active agent called *surfactant*. The alveolar epithelium rests on a thin basement membrane.

When the lung is deflated, the interalveolar septa are thick, but they are thin when it is inflated. The septa are made of a lattice of loose connective tissue rich in elastic fibers as well as in macrophages. Embedded in this lattice is a very fine network of wide-caliber capillaries separated from the overlying alveolar cells only by a basal lamina and bulging into the alveolar cavity. The interalveolar septa often have apertures of 10-15 um in diameter by which the alveoli communicate with one another (*interalveolar pores of Kohn*).

At the opening of each alveolus, besides the collagen and reticular fibers, there is a ring of smooth muscle that regulates the aperture between the cavity of the alveolus and that of the alveolar sac.

URINARY SYSTEM

Kidney

The kidney is composed of tubules each about 40-60 mm in length and numbering one to two million. The *nephron* is the basic unit of the kidney that produces and concentrates urine and transports it to a collecting tubule that excretes the urine from the kidney. The collecting tubules of the kidney form a system of ducts that become wider as they approach their outlet at the apex of the renal papilla. The nephron begins in the periphery of the parenchyma, the *cortex*. At this point it is a blind tubule which holds, almost like a clamp, an intricate capillary network, the *glomerulus*. Together with the associated tubule the glomerulus forms the *renal* (or *Malpighian*) *corpuscle*. The nephrons have their confluence in the collecting ducts which cross the papillae and increase in size to become *Bellini's papillary ducts*. The areas of the nephron that are arranged in straight lines are the region of the parenchyma known as the medulla. The cortex and medulla can be distinguished in a cross section of the kidney, with the medulla being red due to the presence of blood vessels and striated due to the arrangement of the tubules. The cortex has fine red-yellow granules due to the presence of the renal corpuscles.

Organization and structure of the kidney (Plate 8.25). In a longitudinal section from the surface to the center of the kidney the renal capsule is encountered first. This capsule is a thin, tough and transparent covering which can be stripped easily from the parenchyma. It is made of membranous connective tissue with criss-cross bundles of elastic and smooth muscle fibers. Of these, the inner layer abounds in cells while the outer layer has a high concentration of blood vessels.

Beneath the capsule lies the cortex which surrounds the medulla, which is divided into conical or cylindrical regions (*renal pyramids*) whose apical portions (renal papillae) are directed into the center of the organ and project into the renal sinus. Between the renal pyramids the cortex extends to form the so-called *renal columns (of Bertin)*. From the base of the pyramids, medullary tissue extends into the cortex as *medullary rays (of Ferrein)*. Thus, in the cortex the *convoluted part*, consisting of renal corpuscles and twisted tubules, can be distinguished from parallel tubules which form the medullary rays, the *radiate part*. The peripheral part of the cortex is composed solely of convoluted tubules and is called the *cortex corticis*. A lobe of the kidney consists of one pyramid with its medullary rays and corresponding section of cortex. A lobule of the kidney is that part of a lobe consisting of one medullary ray surrounded by the corresponding convoluted part of the cortex. The functional unit of the kidney, however, is not the lobule but the nephron, one of the numerous tubules that constitute the lobule.

The *nephron* (Plates 8.26, 8.27, 8.28, 8.29 A). The first part of each nephron is a blind, double-walled sac (*Bowman's capsule*). This capsule completely surrounds an intricate skein of arterioles (*glomerulus*). The inner, visceral layer of the capsule is closely applied to the glomerular capillaries. The outer or parietal layer consists of simple squamous epithelium while the visceral layer is composed of specialized cells (*podocytes*) which have cytoplasmic processes resting directly on the

on the basal lamina that is shared by the visceral layer of the capsule and the capillary endothelium. In the visceral wall of Bowman's capsule there are slits between the processes of the podocytes, and the endothelium of the glomerular capillaries is highly fenestrated. Between the endothelium and the basal lamina are the *mesangial cells,* which act as phagocytes. Bowman's capsule has a slight constriction at its *neck,* where it is continuous with the uriniferous tubule.

The uriniferous tubule consists first of a contorted segment (*proximal convoluted tubule*), then a U-shaped segment (*Henle's loop*), and finally a second contorted segment (*distal convoluted tubule*) which makes contact with the renal

1 Efferent arteriole
2 Bowman's capsule
3 Glomerulus
4 Renal (or Malpighian) corpuscle
5 Afferent arteriole
6 Proximal convoluted tubule
7 Distal convoluted tubule
8 Collecting duct
9 Thin portion of Henle's loop
10 Minor calyx
11 Major calyx
12 Renal column
13 Renal artery
14 Renal vein
15 Renal pelvis
16 Papilla
17 Medullary substance
18 Cortical substance
19 Ureter
20 Urinary bladder
21 Cortex
22 Medulla
23 Papillary duct

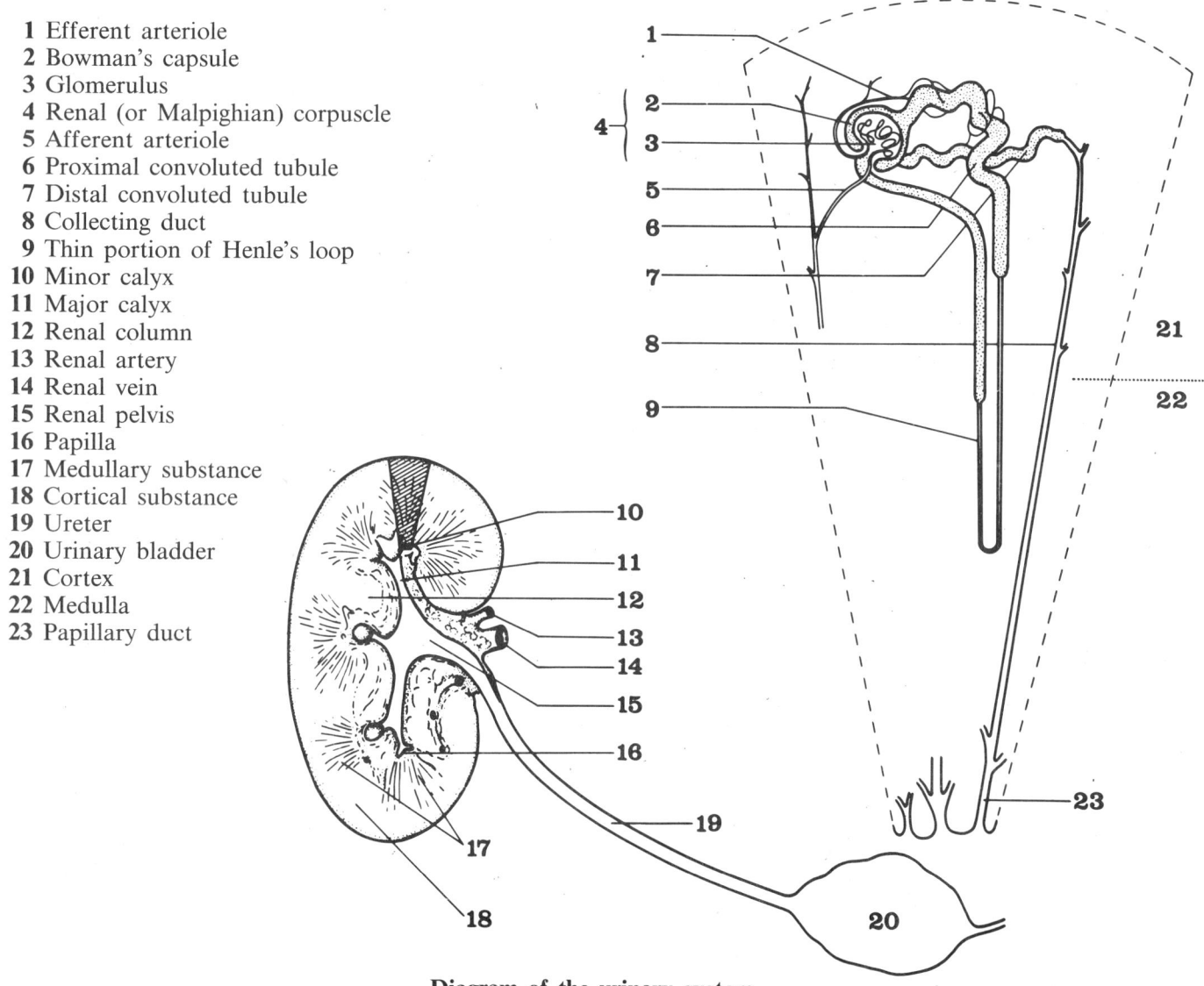

Diagram of the urinary system

The figure on the left shows a human kidney in longitudinal section, with the ureter and urinary bladder. The figure on the right is an enlargement of the shaded portion of the figure on the left and shows a single nephron in its entirety, including the collecting ducts. From P.M. Motta, P.M. Andrews and K.R. Porter. In: *Microanatomy of Cell and Tissue Surfaces. An Atlas of Scanning Electron Microscopy.* Lea & Febiger, Philadelphia, 1977.

corpuscle before emptying into a collecting duct. These three main parts of the tubule can be distinguished by their own structure along the tubule. Each of the epithelial linings rests on a thin basal lamina.

In the proximal convoluted tubule, the thick descending and thick ascending sections of Henle's loop, and in the distal convoluted tubule, the nephron is lined by cuboidal epithelium. In the basal region of the cells lie elongated mitochondria arrayed parallel to one another and perpendicular to the basal surface of the cell. They lie within invaginations of the plasma membrane. There is also a *brush border* of long microvilli at the free surface of the proximal convoluted tubules.

The thin segment of Henle's loop is lined by simple squamous epithelium. The distal convoluted tubule is continuous with the arched collecting tubule, which has a low cuboidal epithelium that stains lightly and has invaginations of the plasma membrane at the base of the cell that rests on the basal lamina.

The distal convoluted tubule returns to the region of the glomerulus. Here it comes into contact with the afferent glomerular arteriole and forms part of a structure called the *juxtaglomerular apparatus.* In this region the epithelial cells of the distal convoluted tubule are specialized to form the *macula densa.* This structure lies very close to the *juxtaglomerular* (JG) *cells,* which are specialized cells of the tunica media of the afferent arteriole. The JG cells secrete renin, an enzyme which acts as a vasoconstrictor.

The distal convoluted tubules lead into collecting ducts which form a drainage system passing through the medullary pyramids and converging at the apices of the papillae, where they open through numerous pores, in a region called the *area cribrosa* (Plate 8.29 B). The epithelium in the collecting ducts is cuboidal, and increases gradually in height towards its more distal parts.

The interlobar arteries branch from the renal artery and, in the region where the cortex and medulla lie next to each other, give rise to the arcuate arteries. From these arteries the interlobular arteries branch at right angles to enter the cortex and extend toward the surface of the organ. At regular intervals the afferent arterioles branch from these arcuate arteries to supply the glomeruli, where they divide to form the capillary network of the glomerulus. This network is drained by the efferent arteriole, which on leaving the renal corpuscle divides into a fine network of capillaries that is in close contact with the convoluted tubules. In the deeper part of the cortex the efferent arterioles leading from their glomeruli pass into a set of straight capillaries (*arteriolae rectae*) which form a network between the tubules of the medulla. Both of these capillary networks are drained by venules that converge to empty into the interlobular veins and from there into the arcuate veins and interlobar veins.

Thus, three systems of capillary circulation exist in the kidney. First, there is the system of glomeruli, whose sole purpose is that of urine filtration. Second, there is the capillary circulation of the cortex, which derives from the efferent arterioles. This circulation has the function of nourishing the tubules, simultaneously gathering water and material reabsorbed from the nephron to be concentrated in the urine. The third system of circulation is that surrounding the medullary tubules. It has a basically nutritive function.

Ureter

The ureter is a long flattened duct which links the renal pelvis to the bladder.

The *wall of the ureter* (Plate 8.29 A) is composed of a mucosa, a submucosa, a muscularis and an adventitia. The mucosa is made up of transitional epithelium and a lamina propria of reticular tissue rich in blood vessels. The mucosa of the ureter is thrown into longitudinal folds which give to the lumen a characteristic star-shaped aspect in cross section. The very thin submucosa is composed of loose connective tissue. The muscularis contains bundles of smooth muscle forming an inner layer running longitudinally and an outer encircling layer. In the distal part of the ureter the muscularis acquires an extra longitudinal layer which derives from the muscle of the bladder. The adventitia is composed of loose connective tissue and contains within it branches of sizable blood vessels and nerves.

Urinary bladder

The urinary bladder is a single organ located medially in the body, and acts as a reservoir. Its function is to collect the urine from the ureters.

Wall of the bladder (Plates 8.29 C, 8.30 B,C). Tissue layers analogous to those of the lower tract of the ureter constitute the bladder wall. The bladder wall is comprised of a mucosa having a transitional epithelium and a lamina propria in which are embedded occasional lymphocytes.

The submucosa is thin and is composed of interwoven smooth muscle fibers separated by elastic fibers of loose connective tissue (Plate 8.30 C); the area of the trigonum vesicae has no submucosa. In the tunica muscularis the bundles of muscle in the inner layer are plexiform; those in the middle layer run in a circular direction, while those in the outer layer run lengthwise. The muscle layers of the bladder, like those of the ureter, have a highly regular arrangement but in their totality form a much tougher layer. On the outer surface of the muscularis are found the adventitia and the serosa. This is part of the peritoneal covering and occurs only in the upper areas of the bladder.

MALE REPRODUCTIVE SYSTEM

Testis

The testis is the organ in which spermatozoa originate and from which male sex hormones are secreted. The testis is ovoid in shape and is contained in a serous sac derived from the peritoneum (*tunica vaginalis*). Its posterior surface is closely associated with the epididymis. In the contact zone between the epididymis and the tunica vaginalis is a deep fissure (*hilum of the testis*) through which the *efferent ductules* exit the testis and the blood vessels and nerves enter it.

Organization and structure of the testis (Plates 8.31 A,B, 8.32). The capsule that covers the testis (*tunica albuginea*) is composed of dense, tough fibrous connective tissue, and from this capsule extend septa of the connective tissue surrounding the compartments which house the numerous tubules sperm-producing. The tunica albuginea adheres firmly to the tunica vaginalis, and at the hilum it is thickened to form a fibrous wedge (*mediastinum testis* or *Highmore body*) from which fibrous septa branch into the testis, forming about 250 pyramidal compartments (*testicular lobules*). Each lobule contains one or more convoluted *seminiferous tubules* between which is loose connective tissue containing nerves and blood vessels.

The blind ends of the seminiferous tubules lie at the periphery of the lobules. They continue on a tortuous course as the *convoluted tubules*. The tubules of each lobule then join at its apex to a short straight *tubulus rectus* which enters the hilum to merge with other tubuli recti from various lobules to form a network (*rete testis*). This network passes through the mediastinum of the testis and becomes a system of efferent ductules constituting the head of the epididymis.

The seminiferous tubules are composed of a laminar layer of connective tissue with elastic fibers and some smooth muscle, and of a basal lamina on which two types of cells rest, the *Sertoli cells* (having supporting and nutritive functions) and *male germ cells* in various stages of maturation (*spermatogonia, primary and secondary spermatocytes, spermatids*), arranged in several layers (see also Chapter 6 and Plates 6.6ff). Between the seminiferous tubules are groups of endocrine cells, the *Leydig interstitial cells* (see p. 183).

Epididymis

The epididymis is an organ that adheres to the posterior margin of the testis and has the shape of a comma. It can be divided into an upper enlarged part, the head, a body in the middle and a tail that turns up to continue as the *ductus deferens*.

Organization and structure of the epididymis (Plates 8.31 A,C, 8.33). The ductuli efferentes, after a short straight course, give rise to a bundle of ductules forming the *head of the epididymis*. The ductuli thus converge in a single collecting duct which is highly convoluted and forms the *body* and *tail* of the epididymis.

The lamina propria of the ductuli efferentes is composed of connective tissue rich in elastic fibers, with some smooth muscle. A simple, ciliated columnar epithelium rests on the basal lamina and includes some paler cuboidal cells that appear to be secretory in function. In some areas the epithelium is pseudostratified.

The *ductus epididymis* is encircled by a muscular layer sandwiched between two layers of connective tissue. Resting on the basal lamina is a pseudostratified columnar epithelium which contains cells having a tuft of stereocilia on their free surfaces, like the bristles of a paint brush (*brush cells*). Between them are *basal cells* (germinative cells) which regenerate the brush cells (Plates 1.32 C).

The epididymis is surrounded by a thin connective tissue capsule which is a continuation of the tunica albuginea of the testis. From this capsule septa extend into the interstitial loose connective tissue surrounding the epididymal tubules.

Ductus deferens

The ductus deferens is a long tube that is a continuation of the ductus epididymis. After its passage through the scrotum and the inguinal canal into the pelvis, the ductus deferens ends in a dilation, the *ampulla*. At this point it is joined by the duct of the ipsilateral seminal vesicle and, passing through the prostate gland, becomes the ejaculatory duct, which empties into the prostatic portion of the urethra.

The wall of the ductus deferens (Plates 8.31 A, 8.34 A) is composed of a mucosa (which has a pseudostratifed epithelium with brush cells rich in stereocilia and basal germinative cells) and a thick submucosa that is folded longitudinally to form evaginations which project into the lumen. Surrounding the mucosa is the muscularis, which is composed of an inner longitudinal layer, a middle spiral layer and an outer longitudinal layer. The adventitia contains elastic fibers and some smooth muscle running lengthwise.

Seminal vesicle

Just beyond the ampulla of each ductus

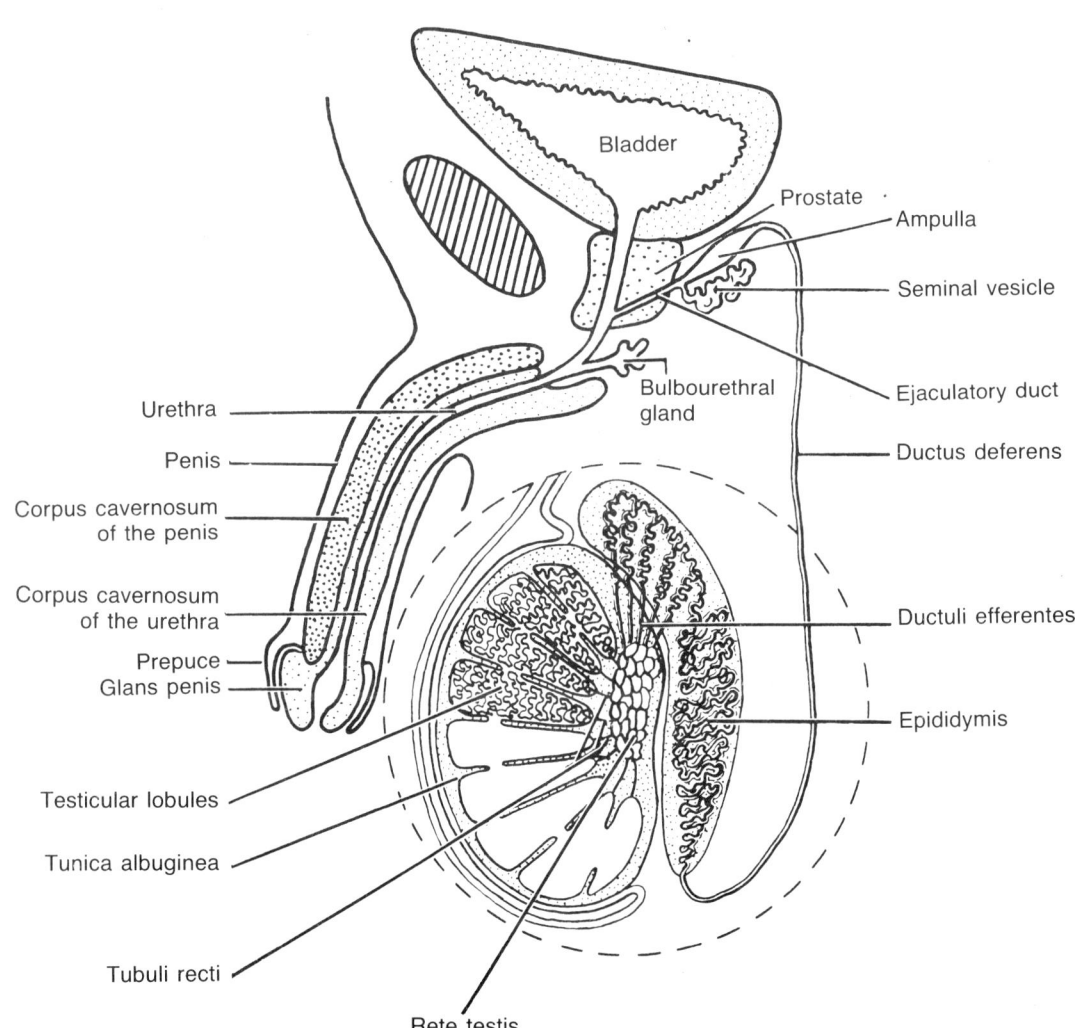

Diagram of the mal genital system. Courtesy of L.C. Junqueira. In: L.C. Junqueira and J. Carneiro. Basic histology 3rd ed. Los Altos, Ca. Lange med. publ., 1980.

deferens is the opening of the the seminal vesicle. This elongated, leaf-shaped gland has within it a single coiled, blind-ended tubule.

The seminal vesicle (Plate 8.34 D) has a highly folded mucosa that forms a complex network of diverticula lined by a simple columnar secretory epithelium that has few basal germinative cells. The lamina propria is rich in elastic fibers and smooth muscle. There is no true submucosa. The muscularis has two layers: an inner longitudinal one and an outer very thin layer containing fibers running obliquely. The adventitia merges with the surrounding connective tissue.

Glands of the urethra

The glands opening into the urethral lumen are classified as *prostatic glands, bulbourethral glands* and *glands of Littré*. These latter are simple branched tubular glands with alveolar dilations linked to the epithelium of the urethra. They produce a secretion containing mucus. Their excretory duct contains either pseudostratified or stratified columnar epithelium. These glands secrete continuously in order to keep the mucosa lubricated. On the contrary, the secretions of the prostate and bulbourethral glands occur during ejaculation.

Organization and structure of the prostate (Plate 8.34 B,C). Associated with the wall of the urethra is the prostate, an organ composed of branched tubulo-alveolar glands, each having its own excretory duct. The prostate consists of a capsule, stroma and glands. The capsule is the external part of the urethra not occupied by the glands. It has three layers: a deep layer composed of muscle, a middle layer of connective tissue fibers and an outer layer rich in blood vessels. The stroma is formed as a thickening of both the connective tissue surrounding the urethral duct and the septa of connective tissue rich in elastic fibers that extend to the capsule at the periphery.

The arrangement of the glands is radial. They are in four groups: one ventral, one dorsal and two lateral. The group of glands located inside the *prostatic utricle* forms the *utricular lobe.* The gland tubules dilate, and have branching diverticula that may anastomose. The tubules are composed of a thin lamina propria on which rest secretory epithelial cells, some of which are tall

and others short. Depending upon the phase of secretion, these cells have varying quantities of lipoid granules.

The secretion of the prostate gland is thick, slightly acid and rich in enzymes. It combines with the secretion of the seminal vesicles to form the liquid part of the ejaculate (seminal fluid), in which the spermatozoa are immersed. Masses of lamellar concretions of prostatic secretions and degenerate cells (*corpora amylacea*) can occur in the tubules. The size of the prostate gland becomes definitive at puberty. In later life the prostate undergoes hypertrophy in the majority of men.

The *bulbourethral glands (of Cowper)* are tubulo-alveolar glands located in a groove of the urogenital diaphragm. These glands are composed of tubules that dilate to form sacs lined with simple columnar epithelium and embedded in connective tissue containing an abundance of elastic fibers, as well as smooth and striated muscle fibers from the sphincter of the urethra. Cowper's glands have long excretory ducts which empty into the bulb of the urethra. Their thick alkaline secretion is thought to have a role in making the ejaculate viscous.

FEMALE REPRODUCTIVE SYSTEM

Ovary

The ova mature in the ovary, and it is this organ that produces the hormones that partially regulate the reproductive cycle in the female. In shape the ovaries are like almonds and in size they vary with age, undergoing a slow atrophy after menopause.

Organization and structure of the ovary; the luteo-follicular complex (Plates 8.35, 8.36, 8.37, 8.38. 8.39). The ovary can be divided into a *cortex* and a *medulla*. The latter is rich in blood vessels and continuous with the *hilum* of the organ.

Both the cortex and medulla are made up of a connective tissue stroma interwoven with bundles of supporting fibers, smooth muscle cells and elastic fibers. The stroma is dense in the medulla but looser in the cortex. At the periphery of the cortex, the collagen bundles of the stroma thicken and interweave to form a surface layer. This layer is analogous to the testis and is called the *albuginea* (or *false albuginea*). The surface of the ovary has a covering of simple cuboidal epithelium (*germinal* or *superficial*) which, at the hilum, is continuous with the peritoneum (*Farre-Waldeyer line*). Embedded in the stroma of the cortex are the *ovarian follicles* in various phases of development, degeneration and transformation (see Chapter 6 and Plates 6.1ff).

The initial developmental stage is represented by *primordial follicles*, in which one oocyte is enveloped by only one layer of flattened follicular cells. These primordial follicles grow to become *primary follicles,* in which the oocyte increases in volume and the follicle cells become at first cuboidal, and then multiply to form a *stratum granulosum* with an increasing number of layers. As the follicle grows the oocyte and follicular cells associated with it secrete a complex polysaccharide material which condenses around the oocyte to form a layer called the *zona pellucida*. As a result of the proliferation and secretion of the granulosa cells, small spherical vesicles form in the stratum granulosum (*Call-Exner bodies*). Subsequently the cells of the stratum granulosum produce a liquid (*liquor folliculi*) that eventually fills a single cavity, the *follicular antrum*. (At this stage the follicle is termed *secondary follicle*). The oocyte remains surrounded by several layers of granulosa cells which form a mound, the *cumulus oophorus,* that projects into the antrum, which is filled by the liquor folliculi. As the liquid accumulates the follicles increase in volume, becoming *mature* or *Graafian follicles.*

The development of the follicle causes changes also in the connective tissue stroma. An envelope (*theca*) of condensed connective tissue develops around the follicle and is composed of a peripheral layer of dense connective tissue (*theca externa*) and an inner layer near the wall of the follicle (*theca interna*). The theca interna is rich in blood vessels and is composed of cords of epithelioid cells with an endocrine function. A basal membrane (*lamina vitrea*) separates the theca from the wall of the follicle.

When fully mature, the follicles bulging under the surface of the ovary rupture (*dehiscence*) and release into the oviduct the oocyte surrounded by the cells of the cumulus oophorus that form a *corona radiata*. This process of liberation of the oocyte from the ovary is termed *ovulation*. Where the surface of the ovary is ruptured (*stigma*), a hemorrhage results, which is

followed by coagulation. At the site of rupture a small depression forms, and the cells of the stratum granulosum and those of the theca migrate and proliferate around this site, although most of the cells remaining from the follicle hypertrophy and form lipid droplets (*granulosa lutein cells*). The yellow mass that results is termed the *corpus luteum*. The corpus luteum acts as an endocrine gland and, during pregnancy, produces specific hormones (see p. 183). It maintains itself for the duration of the gestation period, increasing greatly in volume during the first six months to occupy a large portion of the ovary (*gravidic corpus luteum*), and gradually decreasing in size thereafter. If fertilization does not occur the corpus luteum is smaller (*menstrual corpus luteum*) and degenerates rapidly. In both cases the corpus luteum ultimately undergoes involution and becomes fibrous scar tissue, the *corpus albicans*.

The follicles that do not mature for various reasons also undergo an involution called *atresia* and are slowly and partially resorbed. Groups of hypertrophied cells of the theca interna remain from the larger follicles after atresia. These cells may continue to function as an endocrine gland and, with other cells possibly derived from the stroma cells embedded in the ovary, constitute the *interstitial cells of the ovary* (see p. 183).

Oviducts

The oviducts or fallopian tubes are two ducts extending from the anterolateral region of the fundus of the uterus on each side and ending in a funnel-shaped enlargement (*infundibulum*) with which they clasp the ovaries. A fringed border, the *fimbria*, lines the distal end of the oviduct. Each oviduct has a broad curving portion (*ampulla*), a straight, narrow portion (*isthmus*) and a *uterine* or *interstitial portion* which penetrates the wall of the uterus.

Wall of the oviduct (Plates 8.40 A,B, 8.41). The lumen of the infundibulum and especially the lumen of the ampulla have primary longitudinal folds projecting into it. The folds in turn have secondary and tertiary folds on them that in histological section appear as a complex maze. In the isthmus and interstitial portions of the oviduct the folds gradually diminish. The mucosa of the tube has a characteristic simple columnar ciliated epithelium with intercalated secretory cells resting on a lamina propria. Lymphocytes are fre-

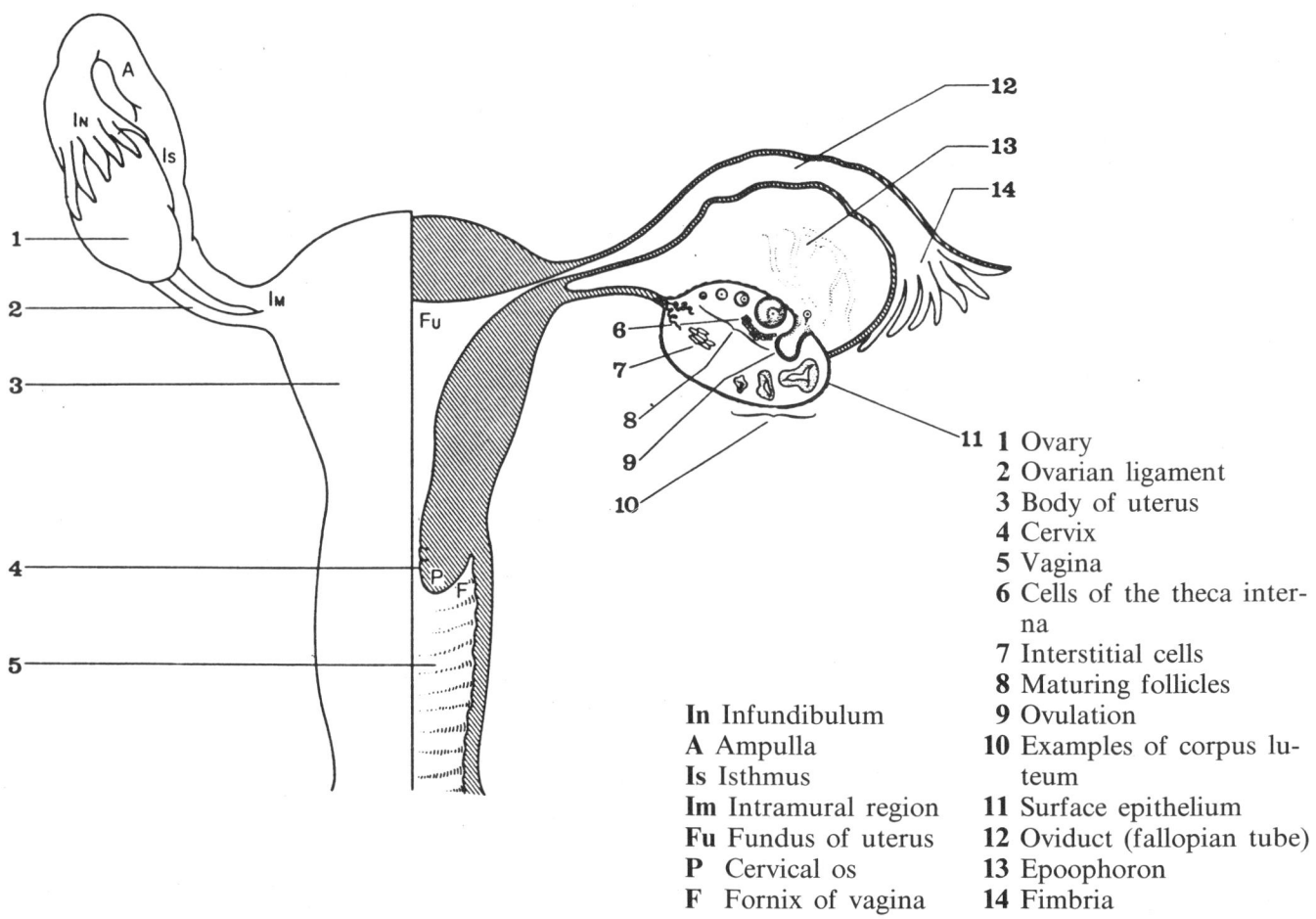

1 Ovary
2 Ovarian ligament
3 Body of uterus
4 Cervix
5 Vagina
6 Cells of the theca interna
7 Interstitial cells
8 Maturing follicles
9 Ovulation
10 Examples of corpus luteum
11 Surface epithelium
12 Oviduct (fallopian tube)
13 Epoophoron
14 Fimbria

In Infundibulum
A Ampulla
Is Isthmus
Im Intramural region
Fu Fundus of uterus
P Cervical os
F Fornix of vagina

Schematic view of the female reproductive system. Drawn by C. Frasier. From P.M. Motta, P.M. Andrews and K.R. Porter. In: *Microanatomy of Cell and Tissue Surfaces. An Atlas of Scanning Electron Microscopy.* Lea & Febiger, Philadelphia, 1977.

quently seen in the lamina propria, which has blood vessels and some smooth muscle. The very thin submucosa is absent in some places. The muscularis is composed of an inner circular layer and an outer longitudinal layer. Where the two layers abut, the cells intermingle and so the two layers are not clearly delineated. A thin subserous layer of loose connective tissue rich in blood vessels and nerves is interposed between the serosa of the peritoneum and the muscularis.

Uterus

The uterus is a single, medially located organ in the abdominal cavity. At its base it is connected with the vagina, and superiorly it is connected with the oviducts, one on each of its sides. The uterus consists of a *body,* with its broad extremity, the *fundus,* and a cylindrical and more narrow lower part, the *cervix.* The two areas are separated by a narrow connection, the *isthmus.*

The *wall of the uterus* (Plates 8.40 C,D, 8.42)

is composed of a mucosa (*endometrium*), a muscularis (*myometrium*) and a peritoneal serosa (*perimetrium*). The appearance of the mucosal surface differs in the body, cervix and the isthmus, and also varies during the different phases of the menstrual cycle. The body of the uterus is lined by low columnar ciliated epithelium, underlain by a lamina propria rich in cells and fibers, highly vascularized and housing numerous simple tubular glands. In the cervix the mucosa is thicker and has a simple columnar epithelium with ciliated cells and mucous cells. Here the lamina propria consists of a coarser network of connective tissue and fewer glands. The mucosa undergoes cyclic growth and disintegration (*menstrual cycle*), culminating in hemorrhage (menstrual bleeding).

The tunica muscularis is thick and consists of an outer layer having both longitudinal and oblique fibers with abundant connective tissue, a discontinuous inner layer with longitudinal, o-

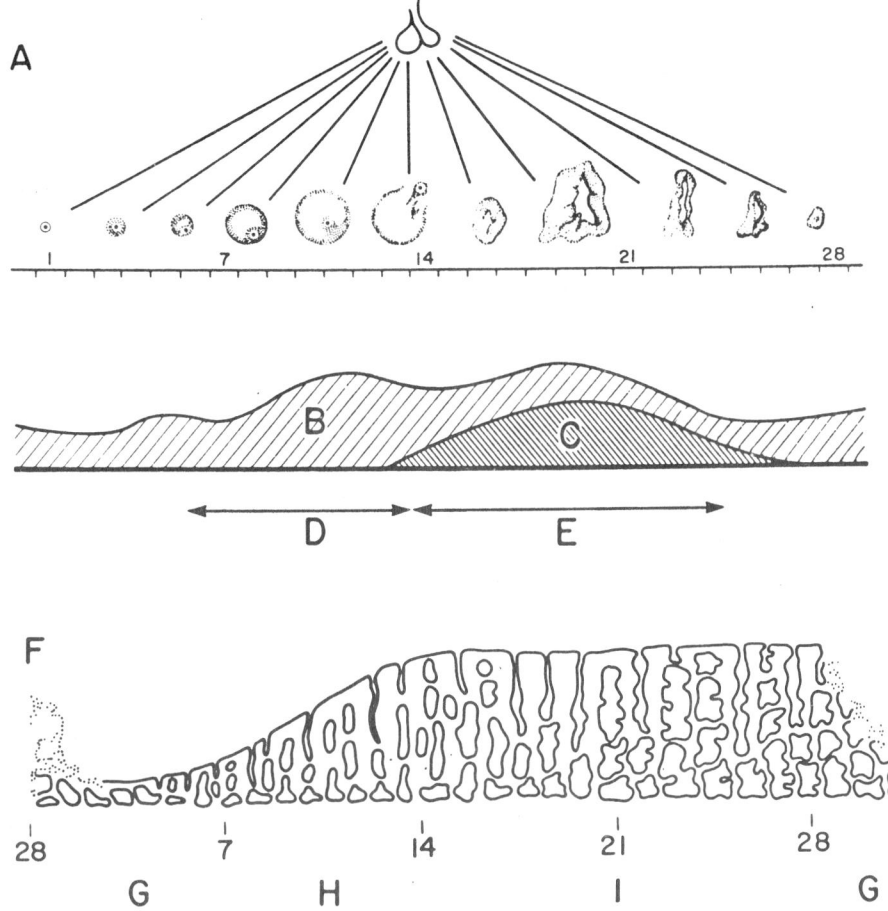

Morphological and functional relationships between the hypophysis, ovary and uterus . In **A** is shown a complete ovarian cycle of 28 days. The cycle includes the growth of the follicle (days 1-14), ovulation (day 14) and the development and degeneration of the corpus luteum (days 14-28). **B** shows the level of estrogens in the blood and **C** the level of progesterone in the blood. **D** represents the follicular phase, **E** the luteal phase. The menstrual cycle in the endometrium is shown in **F**. **G** represents menstruation and repair, **H** the proliferative phase, and **I** the secretory or luteal phase.

blique and circular bundles, and a middle layer which is the thickest and contains a circular network of fibers in which there are many large blood vessels (*stratum vascularis*).

During pregnancy the uterus not only increases greatly in size but both the endometrium and myometrium undergo structural changes.

Upper areas of the uterus are covered not only by the tunica serosa but also by the peritoneum.

LYMPHOID ORGANS

The defense system of an organism is centered in lymphoid tissue. This tissue is composed of a thin web of reticular connective tissue within which are embedded lymphocytes. This type of tissue can be found within the walls of the digestive and respiratory tracts in a form that is either disseminated (*diffuse lymphoid tissue*) or grouped to form rounded bodies, the *lymph nodules or follicles*. Every active lymph nodule contains a *germinal center*. Larger and more complex aggregates of lymphatic follicles sometimes are closely related to the epithelium, as in the *tonsils*. Organs such as the *lymph nodes*, the *spleen* and the *thymus* have specific functions with regard to the immune system, and hence are grouped together as lymphoid organs.

Lymph nodes

Lymph nodes or lymph glands are small masses of lymphoid tissue distributed along the course of lymph vessels. They act to filter the lymph and form new lymphocytes.

Organization and structure of the lymph node (Plates 8.43 C,D, 8.45). The lymph node consists of a cortex containing lymphoid follicles and a *medulla* with thick cords of lymphocytes (*medullary cords*) separated by areas of reticular tissue (*medullary sinuses*), which converge into a terminal sinus at the hilum. The lymph node is enveloped by a dense fibrous capsule of connective tissue. From this tissue arise septa and trabeculae which extend into the cortex to surround the cortical compartments and form partitions among the medullary cords.

In the cortex, just below the fibrous capsule, is a peripheral or *marginal sinus*. The afferent lymph vessels enter the convex surface of the node, pass through the capsule and flow into the peripheral sinus. The lymph passes through the cortex to the medullary sinuses and thence reaches the hilum, where it is discharged into the efferent lymph vessel. The arteries reach the lymph gland at the hilum and are supported by the connective tissue trabeculae. The veins return by a similar route to converge at the hilum.

Tonsils

Lymphocytes forming a continuous layer made up of lymphoid nodules are found in the mucosa of the fauces, the fornix, the superior and lateral walls of the pharynx and almost all of the zones around the nasal and oral openings into the pharynx. The areas of mucosa that contain such aggregations of lymphocytes, not only in the lamina propria but also in the epithelium, are called the *tonsils* (Plate 8.43 A). The epithelium of the tonsil is invaginated to form crypts, furrows or even excretory ducts for abnormally dilated salivary glands. The lymphoid tissue forms a thick, regular but diffuse layer around these invaginations, and extends into the lamina propria of the mucosa. After birth the first lymph nodules in this diffuse lymphoid tissue begin to form, and they are aligned around a depression in the epithelium. The lymphocytes forming these structures lie within the meshwork of reticular connective tissue that is highly vascularized by blood and lymph vessels.

The primary characteristic of the tonsil is the penetration of the epithelium by lymphocytes from the reticular tissue surrounding the crypts.

Tonsils undergo modification during the life-time of the individual. Their maximum development is in childhood, with regression of the organ occuring after puberty.

Tonsils are categorized as *palatine, lingual* and *pharyngeal*. Microscopically these structures appear similar to one another. The fundus of the crypts is ramified and extends almost to the capsule that forms the lower boundary of the organ. The abundance of lymphocytes alters the structure of the epithelium in the palatine tonsils, whereas the epithelium is much less structurally altered in the lingual tonsil. The mucosa of the pharyngeal tonsil is lined by a pseudostratified columnar epithelium at the fundus of the furrows. The opening of the pharyngeal glands is at this point, and a thick layer of lymphoid tissue packed in the lamina propria is gathered into a single row of nodules.

The other diffuse lymphoid tissue embedded in the mucosa of the pharynx constitutes, with the tonsils, the *lymphatic (Waldeyer's) ring of the pharynx*.

Isolated and aggregated lymph nodules in the small intestine (Plate 8.43 B). The lamina propria of the small intestine has abundant lymphocytes in isolated nodules or aggregates immersed in a web of reticular tissue (Plate 8.6 A,B). Where the accumulations of lymphocytes occur, the lamina propria has folds which are visible even with a hand lens. In the mesentery of the small intestine and especially in the ileum the lymph nodules are grouped to form conspicuous lymphatic masses (*Peyer's patches*). These patches, which spread into the submucosa and project onto the surface of the mucosa, are visible to the naked eye.

Spleen

The function of the spleen is to produce lymphocytes and blood platelets. As well as having a general role in the body's defense system, the spleen also destroys old erythrocytes and in many animals acts as a blood reservoir.

Organization and structure of the spleen (Plates 8.44 A,B, 8.46). The peritoneum adheres firmly to the fibrous connective tissue covering the spleen. From this coat trabeculae branch towards the center of the organ and anastomose with one another and with the branches of other trabeculae which extend from the hilum and support the blood vessels. The areas between the trabeculae are filled with splenic pulp. The splenic artery enters the spleen at the hilum and then ramifies into many arterioles which pass along the trabeculae and then penetrate the pulp areas of the organ. The lymphocytes condense to form lymphoid sheaths around the arterioles. At irregular intervals lymph nodules form in this sheath (*splenic* or *Malpighian corpuscles*). After leaving the white pulp the arterioles further divide to form a brushlike array of straight arterioles, the *penicilli*. The continuations of these vessels have a wrapping of macrophages that form a sheath around them (*sheath cells*). These sheathed capillaries lead either into a system of spacious vessels (*sinuses of the spleen*) or directly into the meshwork of the reticular tissue of the red pulp.

Splenic pulp is commonly classified as *white pulp* and *red pulp*. White pulp is made up of lymphoid tissue, whereas red pulp is rich in venous sinuses and therefore in erythrocytes. The stroma of both white and red pulp is made up of reticular connective tissue.

The fibrous capsule and the trabeculae deriving from it have a high content of smooth muscle.

Thymus

The thymus is a lobulated lymphoid-epithelial organ. It functions in the development of certain classes of lymphocytes and also has an endocrine function.

Organization and structure of the thymus (Plate 8.44 C). A thin capsule of loose connective tissue covers the thymus and forms septa which extend into the organ, subdividing it into polygonal *lobules*. Each lobule has a cortical and a medullary region that has a stroma of epithelial cells. In the cortex the stroma is infiltrated by masses of lymphocytes (*thymocytes*) which, however, never contain germinal centers. In the medulla the lymphocytes are fewer and are separated by large numbers of epithelial cells. There are also thymic corpuscles (*Hassal's corpuscles*) in the medulla. These corpuscles are spherical bodies varying in diameter from 50 to 200 um with a core and a peripheral part. The core contains cell debris and shows evidence of degeneration. The periphery is made up of flattened cells in various concentric arrangements.

Shortly before puberty a slow involution of the thymus begins, in which the parenchyma is almost wholly replaced by adipose tissue, the *retrosternal adipose body*. Small aggregations of

lymphocytes and Hassal's corpuscles persist within this fatty body.

ENDOCRINE ORGANS

Pituitary gland

The pituitary gland or *hypophysis* is an endocrine organ attached to the floor of the diencephalon by a stalk (*hypophyseal stalk*) and located in the sella turcica of the sphenoid bone. It consists of an anterior lobe (*adenohypophysis*) which is subdivided into the *pars distalis, pars tuberalis* and *pars intermedia,* and a posterior lobe (*neurohypophysis* or *pars nervosa*).

The pars distalis and the pars intermedia are separated by the *residual cleft,* which is a remnant of the primitive buccal cavity of *Rathke's pouch.* From this pouch the ectoderm of the mouth (*stomodeum*) evaginates during embryogenesis to form the anterior lobe.

The anterior lobe, with its cords of cells, has a structure typical of an endocrine gland, and has follicle formations only in its peripheral and especially dorsal regions. Two kinds of cord cells have been described: small scattered *chromophobe cells,* which stain weakly, and the larger *chromophil cells* that take either acidic or basic stains easily (*acidophils* and *basophils*) (Plates 8.47, 8.48). The hormones secreted by the basophils are glycoproteins, and include FSH (follicle-stimulating hormone), LH (luteinizing hormone) and TSH (thyroid-stimulating hormone). ACTH (adrenocorticotropic hormone) and LPH (lipotropic hormone) are also secreted by basophils, but these are polypeptide hormones, as are the hormones secreted by the acidophils, GH (growth hormone or somatotropic hormone) and PR (prolactin) (Plates 8.47, 8.50).

The cells of the anterior lobe, which are usually closely associated with the wall of the sinusoids, sometimes detach from the walls and surround spaces outside the sinuses in which occasional macrophages can be found. The endothelium of the sinusoids is fenestrated and has the same characteristics as that of other endocrine glands. A typical exocytosis mechanism is thought to be the means by which hormone secretion takes place in these cells.

The pars distalis is usually separated from the pars intermedia (which is not well defined in humans) by a small cleft. The pars intermedia originates from epithelium and has fewer cords but more vesicles (follicles containing colloid) than the pars distalis. Its cells are weakly basophilic with relatively little cytoplasm compared to other cells. They secrete MSH (melanocyte-stimulating hormone or intermedin), a peptide hormone which, in lower vertebrates, stimulates the synthesis and transport of melanin pigments (Plates 8.49, 8.50).

The pars tuberalis can be considered the extension of the pars distalis covering the hypophyseal stalk. Structurally it is similar to the pars distalis, although it usually has fewer active secretory cells.

The posterior lobe or pars nervosa is a continuation of the diencephalon or hypothalamus and develops from neural ectoderm. It is composed of nerve fibers and special glial cells (*pituicytes*), as well as connective tissue trabeculae containing blood vessels. Within the endings of the nerve fibers of the posterior lobe can be identified the secretory granules (*Herring bodies*). These are produced by the neurons of the supraoptic and paraventricular nuclei in the hypothalamus (Plate 8.48). Two hormones having similar chemical composition derive from the neurohypophysis: oxytocin and vasopressin (antidiuretic hormone, ADH).

By means of small aggregates of neurons the hypothalamus also produces releasing or inhibitory factors. These factors are peptides that are discharged into a special portal system of blood vessels and reach the cells of the anterior lobe, where they regulate secretory activity.

Pineal gland

The pineal gland or *epiphysis* is a small conical body covered by the pia mater of the meninges. It is an appendage of the dorsal region of the diencephalon and is located in the posterior extremity of the third ventricle (Plate 8.51 A,B).

Septa of connective tissue penetrate the pineal gland and separate it into irregular lobules. These septa, which originate from the capsule of connective tissue, anastomose and contain blood vessels. The parenchyma consists of glial cells which sometimes have the appearance of epithelium. These *pinealocytes* are embedded in a stroma that is partly reticular and partly neuroglial. After puberty the pineal body tends to diminish

in size and the stromal tissue increases. With age mineralized bodies appear in the stroma, the so-called *brain sand (corpora arenacea)*. The pineal gland produces a hormone, *melatonin*, which in amphibians has an effect on pigmentation. In higher vertebrates it is thought to modulate the daily physiological activity of the gonads.

The pineal gland can be thought of not so much as an endocrine organ as a "neuroendocrine transducer," in that its cells produce a hormone only if stimulated by the nervous system.

Thyroid gland

The thyroid gland is an endocrine organ located on the ventral surface of the trachea. From the highly vascularized fibrous capsule septa enter and divide the parenchyma of the organ into lobules varying in shape and size. In the septa are blood vessels and nerves. Within each lobule the secretory epithelium forms spherical vesicles (*thyroid follicles*) embedded in a web of reticular tissue which is rich in blood vessels and nerves (Plates 8.52, 8.53).

The follicles are limited by a layer of secretory epithelial cells that are usually cuboidal (*thyroid cells*). These cells are attached to a basement membrane and are in close proximity to a dense capillary network. Other cells, fewer in number, are associated with the thyroid cells of the follicle; these cells have the special function of secreting calcitonin and are called *parafollicular cells* or *C cells*. The follicles contain within them a substance (*colloid*) produced by the follicular cells. The colloid contains the precursors of the thyroid hormones (thyroxine and triiodothyronine) and stains weakly.

Parathyroid glands

The four parathyroid glands are small bodies, each about the size of a pea, located on the posterior medial margin and embedded in the connective tissue capsule of the thyroid gland (Plate 8.51 C,D). Each of the glands is contained in a thin capsule of connective tissue from which arise septa that penetrate the organ and through which pass blood vessels and nerves. Irregular compartments are thus formed, and contain cords of cells in a highly vascularized reticular stroma.

There are two types of cells in the parathy-

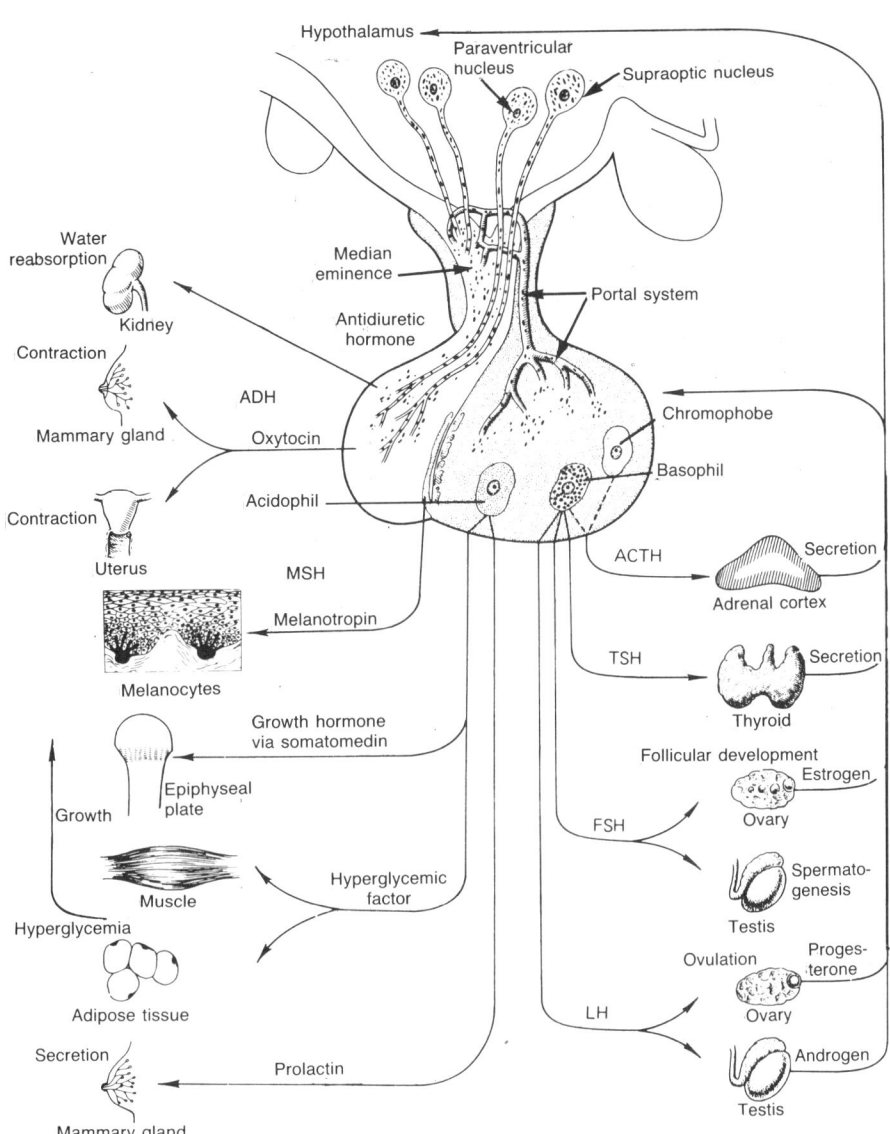

Drawing showing pituitary hormones and their effects on target organs. Courtesy of L.C. Junqueira. In: L.C. Junqueira and J. Carneiro. Basic Histology. 3rd ed. Los Altos, Ca. Lange Med. Publications, 1980.

roid gland: *principal cells,* which have a lightly staining cytoplasm, and *oxyphil* cells, which stain easily with acidic dyes. A third type, the hyaline cell, has been proposed to exist by some investigators; it is considered to be an intermediate between the two other types of cells. The principal (or *chief*) cells predominate in number and produce the parathyroid hormone. The function of the other two types of cells is not definitely known.

Adrenal glands

The two adrenal or suprarenal glands are endocrine organs, each of which is located at the cranial pole of a kidney. They are composed of two parts that differ in origin and function, the *cortex* and the *medulla* (Plates 8.54, 8.55, 8.56).

In the cortex three layers of cells can be distinguished according to their organization: the *zona glomerulosa, zona fasciculata* and *zona reticularis.* The cells of the cortex are polygonal in shape and have abundant cytoplasm rich in lipid droplets, smooth endoplasmic reticulum and mitochondria with many villiform or tubular cristae. These cells produce steroid hormones (mineralocorticoids, glucocorticoids and androgens). The stroma of the organ consists of reticular tissue in which networks of sinusoidal capillaries are embedded.

The medulla is composed of large cells that form a network of anastomosing cords surrounded by a dense network of spacious sinusoidal capillaries. The cells of the medulla are called chromaffin cells and produce the catecholamines, epinephrine and norepineprhine. These cells are the equivalent of modified postganglionic neurons of the sympathetic nervous system.

Pancreas

The endocrine part of the pancreas is composed of groups of cells (*islets of Langerhans*) which are distributed more or less at random within the exocrine part of the gland (Plate 8.7 C,D). The islets of the pancreas, which in the embryonic stage originate from the walls of the pancreatic ducts, lose all connection with the exocrine part during development. The islets constitute approximately 1% of the tissue of the pancreas. In appearance they are small spheroid masses of variable diameter containing cords of anastomosing epithelial cells. Through these cords passes a network of dilated blood capillaries (*sinusoids*). The cords of epithelial cells are made up of 25% *alpha (A) cells*, which secrete glucagon, and 75% *beta (B) cells*, containing granules of insulin or one of its precursors. The granules of beta cells are somewhat smaller than those of alpha cells. Special staining methods have shown the existence of a third type of cell called *delta (D) cells*, which secrete somatostatin and perhaps gastrin (Plate 8.5).

Interstitial cells of the testis

Polyhedral cells with an appearance similar to that of epithelium are encountered in groups among the seminiferous tubules, in close contact with the blood capillaries. These *interstitial or Leydig cells* often contain intricate and abundant smooth endoplasmic reticulum and mitochondria having villiform or tubular cristae. Together these cells constitute the endocrine tissue of the testis (*testicular interstitial cells*). This tissue is interspersed among the seminiferous tubules (*interstitium*) and is responsible for the production of androgens (testosterone) (Plates 8.32 B, 8.58).

Corpus luteum, theca interna and ovarian interstitial cells

The cells of the theca interna, those of the corpus luteum and the interstitial cells all have in common the synthesis of hormones. These cells are characterized by the presence of lipid droplets in the cytoplasm and an abundance of smooth endoplasmic reticulum and mitochondria having villiform or tubular cristae. These cells, which derive from a single cell line, constitute the endocrine tissue (*interstitium*) interspersed among the follicles of the ovary. These cells secrete the ovarian hormones (estrogens and progesterone), which regulate the menstrual cycle and pregnancy (Plates 8.35, 8.36, 8.38 C, 8.59, 8.60, 8.61).

NERVOUS SYSTEM

The nervous system extends as an interconnected system to all the tissues and organs in the body, except for the cartilaginous tissue. Nervous tissue is composed of specialized cells (*neurons*) which originate, disperse and transmit impulses that act as signals for communication by means of special nerve processes. Other cells (*neuroglia*) in this system have a role in supporting and nourishing the neurons.

The nervous system is divided into three fundamental parts. One, the *central nervous system (CNS)*, is composed of centers in which the impulses originating from outside the body are integrated with other impulses. The central nervous system is made up of the brain and spinal cord. The second part, *the peripheral nervous system (PNS)*, includes all of the nerve tissue outside the central nervous system. Specialized endings of nerve cell processes reside in various organs and tissues. Those endings that stimulate muscles and glands to activity are called motor endings, and these two types of tissue are called *effectors*. Each organ also has nerve fibers that act as *receptors* and, acting as transducers, convey information toward the central nervous system.

Spinal cord

A cross section of the spinal cord shows a central H-shaped medullary region (*gray matter*) and a surrounding peripheral region with a pale fibrous appearance (*white matter*) (Plate 8.62). The gray matter consists of the neuroglia which surrounds the perikarya and nerve fibers arriving from the periphery and other regions of the central nervous system. Within the gray matter, the dorsal arms of the H are called the posterior horns, while the ventral arms are called the anterior horns. The area between the horns is termed the *gray commissure.*

The cord and other parts of the central nervous system are surrounded by the meninges, which are thin membranes of connective tissue. The layers of the meninges are the *pia mater,* the *arachnoid membrane* and the *dura mater.*

Cerebellum

If a median sagittal section is taken through the hemispheres of the cerebellum the basic layers that characterize this part of the brain can be seen. On the outside is the *molecular layer,* consisting principally of nerve fibers from neurons lying deeper in the cortex and the arborizations of dendrites of *Purkinje cells,* as well as some interneurons. Beneath this is the *granular layer,* so called because of the abundance of nuclei contained within it. Between the granular and molecular layers is a single row of perikarya belonging to the Purkinje cells and Golgi cells. Below the granular layer is a layer of myelinated nerve fibers which comprise the mass of white matter. This medullary region or *arbor vitae* extends into the axes of each of the lobules that form each hemisphere of the cerebellum (Plate 8.63 A,B).

Cerebral cortex

The cerebral hemispheres of the brain have an irregular surface because of their numerous folds (*cerebral convolutions*). Each hemisphere has a superficial covering of gray matter in a continuous layer (*cerebral cortex*) which surrounds a mass of white matter (*medulla*). The telencephalic cortex consists of cells and nerve fibers arranged in six layers and supported by neuroglia.

The layers of the cortex, starting from the outside, are: 1) the molecular or plexiform layer, 2) the layer of small pyramidal cells (outer granular layer), 3) a layer of medium-sized and larger pyramidal cells, 4) the inner granular layer, 5) the layer of large and deep pyramidal cells, and 6) the layer of polymorphic cells (Plate 8.63 B,C).

The eye

The globe of the eye is a sac whose wall is composed of three concentric coats. The outer fibrous coat of connective tissue is divided into an opaque part, the *sclera,* and a transparent part,

the *cornea.* The middle coat is vascular, being highly pigmented in order to prevent the reflection of light. The innermost coat, the *retina,* is composed of photosensitive nerve tissue. The cavity of the eye contains the diopteric apparatus, which consists of (from front to rear) the *aqueous humor, the crystalline lens* and the *vitreous body.*

The posterior two-thirds of the middle coat adheres to the sclera and is called the *choroid.* The intermediate part of the coat is limited to an area that adheres to the sclera but is modified to produce the aqueous humor and form a point of attachment for the organ by which the crystalline lens is suspended. In this area, called the *ciliary body,* is the ciliary muscle. The anterior portion of the ciliary body forms a septum in front of the lens, the *iris,* which has an opening in the center, the *pupil.*

The entire inner coat of nerve tissue adheres to the middle coat. The internal layer corresponding to the choroid is the *pars optica;* the part covering the ciliary body posteriorly is the *pars ciliaris,* and the part covering the posterior surface of the iris is the *pars iridica* (Plate 8.64). The pars ciliaris and the pars iridica do not have a sensory role and constitute the non-photosensitive sector of the retina.

The retina is composed of two layers that adhere to each other so as to render the fissure between them effectively nonexistent. The outer leaf in contact with the choroid constitutes the *pigmented epithelium* of the retina. In the pars iridica this epithelium is transformed into a type of muscle. The inner leaf of the retina is termed the *retina proper.* Between the photosensitive part and the non-photosensitive part is a clear division in the form of a serrated line, the *ora serrata.* In the retina proper there are three basic cell layers. The outer photosensitive layer consists of *rod and cone cells.* The intermediate layer is made up of *bipolar neurons* associated with special cells of the neuroglia. The third or inner layer is made up of *ganglion cells.* The nerve fibers from the retinal neurons converge to form a bundle, the *optic papilla,* at the posterior pole of the cavity where the optic nerve leaves the optic cavity and passes through all the covering coats (Plates 8.66, 8.67).

In the retina proper the photosensitive cells do not have a uniform distribution. They are lacking at the papilla of the optic nerve. Above and beside the papilla an elliptical zone can be seen, the *macula lutea,* which contains yellow pigment. The macula lutea contains only one type of photosensitive cell, *cone cells.* In the remaining portions of the retina, cone cells alternate regularly with rod cells, with the latter predominating in the ora serrata (Plate 8.66).

The cavity of the eye is divided into two chambers: the *anterior* and *posterior chambers.* The anterior chamber contains the aqueous humor, a transparent colorless fluid, and is delimited in front by the cornea and behind by the iris. A small fissure behind the iris, between the iris and the vitreous body, forms the posterior chamber which communicates with the anterior chamber by means of a circular aperture, the *pupil.* The posterior chamber is delimited in front by the posterior face of the iris, and behind by the anterior face of the lens and the *ciliary zonule,* behind which is the vitreous body. The lens, which is biconvex and is capable of undergoing changes in shape, is composed of epithelial cells that have been transformed into long fibers having the appearance of *hexagonal prisms* (Plates 8.64, 8.65).

The space between the posterior face of the lens, including the apparatus that suspends it, and the inner surface of the retina is occupied by the *vitreous body,* a colorless and transparent gelatinous mass.

The ear

Three distinct parts constitute the ear: the *outer ear,* which is composed of the *auricle* and the *external auditory meatus;* the *middle ear,* which is formed by the *tympanic cavity,* the *mastoid cavities* and the *auditory tube;* and the *inner ear,* which is composed of the *osseous labyrinth* and the *membranous labyrinth* (Plates 8.68, 8.69).

The auricle is a lamina of elastic cartilage covered by skin. The external auditory meatus initially is supported by elastic cartilage. At a deeper level, the meatus passes through a bony canal at the end of which is the tympanic membrane. The skin lining the initial passage contains many ceruminous (wax) glands.

The auditory tube is a duct made up partly of bone tissue and partly of fibrous cartilage, and is completely lined by pseudostratified ciliated epithelium.

The tympanic cavity (which includes the auditory ossicles) and the mastoid cavity are lined

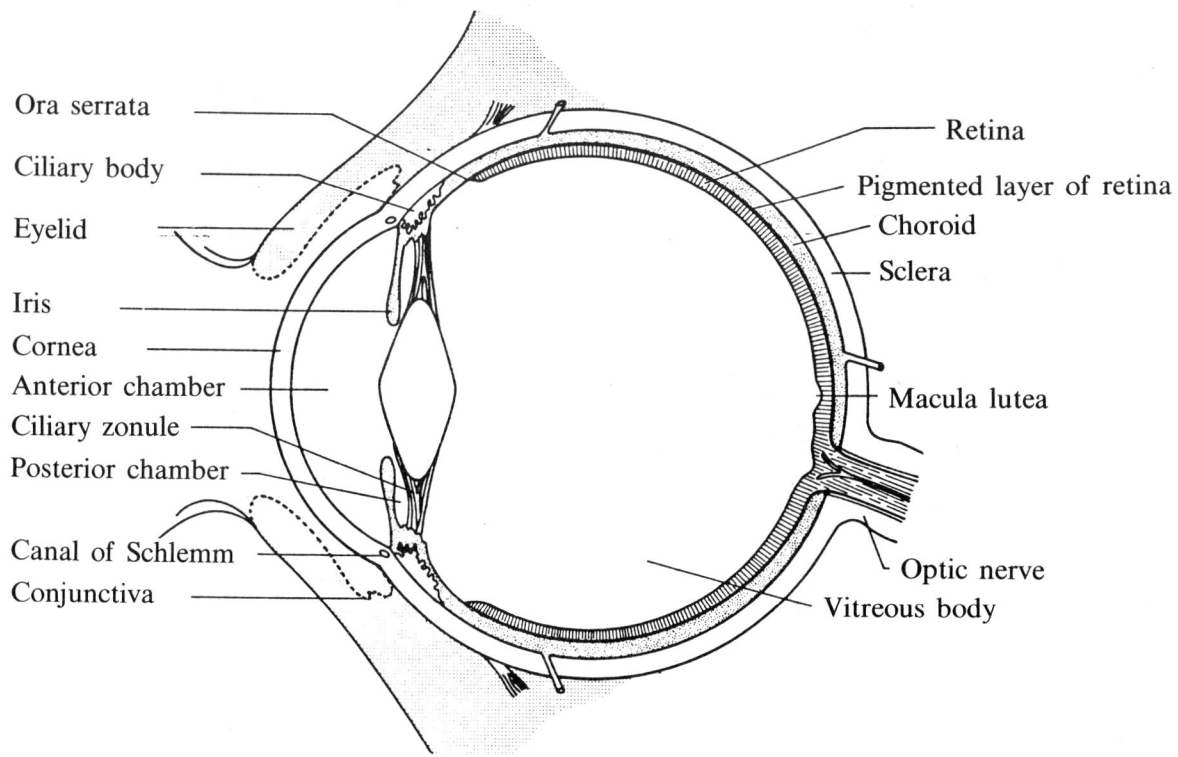

Diagram of the eye in medial longitudinal section. Drawn by C. Frasier. In: P.M. Motta, P.M. Andrews and K.R. Porter. *Microanatomy of Cell and Tissue Surfaces. An Atlas of Scanning Electron Microscopy.* Lea & Febiger, Philadelphia, 1977.

with simple cuboidal epithelium resting on a very thin lamina propria that adheres to the periosteum. The organ of auditory perception is located in the inner ear and is composed of a set of canals forming a membranous labyrinth suspended within a system of bony canals (osseous labyrinth). The perilymphatic fluid circulates between the walls of the osseous labyrinth and those of the membranous labyrinth, while inside the membranous labyrinth is the endolymph. The osseous labyrinth consists of a central cuboid cavity, the *vestibule, semicircular canals* and the *cochlea.* Based on their position, the canals are distinguished as posterior, lateral and superior. The cochlea is a conical mass of compact osseous tissue with a central pillar, the *modiolus,* around which is coiled a tube, the *spiral canal,* containing the *lamina spiralis ossea* that divides the cavity into two scalae, the *scala tympani* and *scala vestibuli.* The parts constituting the membranous labyrinth are the *utricle,* from which the three semicircular canals arise, the *saccule* and the *cochlear duct.*

All these structures have a lining of simple squamous epithelium resting on a basal lamina, and contain endolymph. Specific areas of the membranous labyrinth have differentiated cell formations: the *maculae* in the utricle and saccule, and the *cristae ampullares* in the dilated portion of each semicircular canal. Each macula, which is the sense organ that perceives position, is composed of cylindrical cells that support sensory cells. The latter have a characteristic goblet shape and on their apex are microvilli and cilia. The base of each of these *hair cells* is wrapped by thin nerve processes. On the surface of the macula is a gelatinous substance called the *otolithic membrane,* containing small crystals of calcium carbonate and magnesium (*otoliths*) (Plate 2.7).

The cristae ampullares are the sense organs that perceive rotation, and they resemble the maculae. They are composed of supporting cells and sensory cells embedded in a gelatinous mass, the *cupola* (Plate 8.69 E).

The cochlear duct is the acoustic portion of the membranous labyrinth separating the scala tympani from the scala vestibuli. Between the scala vestibuli and the scala tympani is the osseous *spiral lamina.* The cochlear duct, which is triangular in cross section, extends in a spiral course through the cochlea.

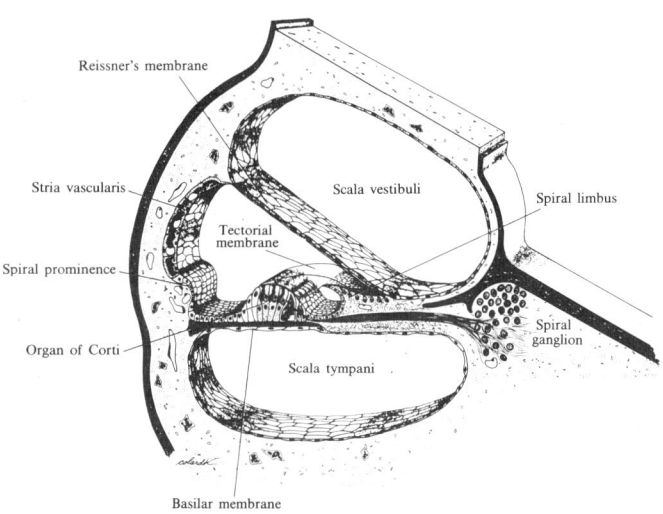

Schematic diagram of a section of a spire of the cochlea. Diagram from S.C. Keen. By courtesy of D.W. Fawcett. In: W. Bloom and D.W. Fawcett. *A Textbook of Histology.* 10th ed. W.B. Saunders Co., Philadelphia/London/Toronto.

On the partition that separates the cochlear duct from the scala tympani is a complex arrangement of cells, the *spiral organ of Corti* (Plate 8.69 A-D). This organ is trapezoid in shape and occupies almost the entire floor of the cochlear duct. It is composed of supporting and sensory cells. Extending throughout the length of its course is the *tunnel of Corti,* a canal delimited by characteristic supporting cells called *inner* and *outer pillar cells.* Next to the inner pillar cells is a row of *inner sensory cells* resting on supporting cells. The inner sensory cells resemble those of the static maculae in that they have an apical surface with a number of ciliary processes. On the outer side of the tunnel, alongside the *outer supporting cells (cells of Deiters),* are tall curved cells, the *cells of Hensen, which lie next to a layer of cuboidal cells of Claudius.* The *outer sensory cells,* wedged between supporting cells, are cylindrical and have on their apices a number of cilia. On the free surface of this spiral organ is a structure resembling a gelatinous ribbon called the *tectorial membrane* (see also Plates 2.6, 2.7).

The wall on the vestibular side of the cochlear duct is thin and covered with a very fine lamina (*Reissner's membrane*). The outer wall of the cochlear duct that adheres directly to the bone has a rounded projection into the lumen (*spiral prominence*) and a highly vascularized tract called the *stria vascularis* from which probably the endolymph is secreted.

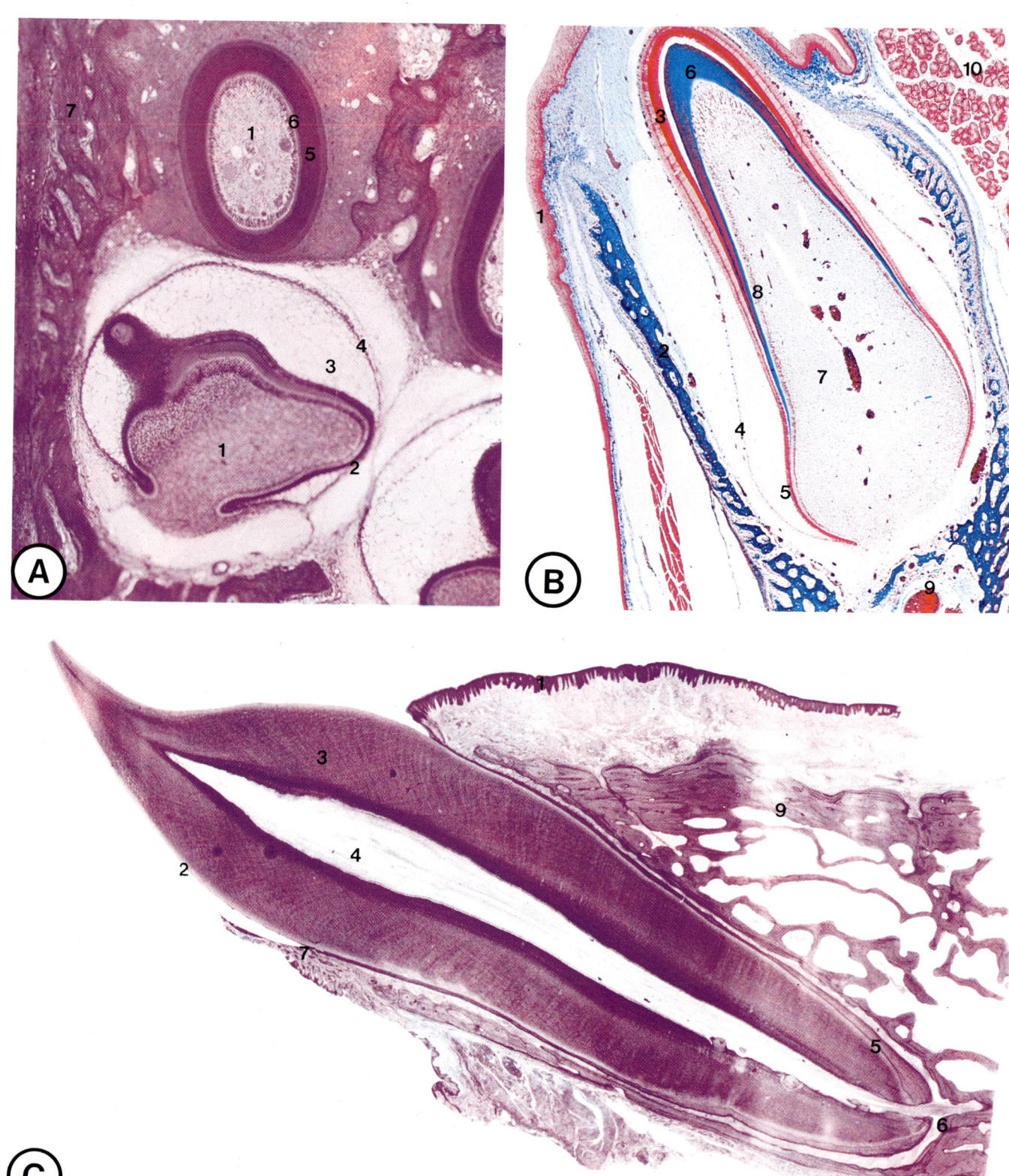

A **Tooth bud of rat (H & E, x20).** Above: cross section of the tooth at the level of the root. Below: oblique section of the tooth bud. **1** = dental papilla. **2** = internal epithelium of the enamel organ (ameloblasts). **3** = pulp of enamel. **4** = external epithelium of enamel organ. **5** = dentin. **6** = odontoblasts. **7** = bone tissue of maxilla.

B **Longitudinal section of the tooth bud of cat (azan-Mallory, x20). 1** = epithelium of gingiva. **2** = bone of alveolus. **3** = enamel with external **(4)** and internal **(5)** epithelia of enamel organ. **6** = dentin. **7** = dental papilla. **8** = odontoblasts. **9** = nerves and vessels of the alveolus. **10** = fragment of the submandibular gland.

C **Sagittal section of fully grown pig tooth fixed within the alveolus (H & E, x30). 1** = gingiva. **2** = enamel. **3** = dentin. **4** = tooth cavity with dental pulp. **5** = cementum. **6** = apical foramen of tooth. **7** = neck of tooth. **8** = periodontium. **9** = alveolar bone.

Plate 8.2   **187**

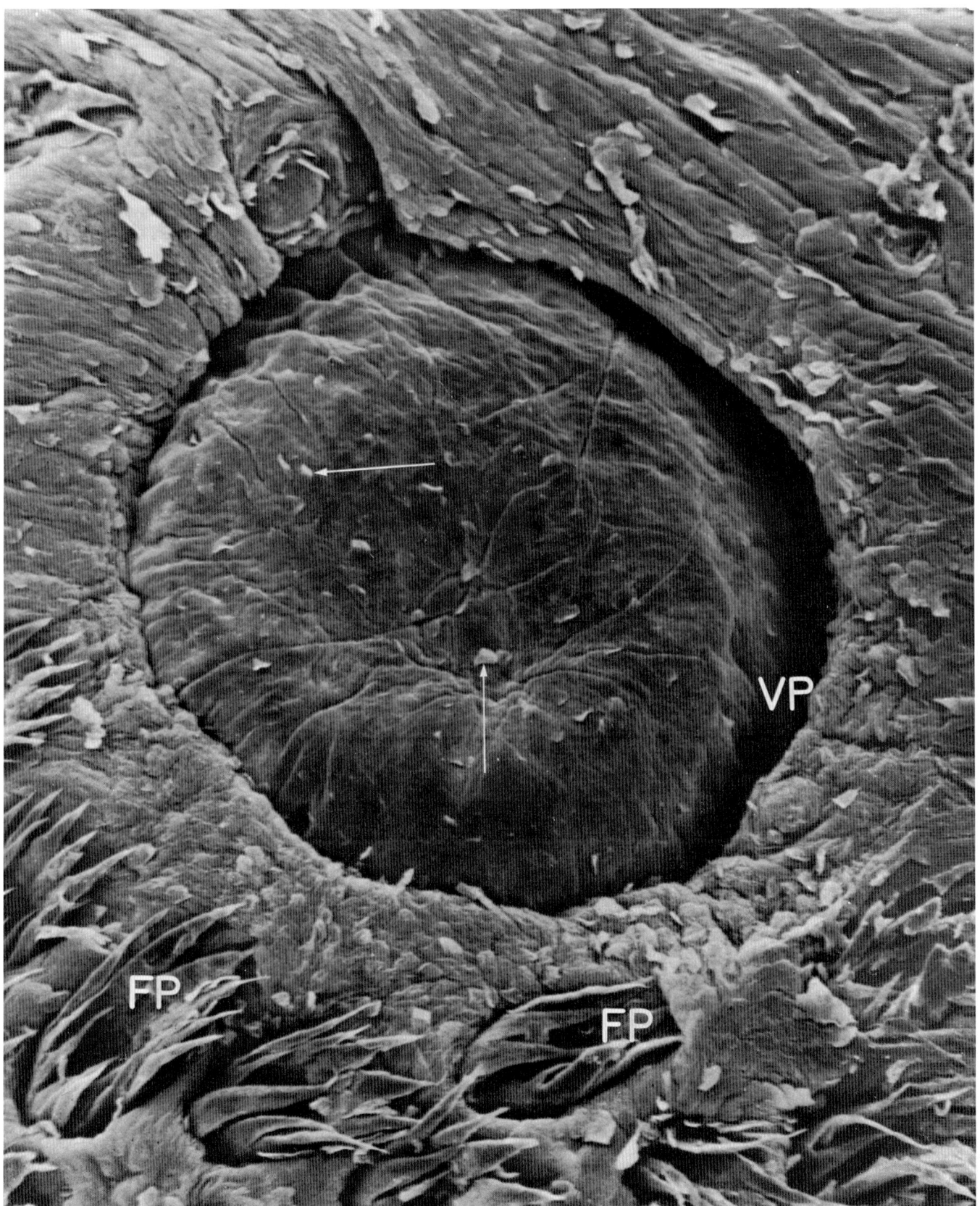

Tongue papillae of monkey (scanning EM, x100). Center: a circumvallate papilla at the V-line of the tongue. The stratified squamous epithelium covering the papilla is partly keratinized and is shedding scales (→). **VP** = vallum of the papilla. A number of filiform papillae **(FP)** are arrayed below the large circumvallate papilla. From P.M. Motta, P.M. Andrews and K.R. Porter. In: *Microanatomy of Cell and Tissue Surfaces. An Atlas of Scanning Electron Microscopy.* Lea & Febiger, Philadelphia, 1977.

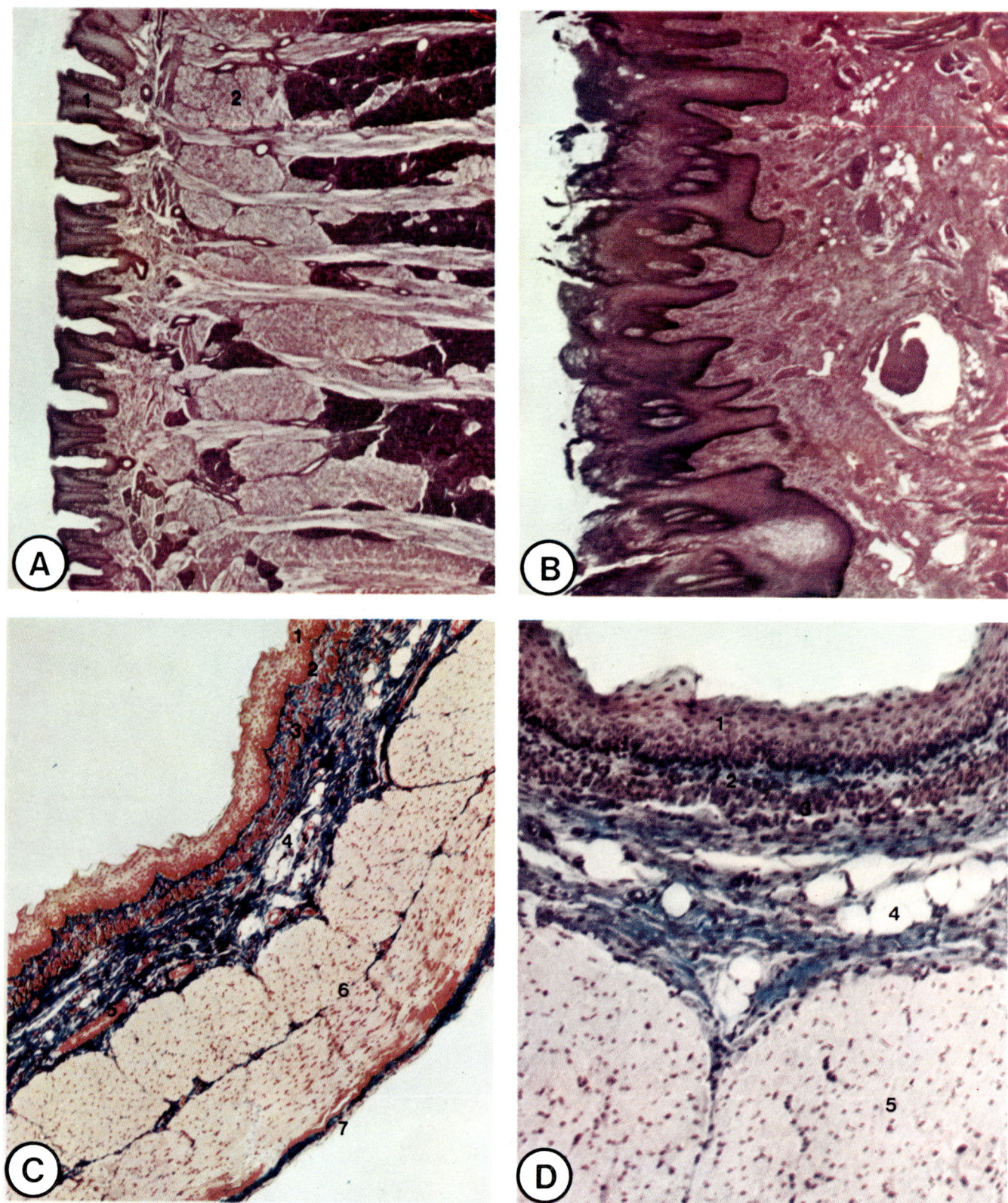

A   **Rabbit tongue (H & E, x40).** The tongue is covered with a mucosa raised to form vallate papillae (1). Beneath the mucosa note the bundles of striated muscle fibers (2). Among these fibers small salivary glands (3) are interspersed.

B   **Rabbit tongue (H & E, x60).** Filiform papillae with partially keratinized epithelium.

C   **Longitudinal section of the esophagus from dog (azan- Mallory, x80).** 1 = stratified squamous epithelium of mucosa. 2 = lamina propria. 3 = muscularis mucosae. 4 = submucosa. 5 = esophageal glands. 6 = muscularis with two distinct layers (the internal circular and the external longitudinal) separated by a thin stratum of connective tissue. 7 = adventitia.

D   **Cross section of esophagus from dog (azan-Mallory, x140).** 1 = epithelium of mucosa. 2 = lamina propria. 3 = muscularis mucosae. 4 = submucosa with adipose cells. 5 = internal circular layer of muscularis.

Plate 8.4   189

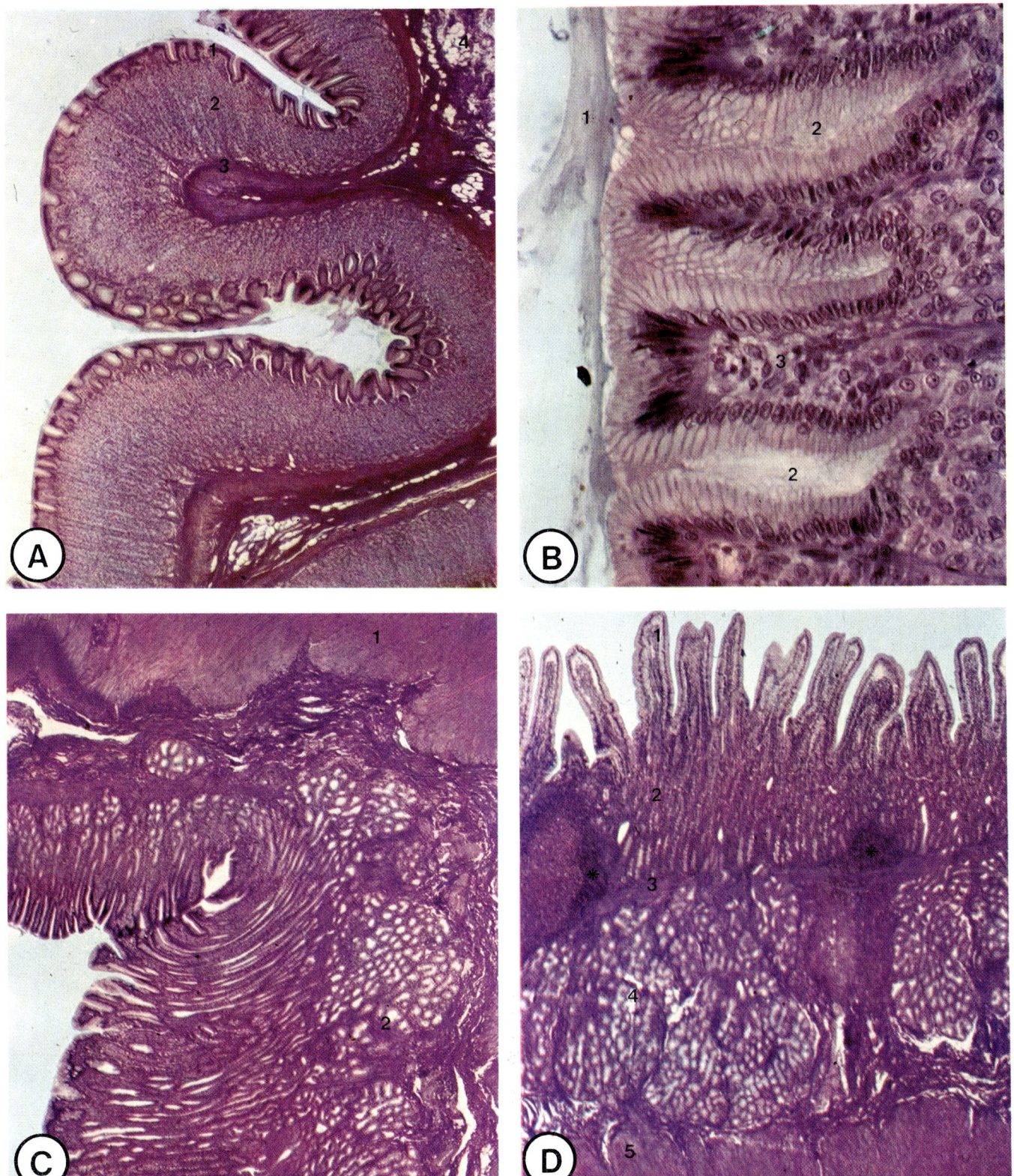

A   **Stomach of cat (H & E, x50). 1** = epithelium with gastric pits. **2** = lamina propria packed with gastric glands. **3** = muscularis mucosae. **4** = submucosa with small lobules of adipose tissue seen as translucent patches.

B   **Detail of mucosa from cat stomach (H & E, x260). 1** = mucus secreted by the epithelium of the mucosa. Simple columnar epithelium covering the surface and lining the gastric pits **(2). 3** = lamina propria with capillaries and smooth muscle cells.

C   **Cat stomach in transitional area between pylorus and duodenum (H & E, x40).** Above: pylorus, below: duodenum. **1** = circular layer of smooth muscle that is thickened to form the pyloric sphincter. **2** = duodenal glands (Brunner's) within the submucosa.

D   **Duodenum from cat (H & E, x50). 1** = villi covered by simple columnar epithelium. **2** = lamina propria with intestinal glands. **3** = muscularis mucosae. **4** = submucosa containing large lobular Brunner's glands. **5** = internal (circular) layer of smooth muscle. ***** = lymph nodules within the lamina propria and submucosa.

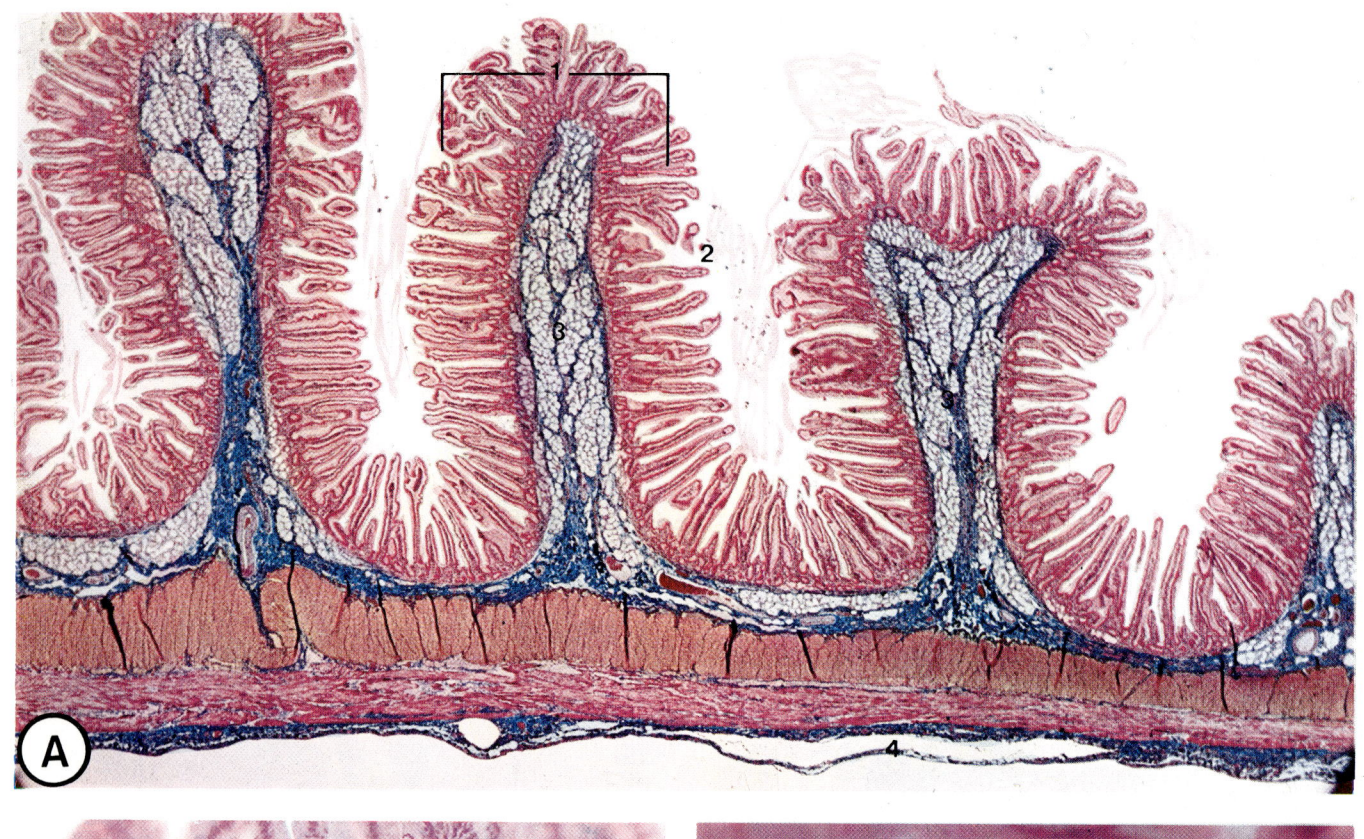

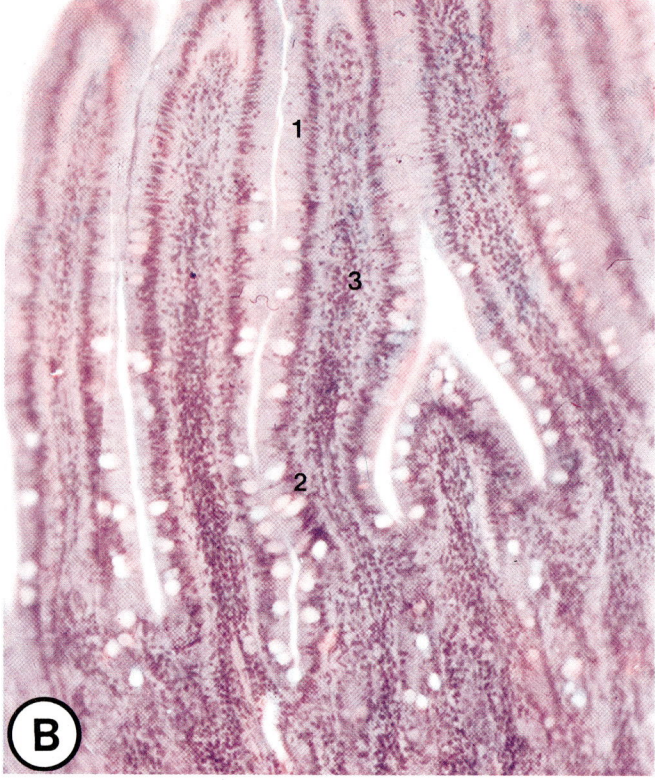

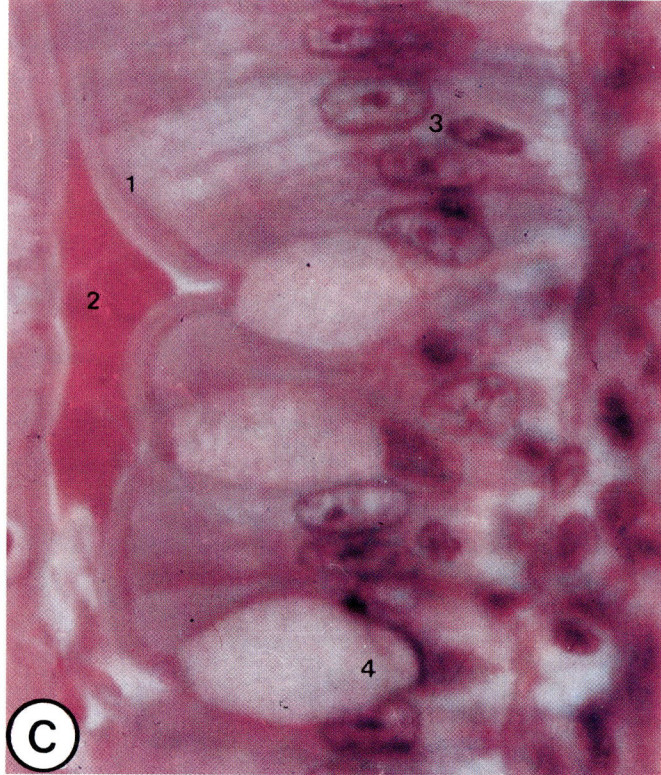

A **Longitudinal section of human duodenum (azan-Mallory, x45). 1 =** circular folds with intestinal villi **(2). 3 =** Brunner's glands in submucosa. **4 =** serosa. Between the submucosa and the serosa a thick muscular layer is present.

B **Longitudinal section of intestinal villi from cat (H & E, x240).** Covering the villi is simple columnar epithelium **(1)** with intercalated mucous goblet cells **(2)** seen as translucent vesicles. The core of the villus contains a richly vascular stroma **(3)**.

C **Epithelium of intestinal villus from cat (H & E, x800). 1 =** apical region of absorptive cell with brush border. **2 =** mucus. **3 =** nuclei of epithelium. **4 =** goblet cell.

Plate 8.6　　　　　　　　　　　　　　　　　　　　　　　　**191**

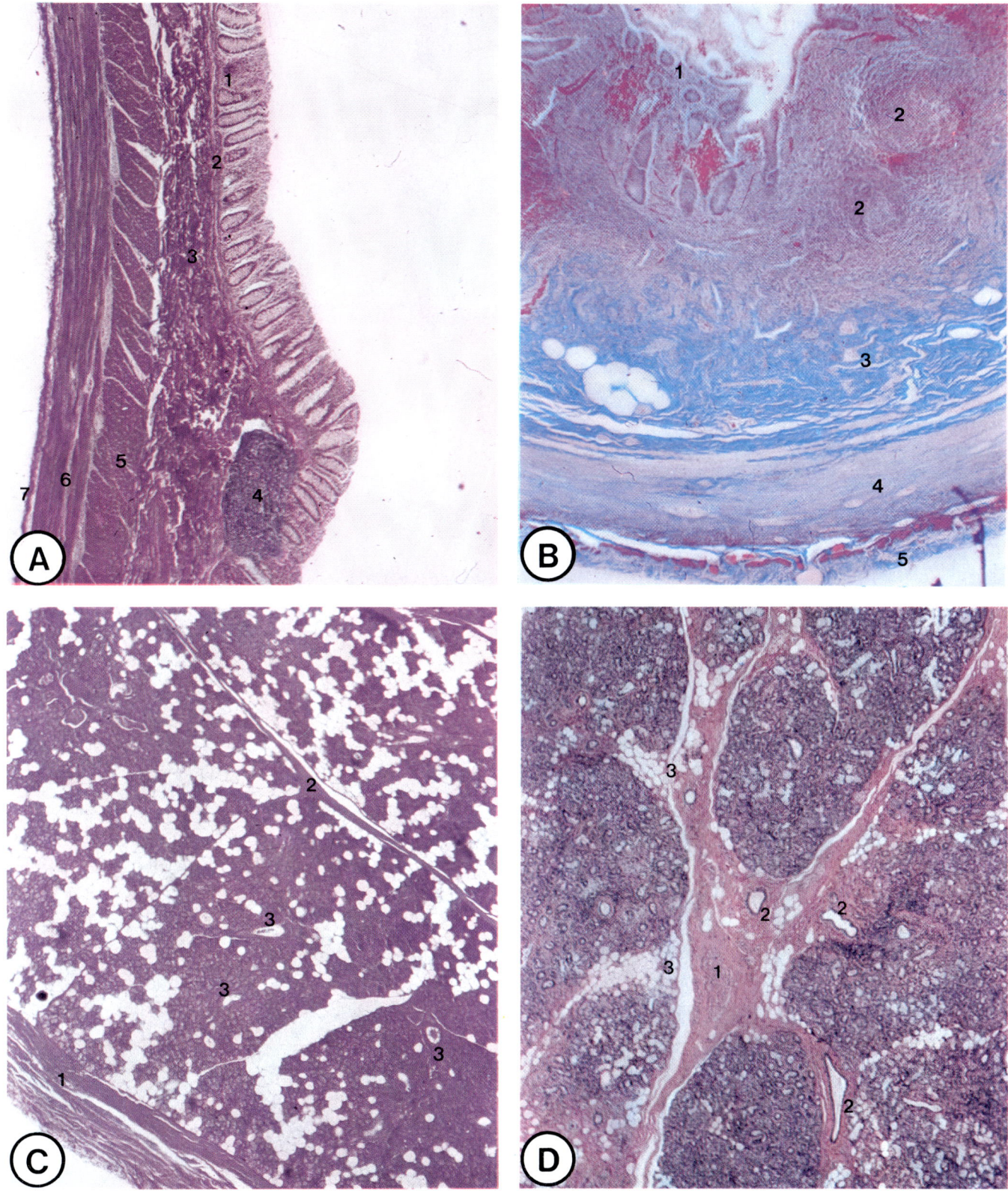

A　**Longitudinal section of human colon (H & E, x50). 1** = mucosa with glands. **2** = muscularis mucosae. **3** = submucosa. **4** = solitary lymph nodule in submucosa. **5** = internal and external **(6)** layers of muscularis. **7** = serosa.

B　**Cross section of human cecum (azan-Mallory, x80). 1** = epithelium. **2** = group of lymphoid follicles that extend the entire width of the mucosa. **3** = submucosa. **4** = muscularis. **5** = serosa.

C　**Parotid gland from cat (H & E, x45). 1** = capsule of connective tissue both surrounding the organ and forming internal septa **(2)** that divide the parenchyma into lobules. **3** = salivary ducts. The numerous transparent areas in the interlobular connective tissue are groups of adipose cells.

D　**Human submandibular gland (H & E, x45). 1** = connective tissue dividing the gland into lobules. **2** = interlobular ducts. A large number of serous acini (violet) and a small number of mucous acini comprise the lobules. In the interlobular connective tissue are accumulations of adipose cells **(3)**.

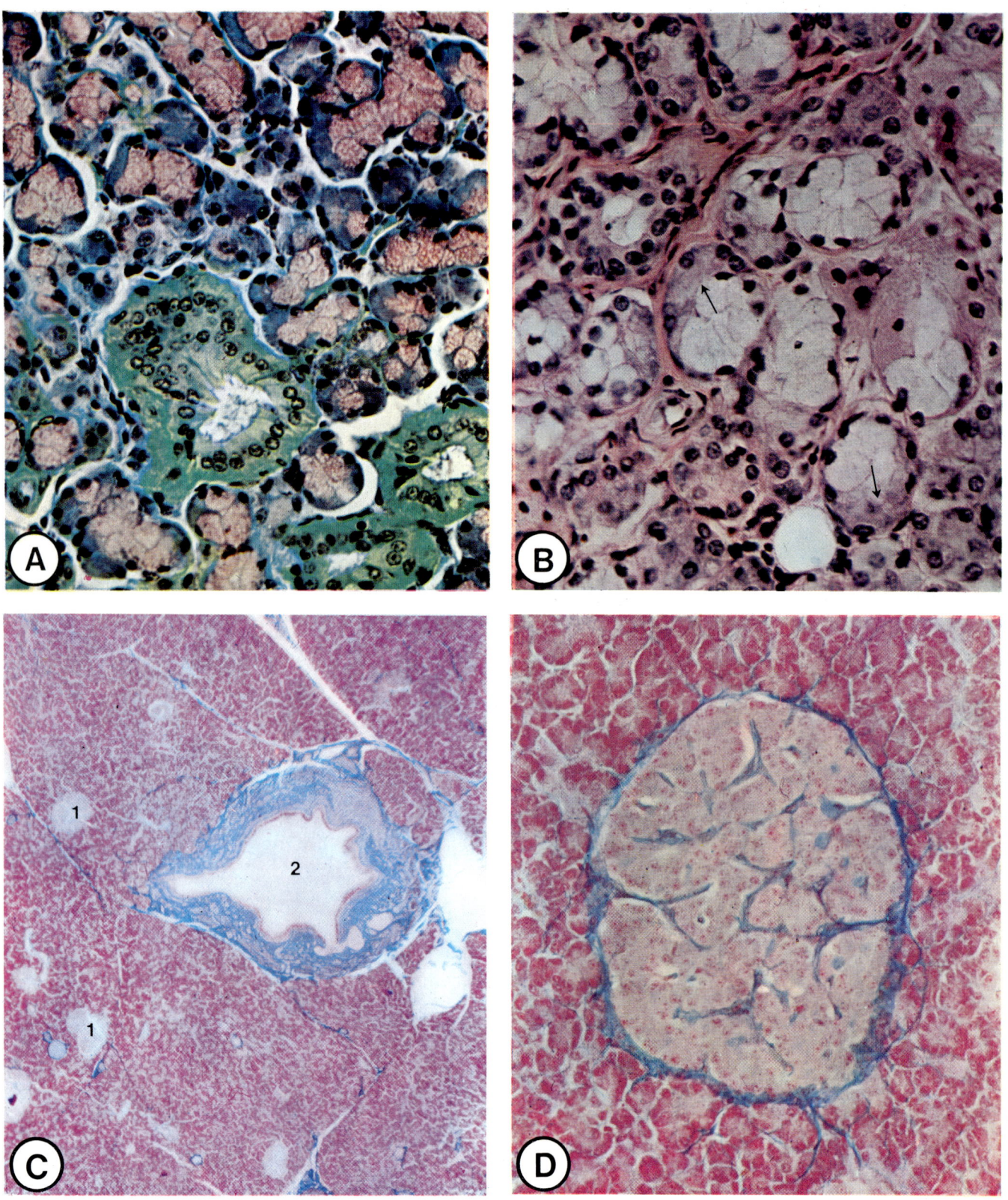

A   **Submandibular gland from calf (safranine orange, Weigert's fast-green/hematoxylin, x220).** Center: an excretory duct (green) surrounded by a number of mixed secretory units. The mucous cells are pink; the serous elements are blue and form demilunes.

B   **Sublingual gland from rat (H & E, x320).** Mucous cells (translucent) and serous cells (dark) are present. The serous cells form Gianuzzi's demilunes (→).

C   **Human pancreas (azan-Mallory, x80).** The interlobular septa of the connective tissue are stained blue. The exocrine area is stained red. The endocrine glands in the pancreas are the islets of Langerhans **(1).** In one interlobular septum is a large excretory duct **(2).**

D   **Human pancreas (azan-Mallory, x260).** Amid the exocrine portion of the gland (red) is an islet of Langerhans covered by a thin capsule of connective tissue (blue). The islets of Langerhans are composed of cords of epithelial cells in an anastomosing network that is interspersed with numerous blood capillaries.

Plate 8.8   **193**

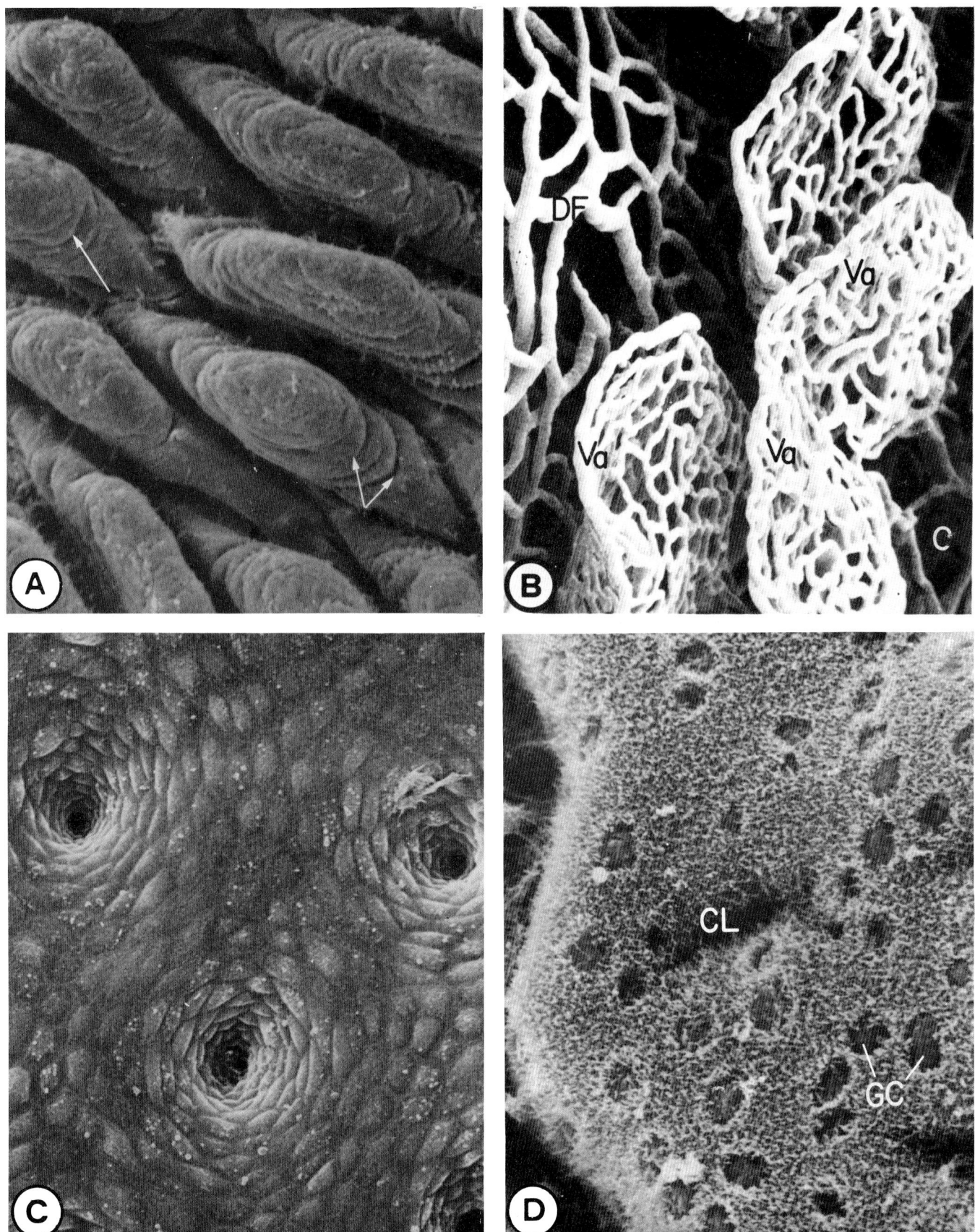

A   **Intestinal villi from monkey duodenum (scanning EM, x125).** Deep furrows (→) in some villi are the result of muscular contraction.

B   **Vascular network of mucosa from ileum of rat (vascular resin injection, scanning EM, x220).** Vascular networks of the villi **(Va)** can be seen as well as those of a gland crypt **(C)** and of a large lymph follicle in a Peyer's patch **(DF)**. By courtesy of T. Murakami and A. Ohtsuka.

C   **Gastric mucosa from monkey (scanning EM, x800).** The epithelium of the mucosa contains invaginations leading to the gastric glands.

D   **Mucosa from monkey colon (scanning EM, x1,000).** Goblet cells **(GC)** are interspersed among absorptive cells covered with microvilli. **CL** = intestinal glands (crypts of Lieberkuhn).

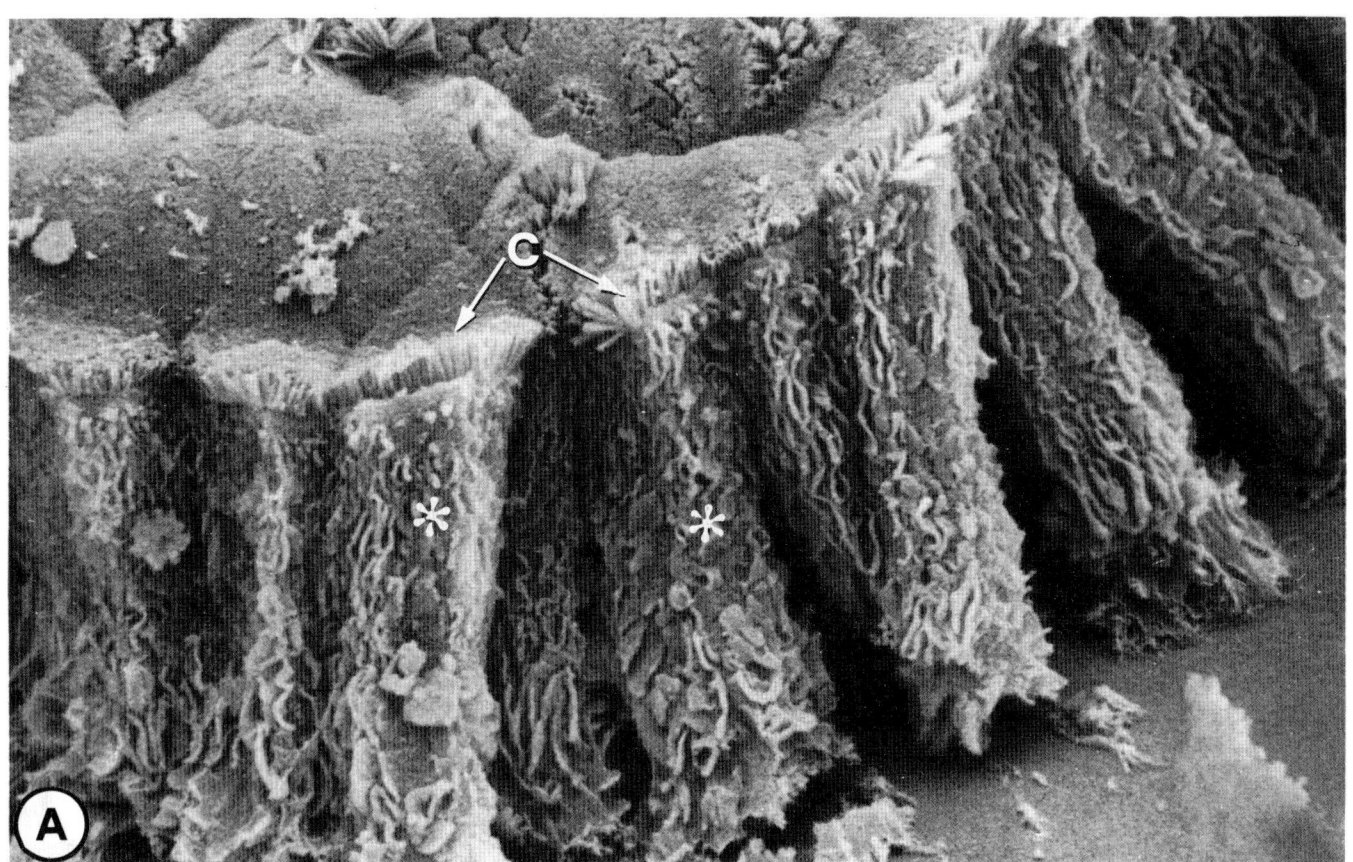

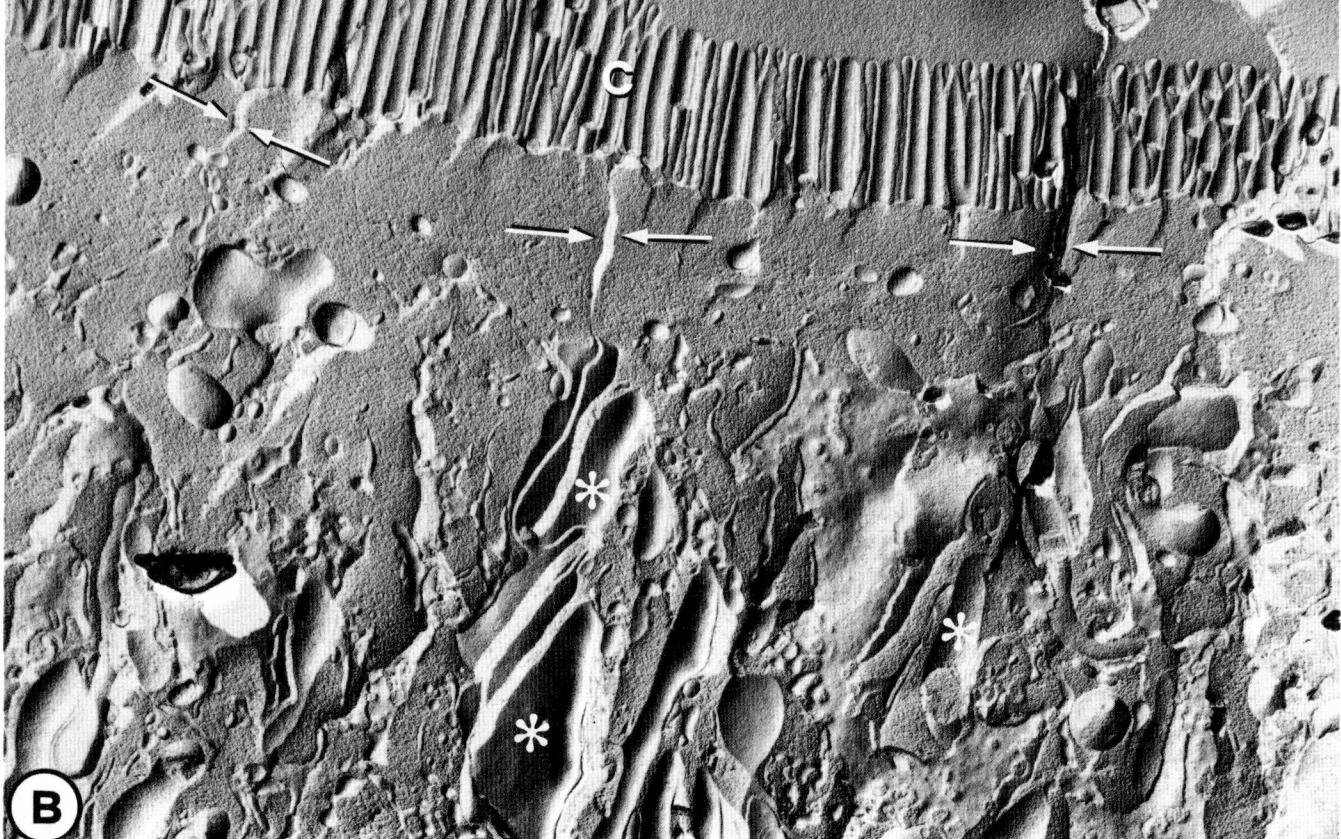

A Absorptive epithelium of rat small intestine (scanning EM, x2,100). The cells of the intestine have been partially stripped from the wall of the mucosa. Their appearance is cylindrical, with microvilli at the surface (brush border) **(C)**. The cells also have lamellar processes on their lateral surfaces **(*)**. These processes provide spaces between the cells through which the absorbed material is conveyed to the underlying lymph and blood vessels. By courtesy of J. Vial.

B Brush border of absorptive cells from rat small intestine (EM, freeze-fracture, x12,500). The cells are firmly bonded by junctional complexes below their apices (→), while in the underlying zone the membranes separate to form sizable intercellular spaces **(*)**. **C** = microvilli of the brush border. By courtesy of L.A. Staehelin.

Plate 8.10 195

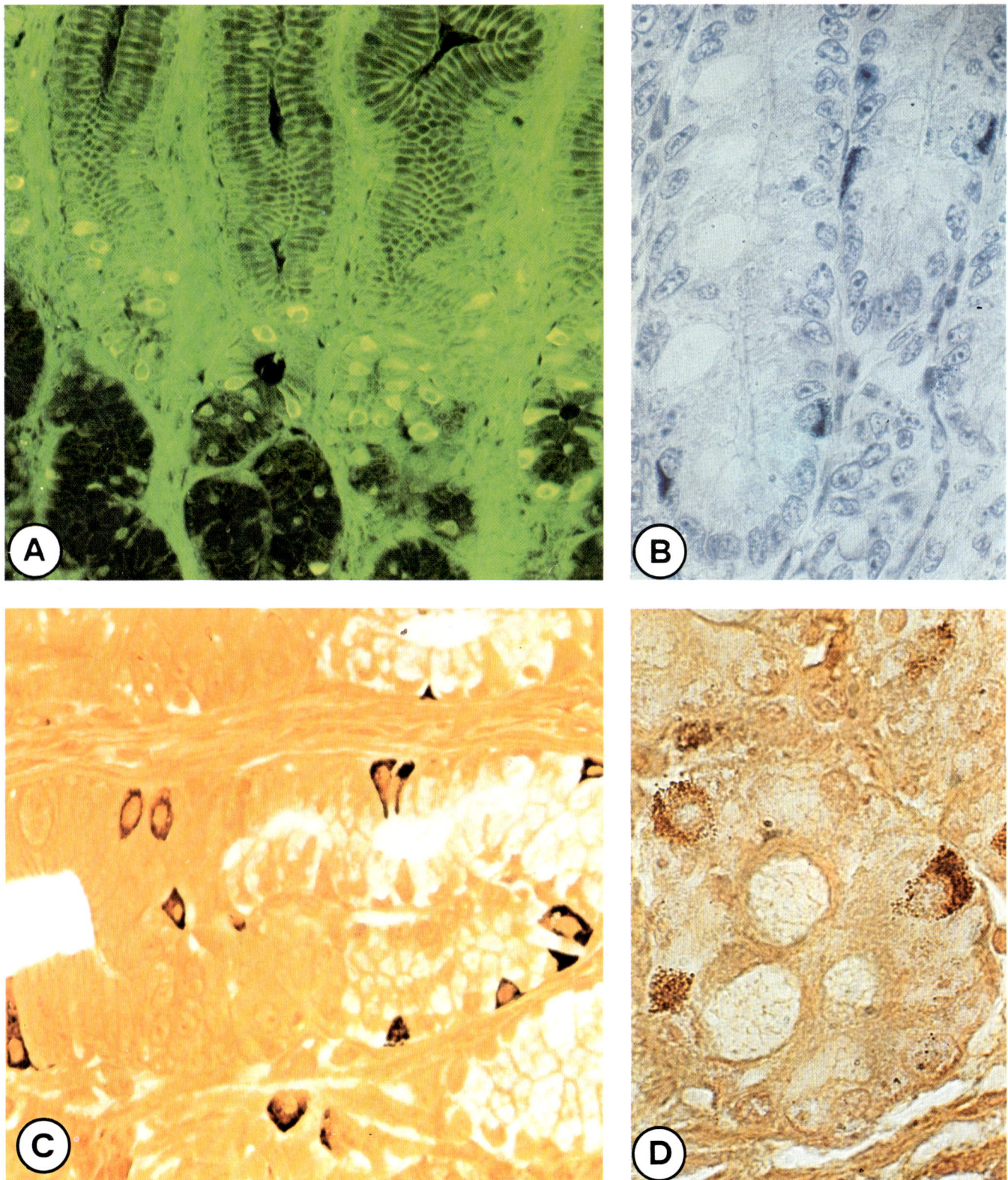

A **Gastrin cells in the pyloric antrum of a dog (indirect immunofluorescence for gastrin, x230).** The G-cells containing gastrin are evident. Original micrograph by T. Fujita.

B **Endocrine intestinal cells from pig duodenum (lead hemotoxylin, McConeil-Solcia method, x230).** In the glandular crypts of the duodenum are endocrine cells with granules concentrated at the basal pole of the cell. Original micrograph by T. Renda.

C **Endocrine cells in duodenum of dog (silver impregnation, Hellman-Hellstrom method, x250).** The endocrine intestinal cells (black) have a characteristic pyramidal shape. They are interspersed among the epithelial cells in the wall of the gland crypts. By courtesy of T. Fujita.

D **Endocrine intestinal cells from pig duodenum (Grimelius' argyrophil method, x820).** Along the wall of the gland are cells containing secretory granules. By courtesy of T. Renda.

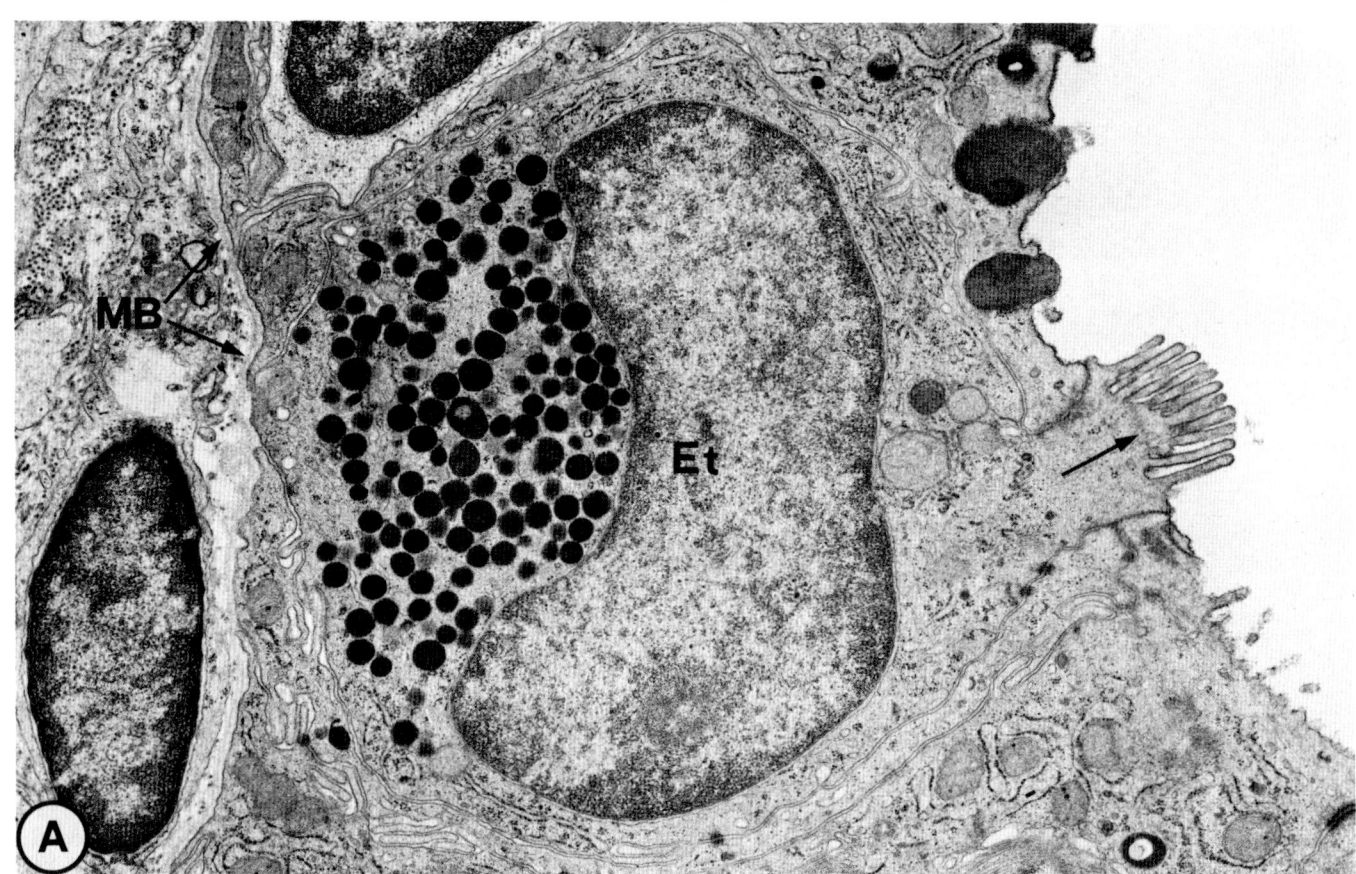

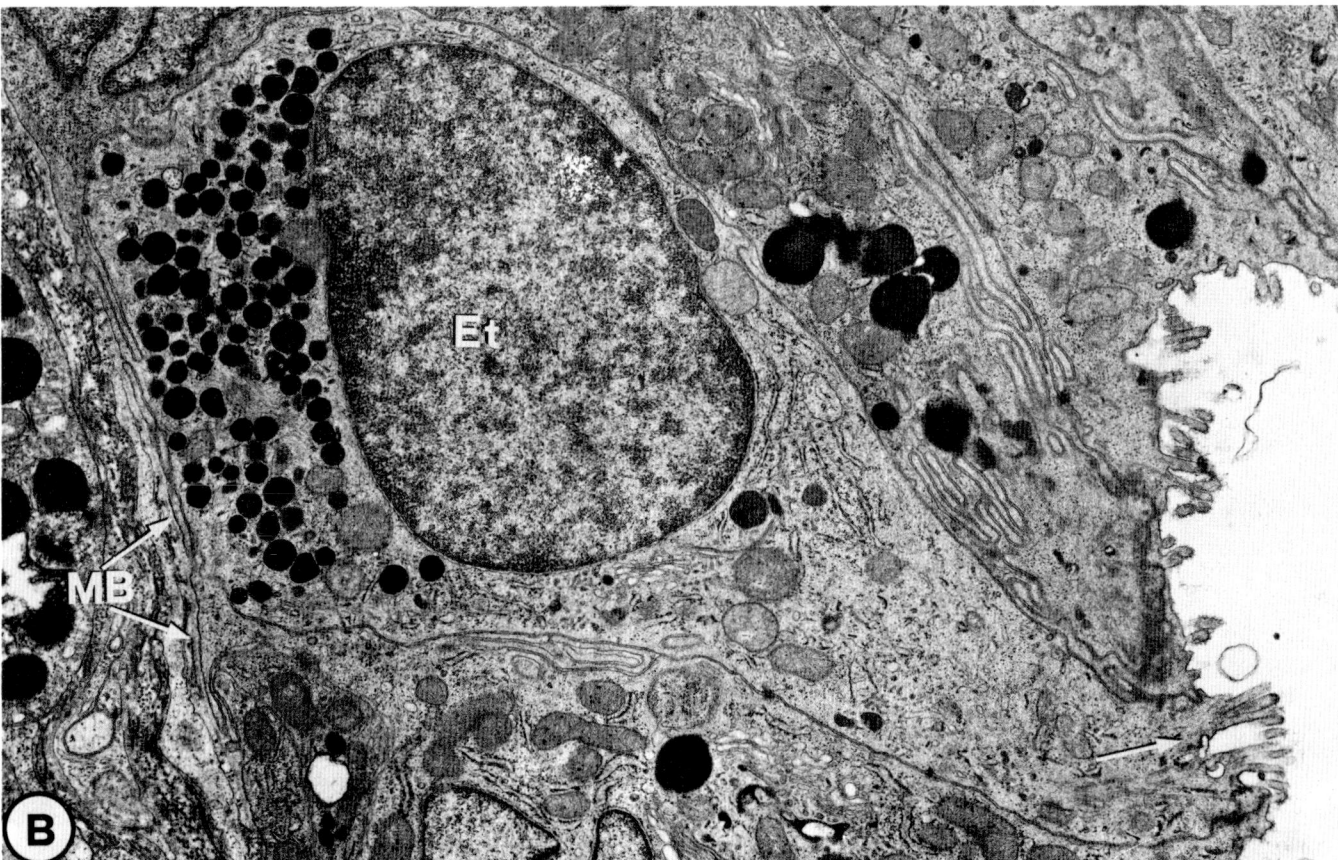

A, B   Endocrine cells from the intestine of human duodenum (EM, x15,000). The endocrine cell **(Et)** in Figure **A** lies among epithelial cells of the duodenal mucosa, whereas the endocrine intestinal cell of Figure **B** is wedged between the epithelial cells of a duodenal gland. Both have secretory granules concentrated in the basal part of the cell that rests on the basement membrane **(MB).** The apices of such cells have a characteristic tuft of microvilli (→). The intestinal cells shown secrete cholecystokinin. By courtesy of S. Kobayashi.

Plate 8.12   **197**

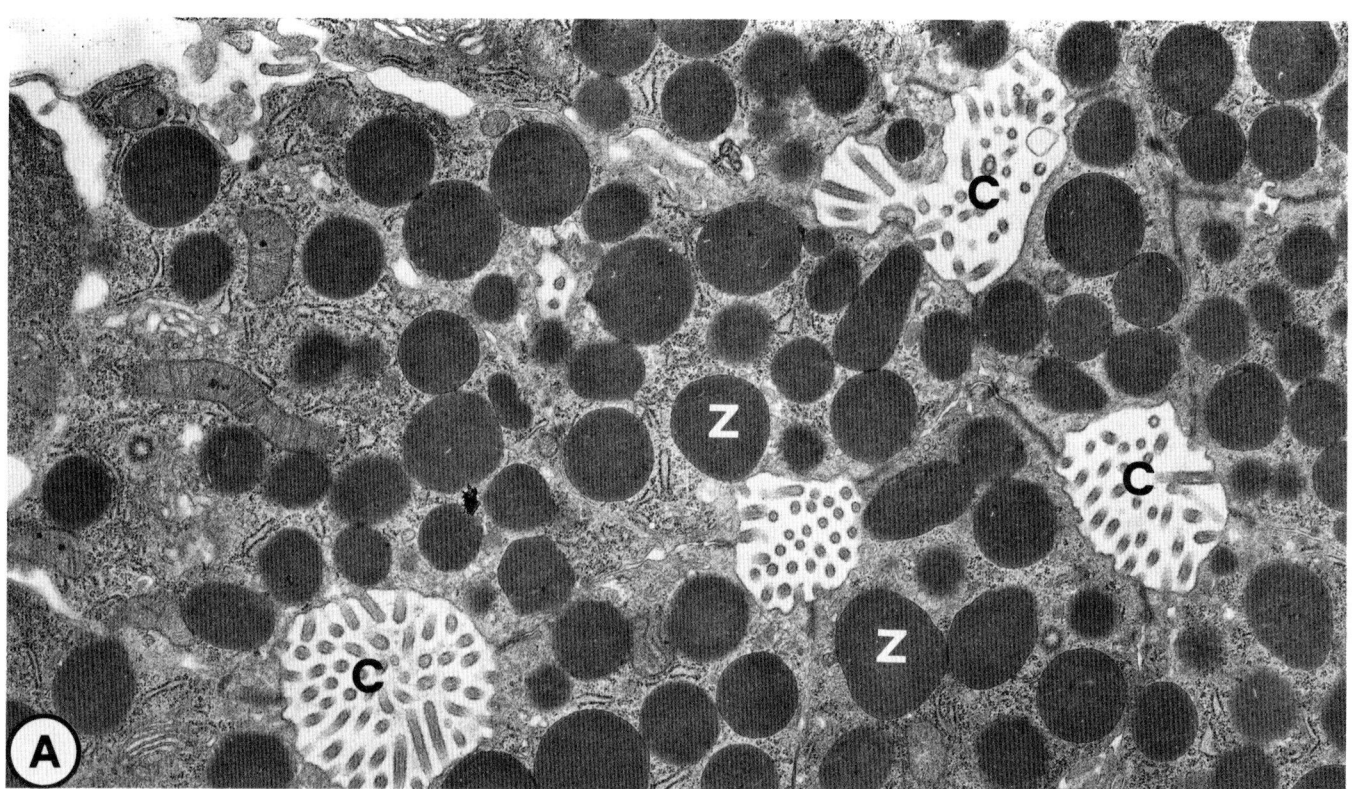

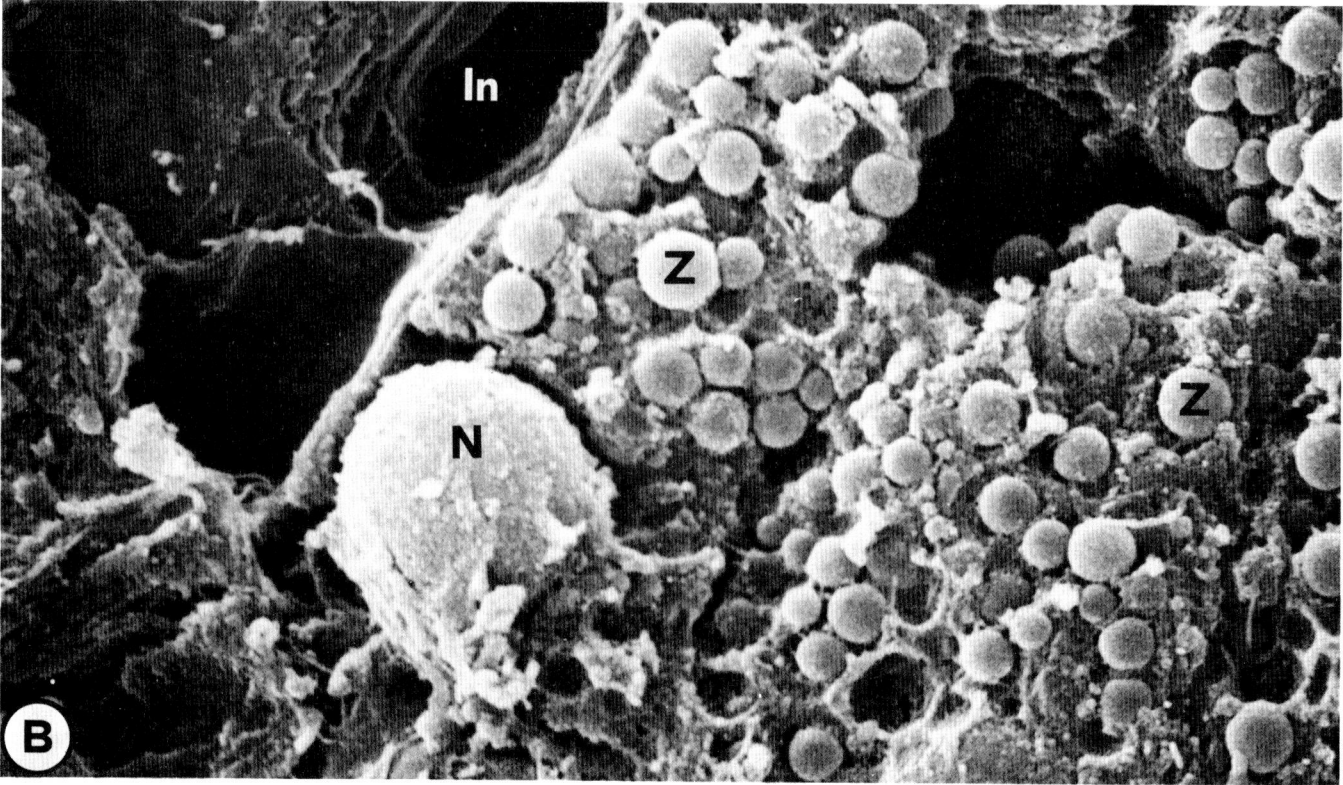

A **Exocrine pancreas from rat (EM, x10,350).** In the cytoplasm of acinar cells zymogen granules **(Z)** can be seen. The apical free surfaces of the cells are covered with microvilli that project into the canaliculi **(C)**.

B **Acinar cells from the exocrine pancreas of monkey (scanning EM, x5,300).** The acinar cells are broken open to reveal many cytoplasmic zymogen granules **(Z). N** = nucleus. **In** = intralobular duct. From P. Motta, P.M. Andrews, F. Caramia and S. Correr. Cell. Tiss. Res. 176: 493, 1977.

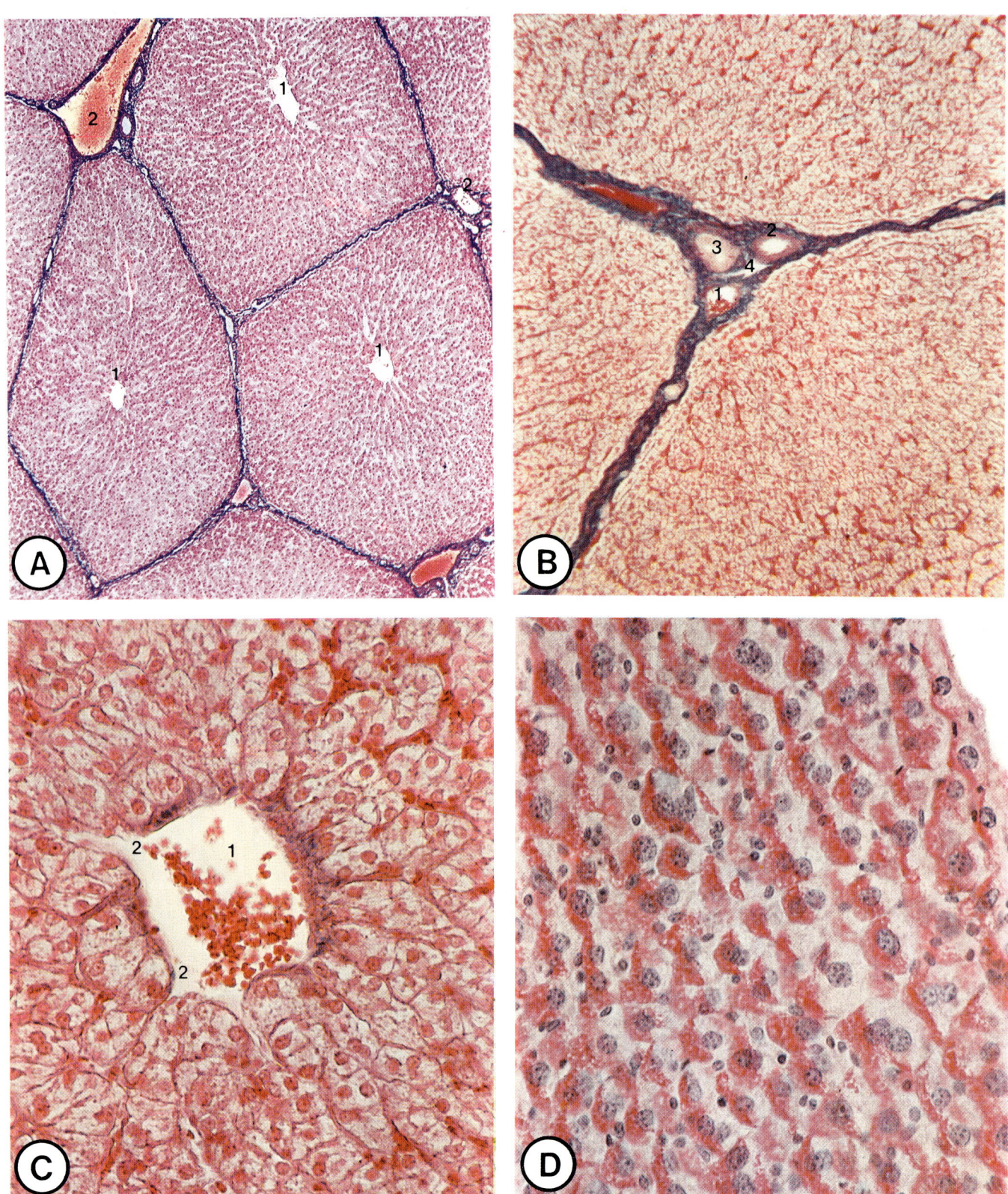

A   **Pig liver (azan-Mallory, x50).** The polygonal liver lobules are bounded by connective tissue septa and are composed of cell plates radiating from the centrolobular vein **(1).** At the corners of the polygons are triangular formations, the portal spaces **(2).**

B   **Pig liver (azan-Mallory, x180).** The portal space contains a branch of the hepatic portal vein **(1),** a branch of the hepatic artery **(2),** a bile duct **(3)** and a lymph vessel **(4).**

C   **Pig liver (azan-Mallory, x300).** The central part of a liver lobule with the centrolobular vein **(1)** contains red blood cells. At the circumference of the vein can be seen the outlets of some sinusoidal capillaries **(2)** which run between the cords of liver cells.

D   **Mouse liver (hematoxylin & Best's carmine, x320).** The glycogen is seen as masses of red granules. The hematoxylin has stained the nuclei violet.

Plate 8.14 199

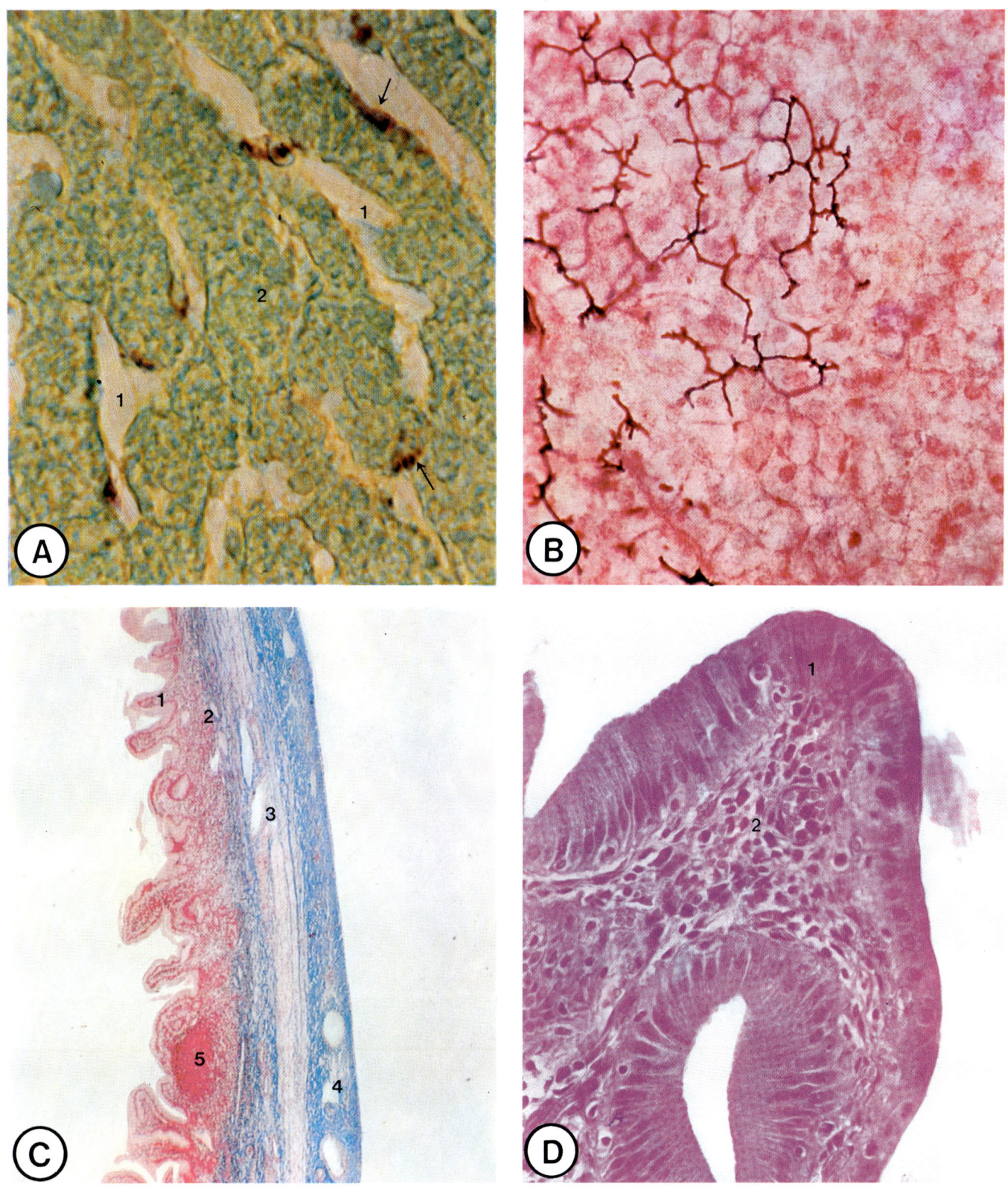

A **Mouse liver (carmine injection with green contrast staining, x800).** On the edge of the sinusoidal capillaries **(1)** can be seen some Kupffer cells, stained violet (→). **2** = cords of liver cells.

B **Mouse liver (India ink injection with carmine contrast staining, x400).** The network of bile canaliculi is enhanced.

C **Longitudinal section of the wall of human gallbladder (azan- Mallory, x50). 1** = mucosa raised in irregular folds and covered with simple columnar epithelium. **2** = lamina propria. **3** = muscular layer. **4** = subserous layer with large vessels. **5** = lymph nodule within the lamina propria.

D **Detail of mucosa of human gallbladder (H & E). 1** = epithelium. **2** = lamina propria.

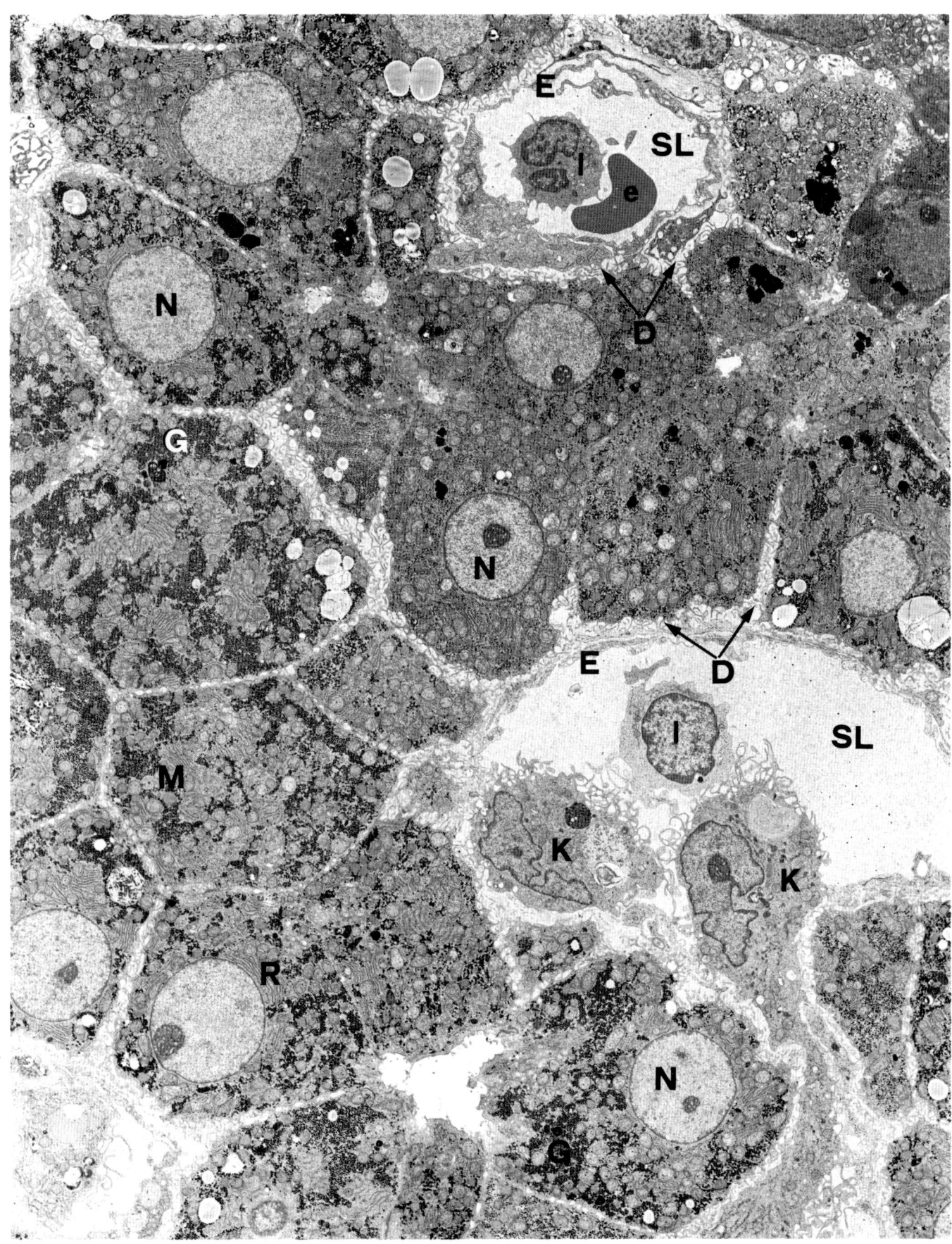

Human liver (EM, x4,600). Liver cells are large and have a typical polyhedral shape. **N** = nucleus. **R** = rough endoplasmic reticulum. **G** = glycogen inclusions. **M** = mitochondria. Sinusoidal lumina **(SL)** containing an erythrocyte **(e)** and leukocytes **(I)** can be seen. **E** = endothelial cells. **K** = Kupffer cells. **D** = spaces of Disse, which continue into broad intercellular spaces (→). By courtesy of F. Caramia et al. In: P.M. Motta and L.J.A. DiDio (eds). Basic and Clinical Hepatology. M. Nijhoff Publishers. The Hague/Boston/London, 1982.

Plate 8.16 201

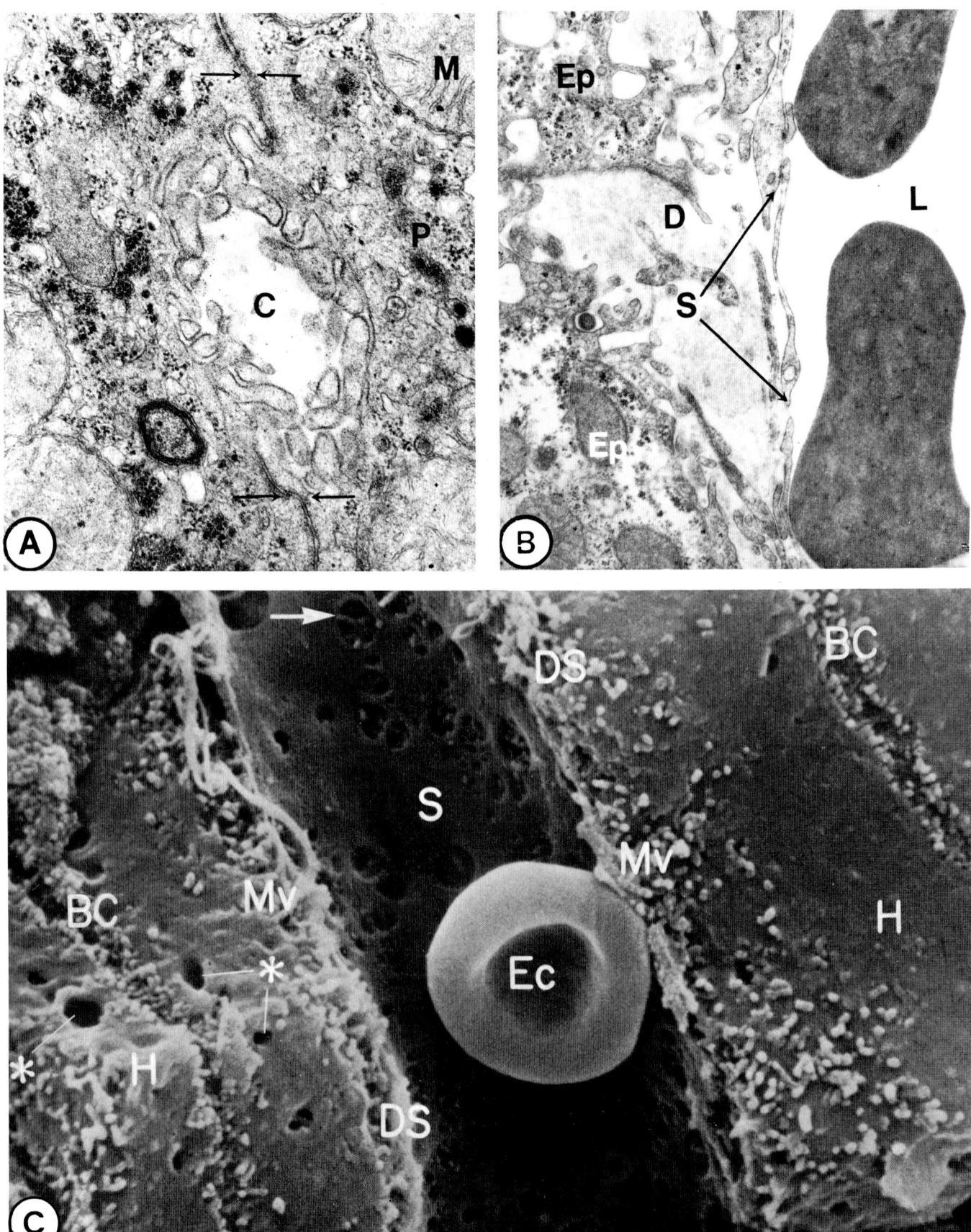

A   **Mouse liver (EM, x38,000).** Two contiguous liver cells can be seen enclosing a typical bile canaliculus (**C**) which has numerous microvilli. The liver cells are joined by junctions (→) and in their cytoplasm are granules of bile pigment (**P**) and mitochondria (**M**).

B   **Rat liver (EM, x18,500).** The surface of the liver cell (**Ep**) is in association with a sinusoid (**S**). Liver cells have a number of irregular microvilli projecting into the subendothelial (Disse) space (**D**). **L** = lumen of sinusoid with erythrocytes.

C   **Rat liver (scanning EM, x8,000).** Center: the fenestrated wall (→) and the lumen of a sinusoid (**S**) containing an erythrocyte (**Ec**). At the sides are two liver cells (hepatocytes) (**H**) with numerous microvilli (**Mv**) projecting into the subendothelial zone (spaces of Disse) (**DS**). The furrows making up one-half of a bile canaliculus (**BC**) can be seen, along with a number of invaginations (*) on the surface of the hepatocytes. From P.M. Motta and K.R. Porter. Cell. Tiss. Res. 148:111, 1974.

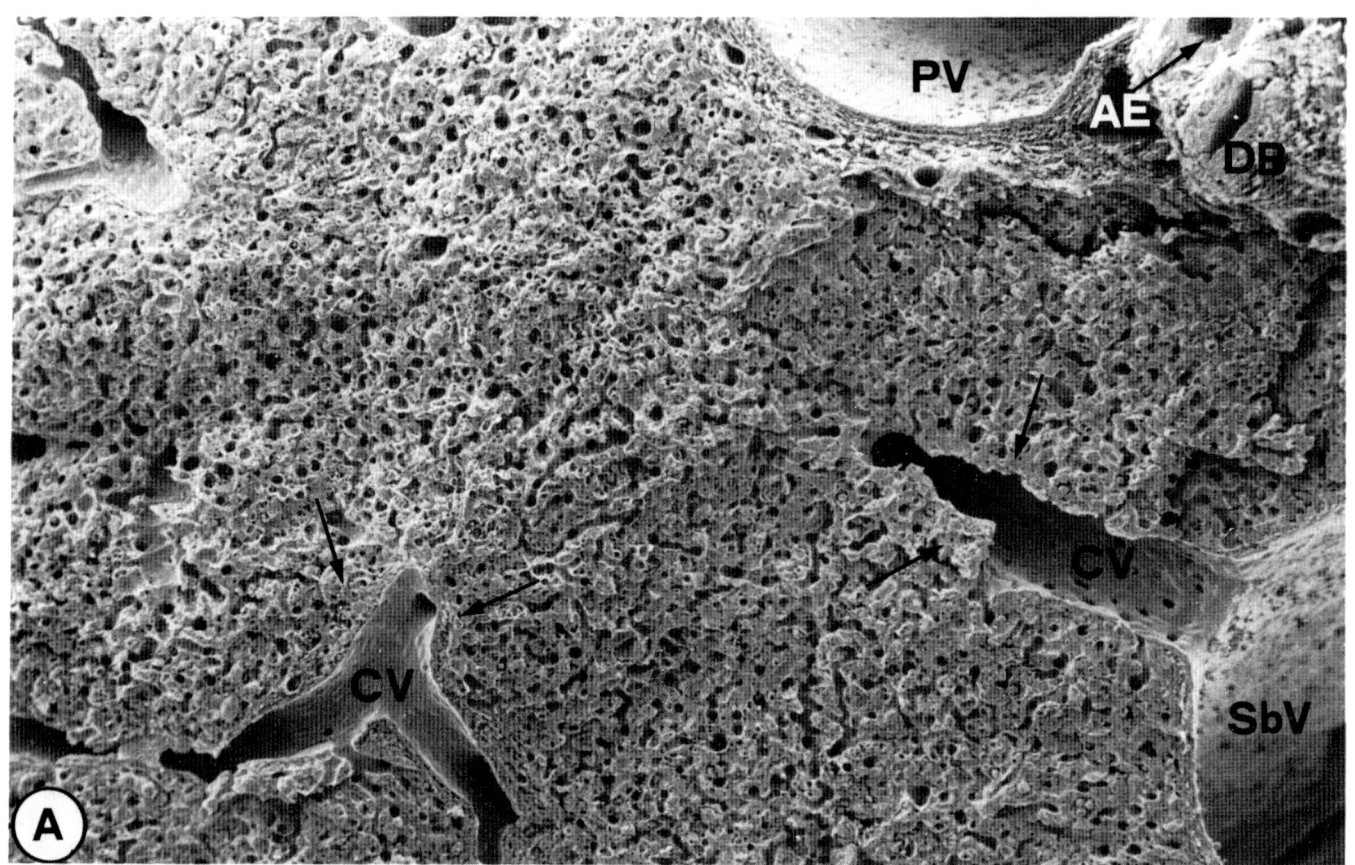

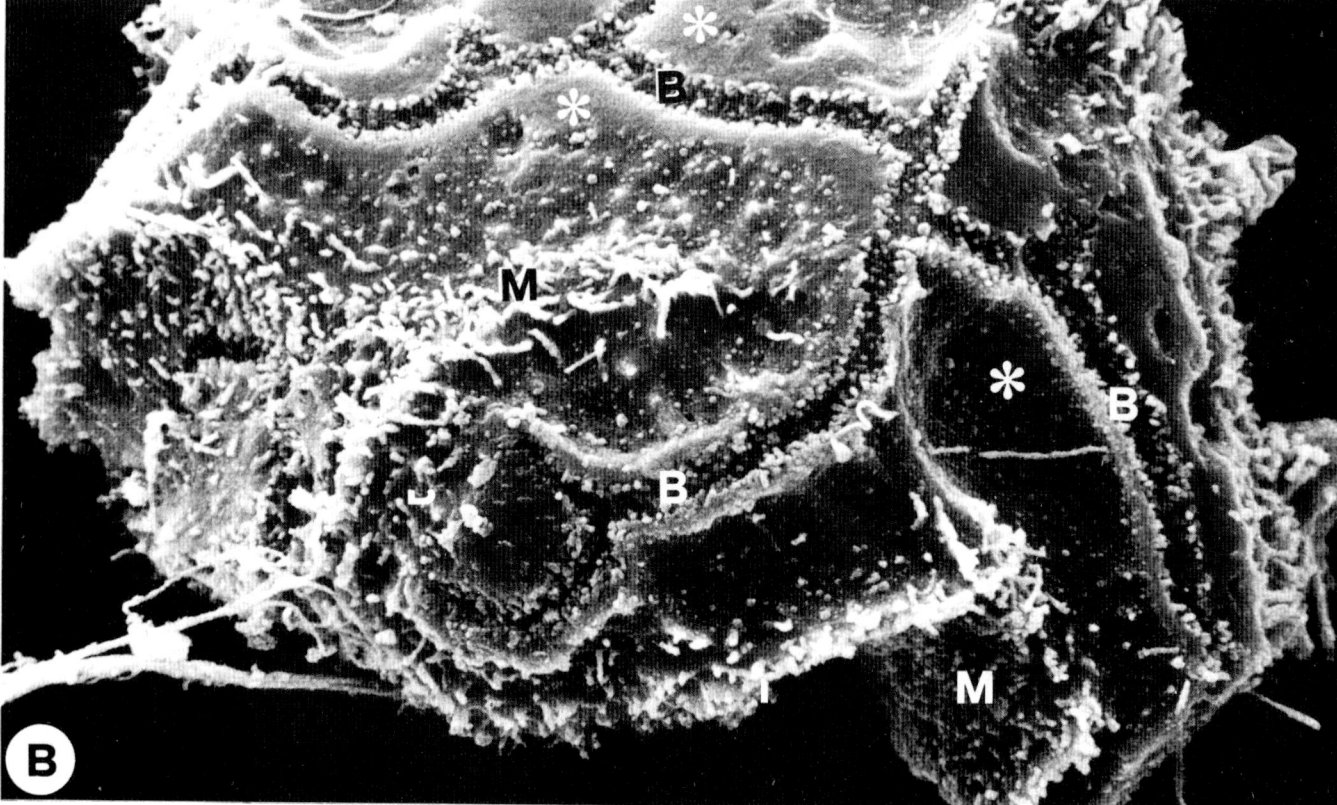

A **Rat liver (scanning EM, x210).** The parenchyma of the liver is composed of cords of hepatocytes and sinusoids radiating from a centrolobular vein **(CV)**. Above: part of the portal area with branches of the portal vein **(PV)**, the hepatic artery **(AE)** and the bile duct **(DB)**. SbV = sublobular vein.

B **Rat hepatocyte (scanning EM, x7,300).** In an isolated cell can be seen the surfaces enclosing the bile furrows **(B)** and those facing the subendothelial space, which is rich in microvilli **(M)**. The smooth surfaces **(*)** mark the areas of the hepatocyte that were joined. From P.M. Motta, M. Muto and T. Fujita. *The Liver. An Atlas of Scanning Electron Microscopy.* Igaku-Shoin, Ltd, Tokyo/New York, 1978.

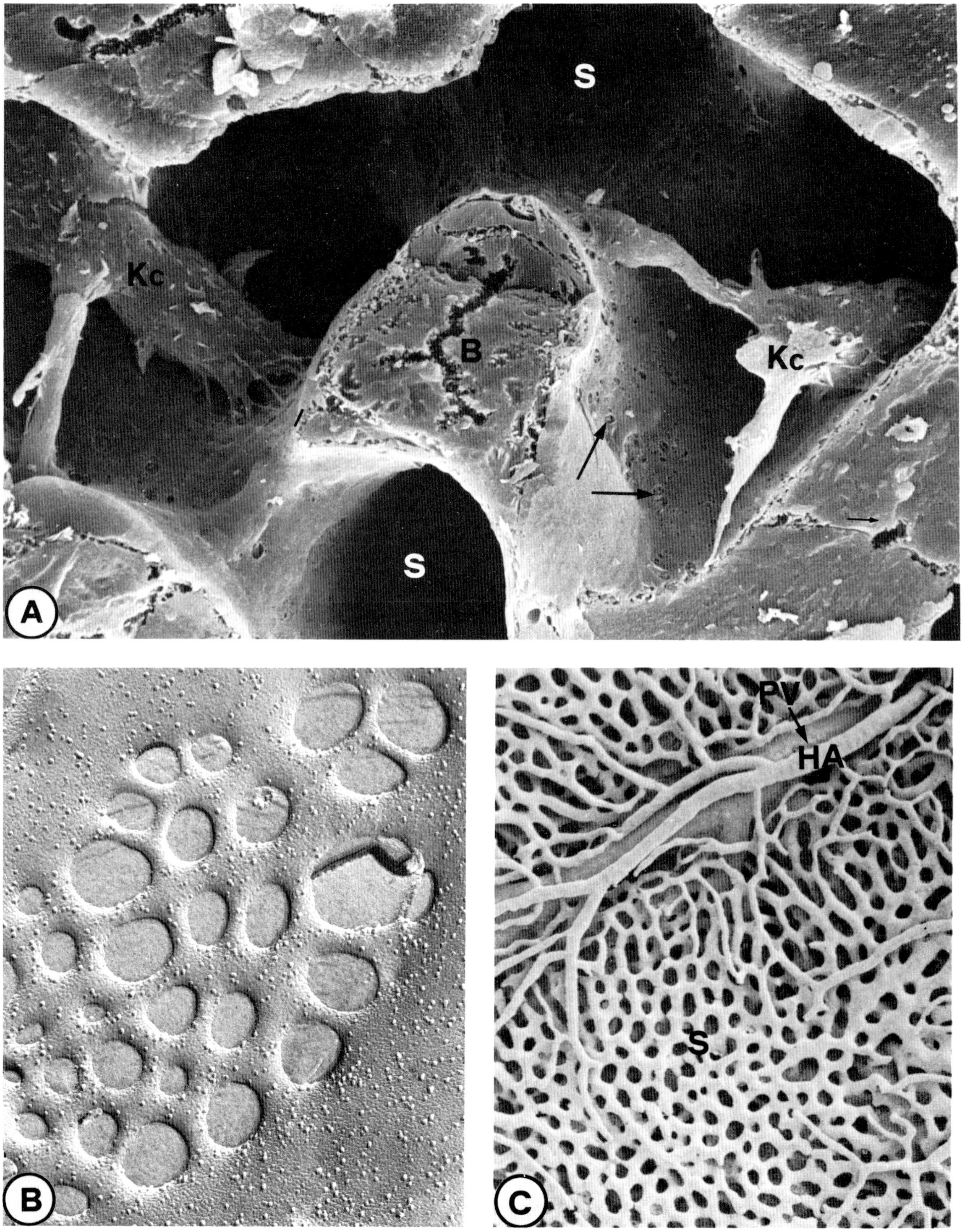

Plate 8.18 203

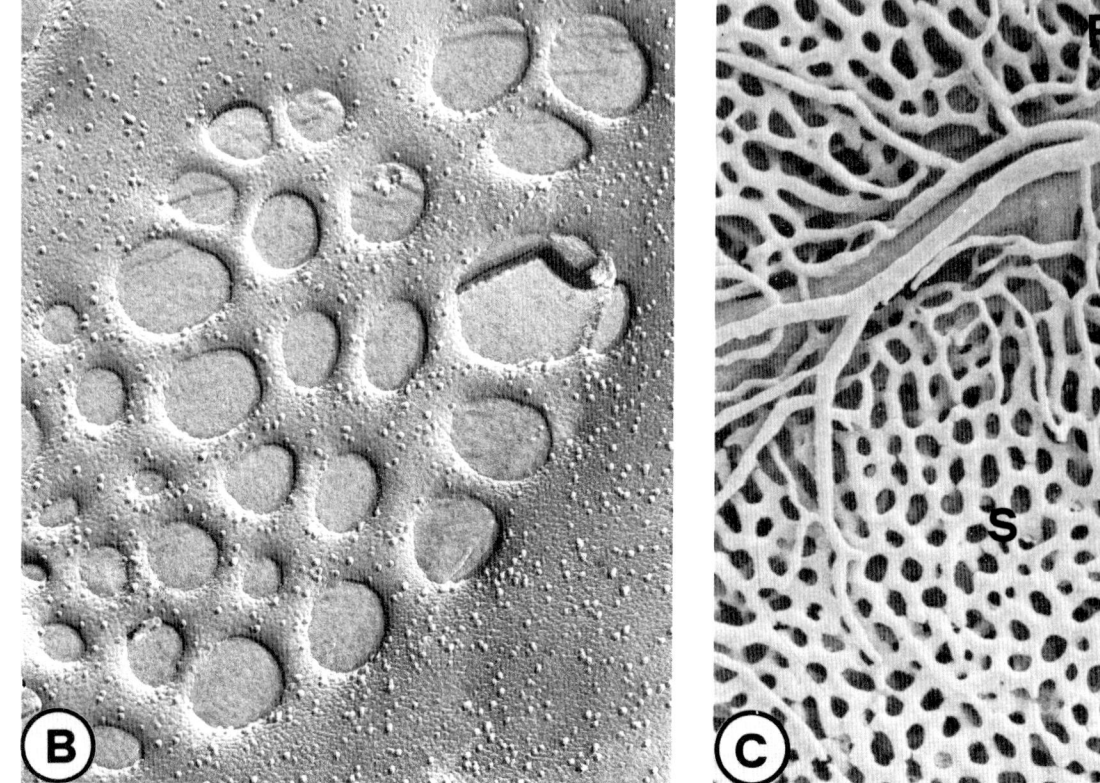

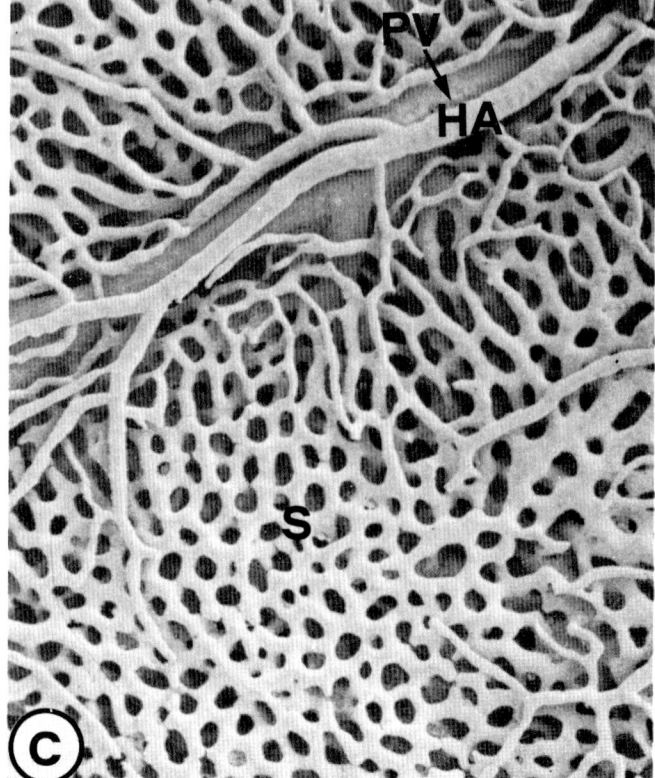

A   **Hepatocytes and sinusoids in guinea-pig liver (scanning EM, x4,200).** The sinusoids have a fenestrated wall (→) and in the lumen are Kupffer cells **(Kc)**. **B** = bile furrows along the surface of a hepatocyte. From P.M. Motta, M. Muto and T. Fujita. *The Liver. An Atlas of Scanning Electron Microscopy.* Igaku-Shoin, Ltd, Tokyo/New York, 1978.

B   **Liver sinusoid from a rat (EM, freeze-fracture, x69,000).** This high resolution image shows the sizable fenestrations of the thin endothelial wall of the sinusoid. By courtesy of R. Montesano and P. Nicolescu. Anat. Rec. 190:861, 1978.

C   **Sinusoidal network from monkey liver (vascular resin injection, scanning EM, x130).** The dense network of sinusoids **(S)** is partly limited by branches of the hepatic portal vein **(PV)** and hepatic artery **(HA).** By courtesy of T. Murakami and O. Ohtani.

Plate 8.19

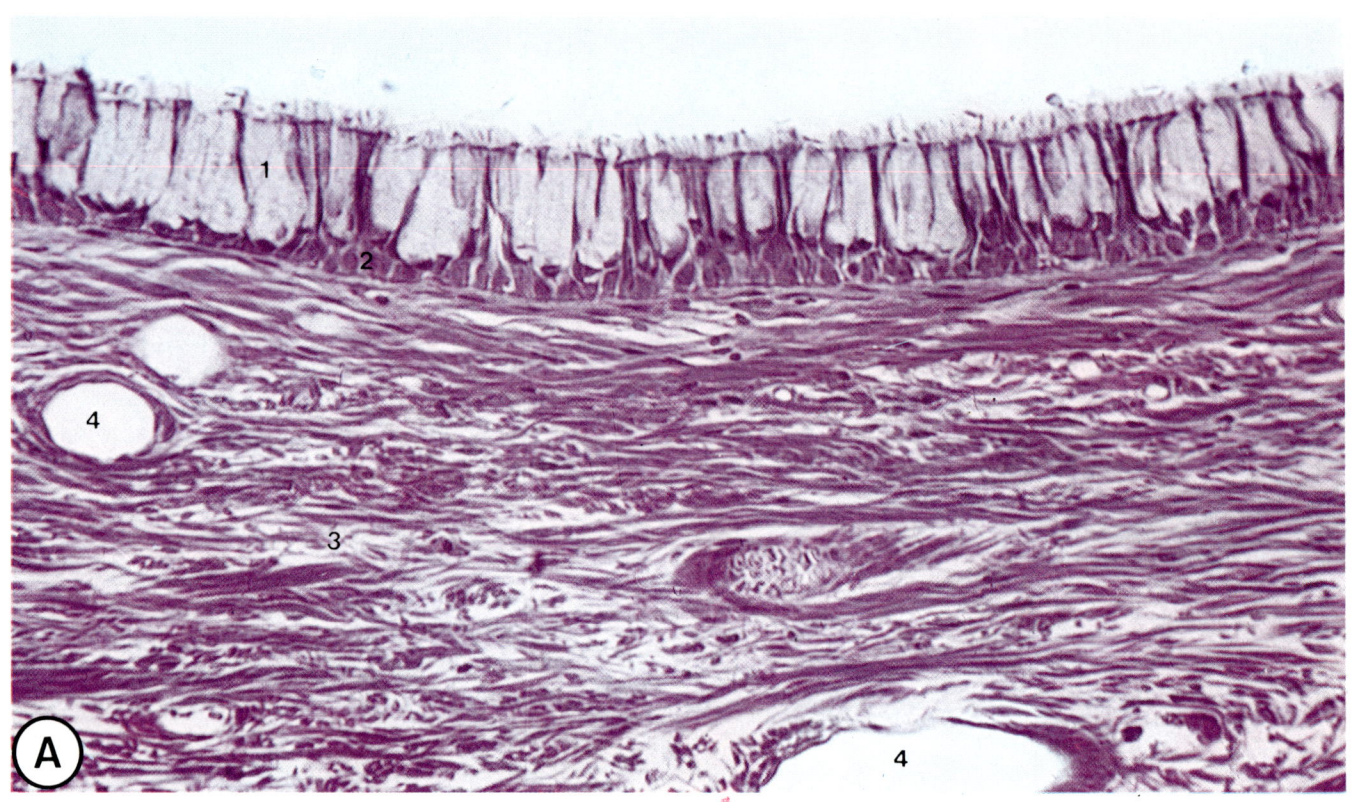

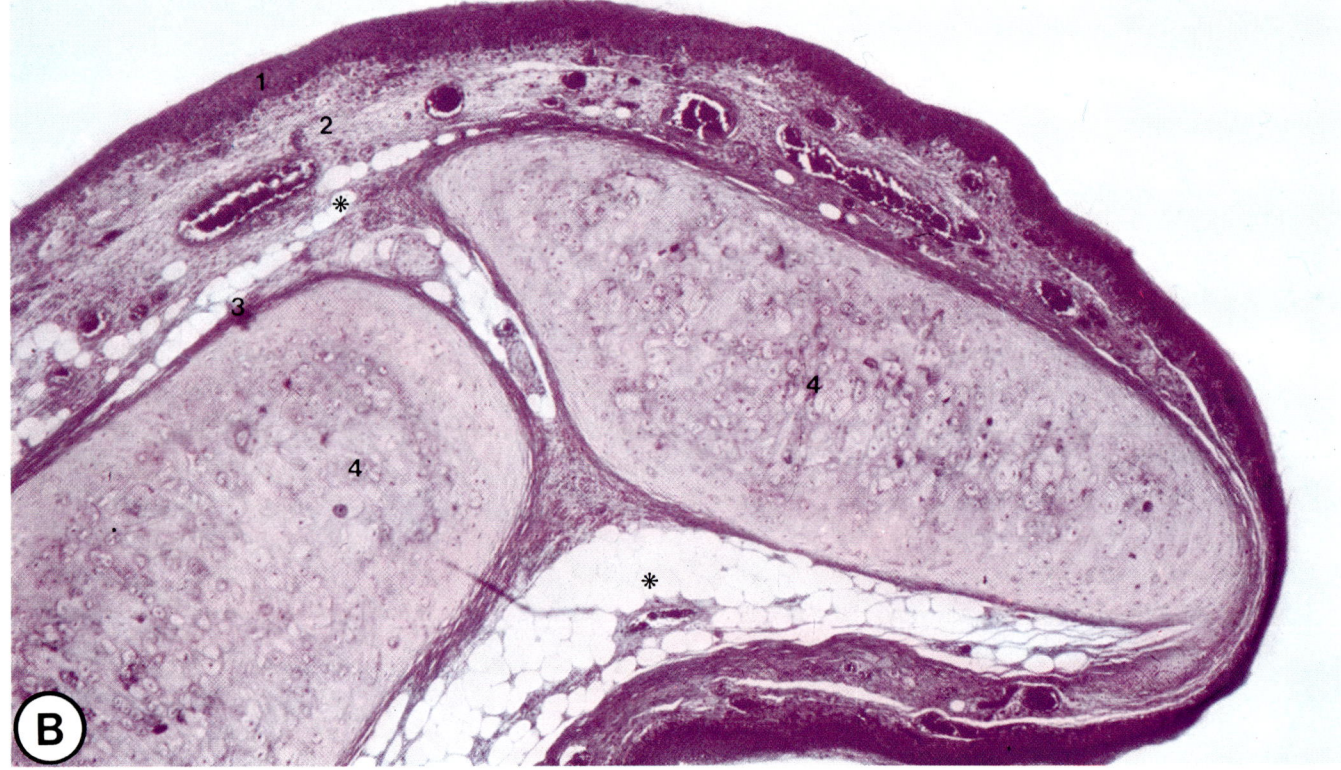

A **Mucosa of human frontal sinus (H & E, x340).** Above: In the mucosa several cell types are present, in addition to the ciliated cells: goblet cells **(1)** having a translucent cytoplasm, and small cells **(2)** bordering the basal lamina. In the underlying lamina propria **(3)** are bundles of collagen and elastic fibers in great numbers with many blood vessels **(4)**. In this section there are no glands present.

B **Apex of human epiglottis (H & E, x30).** **1** = stratified squamous epithelium. **2** = lamina propria with many blood vessels, bundles of collagen fibers and lobules containing adipose tissue (*). **3** = perichondrium. **4** = elastic cartilage.

Plate 8.20 205

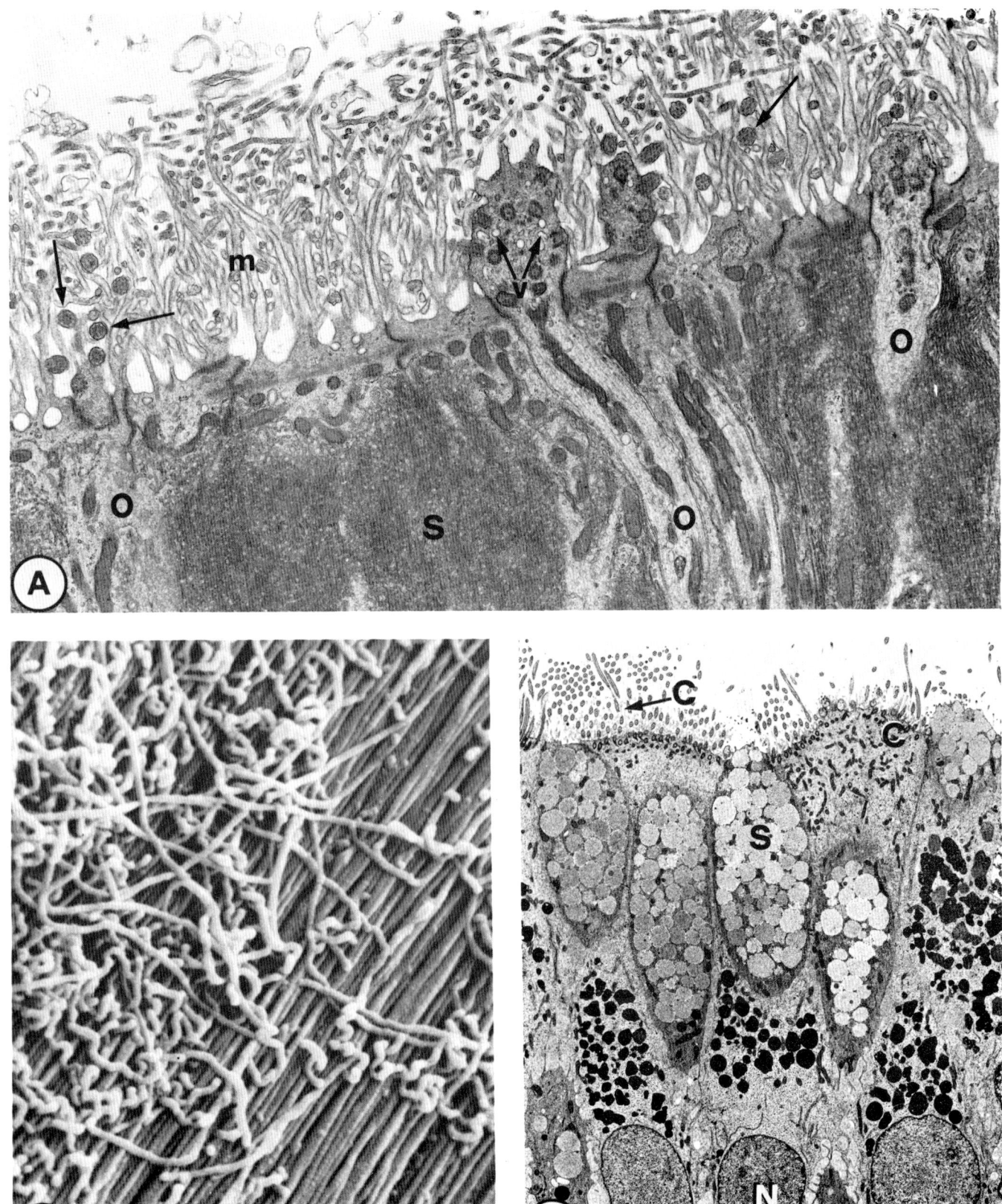

A **Olfactory epithelium of nasal mucosa from rat (EM, x13,200).** Among the supporting cells (**S**), which have long microvilli (**m**), are some olfactory cells (**O**). These are modified neurons with a bulbous surface (olfactory vesicle). From them (→) project a number of long cilia that act as receptors. Original micrograph by F. Caramia.

B **Olfactory cilia from nasal mucosa of rat (EM, x9,000).** The cilia that receive the olfactory stimuli are long processes mingled with microvilli of the supporting cells. By courtesy of P.M. Andrews. Amer. J. Anat. 139:399, 1974.

C **Respiratory mucosa from the trachea of rat (EM, x5,900).** Goblet-shaped secretory cells (**S**) interspersed with numerous columnar cells (**C**) constitute the epithelium of the mucosa. **N** = nuclei. (**C**) = cilia. By courtesy of F. Caramia.

Plate 8.21

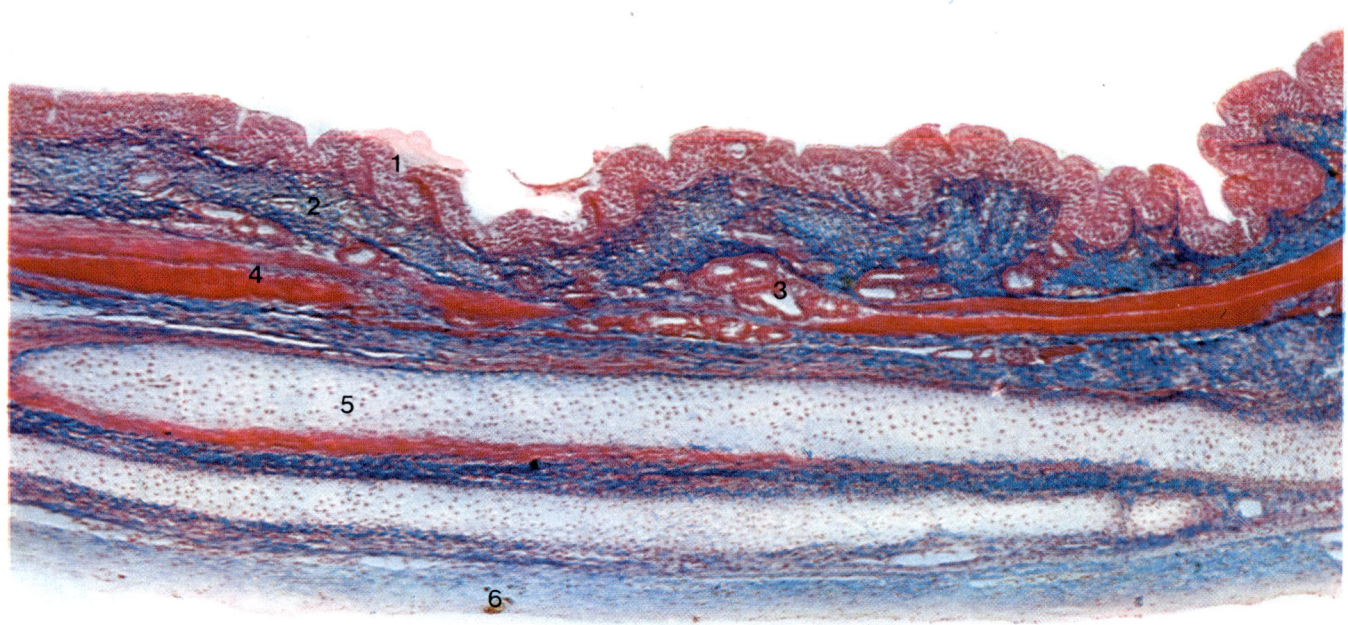

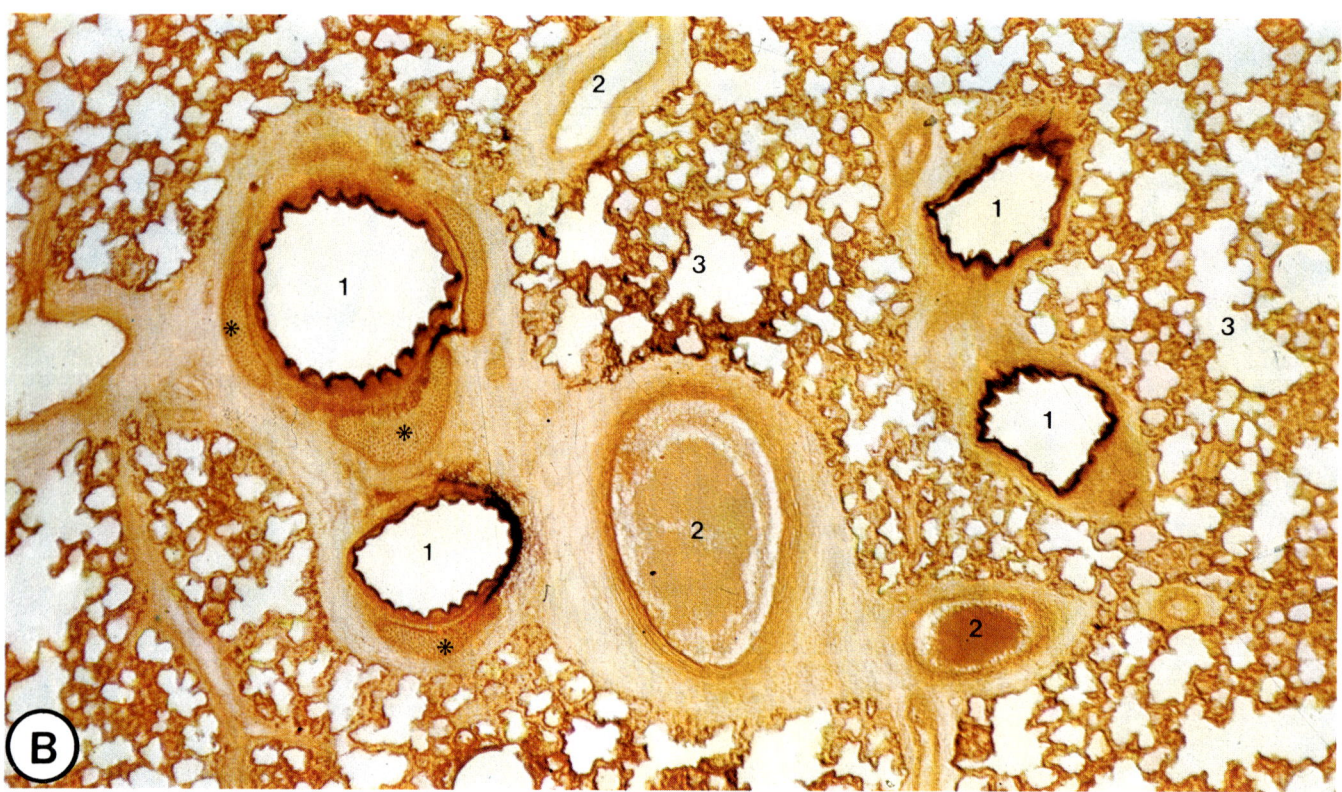

A **Oblique longitudinal section of the trachea from dog (azan-Mallory, x25). 1** = epithelium from mucosa raised in small folds. The epithelium is columnar and contains ciliated cells. **2** = lamina propria. **3** = submucosa with glands. **4** = smooth muscle fibers of the tracheal muscle in the tunica fibrosa. **5** = hyaline cartilage. **6** = adventitia.

B **Lung from cat (silver impregnation, x50).** Center: a number of sectioned interlobular bronchi **(1)** lined with an incomplete ring of cartilaginous plates **(*)** and embedded in the surrounding connective tissue can be seen. In association with the bronchi are blood vessels **(2)**. Inside the lobules are the alveolar ducts containing a large number of openings into the alveoli **(3)**.

Plate 8.22   207

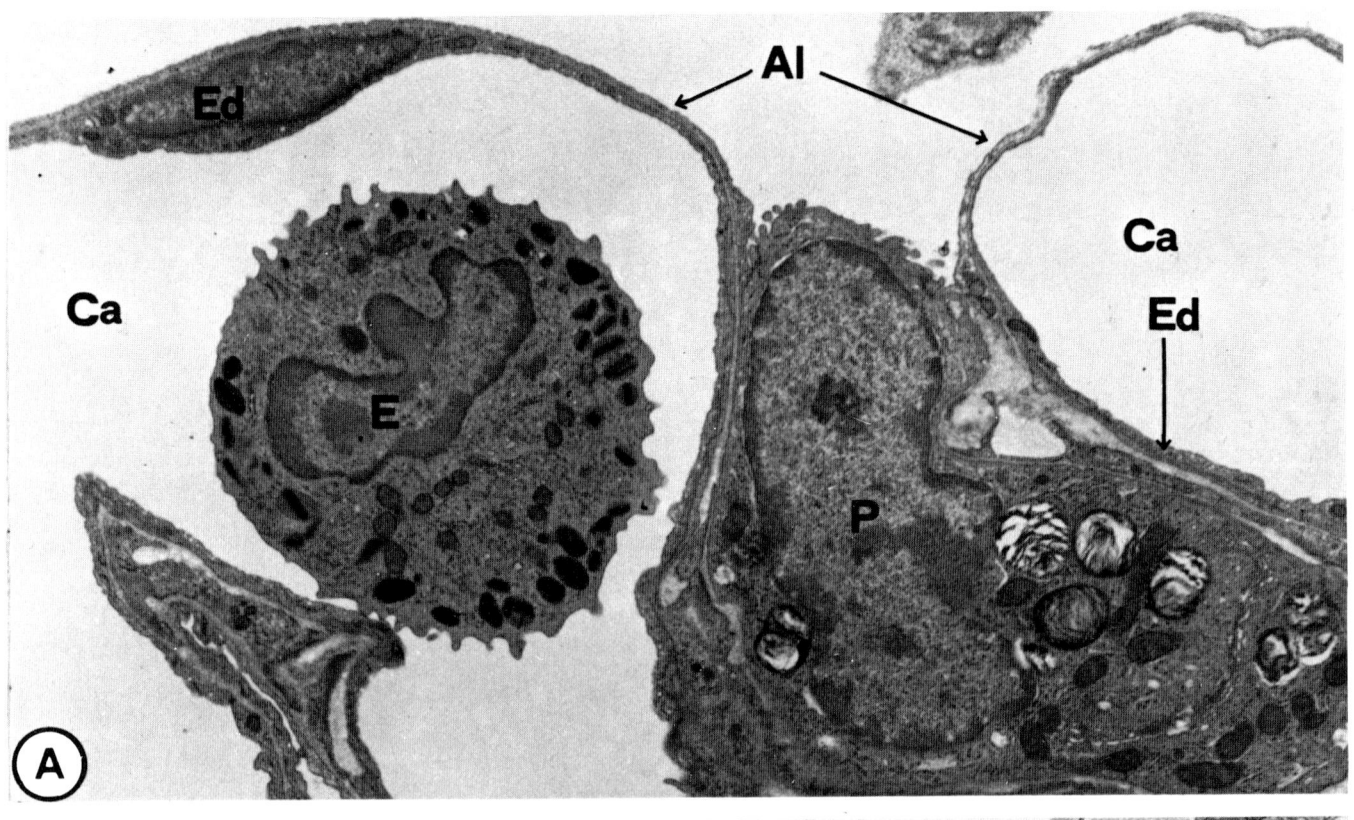

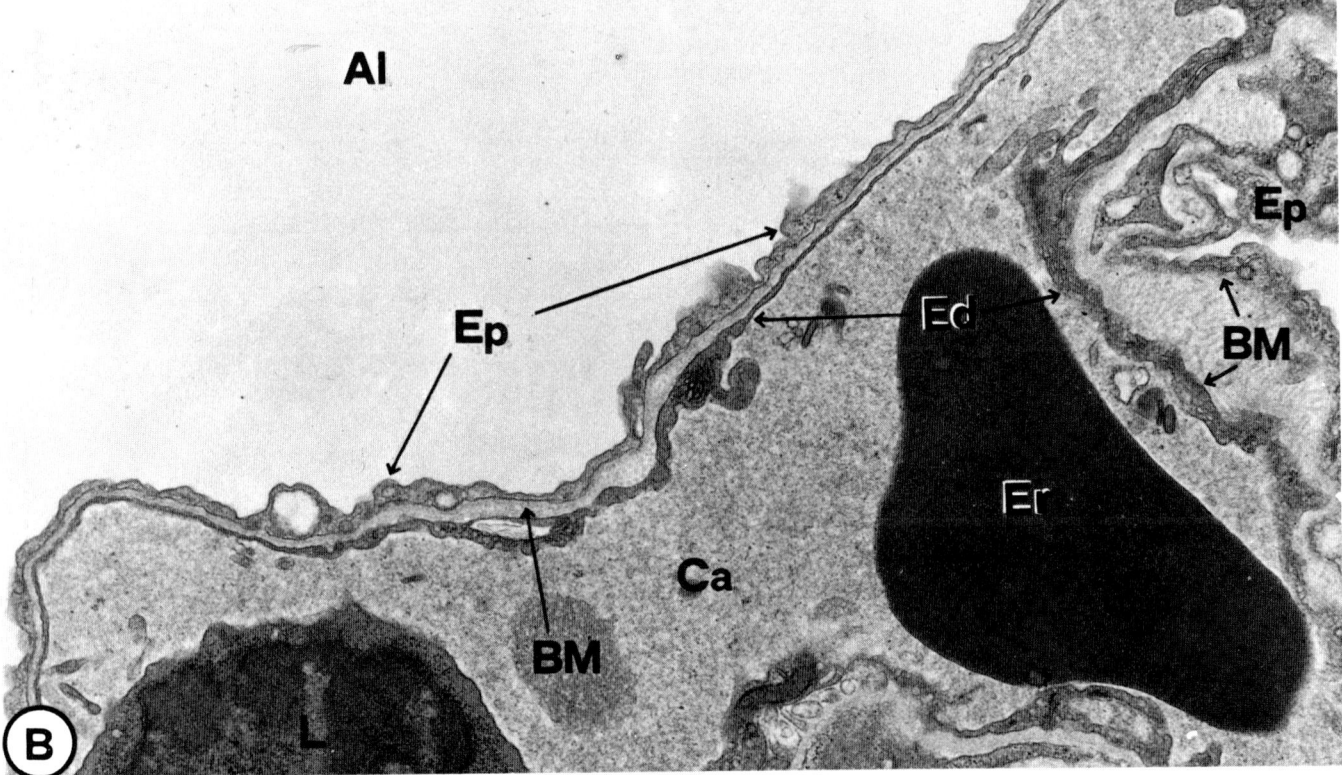

A   **Rat lung (EM, x14,500).** Detail of the wall of an alveolus. **(Ed)** = endothelial cells. **Ca** = blood capillaries. **E** = eosinophilic granulocyte in the lumen of a capillary. The alveolus **(Al)** is lined with flattened cells (*squamous cells*). The lining of the alveolus also contains a *great alveolar cell (septal cell)* **(P)** that has a number of dense lamellar bodies (cytosomes) which contain surfactant.

B   **Wall of alveolus from rat lung (EM, x21,500). Ca** = blood capillary containing an erythrocyte **(Er)** and a leukocyte **(L)**. **(Ed)** = endothelial cells. The wall of the alveolus is lined with flattened epithelial cells that rest on a basement membrane **(BM)**. **Ep** = epithelium of alveolus. **Al** = alveolus. By courtesy of F. Caramia.

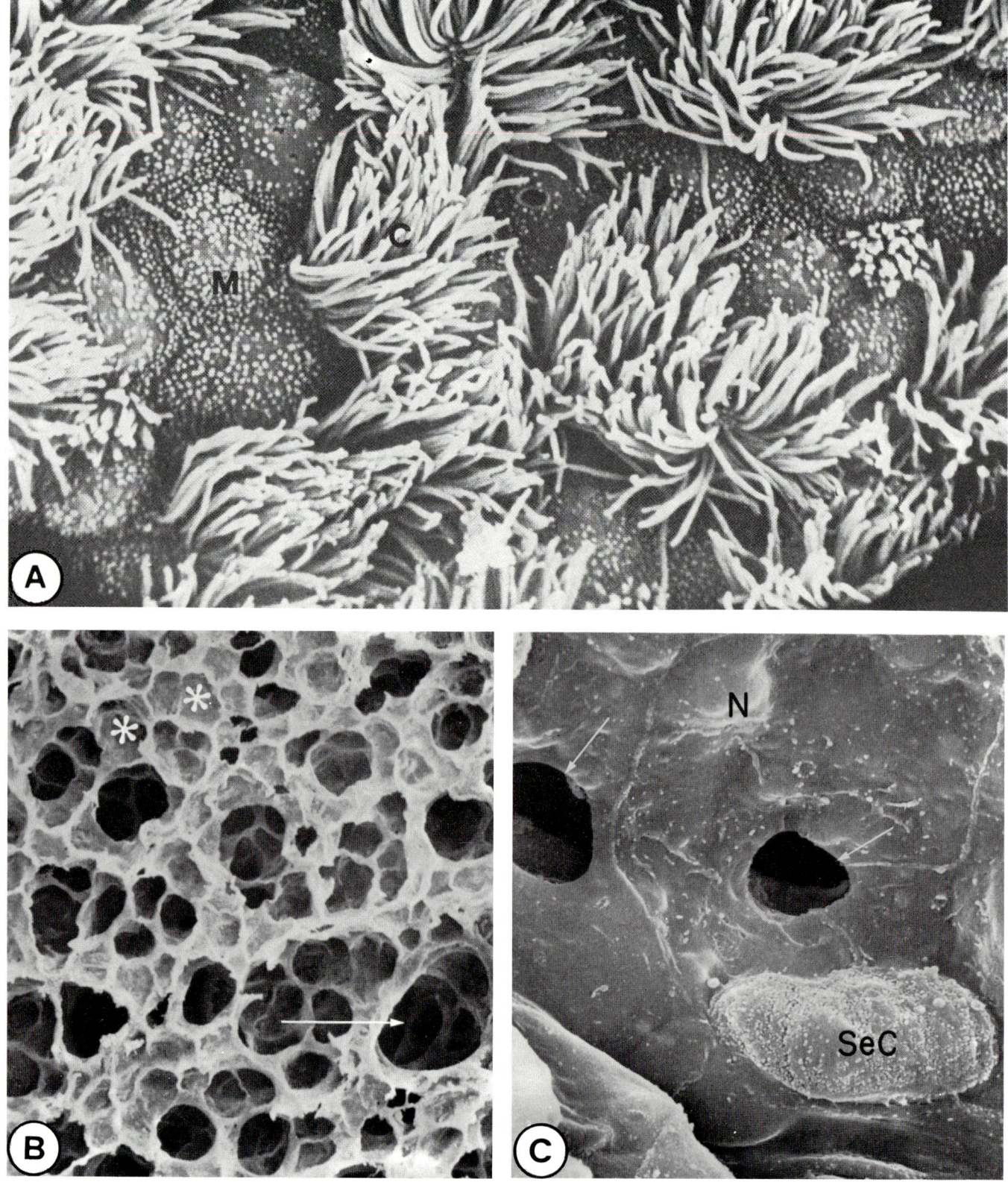

A   **Tracheal mucosa from rat (scanning EM, x5,600).** Ciliated cells **(C)** and secretory cells with microvilli **(M)** can be seen.

B   **Hamster lung (scanning EM, x150).** The section of lung parenchyma shows a number of alveoli **(*)** and some alveolar ducts (→).

C   **Lung alveolus (scanning EM, x5,200).** The lumen of the alveolus is coated with squamous cells. The nucleus **(N)** of one of them is seen bulging into the cavity. A few microvilli on small alveolar cells, and also a great alveolar cell (septal cell) **(Sec)** can be seen. The latter cell projects into the lumen and secretes surface-active substances. The alveolar wall is perforated by two large alveolar pores. (→) By courtesy of P.M. Andrews.

Plate 8.24   **209**

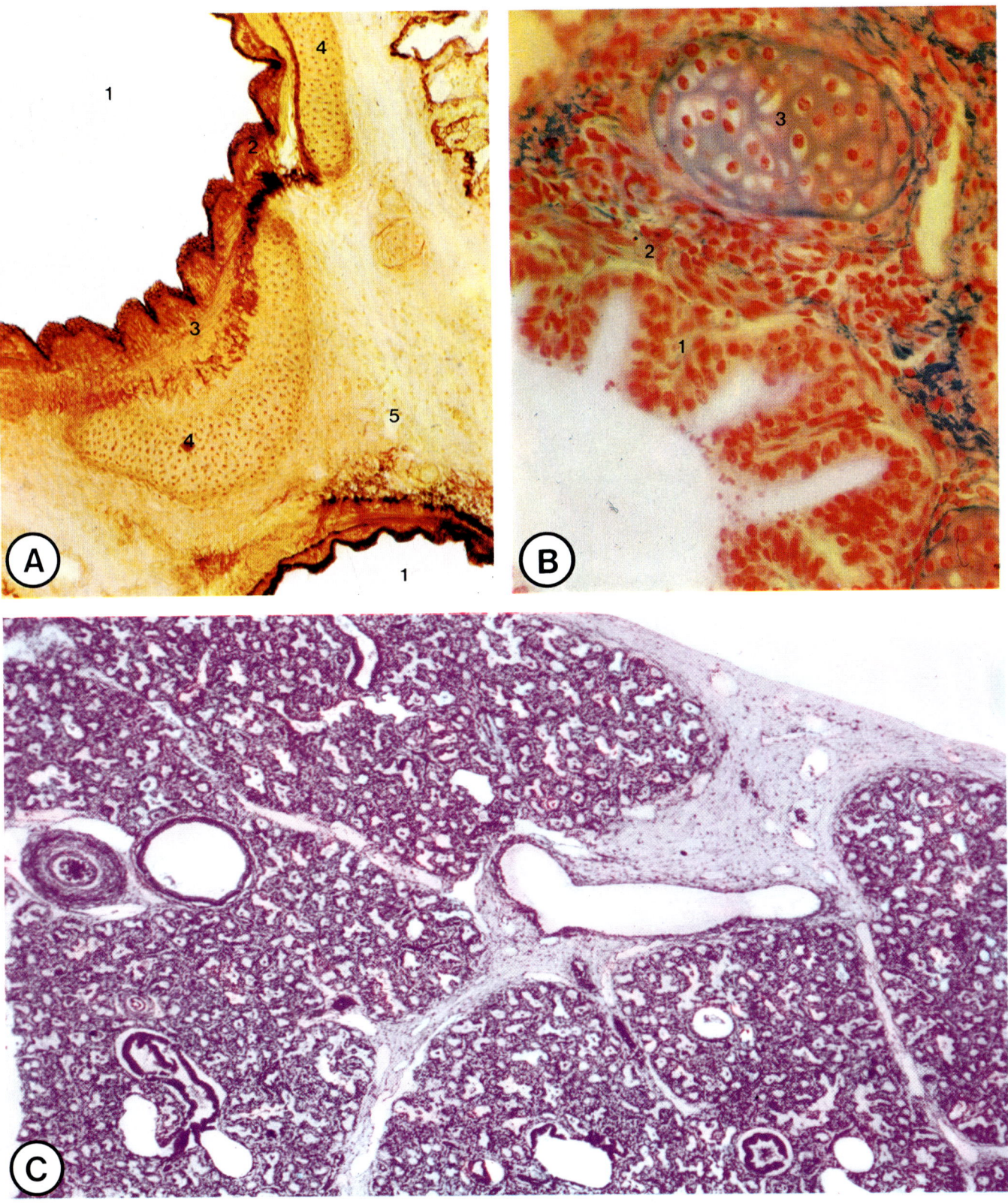

A   Interlobular bronchi from cat lung (silver impregnation, x150). 1 = medium-sized bronchi displaying shallow longitudinal
folds **(2). 3 =** bundles of smooth muscle fibers. **4 =** cartilage plate. **5 =** interlobular connective tissue.

B   Wall of intrapulmonary bronchus from cat (azan-Mallory, x38). 1 = mucosa with small longitudinal folds and covered by
ciliated simple columnar epithelium. In the underlying connective tissue can be seen occasional smooth muscle cells **(2)** and
a cartilage plate **(3).**

C   Lung from human fetus (H & E, x80). The lung parenchyma appears condensed because the alveoli are only partially dilated.
The gland-type architecture of the parenchyma is still apparent. A number of ducts are present, along with intralobular and
interlobular blood vessels which are not yet fully developed and are surrounded by the mesenchyme.

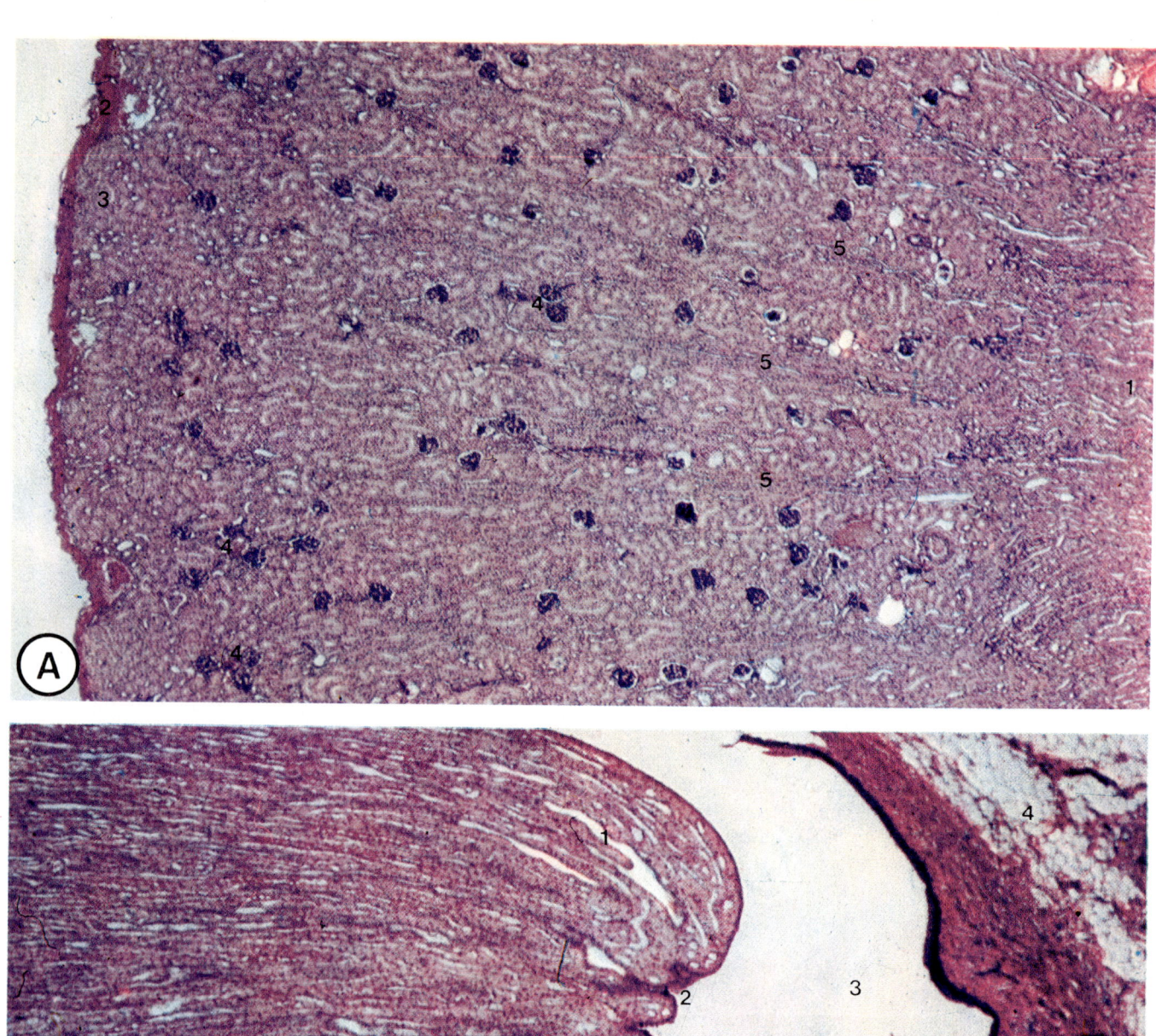

A   **Kidney from cat (H & E, x20).** Most of the figure is taken up by the cortex. Extreme right: the medulla (**1**) is just visible. **2** = renal capsule of connective tissue. **3** = cortex corticis. **4** = glomeruli. **5** = medullary rays radiating from the medulla towards the cortex.

B   **Longitudinal section of renal papilla from cat (H & E, x20).** A number of collecting tubules (**1**) run through the papilla and converge in the papillary ducts (**2**) at the point where the papilla bulges into the cavity of the calyx (**3**). **4** = wall of the calyx.

Plate 8.26   **211**

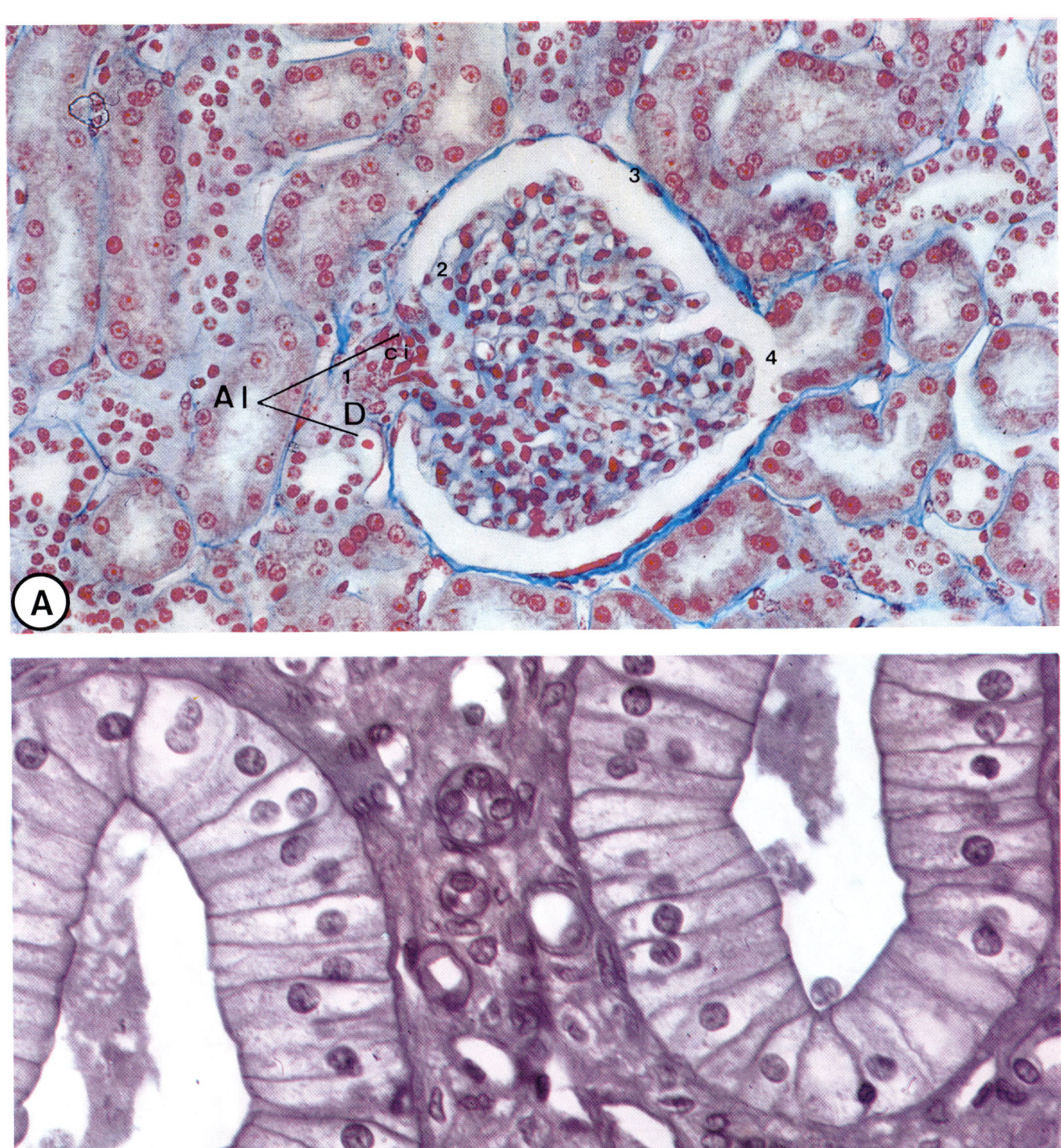

A   **Human renal corpuscle (azan-Mallory, x400).** The arteriole **(1)** gives rise to capillaries inside the glomerulus, which is surrounded by Bowman's capsule. The visceral layer **(2)** adheres to the looped capillaries while the parietal layer **(3)** is continuous with the epithelium of the proximal convoluted tubule in the neck region **(4)**. Around the renal corpuscle are sectioned profiles of the convoluted tubules. **(AI)** = juxtaglomerular apparatus. **D** = macula densa. **ci** = juxtaglomerular cells.

B   **Cross section of renal papilla from rabbit (H & E, x500).** The two papillary ducts are lined by a simple columnar epithelium.

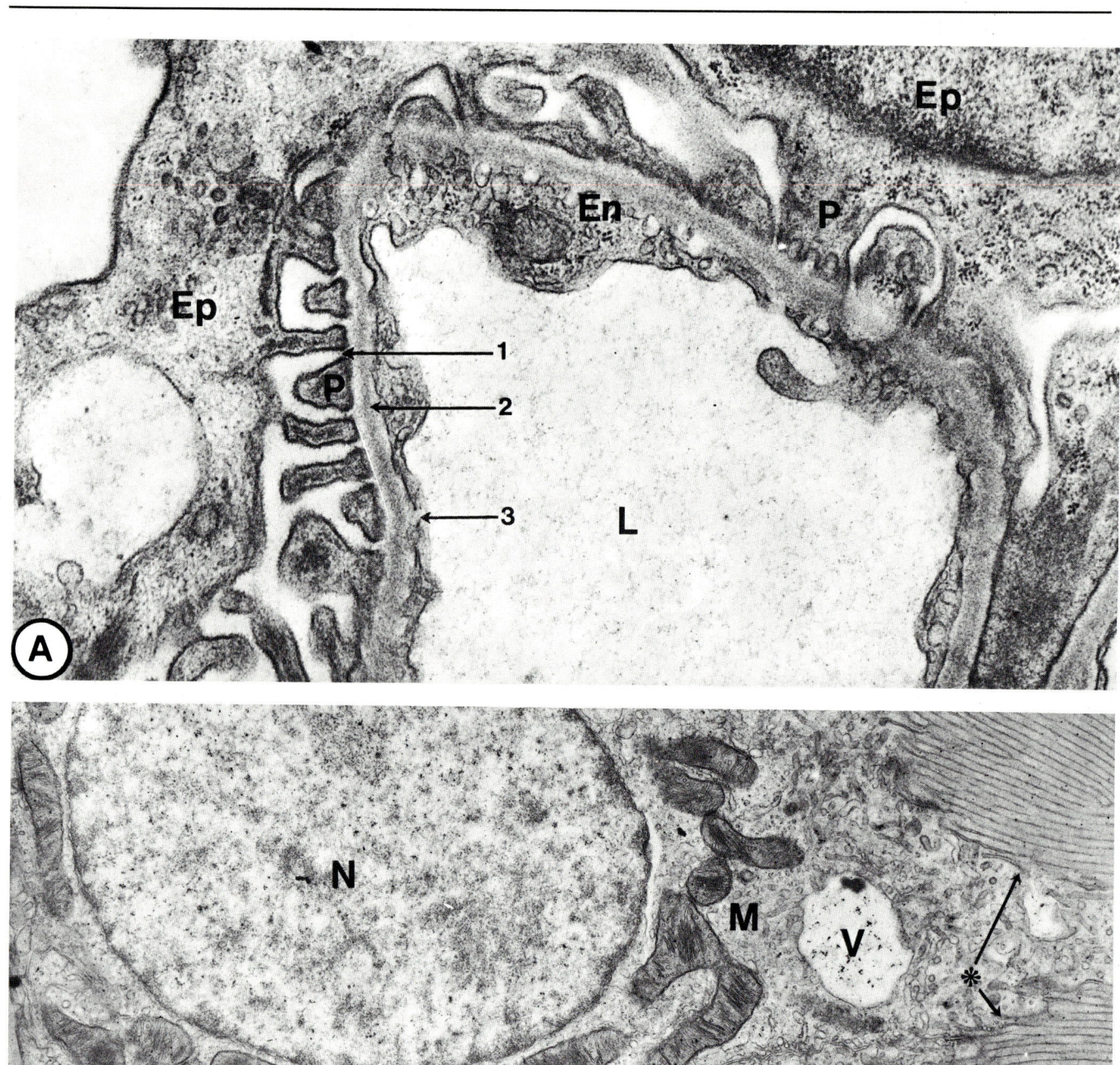

A **Rat glomerulus (EM, x36,000).** Where the visceral layer of Bowman's capsule borders on the endothelium of a blood capillary wall can be seen epithelial cells (podocytes) **(Ep)** with many pedicels (P), endothelial cells **(En)**, a capillary lumen, **(L)**, the urinary slits **(1→)** between the extremities of the pedicels, the basal lamina **(2→)** and endothelial pores **(3→)**.

B **Endothelial cell of the wall of the proximal convoluted tubule from rat kidney (EM, x16,000). N** = nucleus. **M** = mitochondria. **V** = protein reabsorption vesicles. **(*)** = brush border of microvilli projecting into the lumen of the tubule. **B** = basement membrane. By courtesy of C. De Martino.

Plate 8.28   213

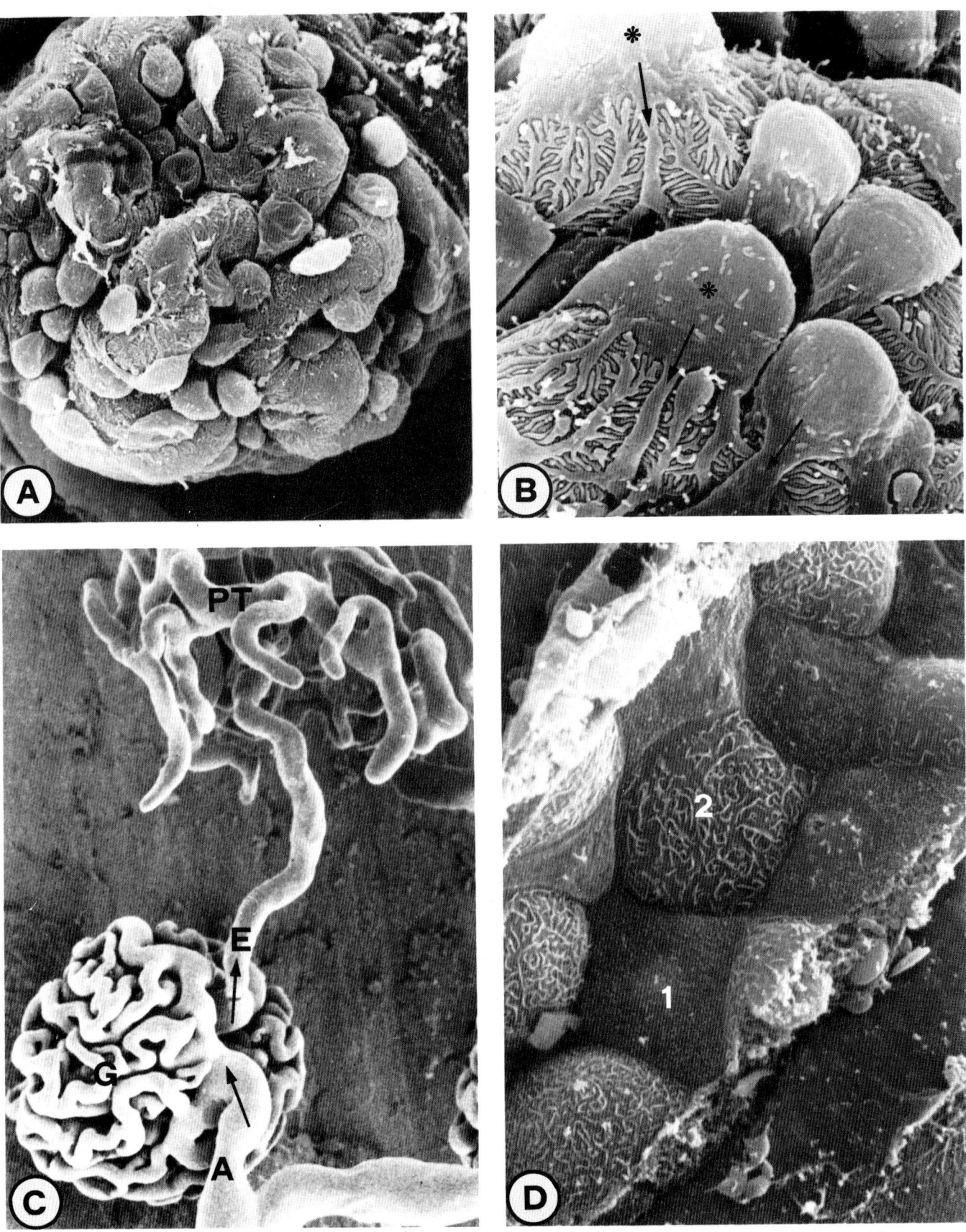

A **Renal corpuscle from rat (scanning EM, x1,000).** The vessels of the glomerulus, covered with podocytes, have been teased apart.

B **The visceral surface of Bowman's capsule from rat renal corpuscle (scanning EM, x4,800).** The bodies (*) of the podocytes, with primary and secondary processes (→), are clearly illustrated.

C **Glomerulus from monkey (vascular resin injection, scanning EM, x300). A** = afferent arteriole leading to the vessels of the glomerulus **(G)**. The narrower efferent arteriole **(E)** leads to a dense network of vessels that surround the cortical tubules **(PT)**. The arrows show the direction of blood flow. Original micrograph by T. Murakami.

D **Collecting duct from rat kidney (scanning EM, x6,000).** Lining the lumen are two types of cells. The first **(1)** are smooth-surfaced, while the second **(2)** have small microvilli and microplicae. Original micrograph by M. Castellucci.

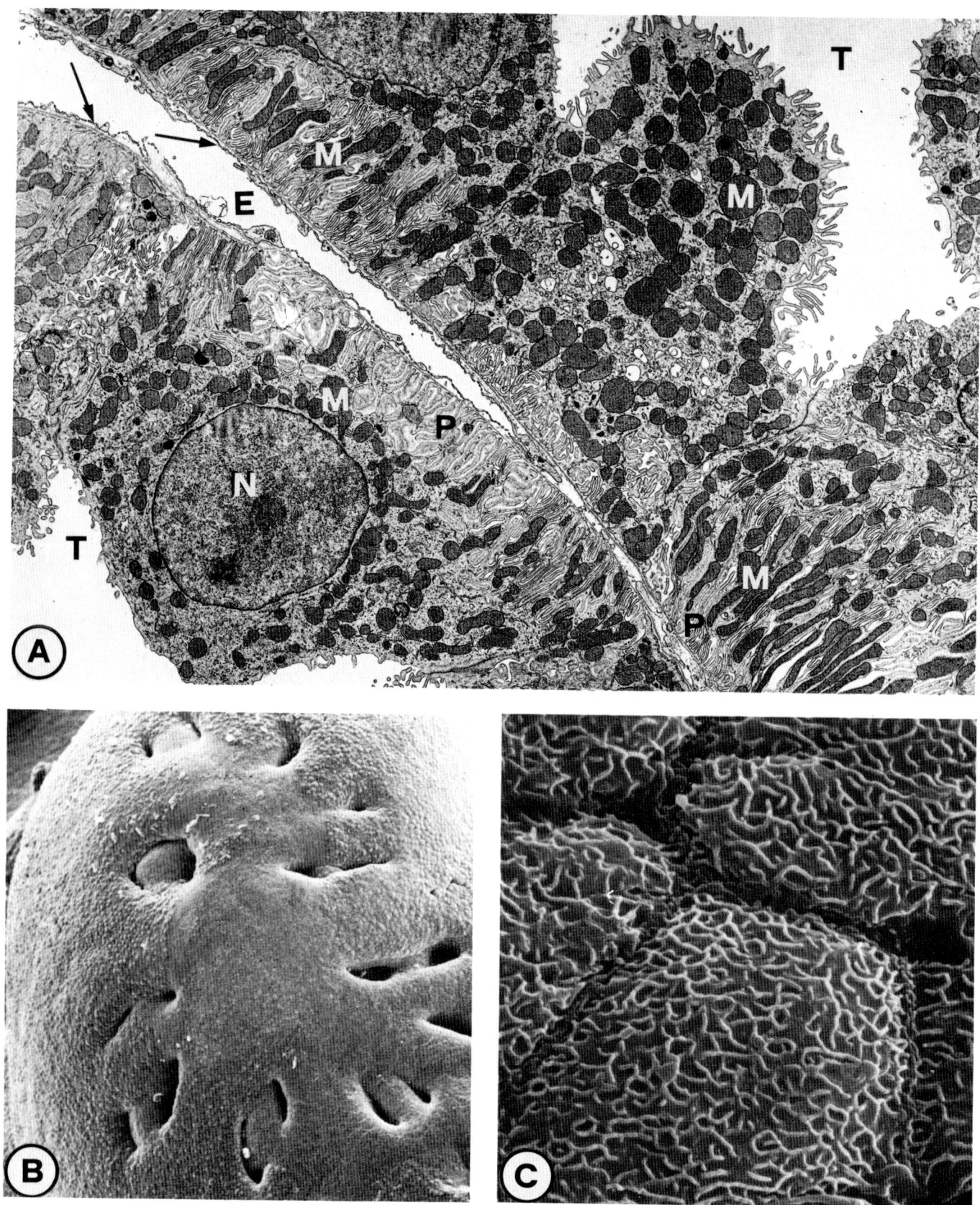

A **Distal convoluted tubule from mouse kidney (EM, x11,500).** The plasma membrane at the basal surface of the cell is invaginated to form numerous folds **(P)**. The folds delimit cytoplasmic areas containing elongated mitochondria **(M)**. **N** = nucleus of epithelial cell. **T** = lumen of tubule. **E** = subtubular capillary with fenestrated endothelial cell (→). Original micrograph by G. Familiari.

B **Area cribrosa in renal papilla from a pig (scanning EM, x60).** The tip of the papilla has a number of slits which are the openings for the papillary (Bellini's) ducts. From M. Castellucci. In: D.J. Allen, P.M. Motta and L.J.A. DiDio (eds). *Three-dimensional Microanatomy of Cells and Tissue Surfaces.* Elsevier/North Holland, New York, 1981.

C **Transitional epithelium of mucosa from pig bladder (scanning EM, x2,800).** The surfaces of these epithelial cells are raised in small characteristic folds. The cell margins are clearly visible. Original micrograph by M. Castellucci.

Plate 8.30   **215**

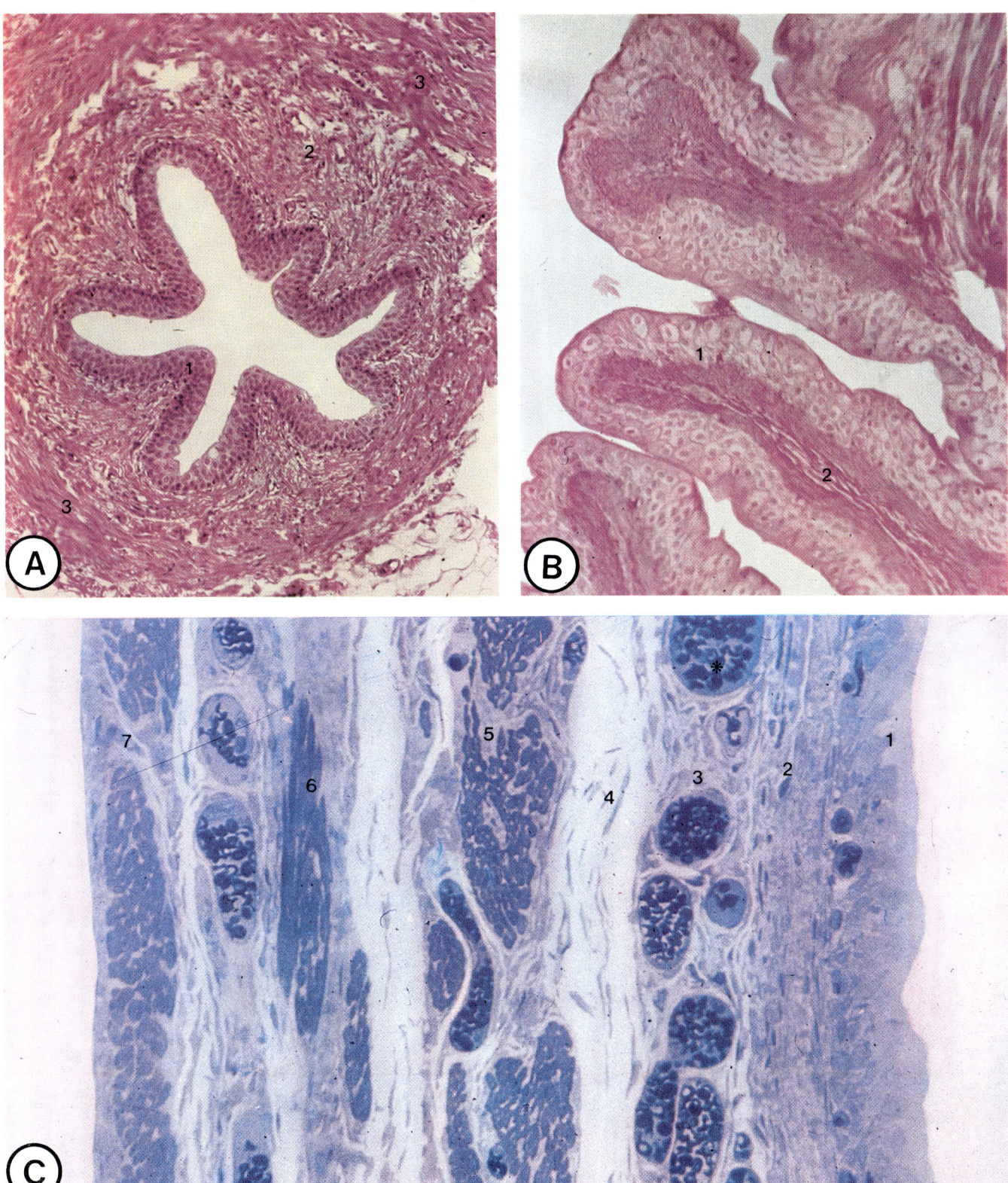

A **Cross section of rabbit ureter (H & E, x50).** The stellate lumen is lined by the transitional epithelium (1) of the mucosa. 2 = lamina propria. **3** = muscularis.

B **Tunica mucosa from rat bladder (H & E, x400).** The mucosa is characterized by large folds. The epithelium at the luminal surface has the characteristic appearance of transitional epithelium (1). 2 = lamina propria. By courtesy of E. Nesci.

C **Semithin section of wall of rat bladder (methylene blue, x500).** From right to left: the covering epithelial layer (1) of the mucosa resting on its lamina propria (2), the submucosa (3) with abundant cross-sectioned blood vessels (*), and the muscularis, composed of smooth muscle fiber bundles separated by loose connective tissue (4). In this tissue, three layers of the muscularis can be distinguished: the inner (5), middle (6) and outer (7) layers. By courtesy of E. Nesci.

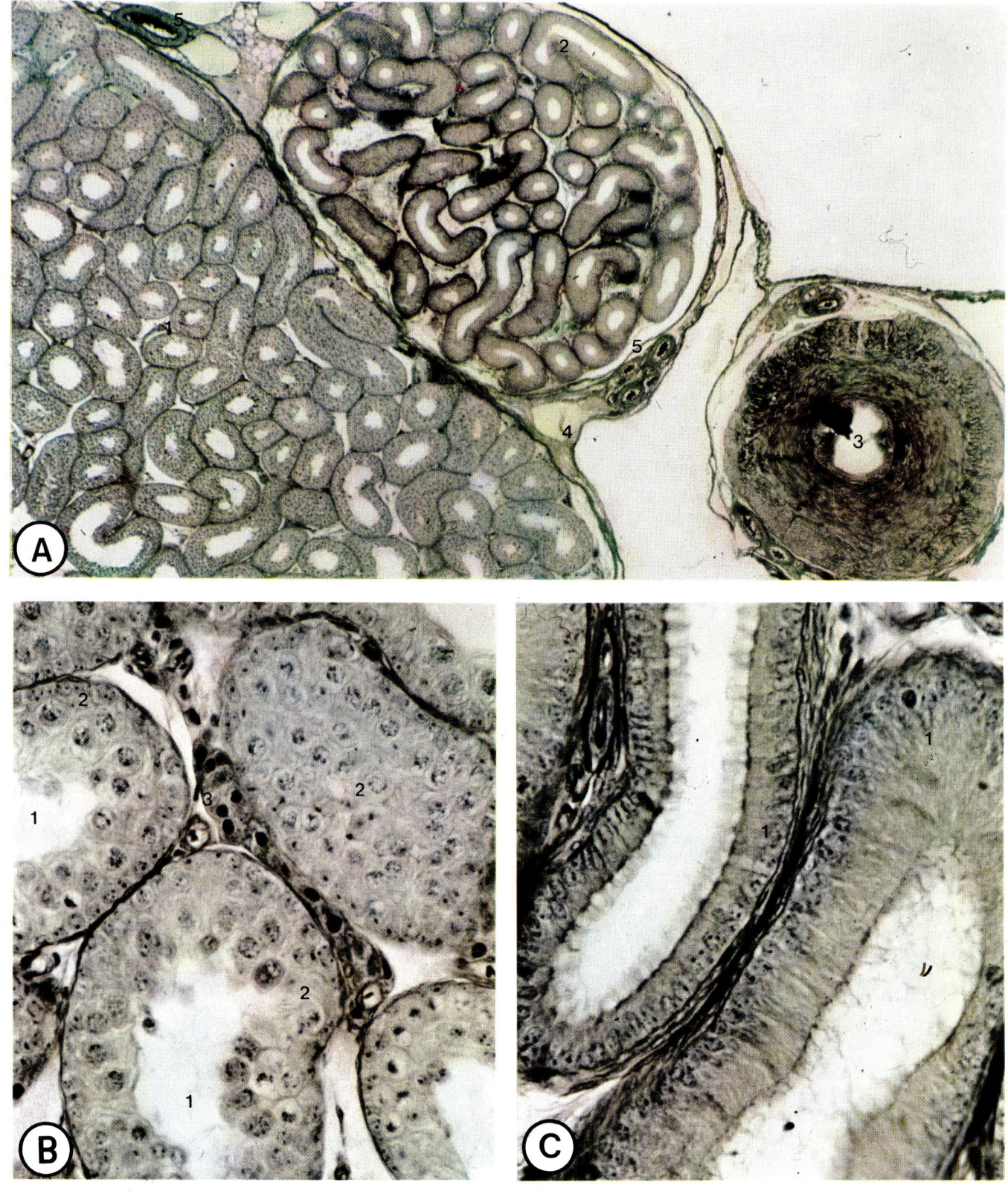

A   **Epididymis and ductus deferens from a guinea-pig (iron hematoxylin, x50). 1** = convoluted seminiferous tubules. **2** = ductus epididymis. **3** = cross section of ductus deferens. **4** = tunica albuginea forming the covering of the epididymis. **5** = blood vessels.

B   **Convoluted seminiferous tubules and interstitial cells (iron hematoxylin, x250). 1** = lumen of seminiferous tubules. **2** = wall of tubules composed of germinal cells and Sertoli cells. **3** = group of Leydig interstitial cells beneath the basal lamina of the seminiferous tubules.

C   **Ductus epididymis of guinea-pig (iron hematoxylin, x250). 1** = epithelium with typical stereocilia. The wall of the ductule is covered by a thin layer of connective tissue.

Plate 8.32 217

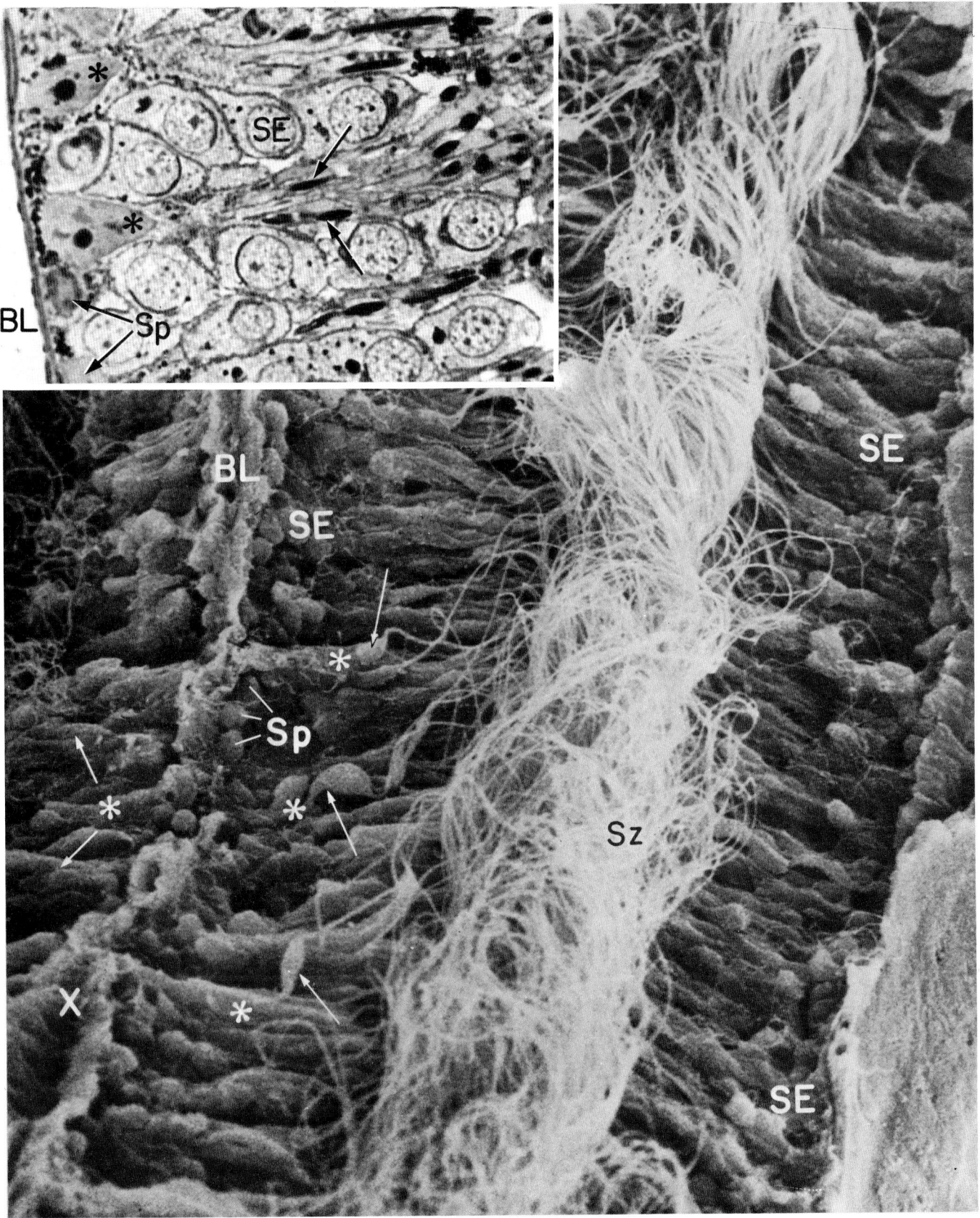

Convoluted seminiferous tubules from rat (scanning EM, x350). Inset: semithin section, methylene blue, x1,200. Inset, above left: seminiferous epithelium (**SE**), composed of germinal cells with large Sertoli cells (*). The epithelium rests on a basal lamina (**BL**). The smaller spherical cells at the base of the tubules are mostly spermatogonia (**Sp**). Many differentiating spermatozoa (**Sz**) are attached by their heads to the surface of the Sertoli cells (→). Original micrograph (inset) by C. Di Martino. Main figure: the tails of a number of spermatozoa (**Sz**) are seen in the lumen. **SE** = seminiferous epithelium. **BL** = region of basal lamina and stroma of connective tissue (**X**). **Sp** = spermatogonia. * = Sertoli cells with differentiating sperm attached (→). From P.M. Motta, P.M. Andrews and K.R. Porter. *Microanatomy of Cell and Tissue Surfaces. An Atlas of Scanning Electron Microscopy.* Lea and Febiger, Philadelphia, 1977.

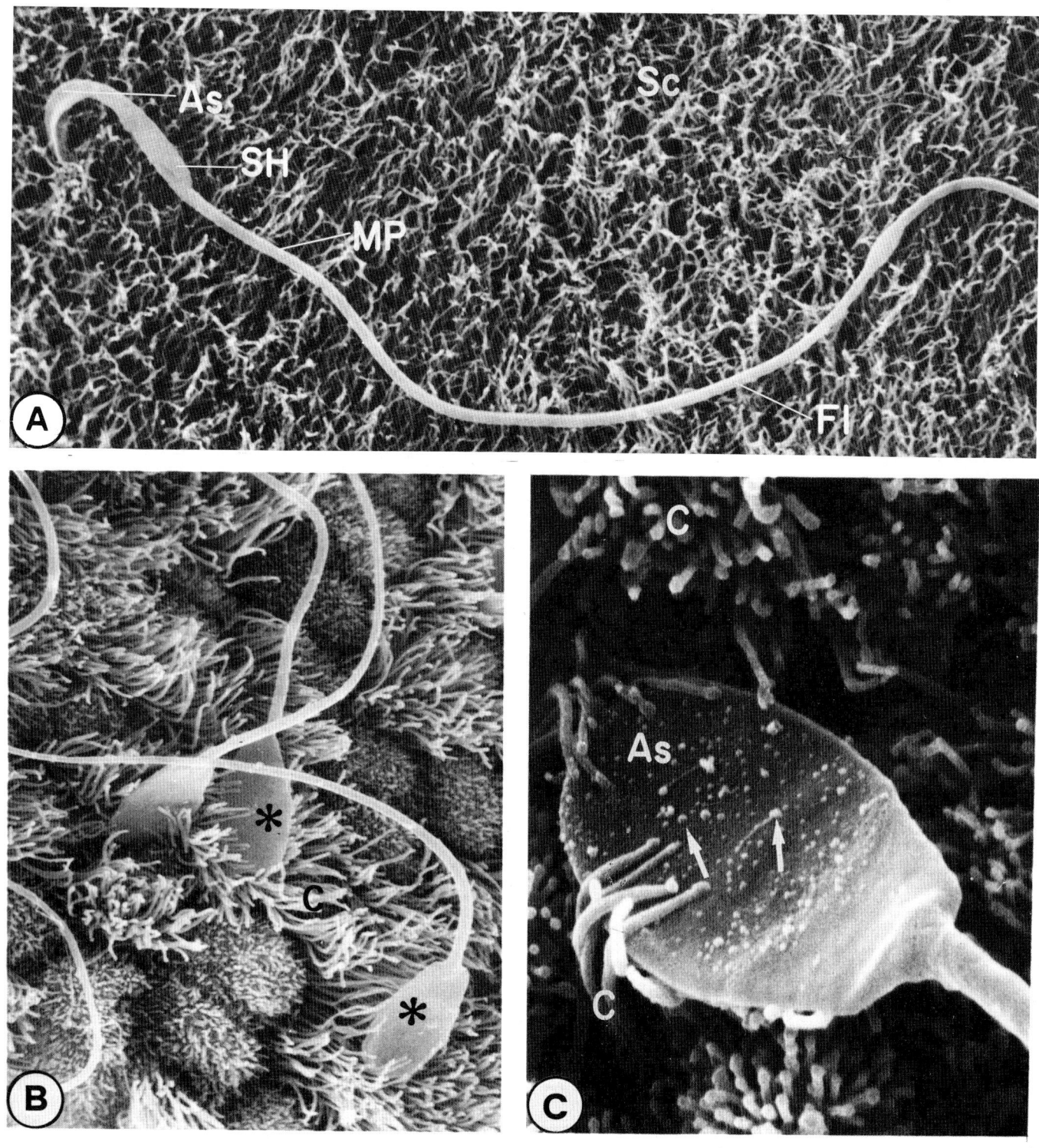

A **Spermatozoon in the lumen of the ductus epididymis from rat (scanning EM, x2,500).** The sperm is lying against the stereocilia **(Sc)** of the ductal epithelium. **As** = acrosome. **SH** = sperm head. **MP** = middle piece. **Fl** = flagellum. Original micrograph by P.M. Andrews.

B, **C Spermatozoa in the uterus of rabbit (scanning EM, x4,200, × 1,000).** The sperm were photographed a few hours after mating. The heads (*) of the sperm (flattened like those of human sperm) are in contact with the ciliated cells of the uterus **(C).** There is an accumulation of small granules and vesicles (→) on the cell membrane which covers the head region containing the acrosome **(As).** The membrane of the cell and of the acrosome will progressively weaken at the site of these granules (acrosome reaction) (Fig. C). From P.M. Motta and J. Van Blerkom. Cell Tiss. Res. 163:29, 1975.

Plate 8.34   **219**

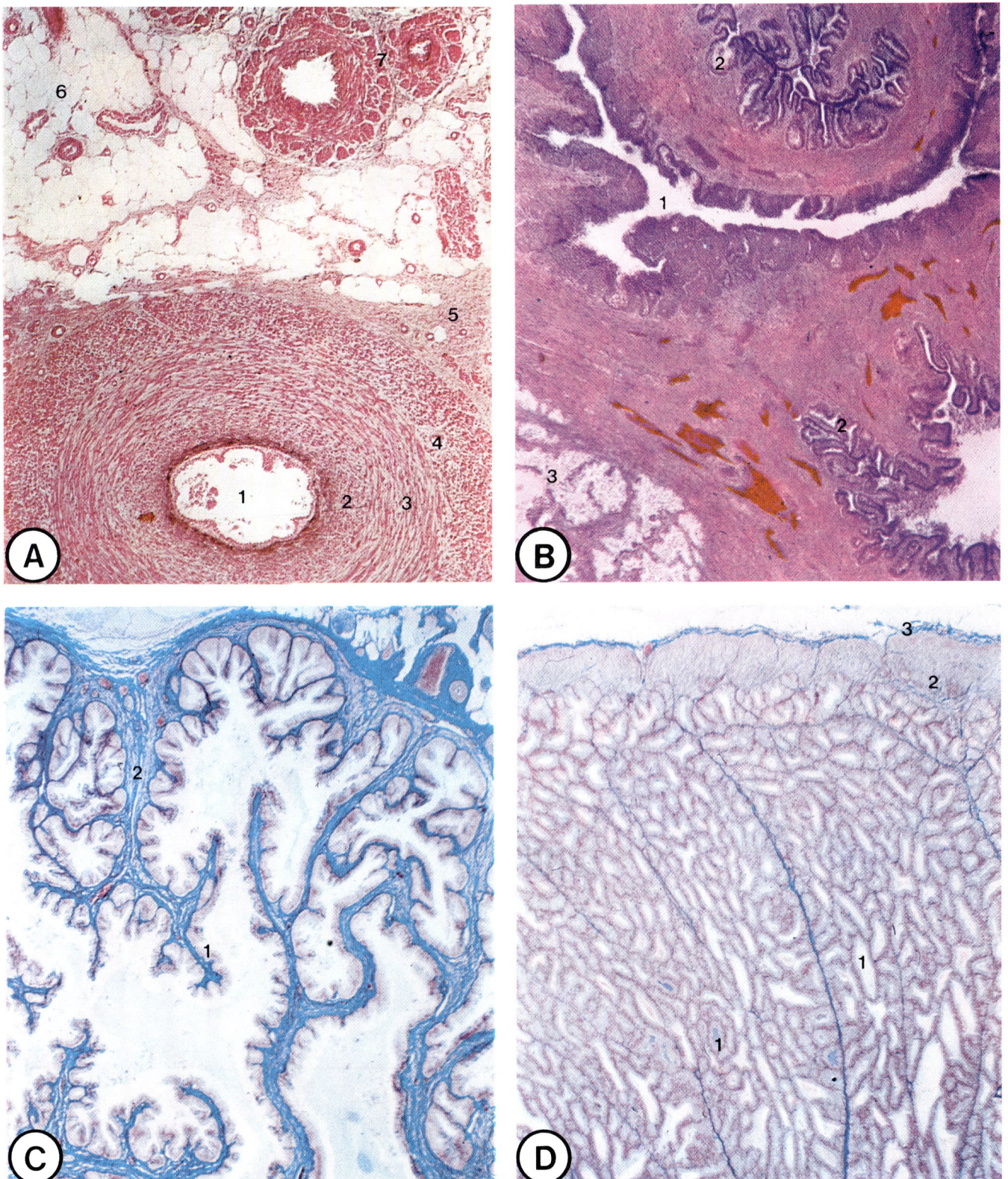

A   **Cross section of human ductus deferens (H & E, x40).** The mucosa and submucosa, both thin and with small folds, surround the lumen of the ductus **(1). 2** = inner longitudinal muscle layer. **3** = middle spiralling muscle layer. **4** = outer longitudinal muscle layer. **5** = adventitia or fibrosa. In the upper part of the micrograph can be seen muscular arteries **(7)** and pampiniform vein plexes among lobules of adipose tissue **(6).**

B   **Human prostate gland (H & E, x25). 1** = section of prostatic urethra. **2** = section of excretory ducts of the prostatic glands in the colliculus seminalis. **3** = prostatic glands.

C   **Detail of human prostate gland (azan-Mallory, × 110).** The number of diverticula makes the gland lumen appear irregular. Occupying the lumen are folds of the mucosa covered by epithelium **(1),** which is supported by connective tissue **(2)** rich in vessels and smooth muscle cells.

D   **Human seminal vesicle (azan-Mallory, x50). 1** = mucosa whose folds form an anastomosing network. **2** = thick muscularis. **3** = tunica adventitia, rich in elastic fibers.

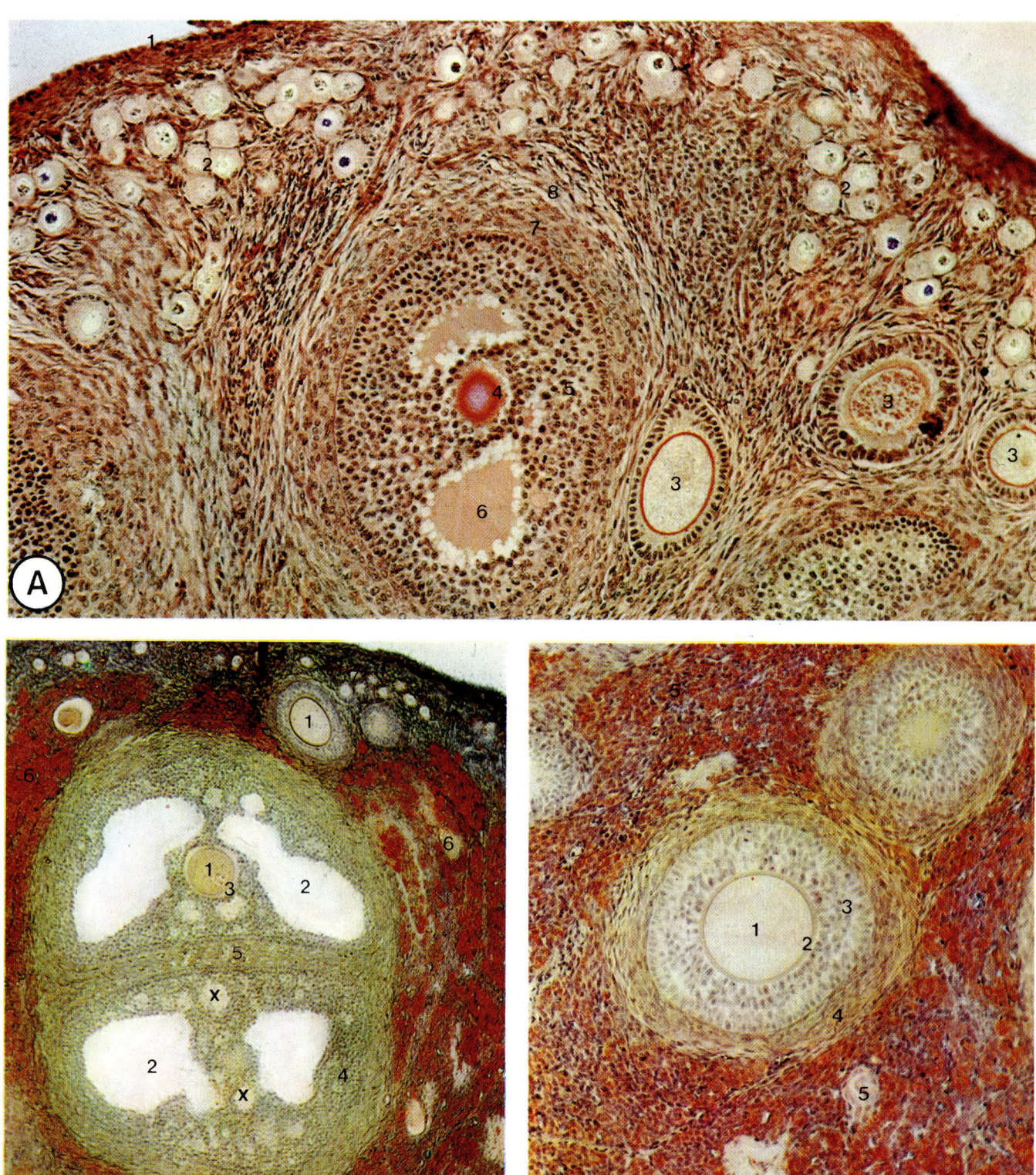

A   **Rabbit ovary (PAS & hematoxylin, x180).** In the ovarian cortex, which is covered by surface epithelium **(1),** are groups of primordial follicles **(2)** and growing follicles **(3).** Center: a more mature follicle in tangential section. **4** = zona pellucida. **5** = stratum granulosum. **6** = liquor folliculi in the antrum. **7** = theca interna. **8** = theca externa.

B   **Growing follicles of rabbit ovary (Sudan III, x110).** Two closely associated follicles can be seen. **1** = oocyte. **2** = liquor folliculi in the antrum. **3** = zona pellucida. **4** = stratum granulosum with Call-Exner bodies (x). **5** = theca interna. The interstitial gland **(6),** which is abundant in rabbits, is stained orange by the Sudan stain and forms cords around the follicles. Above: Cortex of the ovary with primordial and growing follicles **(7).** Original micrograph by P.M. Motta.

C   **Follicles and interstitial gland from rabbit ovary (Sudan III, x240).** The follicles are surrounded by abundant interstitial tissue, which is stained orange. **1** = oocyte of growing follicle. **2** = zona pellucida. **3** = stratum granulosum. **4** = theca. **5** = groups of interstitial cells.

Plate 8.36   **221**

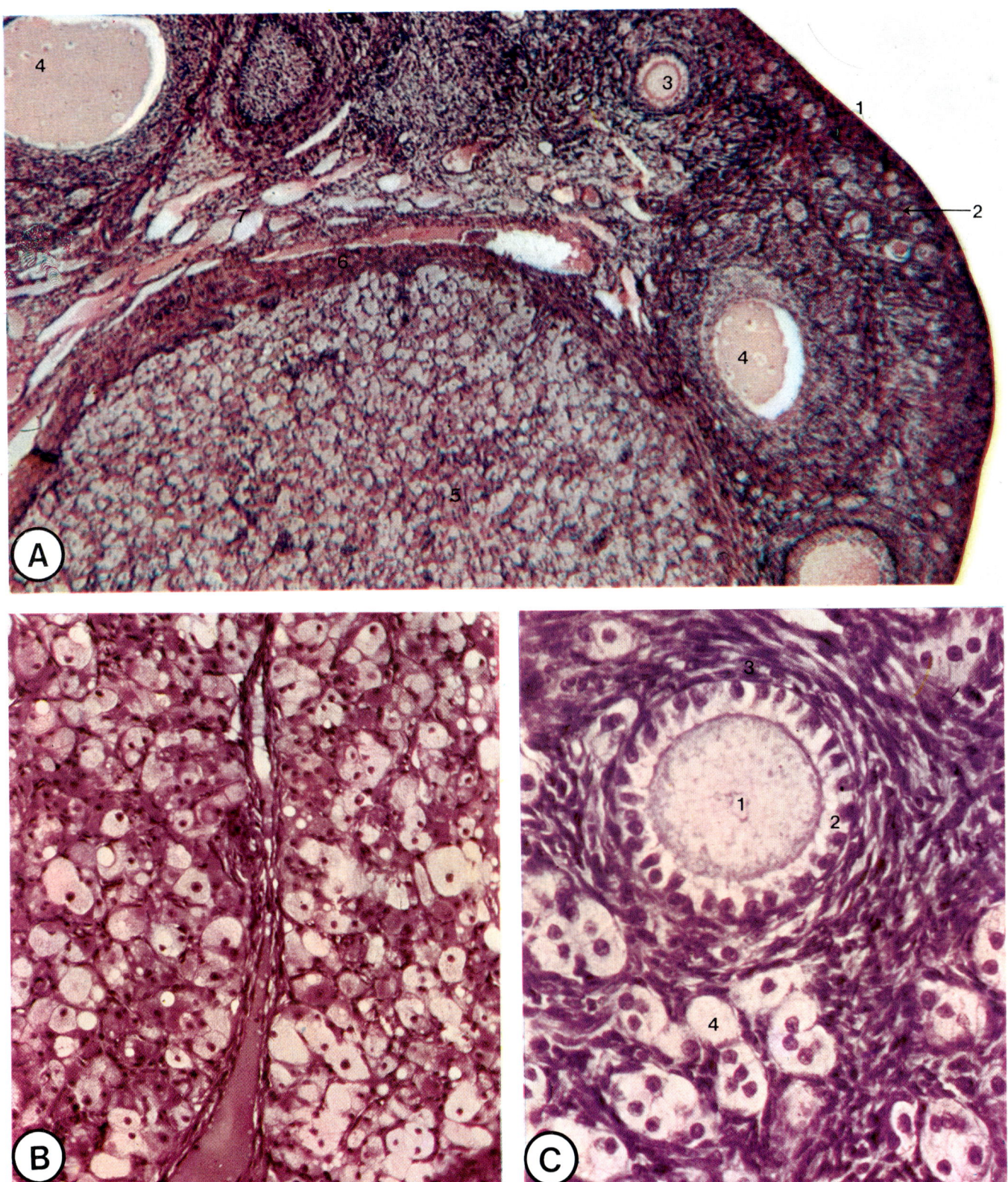

A **Cat ovary (H & E, x70). 1** = surface epithelium. **2** = primordial follicles in the cortex. **3** = maturing secondary follicle. **4** = follicles in atresia with degeneration of antrum and hypertrophy of theca interna. **5** = large corpus luteum with thick covering capsule of connective tissue **(6). 7** = blood vessels.

B **Corpus luteum of cat (H & E, x320).** Center: septum of connective tissue containing dilated blood vessels. The lightly staining cells with abundant cytoplasm are granulosa lutein cells; the smaller dark cells are theca lutein cells. Among the cells are a number of sinusoids.

C **Primary follicle and interstitial cells from rabbit ovary (H & E, x425). 1** = oocyte covered with simple columnar follicle cells **(2). 3** = forming theca interna. In the surrounding stroma are numerous groups of interstitial cells **(4).**

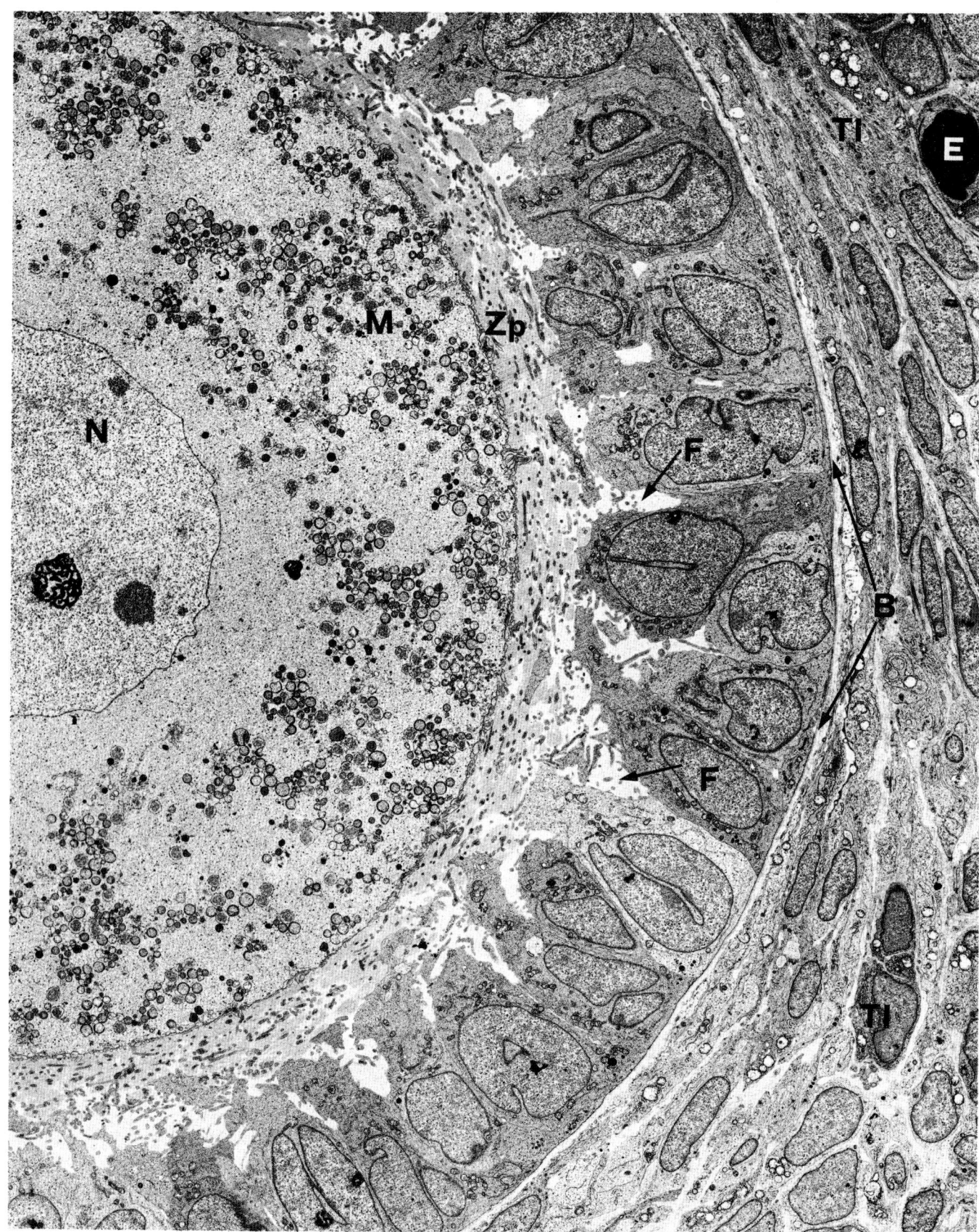

Growing follicle from rabbit ovary (EM, x4,800). The cytoplasm of the oocyte contains many mitochondria (**M**) and a large nucleus (**N**). Running through the zona pellucida (**Zp**) are a number of microvilli from the oocyte and the follicle cells (**F**). The liquor folliculi is beginning to accumulate in the spaces between the follicle cells (→). **B** = basal lamina. **TI** = theca interna. **E** = erythrocyte in the lumen of a small capillary. The theca interna cells of antral follicles form an endocrine gland (thecal gland) capable of synthesizing and secreting steroid hormones.

Plate 8.38   **223**

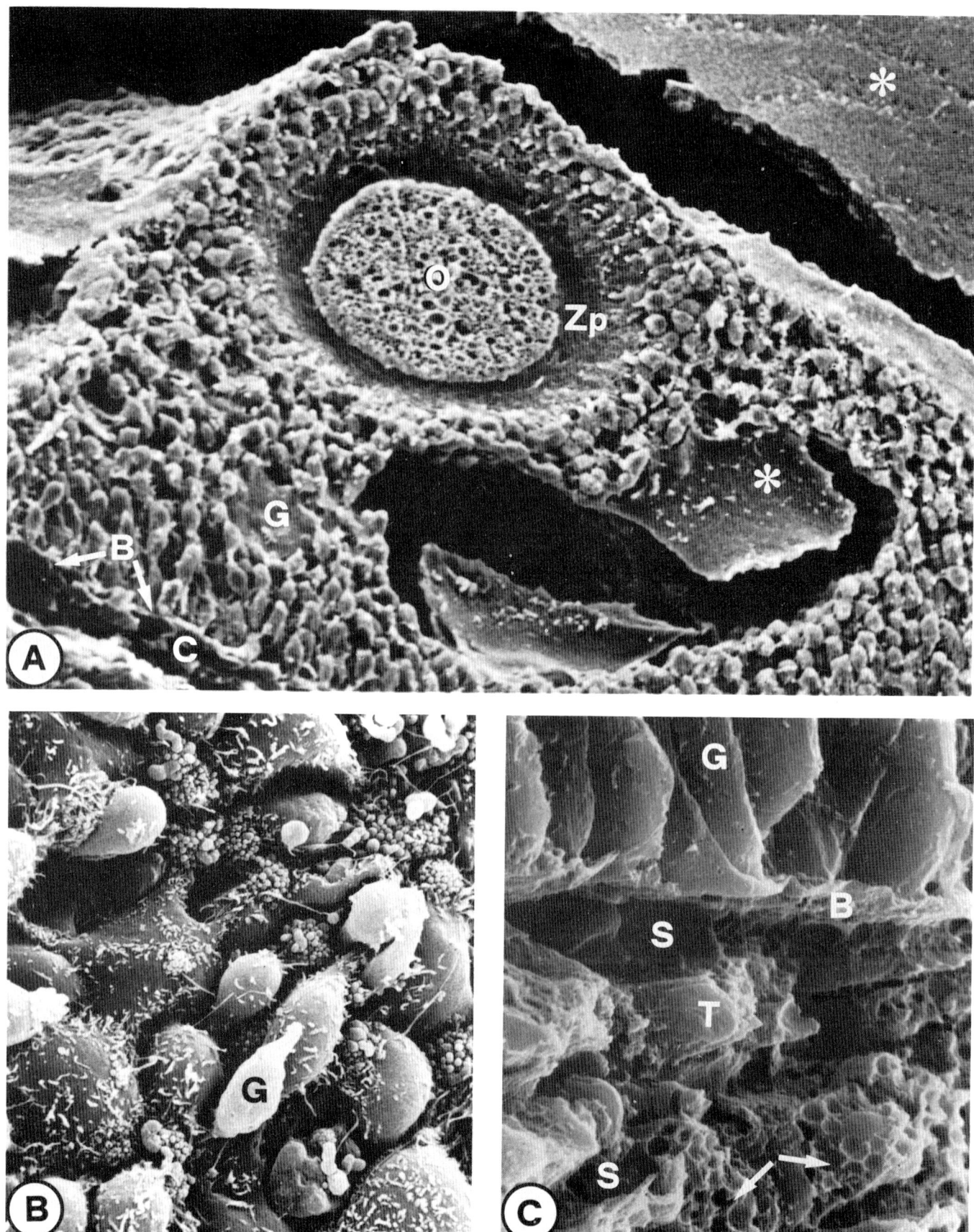

A Cumulus oophorus in Graafian follicle from dog (scanning EM, x3,100). **O** = oocyte. **Zp** = zona pellucida. **G** = cells of stratum granulosum. **B** = basement membrane. **C** = capillary of theca interna. The antrum is filling with liquor folliculi (*).

B Cells of stratum granulosum in human Graafian follicle (scanning EM, x12,800). The cells of the stratum granulosum face the antrum of the follicle. These polymorphic cells proliferate actively and their surfaces are rich in microvilli and blebs. From P.M. Motta and S. Makabe. In: K. Tanaka and T. Fujita (eds). *Scanning Electron Microscopy in Cell Biology and Medicine.* Excerpta Medica, Amsterdam/Oxford, 1981.

C Theca interna and stratum granulosum of mature follicle from dog (scanning EM, x8,200). This photograph is an enlargement showing the boundary between stratum granulosum **(G)** and theca interna **(T)**. The cells of the theca are partially fractured to show a number of vacuoles (→), which probably contain lipid droplets. **B** = region of the basal lamina of follicle. **S** = sinusoids among the cells of the theca interna. From P.M. Motta and J. Van Blerkom. In: P.M. Motta and E.S.E. Hafez (eds). *Biology of the Ovary.* M. Nijhoff Publishers. The Hague/Boston/London, 1980.

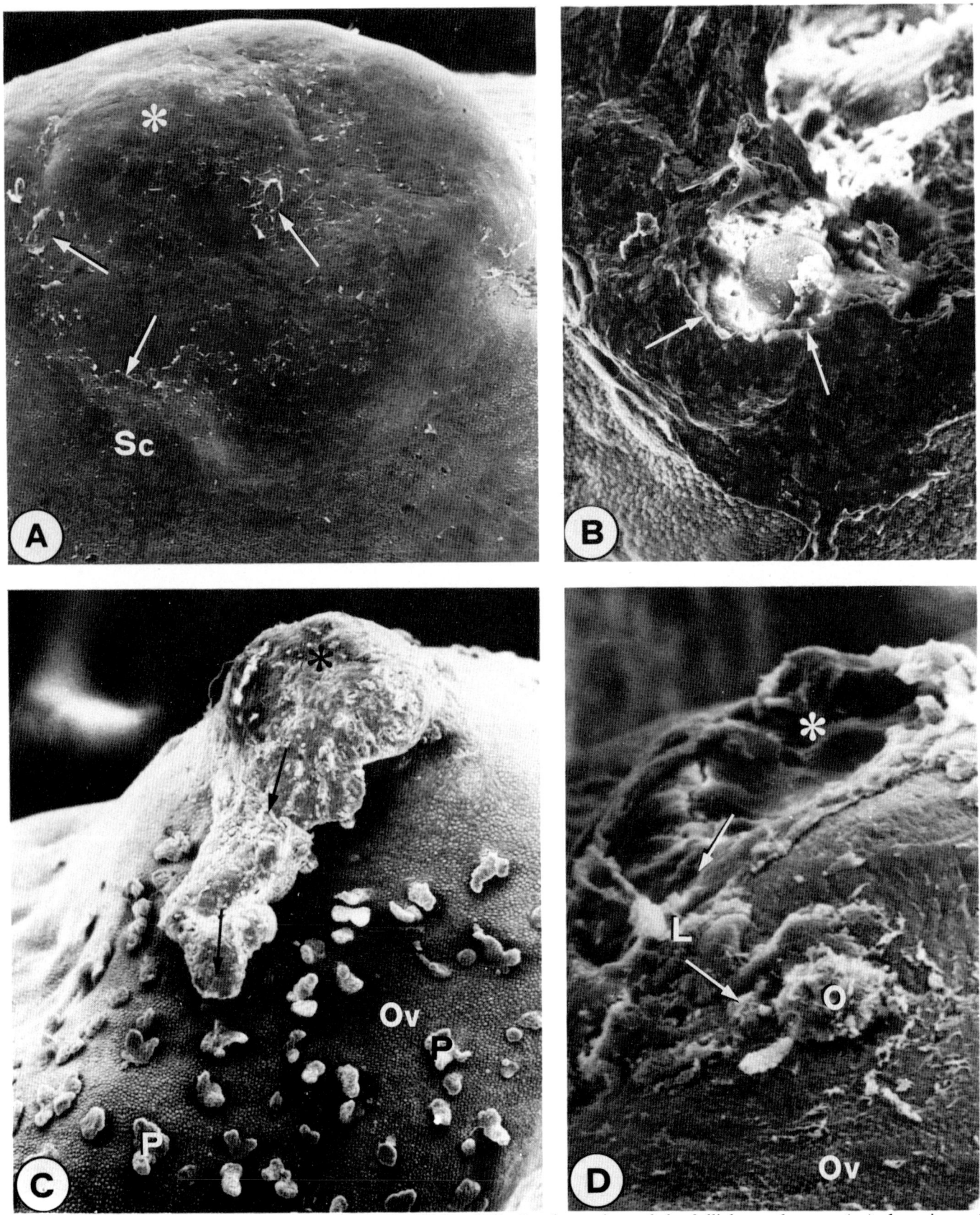

A   **Rabbit follicle just prior to ovulation (scanning EM, x120).** On the surface of the follicle can be seen (→) clear signs of erosion in the epithleium covering the ovary (Sc). The dome of the follicle (*) is the area where the wall will rupture (stigma).

B   **Ovulation in mouse (scanning EM, x230).** The oocyte emerging from the surface of the follicle (→) during ovulation is partially masked by the remains of the liquor folliculi.

C   **Surface of rabbit follicle after ovulation (scanning EM, x120).** The material from the apex (*) of the follicle spreading (→) onto the ovary (Ov) consists of liquor folliculi, blood and cell residue from the ruptured follicle. The surface of the ovary is raised to form papillae (P).

D   **Follicle from rabbit after ovulation (scanning EM, x110).** Above: the opening in the follicle after ovulation can still be seen (*). The liquor folliculi (L) spreading (→) onto the surface of the ovary (Ov) surrounds a small spherical mass. This mass is the corona radiata and contains the oocyte (O) surrounded by the zona pellucida. From P.M. Motta and J. Van Blerkom. Amer. J. Anat. 143:241, 1975.

Plate 8.40 225

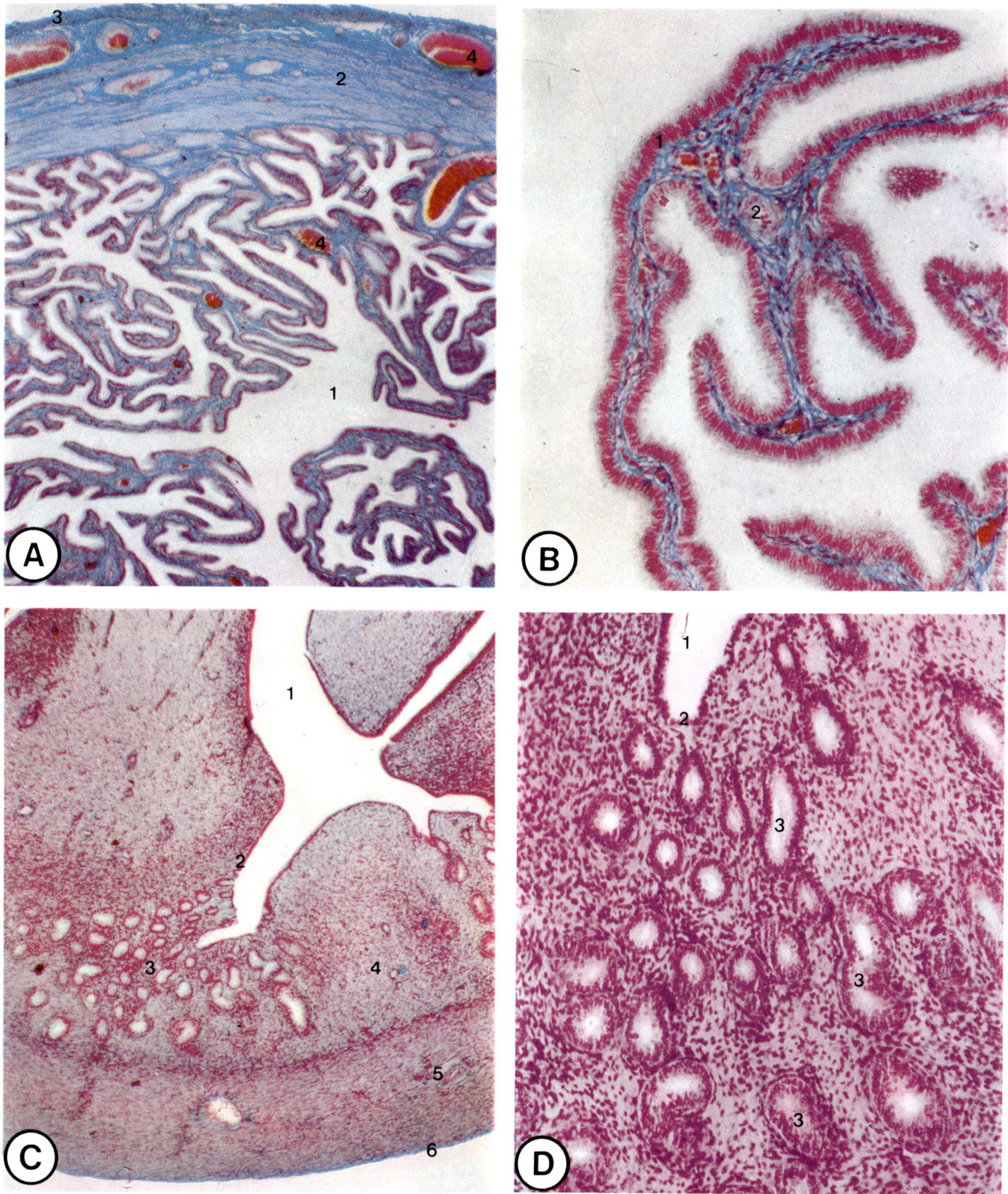

A Cross section of ampulla of human oviduct (azan-Mallory, x40). 1 = lumen, irregular in outline because of the many folds in the mucosa. 2 = muscularis. 3 = serosa. 4 = blood vessels.

B Fold in mucosa of human oviduct (azan-Mallory, x220). 1 = columnar epithelium with ciliated cells and secretory cells. 2 = lamina propria with blood vessels.

C Cross section of sheep uterus in proliferative phase (azan-Mallory, x60). 1 = cavity of the uterus. 2 = epithelium, invaginated to form numerous glands (3). 4 = lamina propria. 5 = muscularis. 6 = serosa.

D Detail of mucosa of sheep uterus in the proliferative phase (azan-Mallory, x125). 1 = cavity of uterus. 2 = epithelium of mucosa. The tortuous course of the glands with dilated lumens (3) can be seen crowded together in the mucosa.

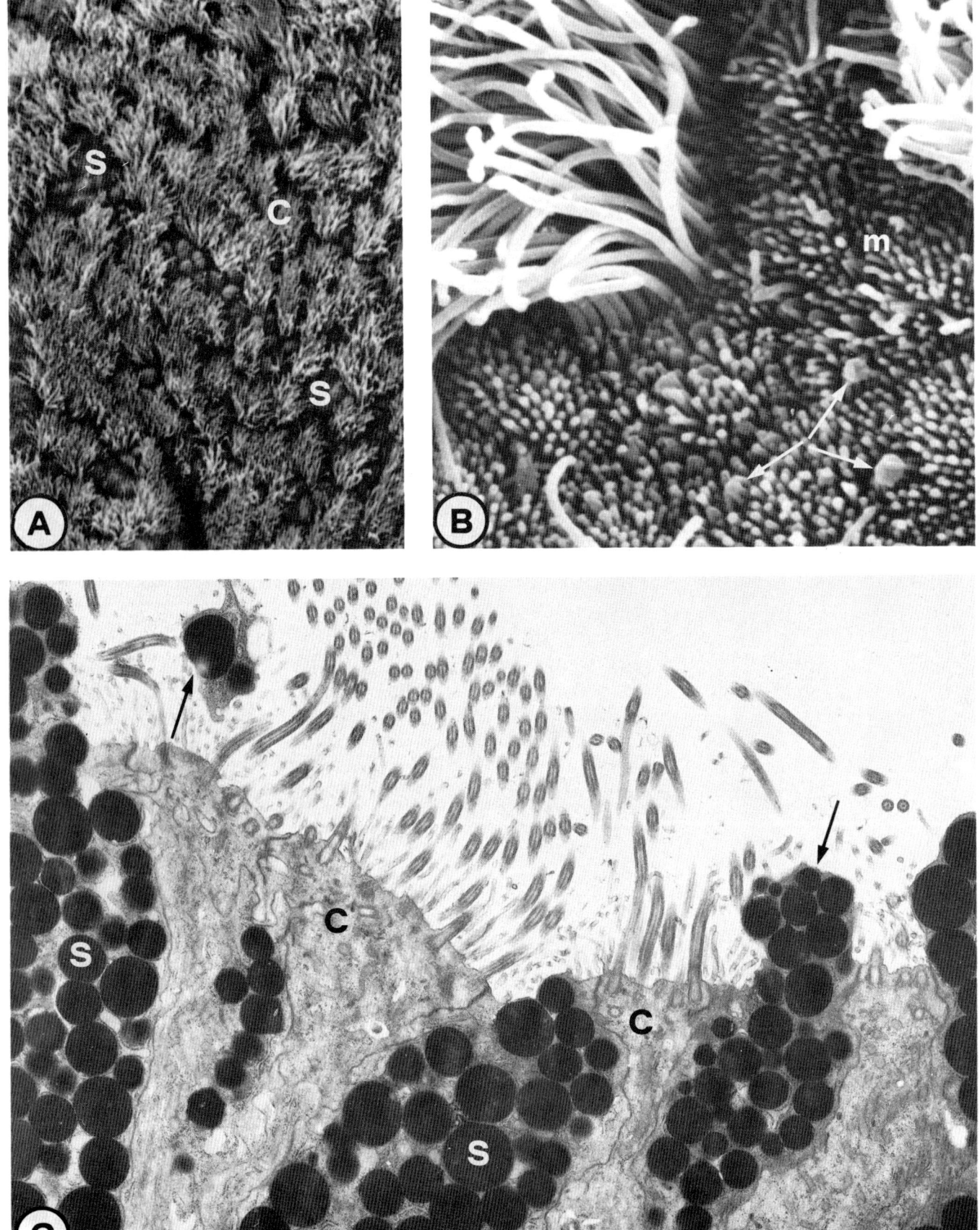

A, **B Isthmus of rabbit oviduct (scanning EM, x1,880, x10,800).** Secretory cells **(S)** alternate with the many ciliated cells **(C)**. The higher magnification of Figure **B** shows the surface of the secretory cells covered by microvilli **(m)** and having small blebs (→) which are secretion droplets (exocytosis).

C **Rabbit oviduct taken at the isthmus (EM, x18,000).** Ciliated cells **(C)** and cells containing secretory granules **(S)** can be seen. Some of these granules are being extruded from the cell (exocytosis) (→). Original micrograph by J. Van Blerkom.

Plate 8.42

227

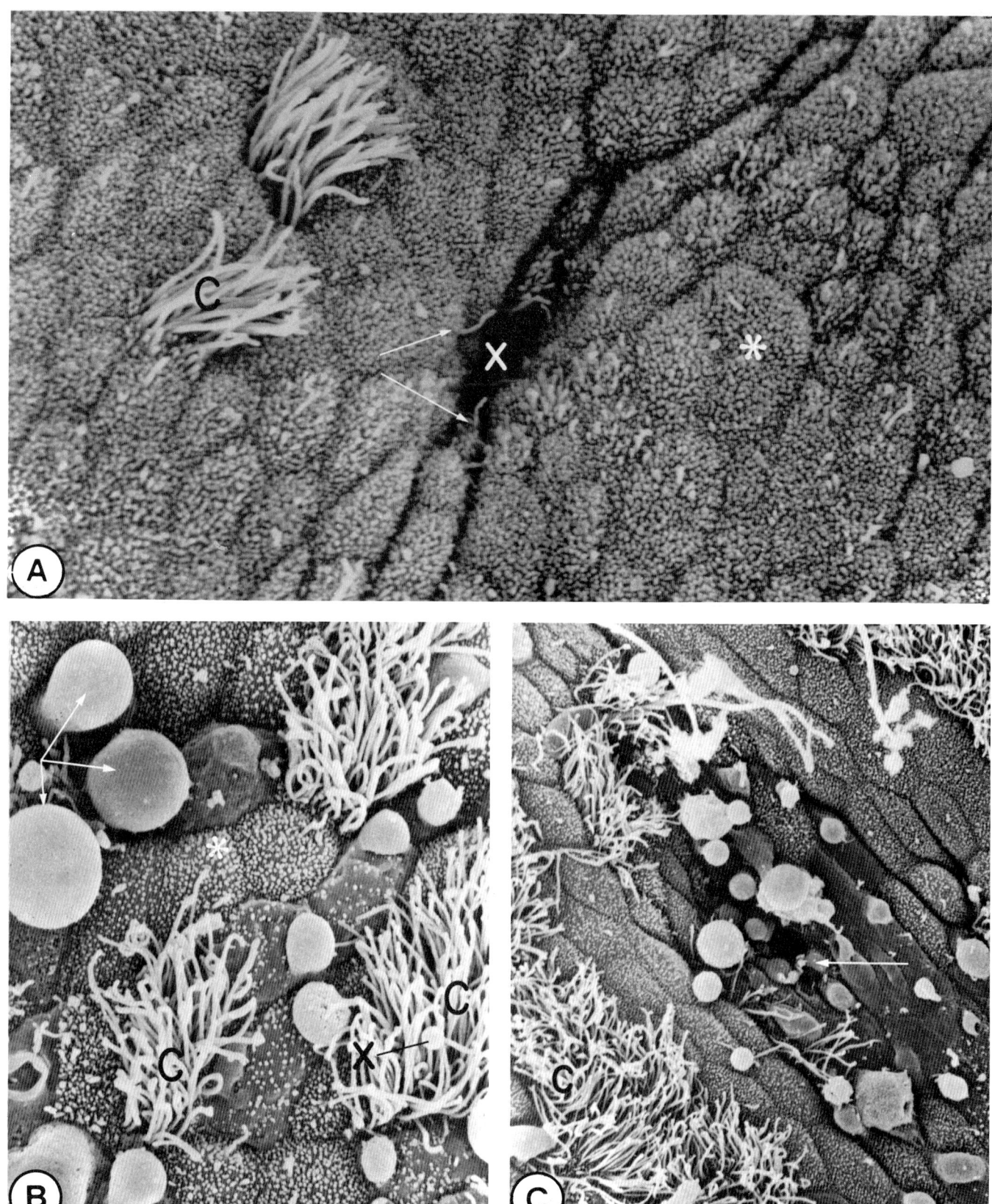

A **Rabbit endometrium (scanning EM, x3,800).** The epithelium of the mucosa consists of ciliated cells **(C)** and cells rich in microvilli **(*)**. Center: note the orifice of the gland **(x)** lined with cells having microvilli and single cilia **(→)**.

B, C **The secretory phase in the endometrium and glands from rabbit (scanning EM, x2,200, x3,800).** The epithelium surrounding the gland openings is overlain by secretions in the form of large vesicles **(→)**. Smaller secretory droplets are also found in contact **(x)** with a number of ciliated cells **(C)**. From P.M. Motta and P.M. Andrews. J. Anat. (London) 122:325, 1975.

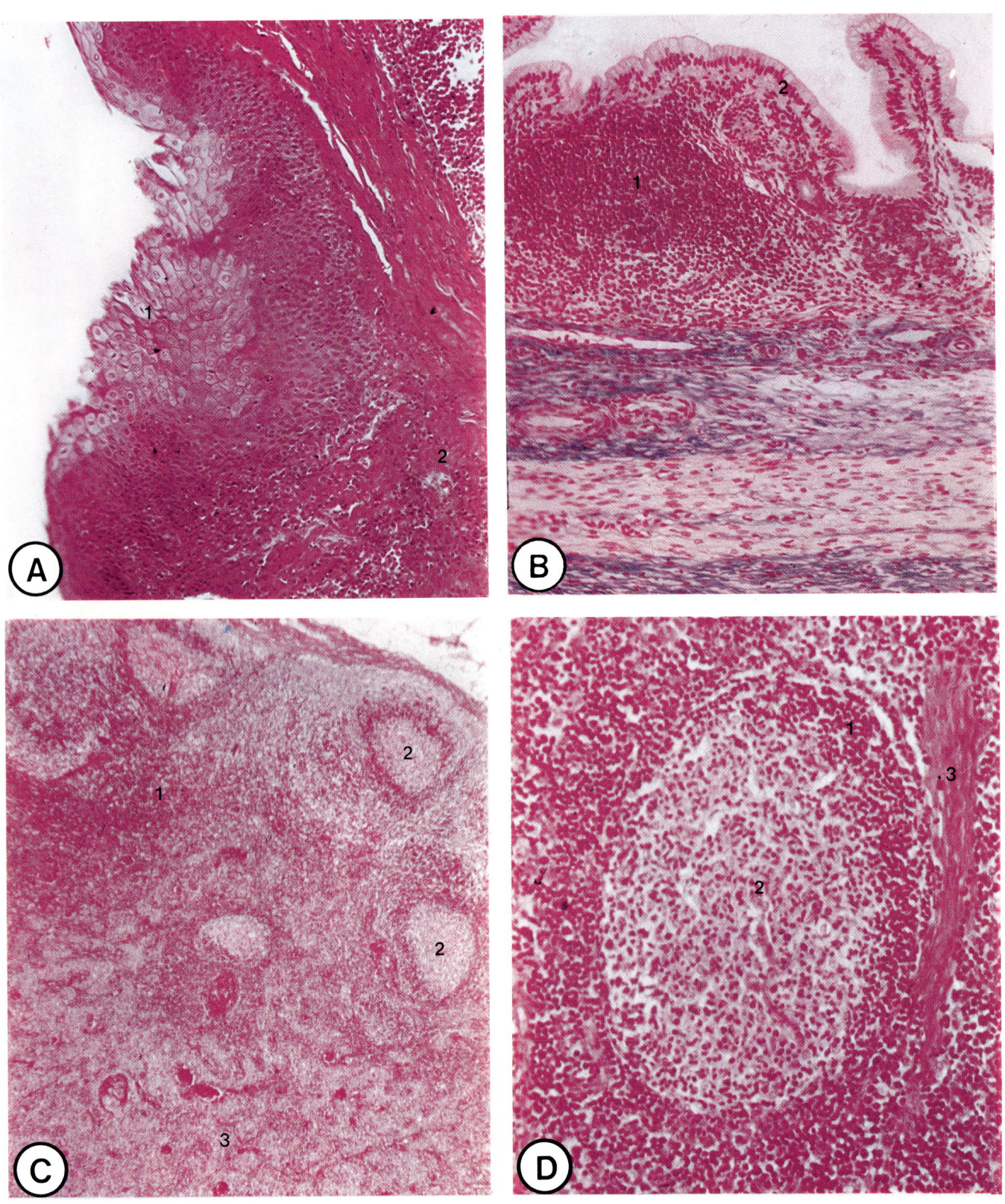

A **Lingual tonsil from dog (H & E, x210).** In both the stratified squamous epithelium **(1)** and the lamina propria **(2)** are embedded many lymphocytes (lympho-epithelial symbiosis).

B **Isolated lymph nodule from canine small intestine (azan- Mallory, x175).** The entire width of the lamina propria is occupied by the lymph nodule **(1). 2** = epithelium.

C **Lymph node from dog (H & E, x80). 1** = cortex of lymph node with many lymph follicles **(2). 3** = medulla of lymph node containing anastomosing cords of lymphocytes and blood vessels.

D **Lymph follicle of dog lymph node (H & E, x220).** The lymph follicle is oval in shape and consists of a peripheral part with concentrations of small lymphocytes **(1)** and a light-staining center (germinal center) **(2). 3** = trabecula of connective tissue between the follicles.

Plate 8.44 229

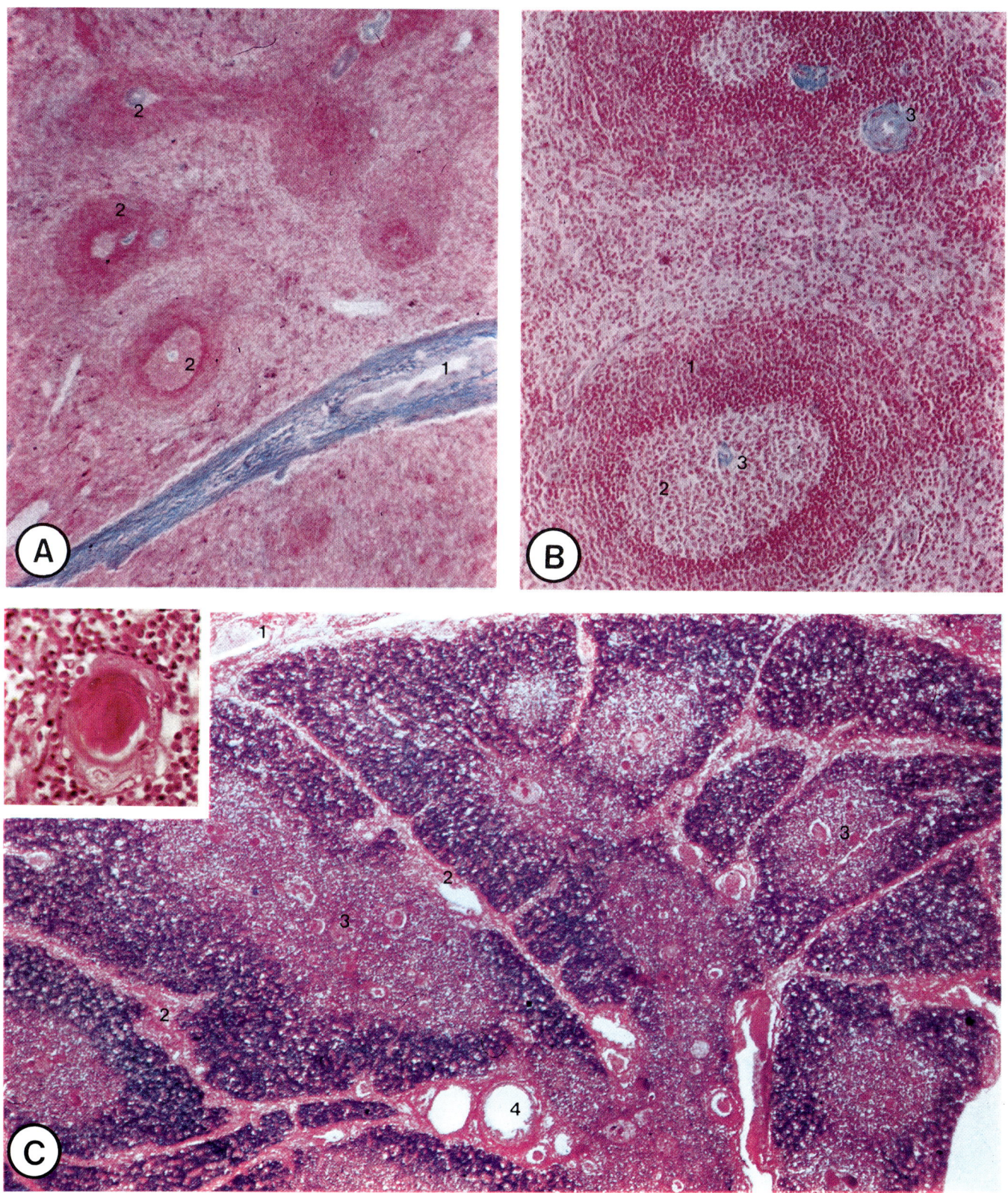

A   **Human spleen (azan-Mallory, x65). 1** = large trabecula of connective tissue with blood vessels. An arteriole is passing through the lymph follicles (splenic corpuscles) **(2)**. Between the follicles is the red pulp.

B   **Human spleen (azan-Mallory, x175).** Splenic corpuscles consisting of a peripheral concentration of small lymphocytes **(1)** and a lighter-staining germinal center **(2)** containing an arteriole **(3)** can be seen.

C   **Human thymus (H & E, x60). 1** = capsule from which derive the septa **(2)** that divide the organ into lobules. Each lobule **(3)** has a darker-staining cortex and a lighter center in which many Hassal's corpuscles can be seen. **4** = blood vessels. Inset: **Hassal's corpuscle (x300).**

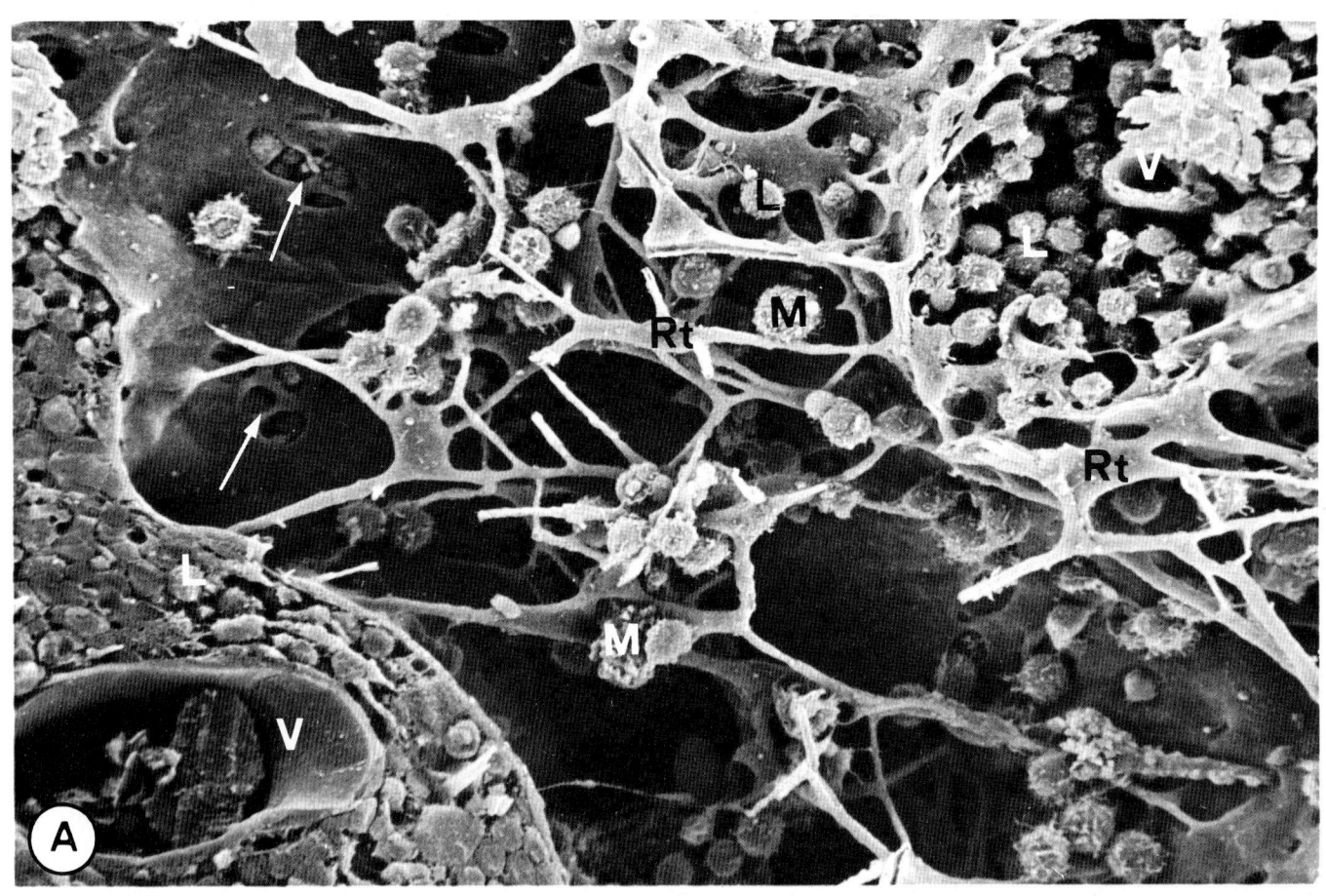

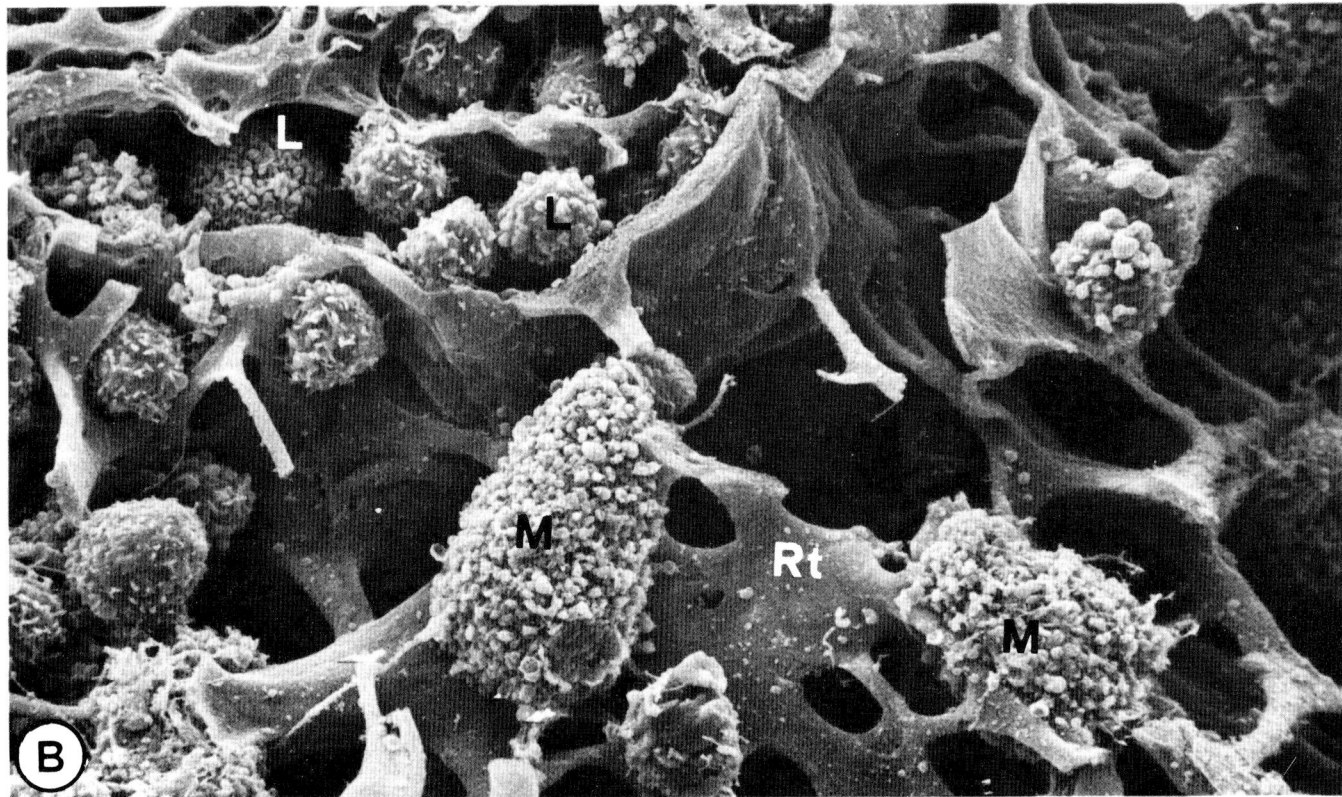

A **Lymph node from dog mesentery (scanning EM, x1,000).** Center: the lymph sinus is formed by a thin fenestrated endothelium (→). Thin cytoplasmic processes from the reticular cells **(Rt)** run through the lumen of the sinus. Among these cells are lymphocytes **(L)** and macrophages **(M)**. Along the walls of the sinus is the pulp of the lymph node with large vessels **(V)** and numerous lymphocytes.

B **Lymph node in axilla of guinea-pig (scanning EM, x2,000).** Along the fenestrated wall of the lymph sinus, which is covered with thin reticular cells **(Rt)**, can be seen large macrophages **(M)**. Above left: pulp of lymph node with many lymphocytes **(L)**. By courtesy of T. Fujita. In: T. Fujita, K. Tanaka and J. Tokunaga. *Scanning Electron Microscopic Atlas of Cells and Tissues.* Igaku-Shoin Ltd, Tokyo/New York, 1981.

Plate 8.46   **231**

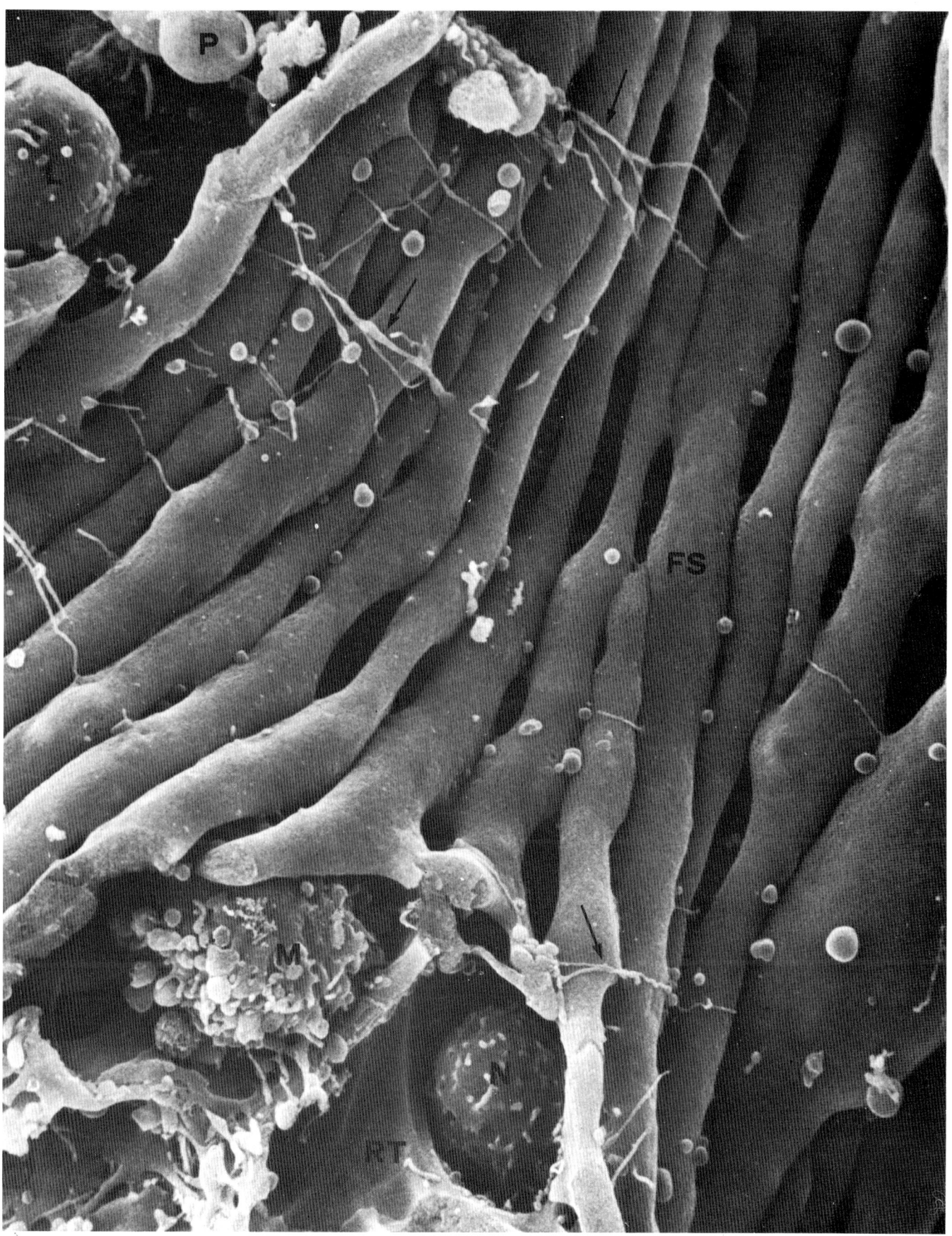

Cross section of a venous sinus of human spleen (scanning EM, x5,800). The endothelial wall of the sinus is composed of fusiform spindle cells **(FS)**. Thin cytoplasmic processes connect the endothelial cells of the sinus (→). A Billroth cord around the sinus is composed of thin reticular cells **(RT)** with a smooth surface. These cells delimit spaces in which are neutrophilic granulocytes **(N)**, platelets **(P)**, lymphocytes **(L)** and macrophages **(M)**. The tissue was prepared by vascular perfusion, thus the erythrocytes that normally occur in the spaces are not seen. By courtesy of T. Fujita. Arch. Histol. Jap. 37:187, 1974.

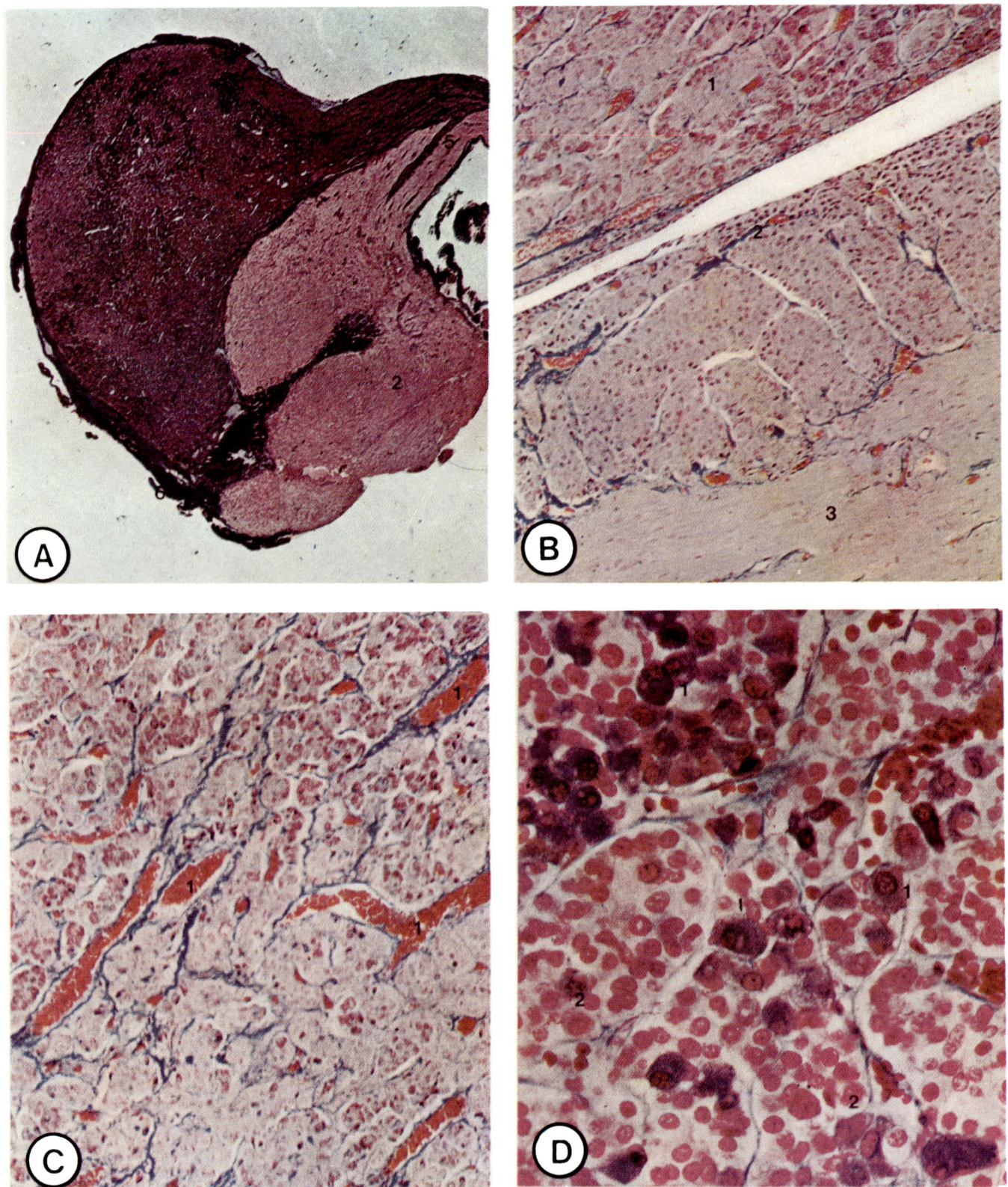

A   **Human pituitary gland (azan-Mallory, x15). 1** = anterior lobe (adenohypophysis). **2** = posterior lobe or pars nervosa (neurohypophysis). **3** = pars intermedia. **4** = pars tuberalis. **5** = hypophyseal stalk. **6** = connective tissue capsule derived from the dura mater of the meninges.

B   **Human pituitary gland (azan-Mallory, x120). 1** = anterior lobe with cords of epithelial cells. **2** = cells of pars intermedia. **3** = pars nervosa.

C   **Anterior lobe of human pituitary gland (azan-Mallory, x220).** Cords of epithelial cells are in contact with spacious sinusoids containing red blood cells **(1).**

D   **Anterior lobe of human pituitary gland (azan-Mallory, x380). 1** = basophilic cells. **2** = acidophilic cells. The cells with translucent cytoplasm are chromophobe cells.

Plate 8.48   **233**

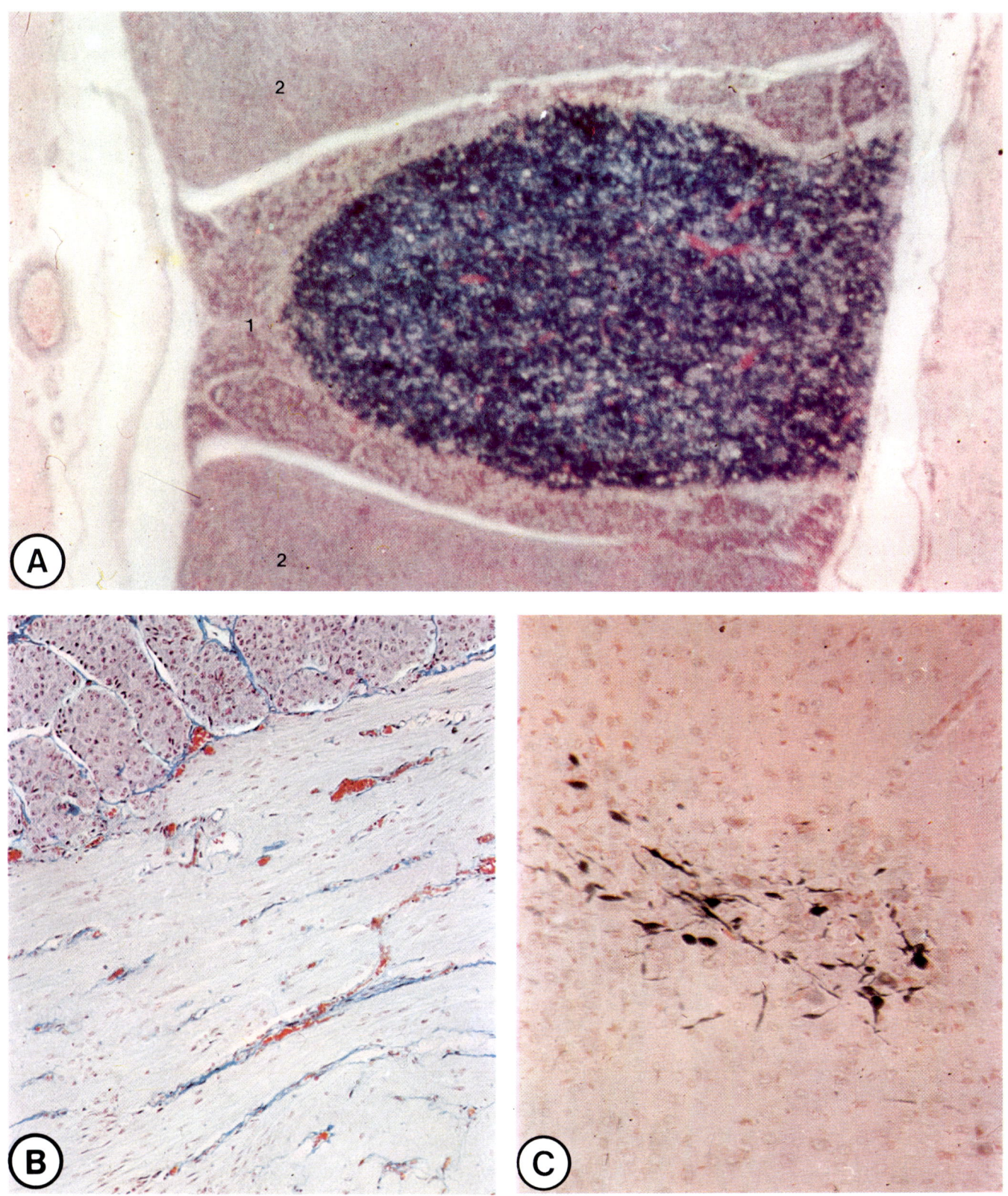

A   **Cross section of rat pituitary gland (chrome hematoxylin and phloxin method, x70).** Center: pars nervosa containing neurosecretory material. The pars nervosa is surrounded by the pars intermedia **(1)** with the foremost region of the anterior lobe **(2)**.

B   **Human pars nervosa (azan-Mallory, x220).** Above: pars intermedia. Center: pars nervosa with nerve fibers, glial cells and connective tissue containing small blood vessels.

C   **Paraventricular nucleus from rat (chrome hematoxylin and phloxin method, x180).** Neurosecretory granules are present (dark brown) within the nerve fibers running between other cells of the tissue. By courtesy of A. Pasqualino.

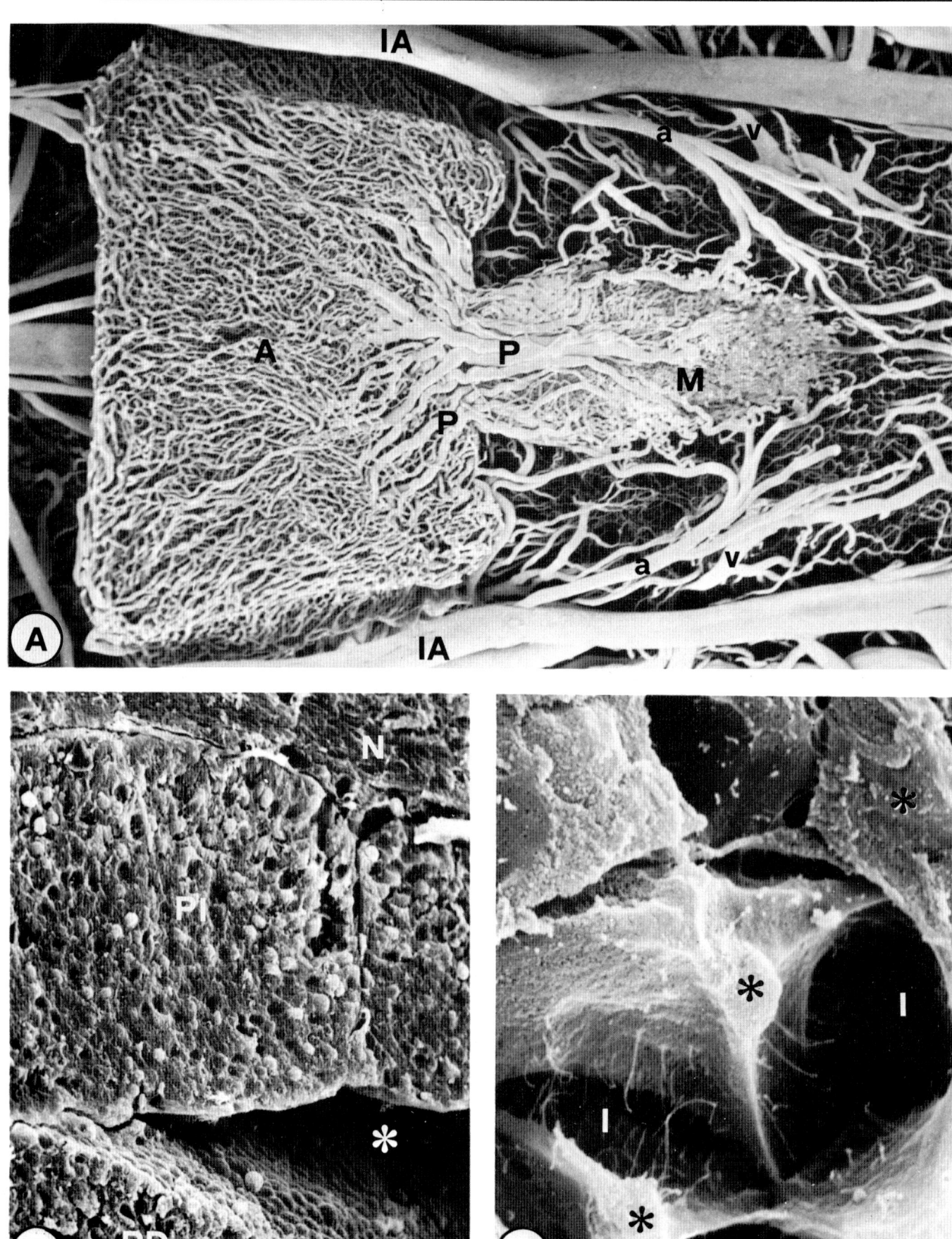

A   **Blood vessel network in rat pituitary gland (vascular resin injection, scanning EM, x42). A** = anterior lobe. **1A** = internal carotid artery with branches **(a). M** = median eminence. **P** = portal system. **v** = venules. By courtesy of T. Murakami.

B   **Rat pituitary gland (scanning EM, x1,250). N** = pars nervosa. **PI** = pars intermedia. **PD** = The pituitary cleft derived from the pars distalis. Rathke's pouch (*) can be seen at the center of the gland. From S. Correr and P.M. Motta. Cell Tiss. Res. 215:515, 1981.

C   **Cells from anterior lobe of rat pituitary gland (scanning EM, x18,000).** Star-shaped cells (*) can be seen in the pars intermedia, which has been fractured. The surfaces of these cells project long, thin microvilli into the intercellular spaces (I). From S. Correr and P.M. Motta. In: K. Tanaka and T. Fujita (eds). *Scanning Electron Microscopy in Cell Biology and Medicine.* Excerpta Medica, Amsterdam, 1981.

Plate 8.50 235

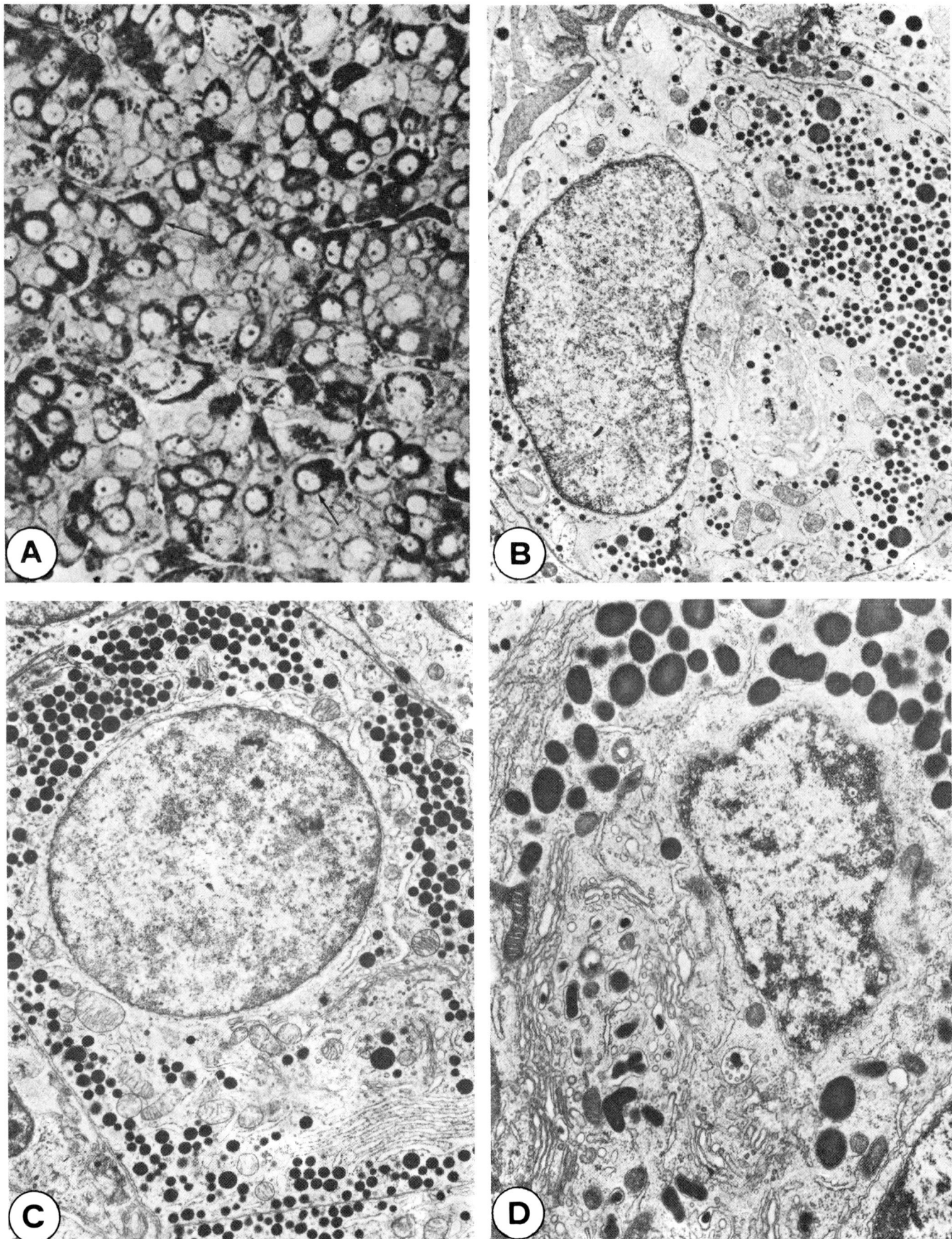

A **Anterior lobe of rat pituitary gland (H & E, x600).** Cords of chromophilic (→) and chromophobe cells with interspersed blood vessels are visible.

B **Gonadotropic cell from rat (EM, x12,500).** In this cell the granules are polymorphic (diameter 200-250 nm) and the endoplasmic reticulum appears dilated.

C **Somatotropic cell from rat (EM, x12,800).** Around the nucleus can be seen typical granules (diameter 350 nm) and a well-developed rough endoplasmic reticulum.

D **Mammotropic cell from rat (EM, x14,000).** The specific granules of this cell are large (diameter 700-750 nm) and some are in association with the maturing face of the Golgi complex. By courtesy of M. Farquhar.

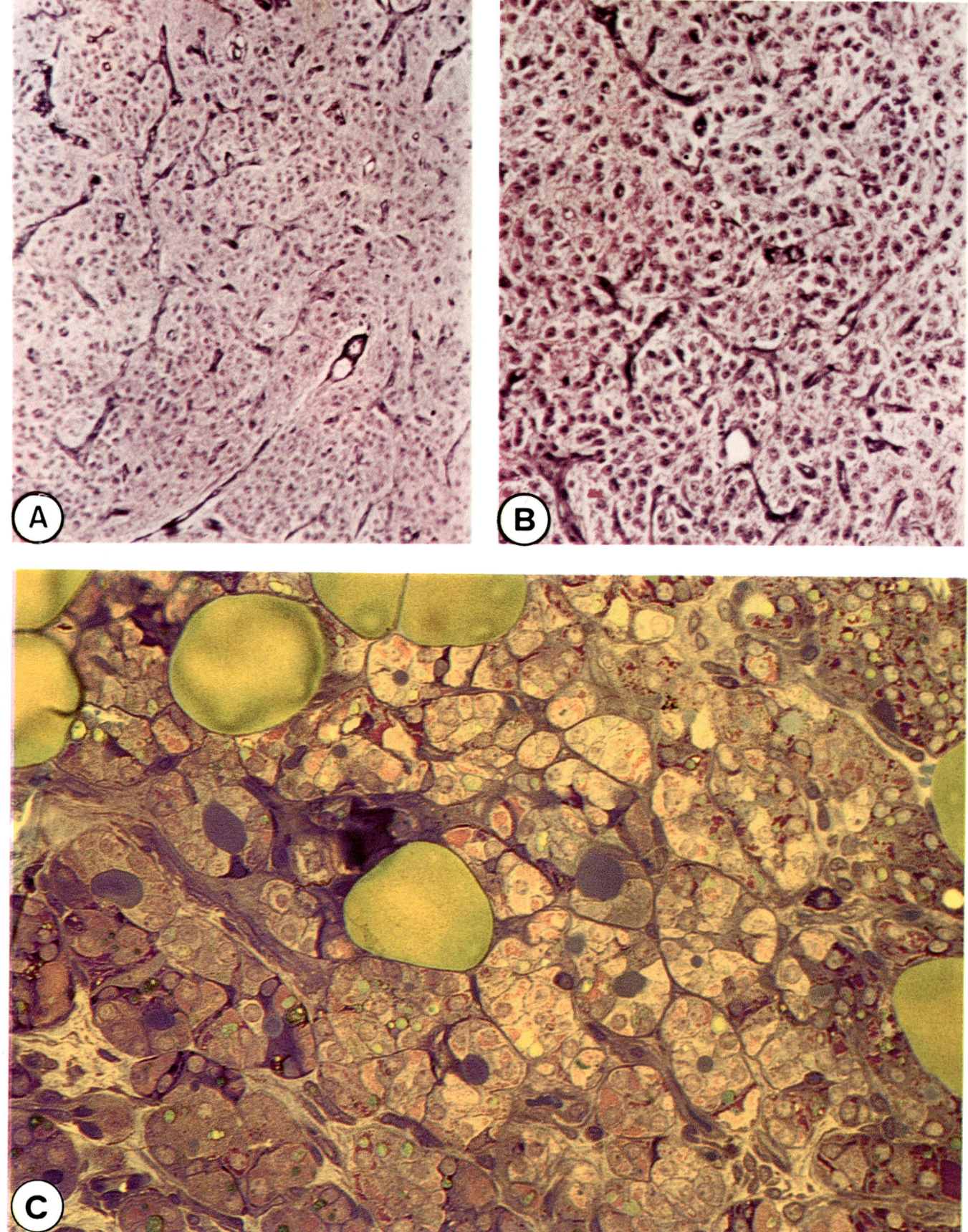

A   **Human pineal gland (azan-Mallory, x75).** Narrow septa separating the stroma cells of the glands are stained blue.
B   **Detail of human pineal gland (azan-Mallory, x420).**
C   **Human parathyroid gland (PAS, x1,250).** An area of follicles is visible at bottom left, as well as non-follicular area, at upper right. Note the presence of adipose cells (in yellow). By courtesy of S. Cinti, S.G. Balercia, et al. J. Submicr. Cytol. 15:661, 1983.

Plate 8.52

237

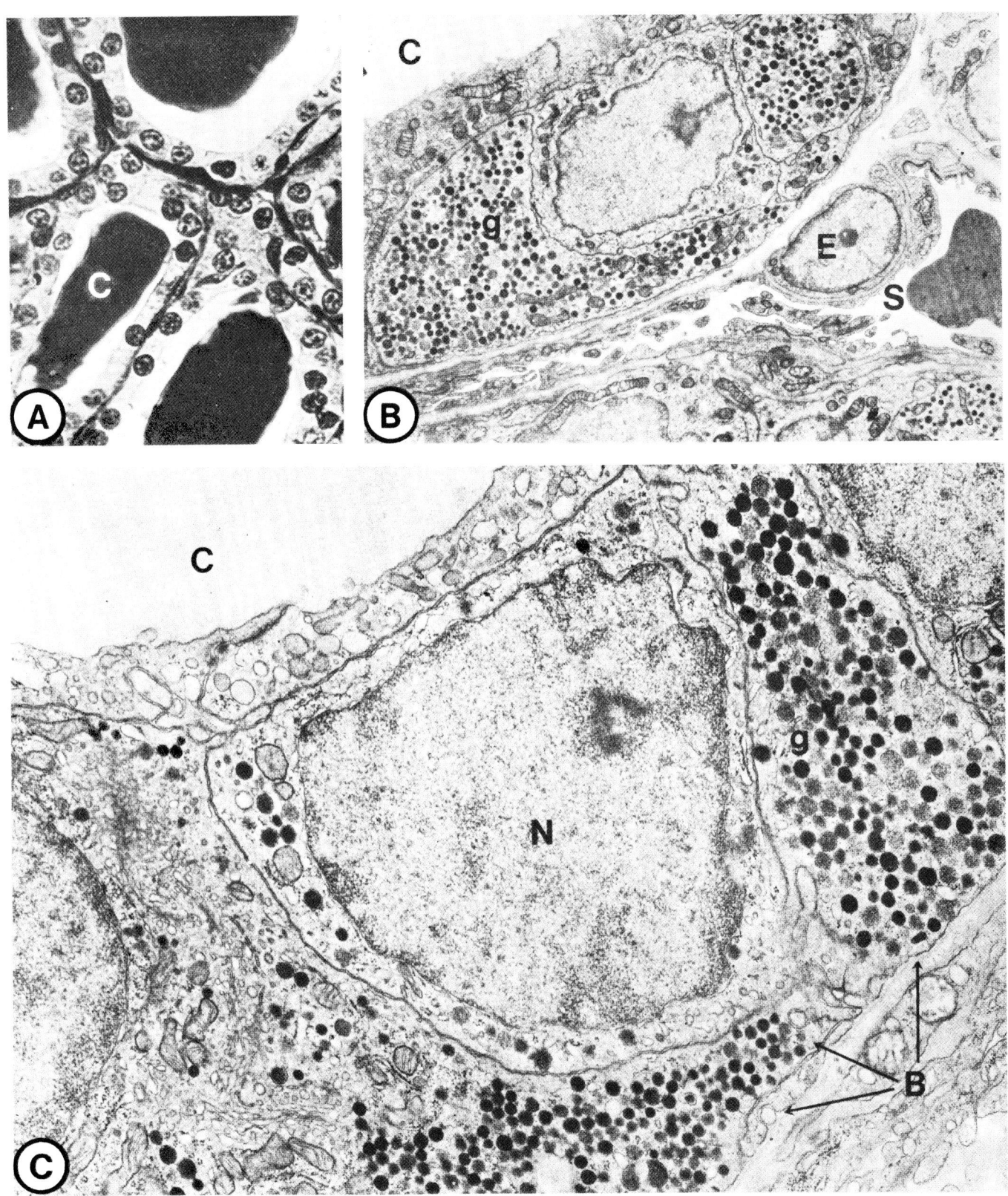

A   **Thryoid gland from dog (H & E, x420).** Thyroid follicles with cuboidal epithelium and colloid **(C)** filling the cavity can be seen.

B   **Thyroid gland from bat: a portion of the wall of the thyroid follicle (EM, x7,800).** Some parafollicular cells containing secretory granules **(g)** are in proximity to the thyroid epithelial cells. **C** = cavity of the follicle. **E** = endothelial cell of a blood vessel **(S)**.

C   **Thyroid gland from bat: detail of follicular epithelium (EM, x22,000).** Center: the cell with the large nucleus **(N)** and the cells with secretion granules **(g)** are the parafollicular cells. Small portions of follicle cells facing the cavity of the follicle **(C)** can be seen. **(B)** = basal lamina. By courtesy of G. Azzali.

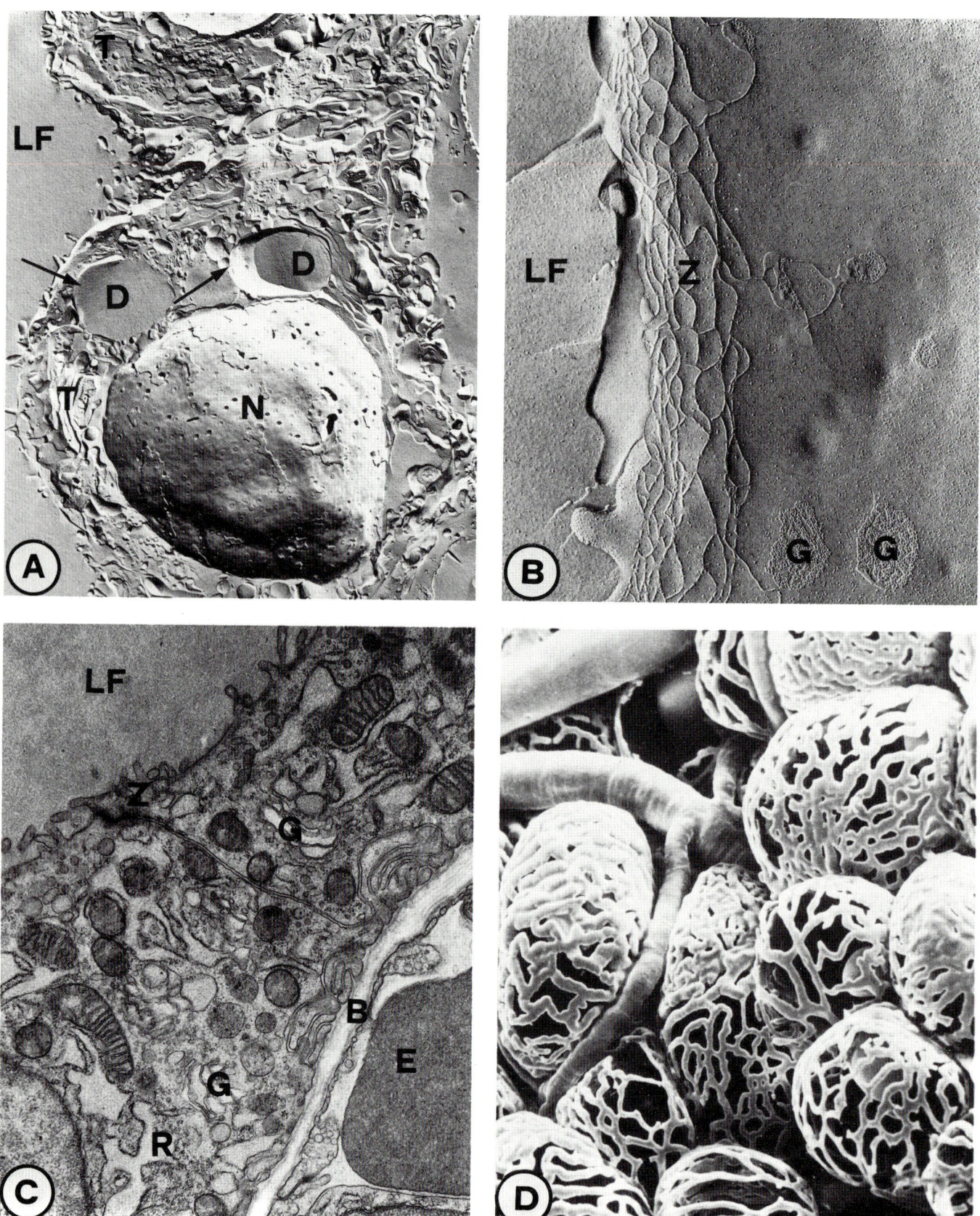

A,   B **Thyroid cells from mouse (EM, freeze-fracture, x9,000, x36,000). LF** = lumen of thyroid follicle. **T** = thyroid cells. **D** = droplets of resorbed colloid (→) in the cytoplasm. **N** = nucleus. Figure **B** is a higher magnification of the apical and lateral regions of a thyroid cell. The delicate network represents a complex zonula occludens (**Z**). **G** = gap junctions. By courtesy of H. Fujita and K. Ishimura. Cell. Tiss. Res. 198:15, 1979.

C   **Thyroid follicle from mouse (EM, x14,000). LF** = lumen of follicle. **B** = basal lamina and underlying connective tissue. **E** = erythrocyte in the lumen of a capillary. The cytoplasm of thyroid cells has a Golgi complex (**G**), highly dilated membranes of rough endoplasmic reticulum (**R**), and many mitochondria. **Z** = junctional zone between two thyroid cells.

D   **Vascularization of monkey thyroid follicles (vascular resin injection, scanning EM, x330).** A profuse network of vessels can be seen surrounding each follicle. By courtesy of H. Fujita and T. Murakami. Arch. Histol. Jap. 36:181, 1974.

Plate 8.54   239

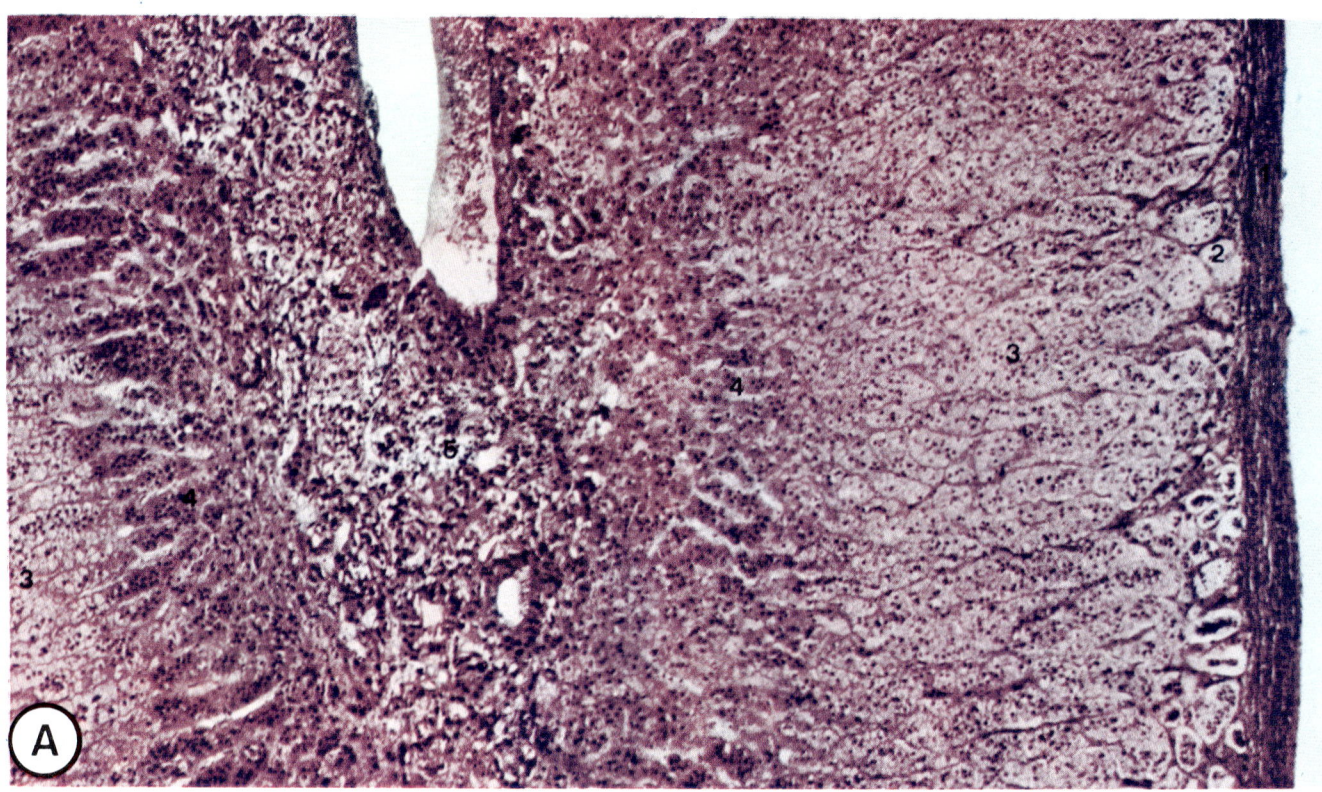

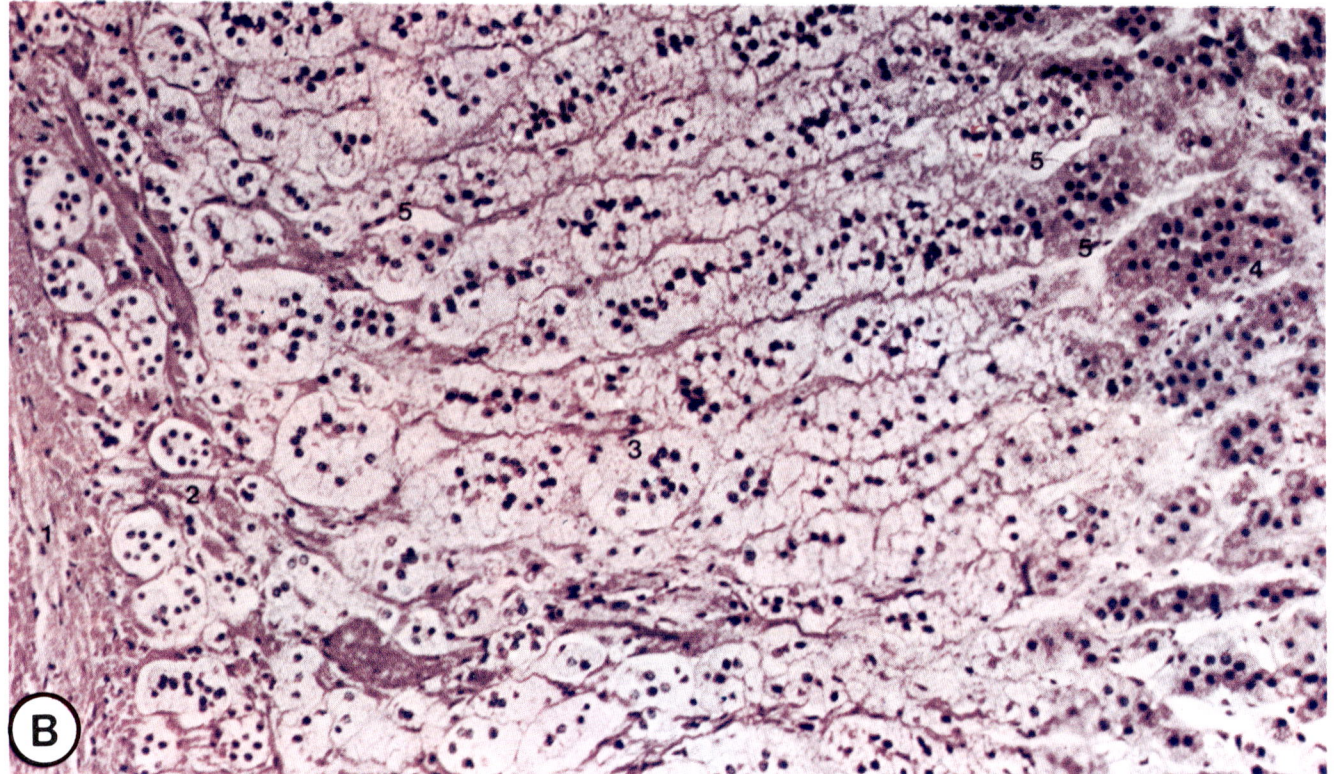

A   **Human adrenal gland (H & E, x80). 1** = connective tissue capsule. **2** = zona glomerulosa. **3** = zona fasciculata. **4** = zona reticularis of cortex. **5** = medulla.

B   **Human adrenal cortex (H & E, x220). 1** = connective tissue capsule. **2** = zona glomerulosa. **3** = zona fasciculata. **4** = zona reticularis. **5** = sinusoids.

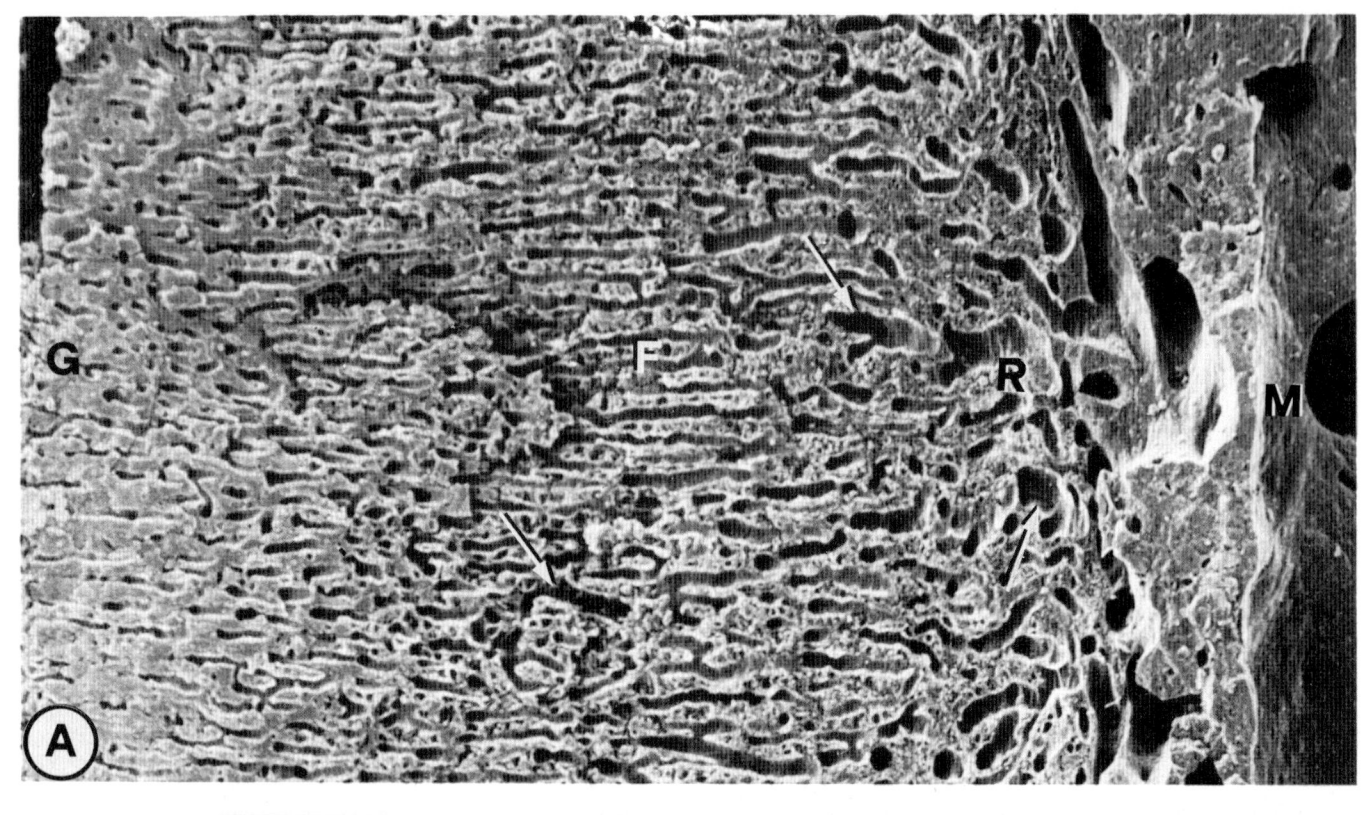

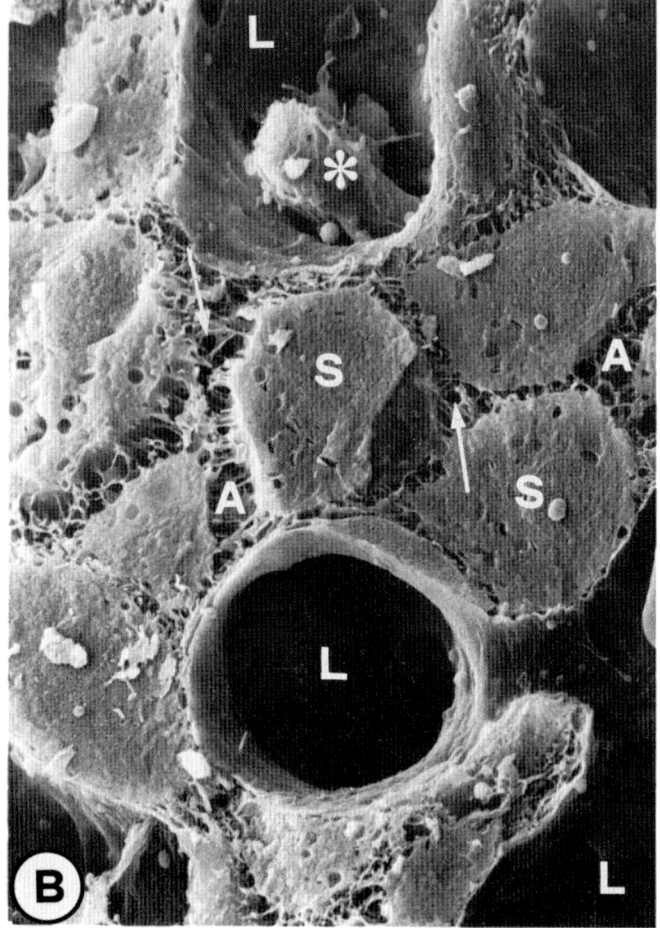

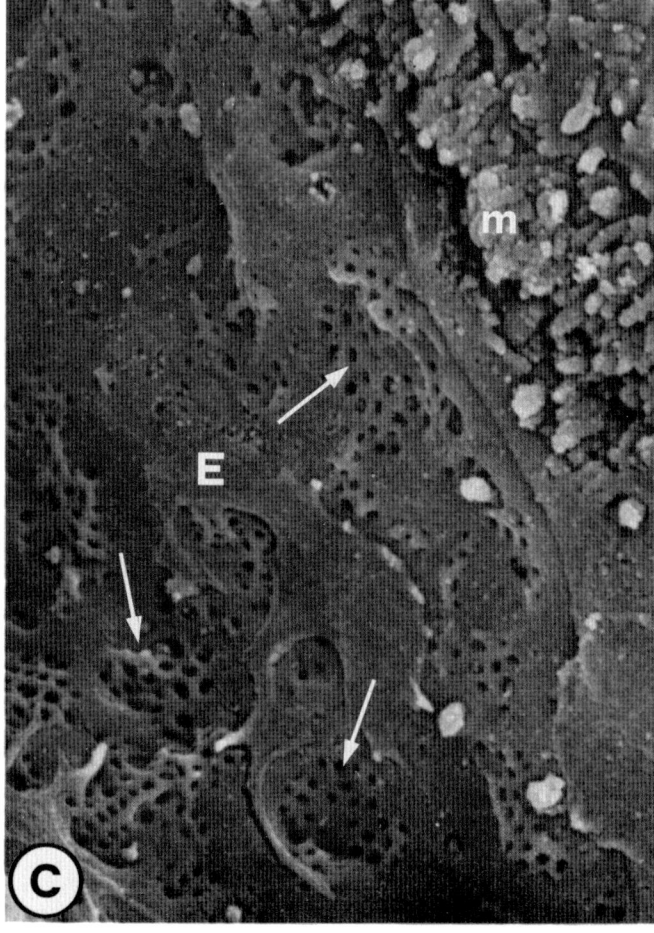

A **Rat adrenal gland (scanning EM, x320). G** = zona glomerulosa. **F** = zona fasciculata. **R** = zona reticularis. **M** = medulla with large vessels. The capillary network crossing the cortex has an irregular course and is formed of sinusoids and larger vessels (→).

B **Zona reticularis from pig adrenal cortex (scanning EM, x6,200).** Sinusoids **(L)** and secretory cells **(S)** are separated by spacious lacunae **(A)** into which the cells project numerous microvilli (→). There is a macrophage in the lumen of one sinusoid **(*)**.

C **Capillary of zona reticularis from pig adrenal gland (scanning EM, x52,000).** In this sinusoid the wall of the endothelium **(E)** is highly fenestrated (→). **m** = microvilli of a secretory cell. From P.M. Motta, M. Muto and T. Fujita. Cell Tiss. Res. 196:23, 1979.

Plate 8.56   241

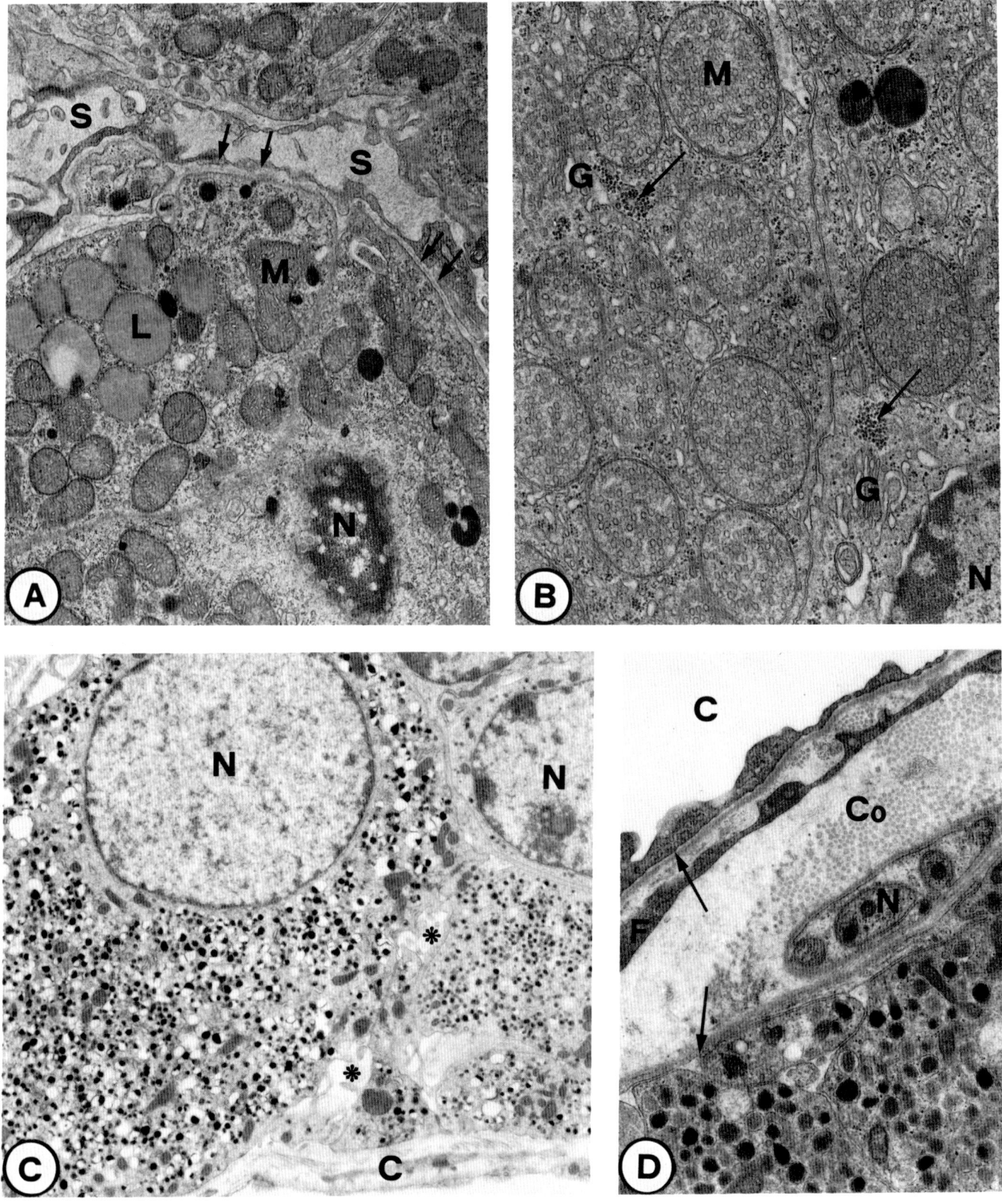

A   Cells from zona glomerulosa of rat adrenal cortex (EM, x12,000). N = nucleus. L = lipid inclusions. M = mitochondria with tubular cristae. S = sinusoids surrounding the cell. Arrows show the basal lamina. By courtesy of G.G. Nussdorfer, V. Meneghelli and G. Mazzocchi.

B   Cells from zona fasciculata of rat adrenal cortex (EM, x19,500). M = mitochondria with tubular cristae. G = Golgi complex. N = nucleus. The arrows show glycogen granules. By courtesy of G.G. Nussdorfer, V. Meneghelli and G. Mazzocchi.

C   Chromaffin cells from adrenal medulla of mouse (EM, x6,630). Many catecholamine granules are visible in the cytoplasm. N = nuclei. Narrow intercellular spaces (*) are seen between the cells, which are adjacent to a blood capillary (C). By courtesy of R.E. Coupland.

D   Chromaffin cell from adrenal medulla of marmoset (EM, x15,640). Chromaffin cells, rich in secretory granules, are associated with a blood capillary (C). In the subendothelial space bounded by the basal lamina of the chromaffin cell and of the capillary (→) can be seen bundles of collagen fibers (Co), the cytoplasmic process of a fibroblast (F) and an unmyelinated nerve fiber contained in a Schwann cell (N). By courtesy of R.E. Coupland. In: P.M. Motta (ed). *Ultrastructure of Endocrine Cells and Tissues.* M. Nijhoff Publishers, The Hague/Boston/London, 1984.

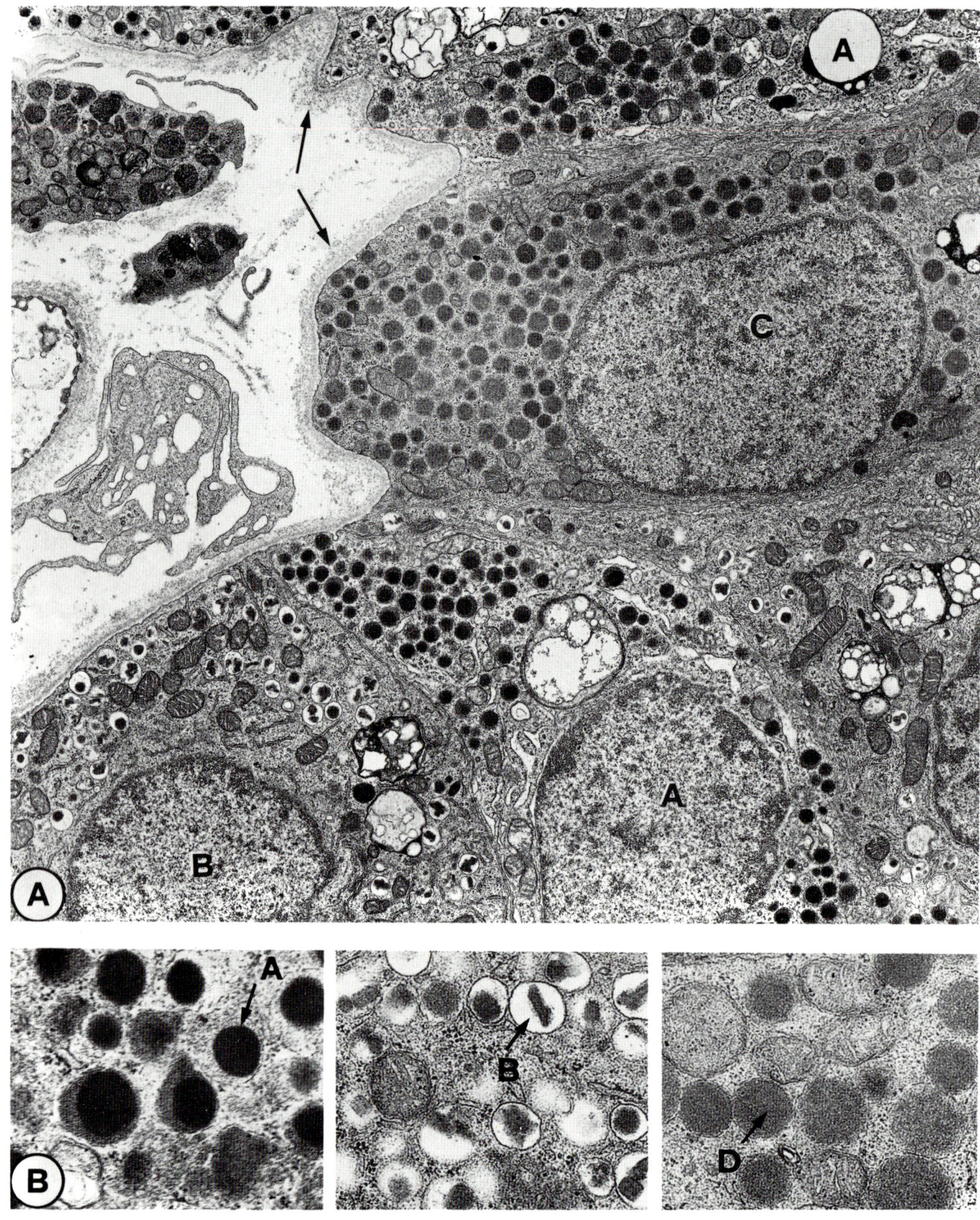

A   **Human endocrine pancreas (EM, x10,500).** An islet of Langerhans bounded by a basal lamina (→) can be seen. Note the **A** (alpha) cells, the **B** (beta) cells and the **D** (delta) cells, each with characteristic granules.

B   **Endocrine cells of human pancreas (EM, x35,000).** From left to right can be seen the granules of **A,B** and **D** cells, respectively. These cells differ from one another in the appearance of their granules. By courtesy of F. Caramia.

Plate 8.58   **243**

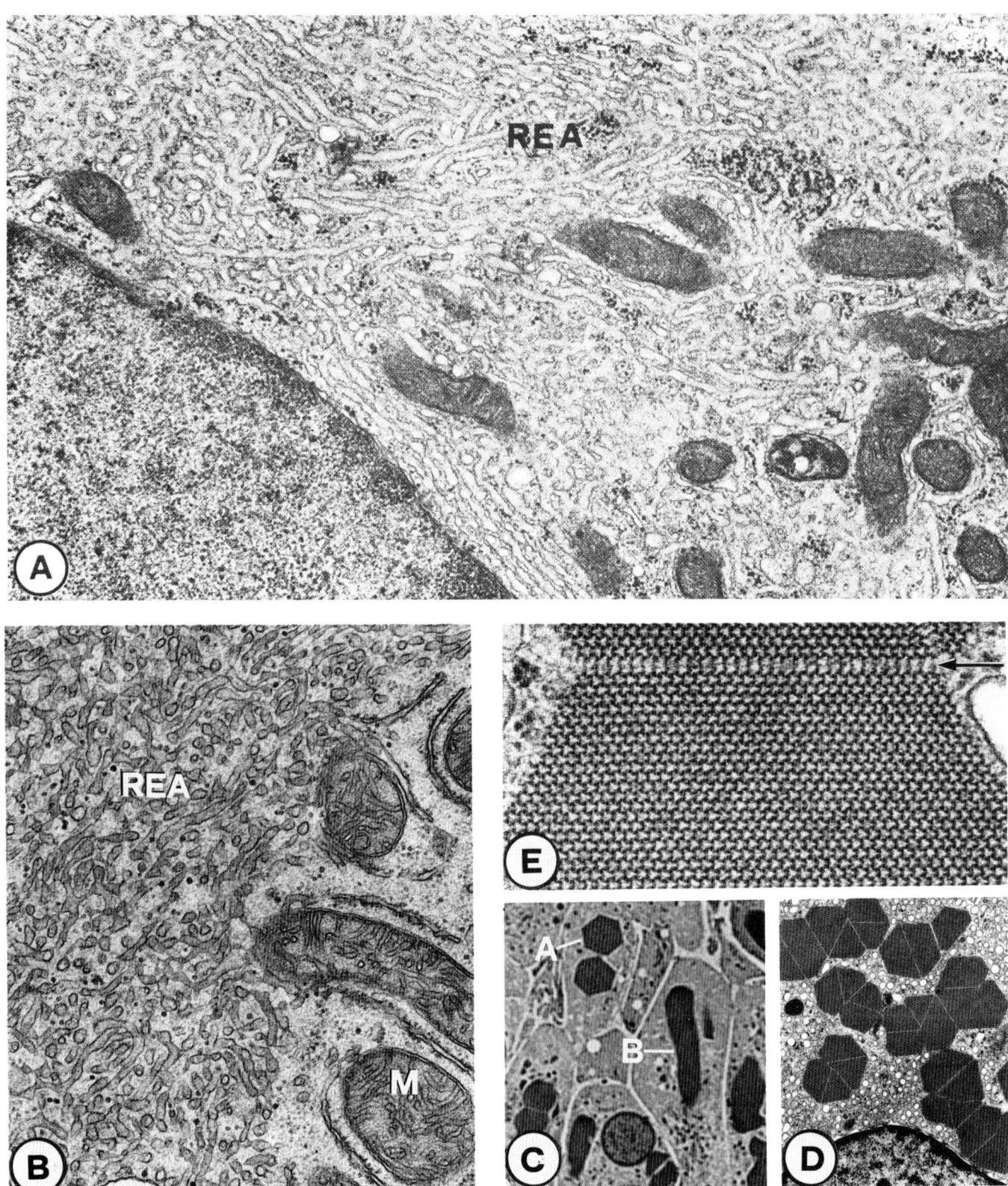

A   **Interstitial cell from guinea-pig testis (EM, x32,000).** The cytoplasm of this steroid-producing cell has abundant agranular endoplasmic reticulum (**REA**). Some of the enzymes having a role in the synthesis of the male hormones are associated with this cell component. The mitochondria have a dense matrix and tubular or villiform cristae. By courtesy of A.K. Christensen. J. Cell Biol. 26:911, 1965.

B   **Interstitial cell from human testis (EM, x32,000).** The abundant agranular endoplasmic reticulum (**REA**) is composed of tubules which anatomose to form a complex network. The mitochondria have tubular cristae. By courtesy of H. Mori.

C,   **D,E Reinke's crystals in the interstitial cells of human testis. Figure C (x1,000)** is a semithin section stained with Heidenheim's iron hematoxylin. Here, Reinke's crystals can be seen in cross (white A) and longitudinal (white B) section in the cytoplasm of the Leydig cell. In **Figure D (EM, x6,800)** Reinke's crystals can be seen in cross section. In **Figure E (EM, x68,000)** the honeycomb structure of the crystal cut in cross section is clear in a magnified segment. The arrow shows the junction between two adjacent crystals. By courtesy of H. Mori. In: P.M. Motta (ed). *Ultrastructure of Endocrine Cells and Tissues.* M. Nijhoff Publishers, The Hague/Boston/London, 1984.

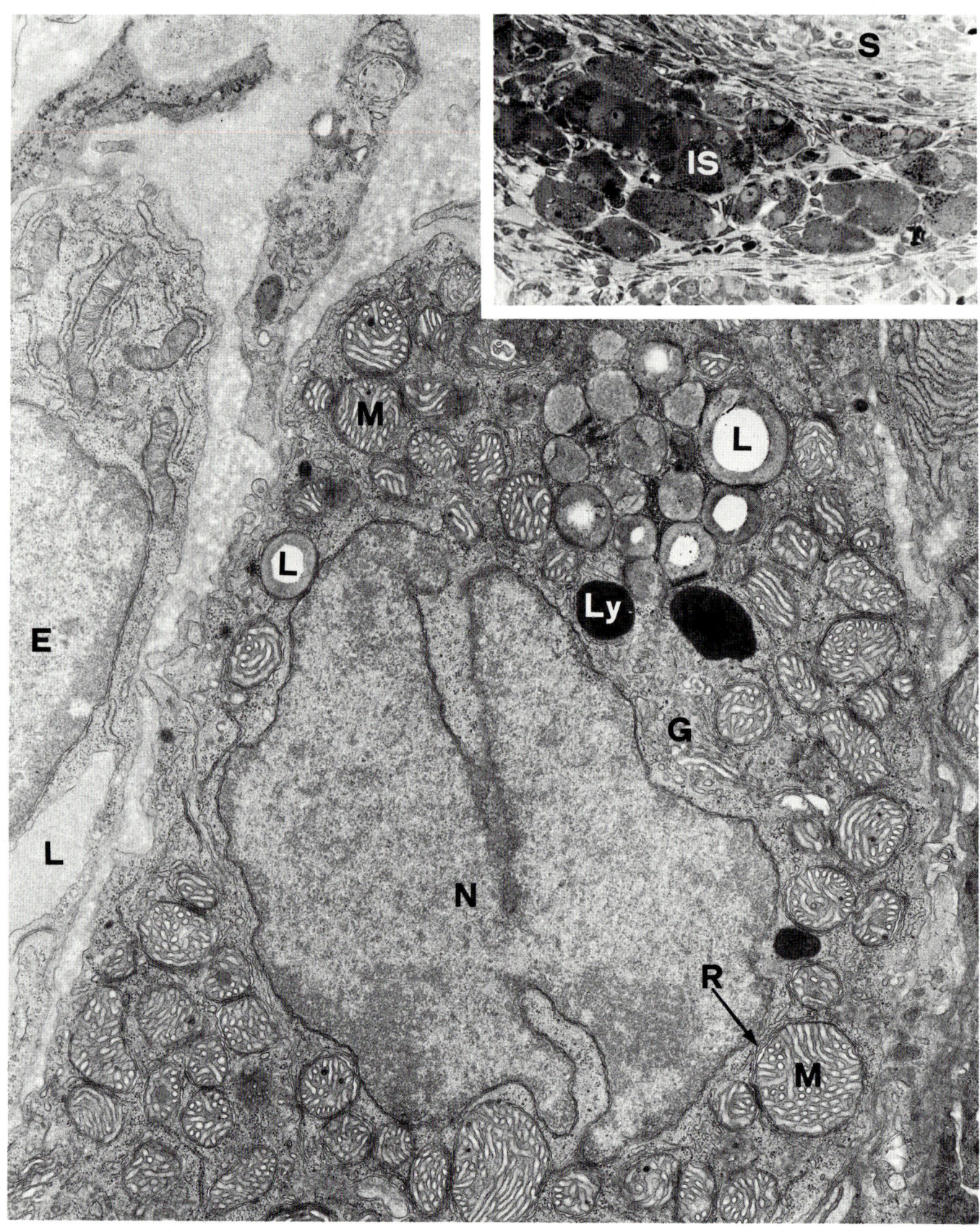

Interstitial cells from rabbit ovary (Semithin section, basic fuchsin, LM x680; EM, x24,200). In the inset are seen scattered interstitial cells **(IS)** in the stroma **(S)** of the ovary. Most of these cells are derived from the theca interna of mature follicles during atresia. The interstitial cells constitute an ovarian endocrine gland (interstitial gland) whose function is to produce steroids. The main figure shows an interstitial cell in detail. The characteristics of this cell are a cytoplasm rich in mitochondria having villiform and tubular cristae **(M)**, lipid droplets **(L)** and smooth endoplasmic reticulum which is at some points in close association with the mitochondria **(R)**. Ly = lysosome. **G** = Golgi complex. **N** = nucleus. **E** = endothelial cell in the lining of a blood capillary **(L)**. Original micrograph by K.R. Porter and P.M. Motta.

Plate 8.60   245

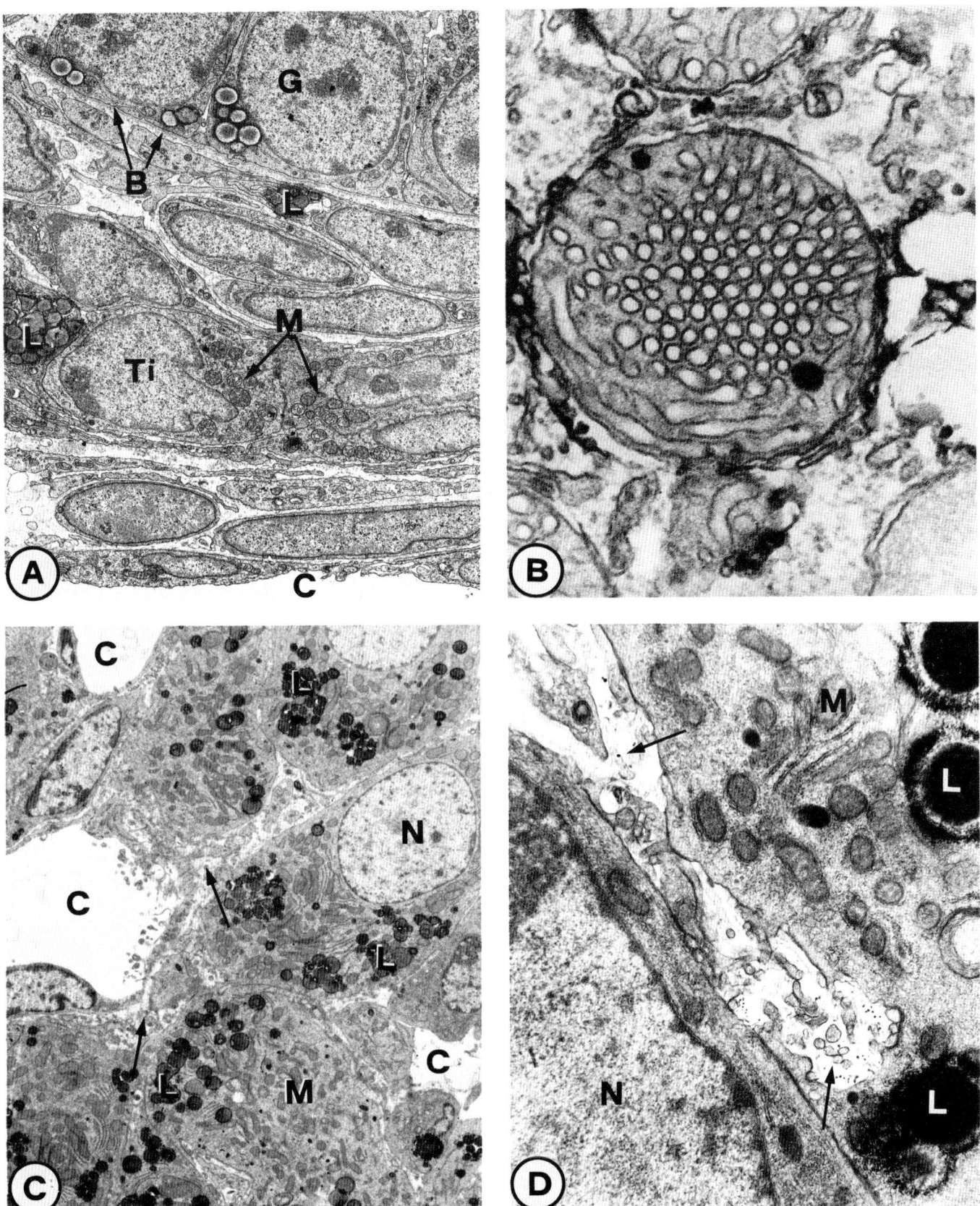

A,B   **Cells from the theca interna of mouse ovary (EM, x43,000, x78,000).** The cells of the theca interna **(Ti)** constitute an endocrine gland as a part of the follicle and have the function of secreting steroid hormones. Their cytoplasm contains lipid droplets **(L)**, smooth endoplasmic reticulum and mitochondria with characteristic tubular or villiform cristae **(M)**. Figure **B** is an enlargement of one of these mitochondria. The cells of the theca interna are separated from the stratum granulosum **(G)** of the follicle by an intervening basal lamina **(B)**. Original micrograph by G. Familiari.

C,D   **Human lutein cells (EM, x5,200, x16,200).** The lutein cells are large and polyhedral with an ovoid nucleus **(N)** and cytoplasm rich in mitochondria with villiform cristae **(M)**. The mitochondria are interspersed among smooth endoplasmic reticulum and lipid droplets **(L)**. The plasmalemma of the lutein cells has microvilli which project into the intercellular spaces (→) and expand the surfaces of the cells facing intercellular canaliculi and capillaries **(C)**. In figure **D** is a deep recess between two lutein cells (intercellular canaliculus). Original micrograph by G. Familiari and R.M. Gualtieri.

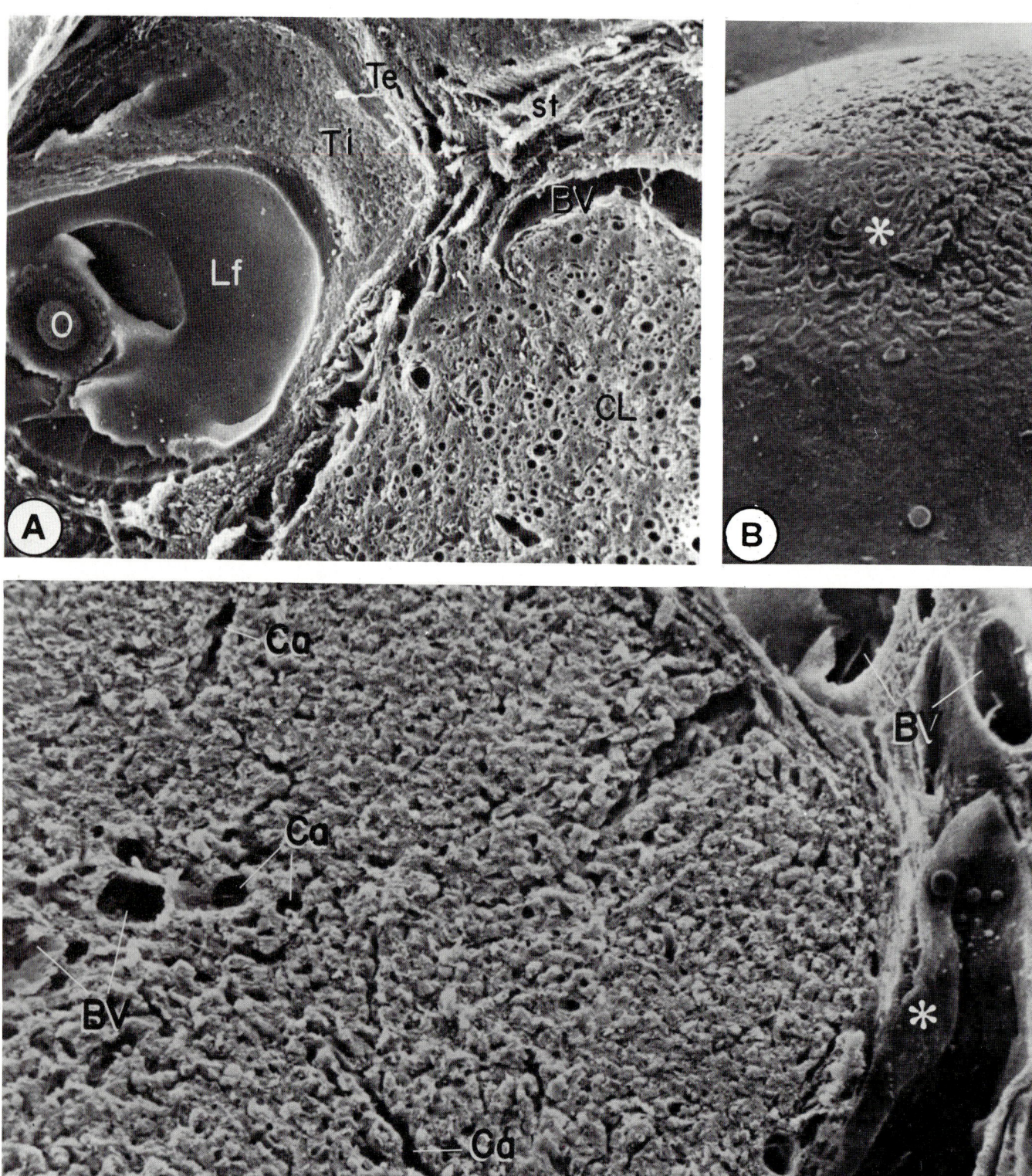

A **Follicle and corpus luteum from dog (scanning EM, x180). O** = oocyte with corona radiata in the antrum which contains liquor folliculi (**Lf**). **Ti** = theca interna. **Te** = theca externa. **st** = stroma. **CL** = corpus luteum perforated by numerous blood capillaries and covered by a capsule containing large vessels (**BV**). Original micrograph by J. Van Blerkom and P.M. Motta.

B **Corpus luteum on the surface of rabbit ovary (scanning EM, x60).** In the zone where the corpus luteum is maturing within the ovary the surface epithelium is raised to form a large number of papillae (*).

C **Corpus luteum in a rat (scanning EM, x220).** The anastomosing cords of large lutein cells have between them blood capillaries (**Ca**) that give the structure its typical spongy appearance. Large blood vessels occur in the center of the corpus luteum (**BV**) and against the capsule of connective tissue (*). From P.M. Motta, P.M. Andrews and K.R. Porter. *Microanatomy of Cell and Tissue Surfaces. An Atlas of Scanning Electron Microscopy.* Lea & Febiger, Philadelphia, 1977.

Plate 8.62   **247**

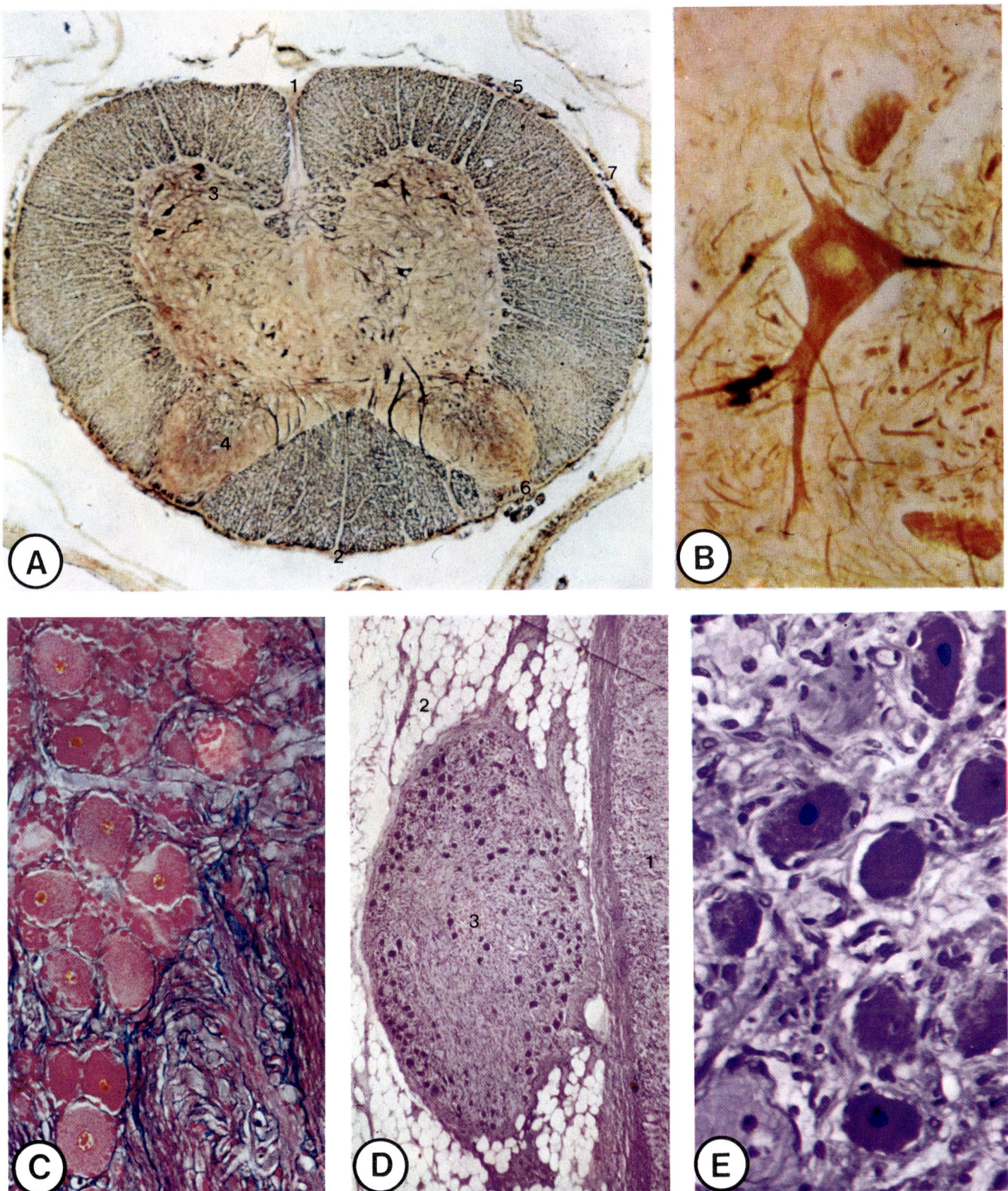

A **Cross section of human spinal cord from lumbar region. (Weigert's method, x12). 1** = anterior longitudinal sulcus. **2** = posterior longitudinal sulcus. **3** = anterior horn with groups of nerve cells (black). **4** = ventral horn. **5** = anterior root in cross section. **6** = Branches of posterior root in cross section. **7** = meninges.

B **Motor neuron from anterior horn of human spinal cord (silver impregnation, x180).** The oval nucleus has a characteristic bladder-like appearance.

C **Spinal ganglion from cat (azan-Mallory, x330).** Large ganglionic neurons are surrounded within a web of fibrous satellite cells whose small nuclei can be seen encircling the perikarya of the neurons. Bottom right corner: nerve fibers gathered in a bundle.

D **Prevertebral ganglion from human sympathetic nervous system (H & E, x80).** In these ganglia the small vertebral ganglionic cells are scattered among nerve fibers. A connective tissue capsule surrounds the ganglion. The ganglionic cells receive preganglionic fibers from the central nervous system and project dendrites to the organs they innervate. Right: adrenal cortex **(1)** with the ganglion **(3)** embedded in the adipose tissue of the adrenal capsule **(2)**.

E **Visceral ganglion cells (H & E, x325).** The ganglionic cells are surrounded by satellite cells and embedded within a web of fibers. Many capillaries are present.

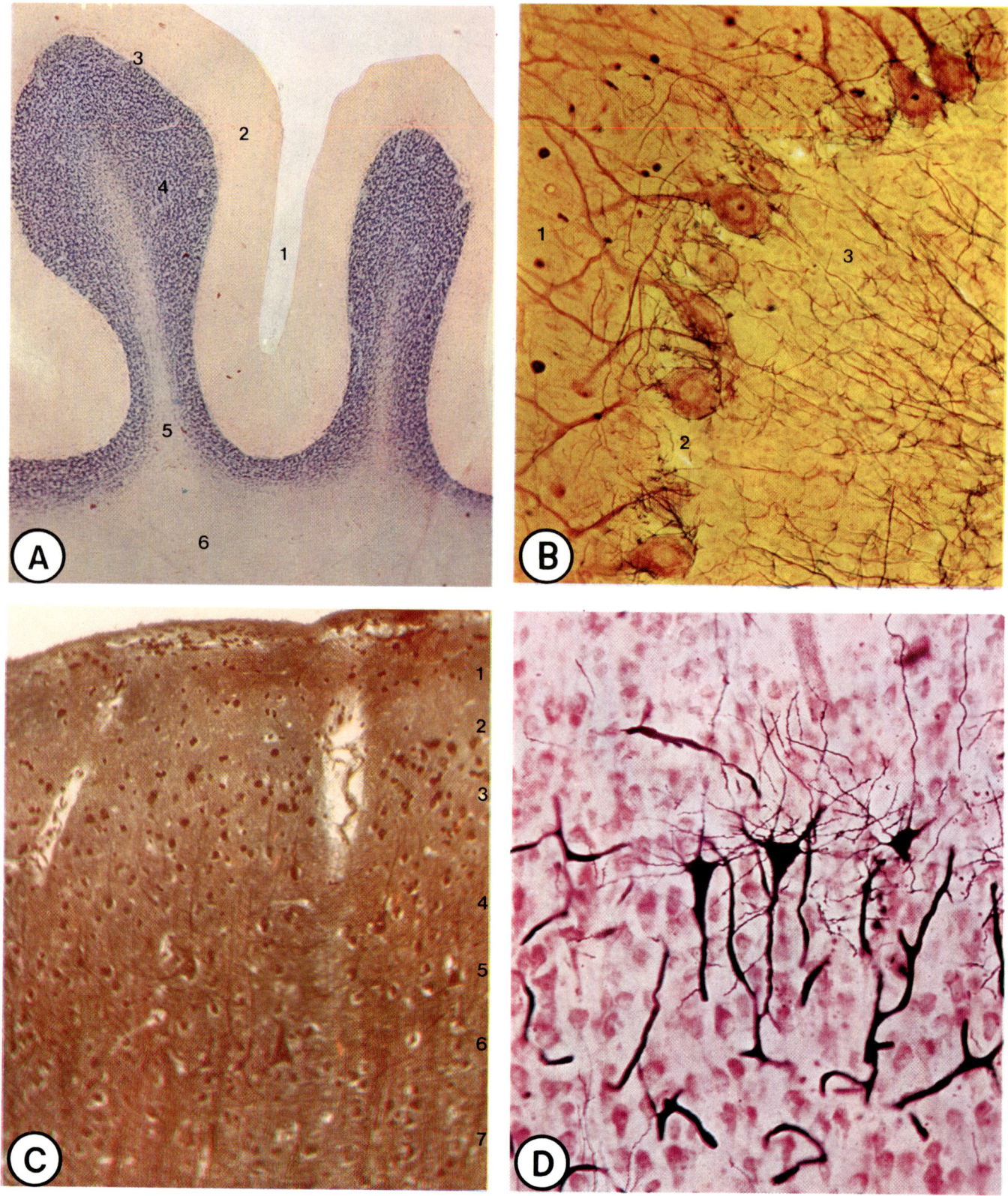

A   **Cerebellum of a mouse (Nissl method, x75). 1** = interlobular fissure. **2** = molecular layer. **3** = layer of Purkinje cells. **4** = granular layer. **5** = white matter of lobule. **6** = medulla.

B   **Human cerebellum (silver impregnation, x140). 1** = molecular layer with dendrites of Purkinje cells. **2** = layer of Purkinje cells with nerve endings of basket cells. **3** = granular layer.

C   **Cerebral cortex of guinea-pig (silver impregnation, x85). 1** = plexiform layer. **2** = layer of small pyramidal cells. **3 & 4** = layer of medium-sized and more superficial large pyramidal cells. **5** = inner granular layer. **6** = layer of deep pyramidal cells. **7** = layer of polymorphic cells bordering the white matter (below).

D   **Cerebral cortex of ox (silver impregnation, x220).** Center: large pyramidal cells (black) with dendrites from the base and the apex. Above: The inner granular layer is visible.

Plate 8.64

249

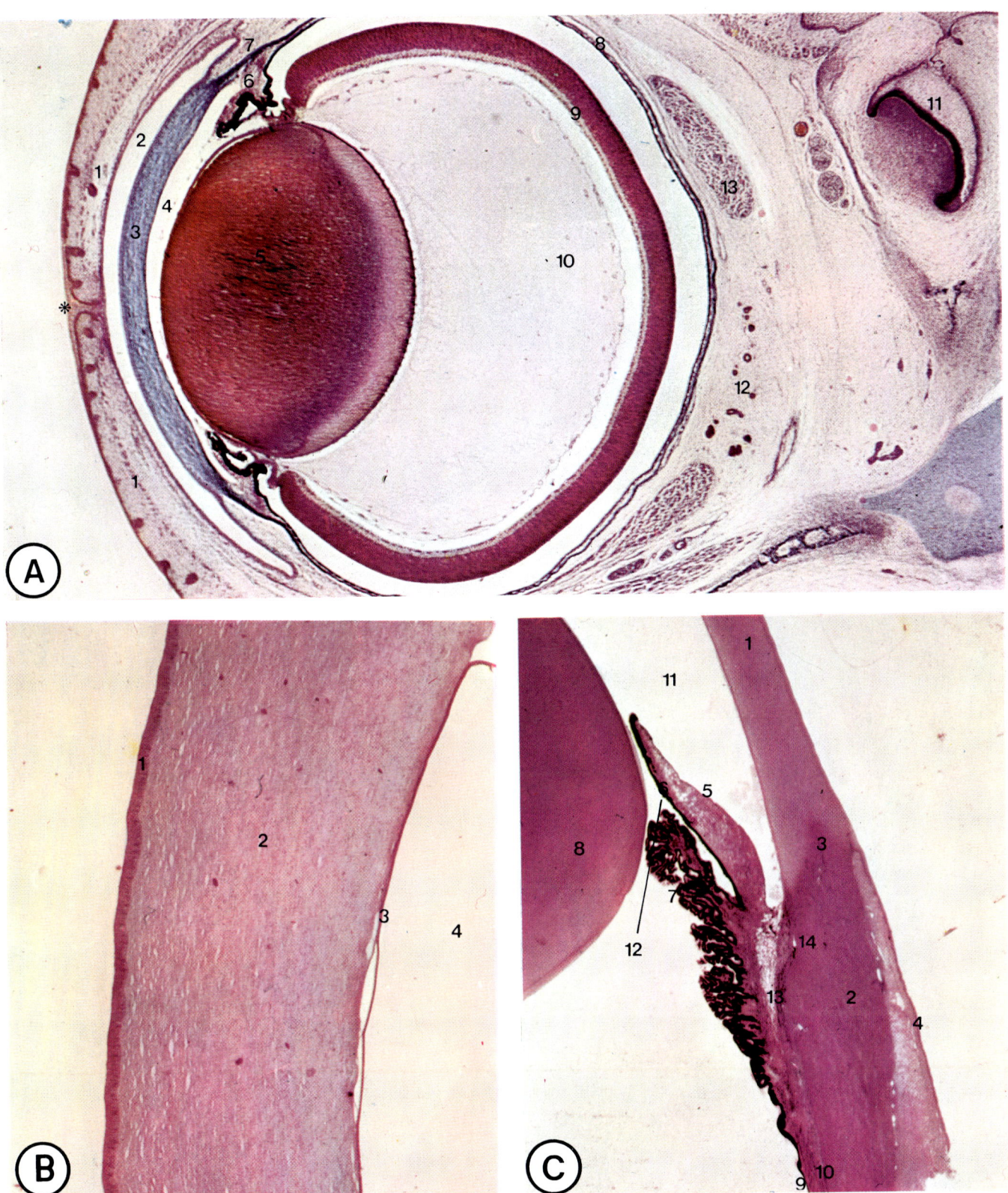

A **Sagittal section of eye from rat fetus (azan-Mallory, x20). 1** = eyelid, still unperforated (*). **2** = conjunctival sac. **3** = cornea. **4** = anterior chamber of eye. **5** = crystalline lens. **6** = iris with ciliary body still at bud stage. **7** = sclera. **8** = choroid, artificially detached. **9** = retina. **10** = vitreous body. **11** = tooth bud in superior maxilla. **12** = blood vessels. **13** = muscle fibers.

B **Pig cornea (H & E, x60). 1** = epithelium of cornea (stratified squamous). **2** = stroma of cornea. **3** = Descemet's membrane, partly detached and resting on the basal lamina. **4** = anterior chamber of the eye.

C **Sagittal section of ciliary body, iris and lens from pig (H & E, x40). 1** = cornea. **2** = sclera. **3** = transition zone between cornea and sclera. **4** = conjunctiva. **5** = anterior face of iris. **6** = posterior face of iris, covered with pigmented epithelium. **7** = ciliary processes. **8** = lens. **9** = non-photosensitive part of the retina. **10** = choroid. **11** = anterior chamber. **12** = posterior chamber. **13** = trabecular meshwork and canal of Schlemm **(14)**.

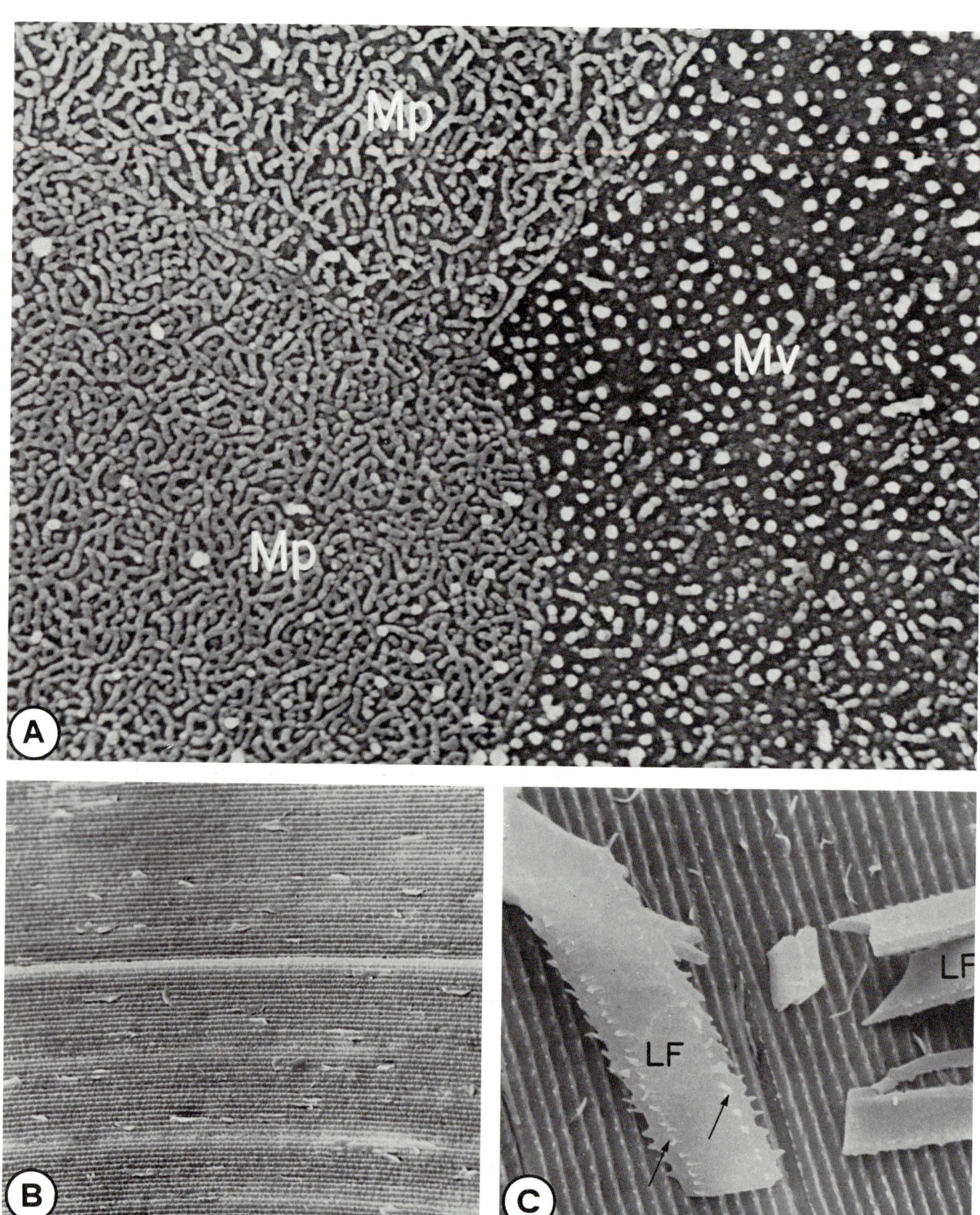

A   **Mouse cornea (scanning EM, x7,500).** On the free surface of the cornea can be seen adjacent corneal cells covered with microvilli **(Mv)** and microplicae **(Mp)**.

B   **Crystalline lens from rabbit (scanning EM, x450).** The lens has been fractured in this section in order to show the regular arrangement of the fibers.

C   **Fibers of rabbit lens (scanning EM, x2,000).** Some fibers **(LF)** of the lens have been isolated and appear as large hexagonal cells with a sawtooth outline (→). From P.M. Motta, P.M. Andrews and K.R. Porter. In: *Microanatomy of Cell and Tissue Surfaces. An Atlas of Scanning Electron Microscopy.* Lea & Febiger, Philadelphia, 1977.

Plate 8.66   251

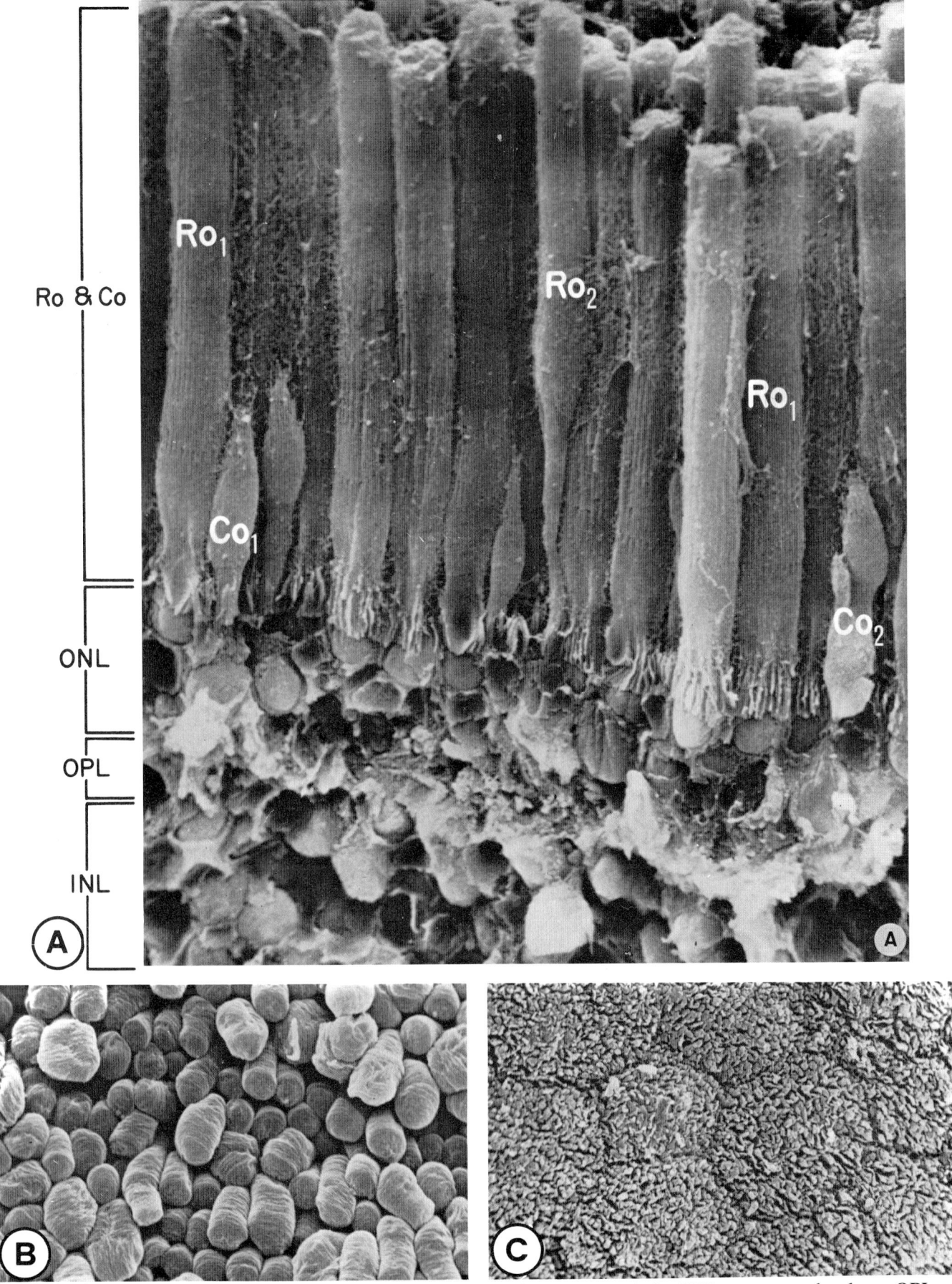

A   **Frog retina (scanning EM, x2,300). Ro & Co** = layer of rods and cones, respectively. **ONL** = outer nuclear layer. **OPL** = outer plexiform layer. **INL** = inner nuclear layer. Four types of photoreceptors are found in this zone: a red rod **(Ro1)**, a green rod **(Ro2)**, a single cone **(Co1)** and a double cone **(Co2)**. By courtesy of R.H. Steinberg. Z. Zellforsch. Mikrosck. Anat. 193:451, 1973.

B   **Rods from rat retina (scanning EM, x1,500).** The apices of rods with surface furrows formed by the characteristic folds of the plasmalemma can be seen.

C   **Pigmented epithelium from rat retina (scanning EM, x43,000).** The inner surface of the pigment cells has many interdigitations among which are embedded the outer segments of the rod and cone cells.

Plate 8.67

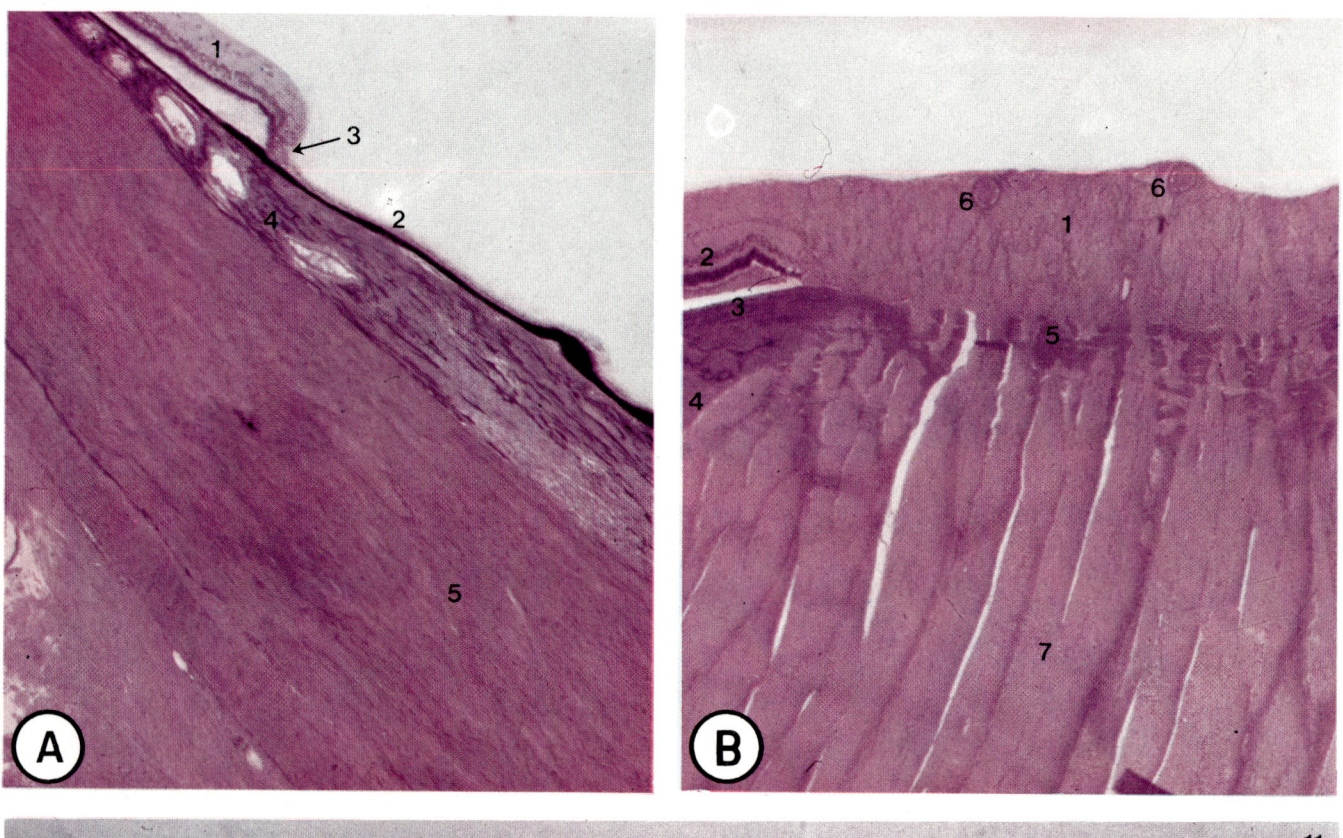

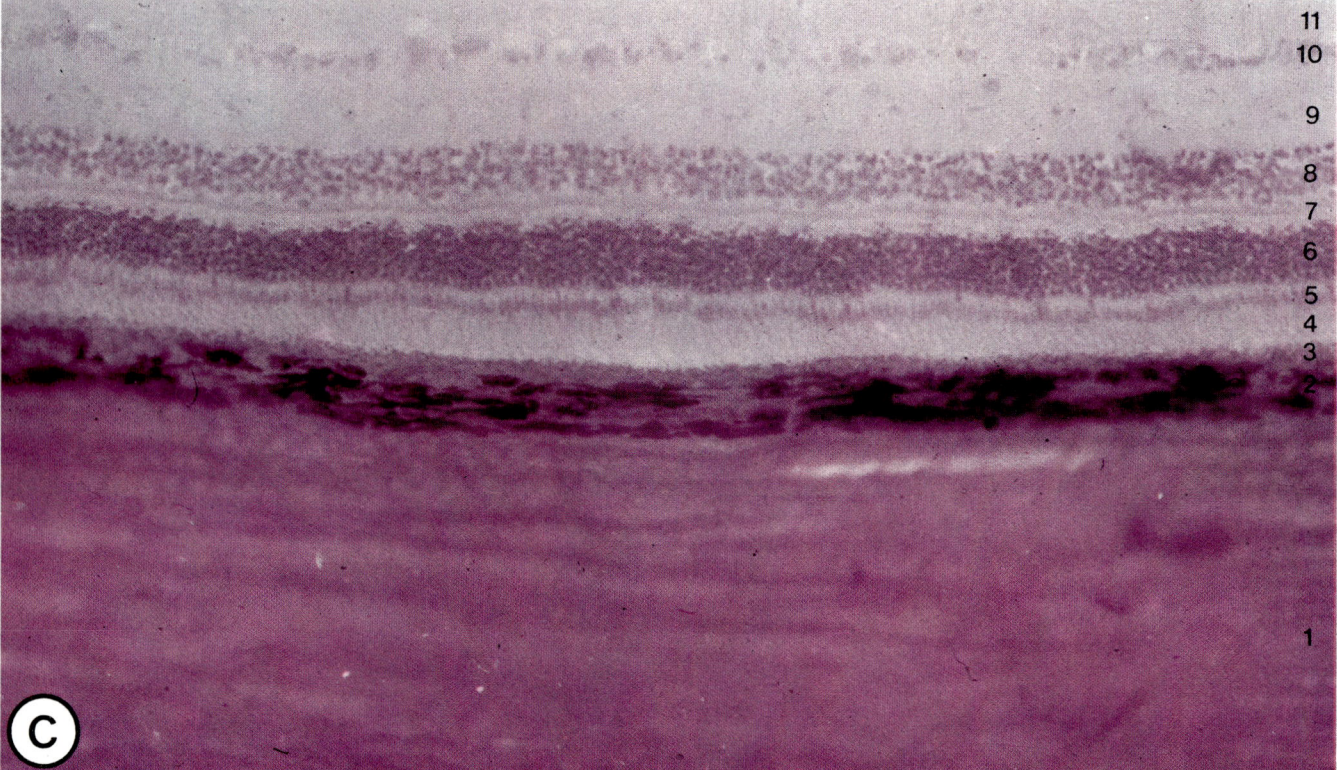

A **Pig retina (H & E, x30).** Transition zone between photosensitive (**1**) and non-photosensitive regions (**2**) of the retina can be seen. **3** = ora serrata. **4** = choroid. **5** = sclera. The retina has been artificially detached.

B **Papilla of optic nerve from a pig (H & E, x40). 1** = papilla of optic nerve. **2** = retina. **3** = choroid. **4** = sclera. **5** = lamina cribrosa of sclera. **6** = central blood vessels of the retina. **7** = fibers of the optic nerve.

C **Pig retina (H & E, x300). 1** = sclera. **2** = choroid. **3** = pigmented epithelium. **4** = layer of rods and cones. **5** = external limiting membrane. **6** = outer granular layer. **7** = outer plexiform layer. **8** = inner granular layer. **9** = inner plexiform layer. **10** = layer of ganglionic cells. **11** = layer of nerve fibers of internal limiting membrane, only partially visible in this section.

Plate 8.68 253

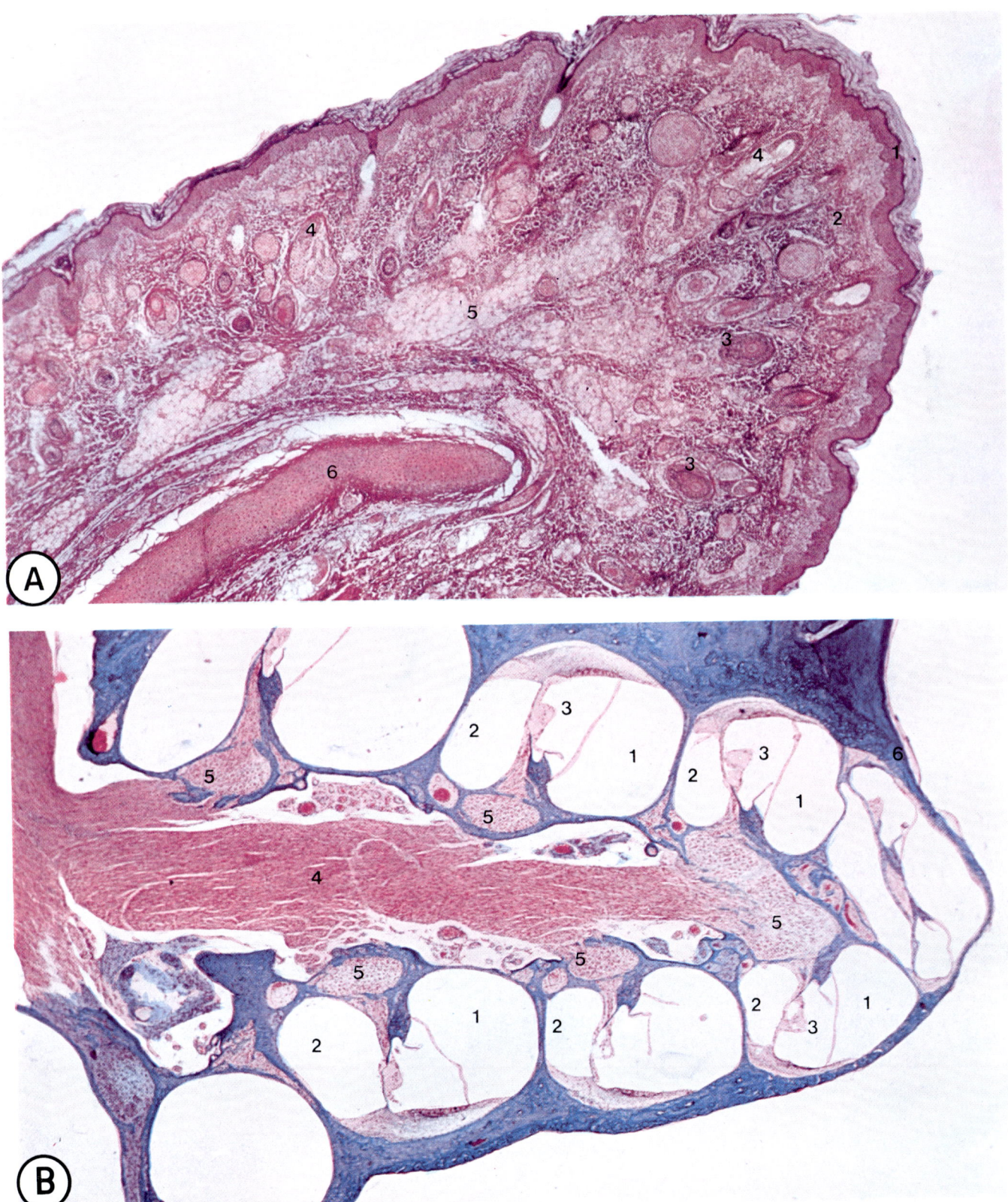

A **Human ear (H & E, x10). 1** = epidermis with thick keratinized epithelial layer. **2** = dermis with hair follicles in cross section (**3**) and a number of sebaceous glands (**4**). **5** = accumulations of adipose tissue in the hypodermis. **6** = lamina of cartilage (elastic cartilage of the ear).

B **Cochlea of guinea-pig, axial section parallel to the longitudinal axis (azan-Mallory, x50). 1** = scala vestibuli. **2** = scala tympani. **3** = cochlear duct. **4** = cochlear nerve within the axis of modiolus. **5** = spiral ganglion of Corti. **6** = bony covering of the cochlea.

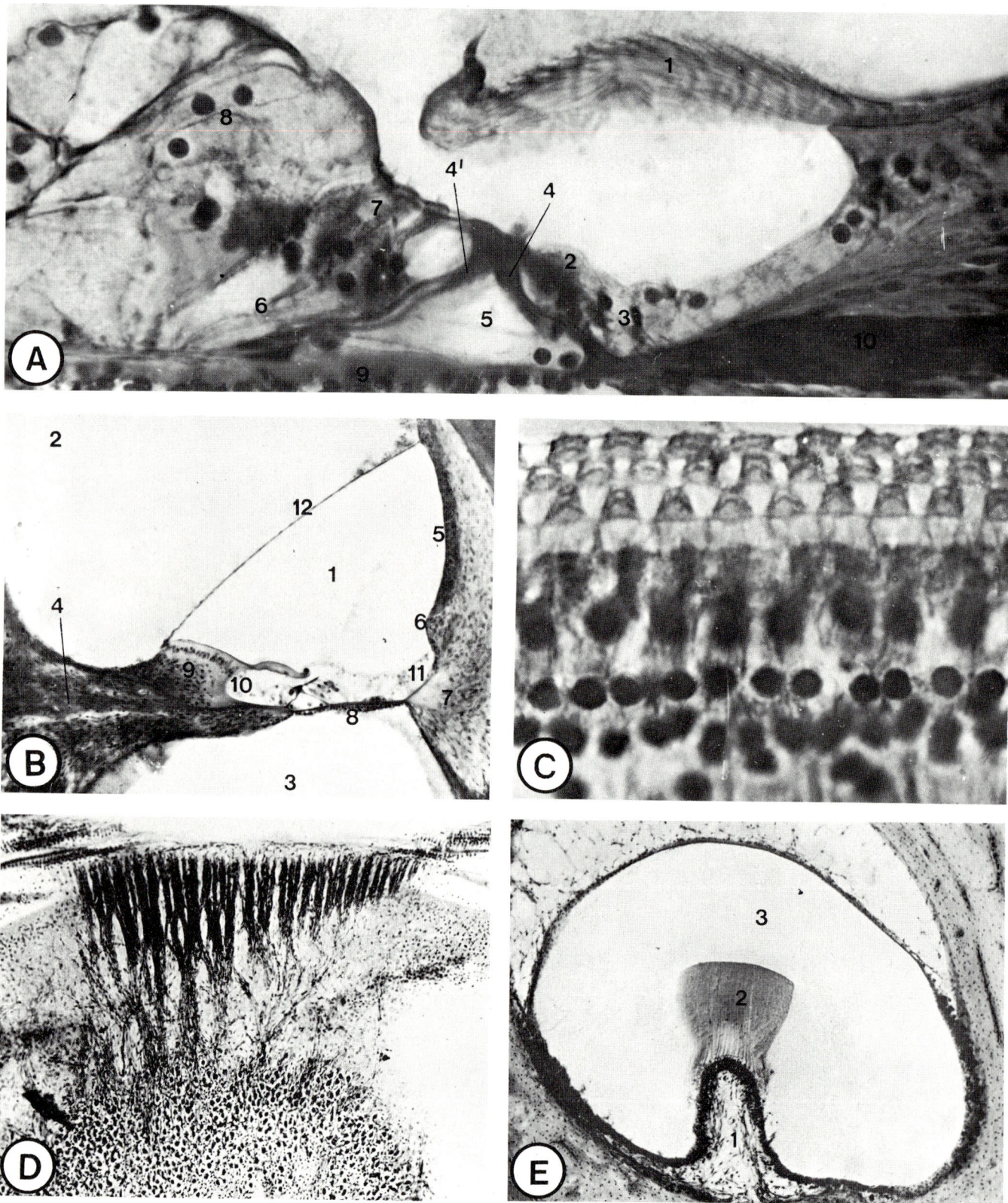

A   **Organ of Corti from rabbit (iron hematoxylin, x380). 1 =** tectorial membrane. **2 =** internal acoustic (sensory) cells. **3 =** internal supporting cells. **4 & 4' =** inner and outer pillar cells. **5 =** internal spiral tunnel. **6 =** external supporting cells (Deiters). **7 =** external acoustic cells. **8 =** cells of Hensen resting on the basilar membrane **(9).** Below right: bundles of nerve fibers **(10).**

B   **Cochlear duct from rabbit (iron hematoxylin, x180). 1 =** cochlear duct. **2 =** scala vestibuli. **3 =** scala tympani. **4 =** osseous spiral lamina with cochlear nerve. **5 =** stria vascularis. **6 =** prominence of the spiral duct. **7 =** ligamentum spirale (crista basilaris). **8 =** basilar membrane. **9 =** limbus of lamina spiralis. **10 =** inner sulcus spiralis. **11 =** outer sulcus spiralis. **12 =** Reissner's membrane.

C   **Surface portion of the organ of Corti from a rabbit (iron hematoxylin, x420).** From top to bottom: supporting cells of Hensen, phalangeal processes of cells of Deiters, outer sensory cells, heads of pillar cells.

D   **Spiral ganglion of Corti with limbus of lamina spiralis and bundles of nerve fibers (iron hematoxylin, x220).**

E   **Crista ampullaris from semicircular canal of rabbit (iron hematoxylin, x180). 1 =** crista ampullaris. **2 =** cupola. **3 =** cavity of the ampulla. By courtesy of E. Borghesan.

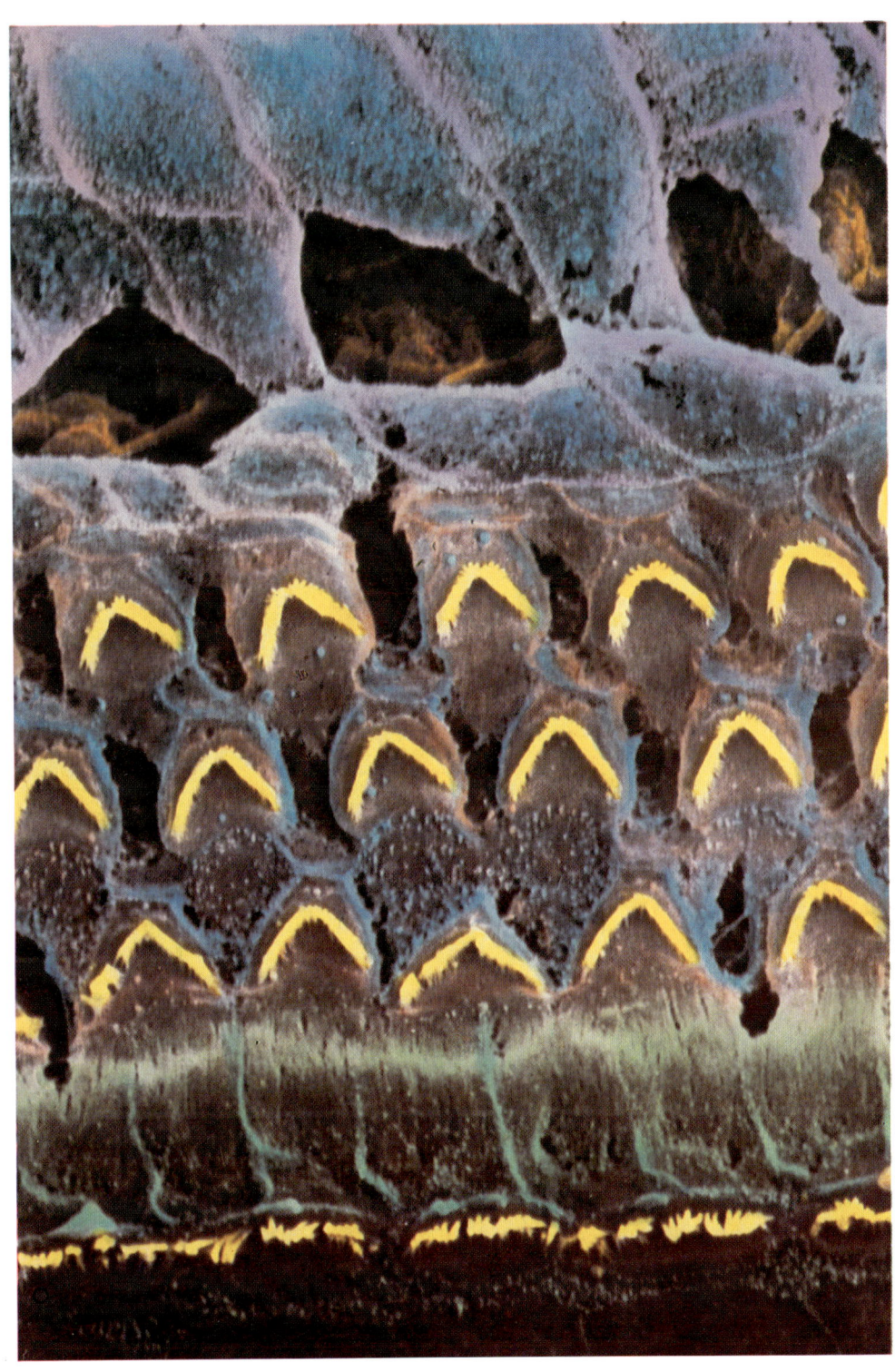

Overview of surface of the organ of Corti in the inner ear. Rows of V-shaped outer hair cells (top) and a single row of inner hair cells (bottom) are evident. Intermingled with these are, from the bottom, the phalangeal cells of Deiters, and some pillar cells. (Colored SEM; 2,100 x).

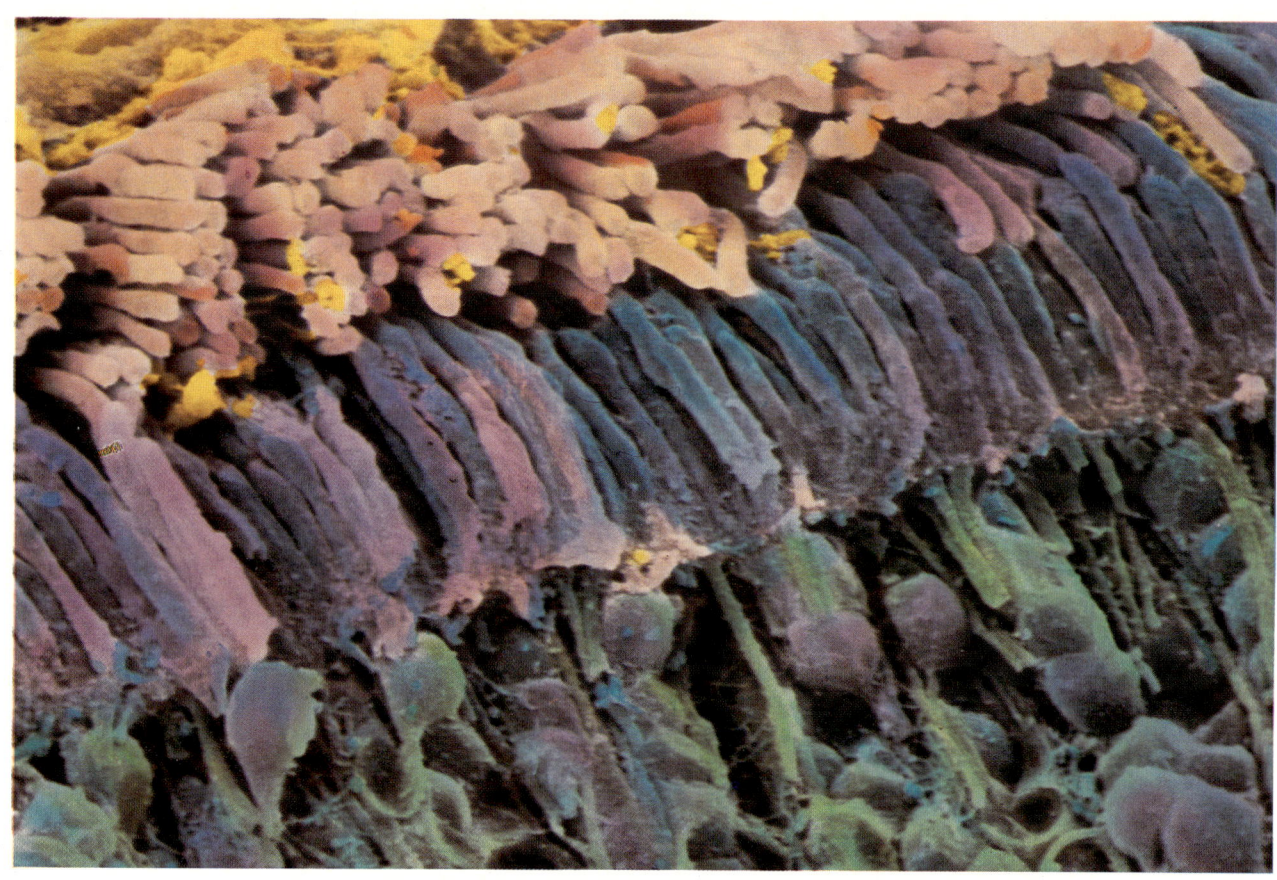

Overview of layer from rat retina. Most of the preparation, from the top down, is occupied by the layer of rods and cones. The nuclei belonging to the cell bodies of visual cells (outer granular layer) can be seen below. (Colored SEM; 2,850 x).

Bibliography

Angela P., Motta P.: Viaggio nel corpo umano. Milano, Garzanti, 1986.

Acosta-Vidrio E., Galina M.A. (Editors): *Advances in the Morphology of Cells and Tissues.* New York, A.R. Liss, Inc. 1981.

Allen D.J., Motta P.M., Di Dio L.J.A. (Editors): *Three- Dimensional Microanatomy of Cells and Tissue Surfaces.* New York/Amsterdam/Oxford, Elsevier/North Holland, 1981.

Balboni G.C. et Al.: *Anatomia Umana.* 2a Ed. Milano, Edi Ermes, 1980.

Bevelander G., Ramaley J.A.: *Essentials of Histology.* 8th Ed. St. Louis/Toronto/London, Mosby Co., 1979.

Bloom W., Fawcett D.W.: *Textbook of Histology.* 10th ed. Philadelphia/London/Toronto, W.B. Saunders, 1975.

Bourne G.H., Danielli J.F. (Editors): *International Review of Cytology.* Series, New York/London, Academic Press, 1960-85.

Bourne G.H.: *Division of Labor in Cells.* 2nd Ed. New York/London, Academic Press, 1970.

Brinkley B.R., Porter K.R. (Editors): *International Cell Biology.* New York. The Rockefeller University Press, 1977.

Cattaneo L., Grossi C., Zaccheo D.: *Anatomia Microscopica.* Torino, U.T.E.T., 1974.

Clara M., Herschel K., Ferner H.: *Atlas der Normalen Mikroscopischen Anatomie der Menschen,* Leipzig, J.A. Barth, 1974.

Czyba J.C., Girod C.: *Histologie.* 3e Ed. Lyon, Simep, 1979.

DiDio L.J.A.: *Synopsis of Anatomy.* St. Louis, Mosby, 1970.

DiFiore M.S.H.: *Atlas of Human Histology.* 5th Ed. Lea & Febiger, 1981.

Ebe T., Kobayashi S.: *Fine Structure of Human Cells and Tissue.* Tokyo, Igaku-Shoin, 1972.

Elias H., Pauly J.E., Burns E.R.: *Histology and Human Microananatomy.* 4th ed. Padova, Piccin Medical Books, l978.

Fawcett, D.W.: The Cell. 2nd Ed. Philadelphia, Saunders, 1981.

Fujita T., Tanaka K., Tokunaga J.: *Scanning Electron Microscopy. Atlas of Cells and Tissues.* Tokyo/New York, Igaku-Shoin, 1981.

Fumagalli Z.: *Guida allo Studio dell'Istologia.* Milano, Vallardi, 1969.

Gall J.G., Porter K.R., Siekevitz P. (Editors): *Discovery in Cell Biology.* New York, The Rockefeller University Press, 1981.

Girod C., Czyba J.C.: *Biologie de la Reproduction.* 2e Ed. Lyon, Simep, 1977.

Girod C.: *Introduction à l'Etude des Glandes Endocrines.* 2e Ed. Lyon, Simep, 1980.

Hadjoloff A.I.: *Histologhia y Embryologhia.* 4th Ed. Sofia, Press de l'Academie, 1973.

Hafez E.S.E. (Editor): *Scanning Electron Microscopy. Atlas of Mammalian Reproduction.* Tokyo, Igaku-Shoin, 1975.

Ham W.: *Histology.* 8th Ed. Philadelphia/Toronto, Lippincott, 1979.

Hayat M.A. (Editor): *Introduction to Biological Scanning Electron Microscopy.* Baltimore, University Park, 1978.

Holstein A.F., Roosen-Runge E.C.: *Atlas of Human Spermatogenesis.* Berlin, Grosse Verlag, 1981

Johannessen J.V. (Editor): *Electron Microscopy in Human Medicine.* Series, New York, McGraw-Hill, 1970-80.

Junqueira L.C., Carneiro J., *Basic Histology.* 3rd ed. Los Altos, Ca. Lange Medical Publications, 1980.

Kessel R.G., Kardon R.H.: *Tissue and Organs. A Text-atlas of Scanning Electron Microscopy.* San Francisco, W.H. Freeman, 1979.

Krstic R.V.: *Die Gewebe des Menschen und der Säugetiere.* Berlin / Heidelberg / New York, Springer, 1979.

Krstic R.V.: *Ultrastructure of the Mammalian Cell. An Atlas.* Berlin/Heidelberg/New York, Springer, 1979.

Laguens R.P., Gomez-Dumm, C.L.A.: *Atlas of Human Electron Microscopy.* St. Louis/Toronto/London, Mosby Co., 1969.

Langman J.: *Medical Embryology. 4th ed. Williams & Wilkins Baltimore/London, 1981.*

Leeson T.S., Leeson C.R.: *A Brief Atlas of Histology.* Philadelphia, Saunders, 1979.

Lentz T.L.: *Cell Fine Structure. An Atlas of Drawings of Whole-cell Structure.* Philadelphia/London/Toronto, Saunders, 1971.

Matthews J.L., Martin J.H.: *Atlas of Human Histology and Ultrastructure.* Philadelphia, Lea & Febiger, 1971.

Monesi V.: *Istologia,* 2a Ed. Padova, Piccin, 1980.

Motta P.M. (Editor): *Ultrastructure of Endocrine Cells and Tissues. Series in Electron Microscopy.* Vol I. The Hague/Boston/London. M. Nijhoff Publishers, 1984.

Motta P.M., Andrews P.M., Porter K.R.: *Microanatomy of Cell and Tissue Surfaces. An Atlas of Scanning Electron Microscopy.* Philadelphia, Lea & Febiger, 1977.

Motta P.M., DiDio L.J.A. (Editors): *Basic and Clinical Hepatology.* The Hague/Boston/London, M. Nijhoff Publishers, 1982.

Motta P.M., Hafez E.S.E. *(Editors): Biology of the Ovary.* The Hague/Boston/London, M. Nijhoff Publishers, 1980.

Motta P.M., Muto M., Fujita T.: *The Liver. An Atlas of Scanning Electron Microscopy.* Tokyo/New York, Igaku-Shoin, 1978.

Mountcastle V.B. (Editor): *Trattato di Fisiologia Medica.* Piccin, Padova, 1980.

Novikoff A.B., Holtzman E.: *Cells and Organelles.* New York, Holt, Rinehart and Winston, Inc., 1970.

Olah I., Roulich P., Toro I.: *Ultrastructure of Lymphoid Organs. An Electron Microscopic Atlas.* Budapest, Akademiai Kiadu, 1975.

Olivo O.M., Toni G.: *Atlante di Anatomia Microscopica.* 2a Ed. Milano, Vallardi, 1973.

Orci L., Perrelet A.: *Freeze-etch Histology. A Comparison Between Thin Sections and Freeze-etch Replicas.* Berlin/Heidelberg/New York, Springer, 1975.

Passmore R., Robson J.S. (Editors): *Companion to Medical Studies.* 2nd Ed. Oxford/London, Blackwell Scientific Publications, 1976.

Porter K.R., Bonneville M.A.: *Fine Structure of Cells and Tissues.* 4th Ed. Philadelphia, Lea & Febiger, 1973.

Reale E.: *Elektronenmikroscopie der Zellen und Gewebe.* Stuttgart, Fischer, 1973.

Rhodin J.A.G.: *Histology. A Text and Atlas.* London/Toronto, Oxford University Press, 1974.

Rizzoli C., Brunelli M.A., Castaldini C.: *Guida Illustrata all'Istologia.* Padova, Piccin, 1982.

Rosati P. et Al.: *Istologia.* Milano, Edi Ermes, 1981.

Rosenbauer K.A., Kegel H.B.: *Rasterelektronmikroskopische. Technick.* Stuttgart, Thieme, 1978.

Sandborn E.B.: *Cells and Tissues by Light and Electron Microscopy.* London, Academic Press, 1970.

Tanaka K., Fujita T. (Editors): *Scanning Electron Microscopy in Cell Biology and Medicine.* Amsterdam/Oxford/ Princeton, Excerpta Medica, 1981.

Tanikawa K.: *Ultrastructural Aspects of the Liver and its Disorders.* 2nd Ed. Tokyo/New York, Igaku-Shoin, 1979.

Toner P.G., Carr K.E.: *Cell Structure. An Introduction to Biological Electron Microscopy.* 2nd Ed. Edinburgh/ London, Livingstone, 1982.

Van Blerkom J., Motta P.M.: *The Cellular Basis of Mammalian Reproduction.* Munich/Baltimore, Urban & Schwarzenberg, 1979.

Van Blerkom J., Motta P.M. (Editors): *Ultrastructure in Reproduction. Series in Electron Microscopy.* Vol. II. The Hague/Boston/London, M. Nijhoff Publishers, 1984.

Weiss L., Greep O.R.: *Histology.* 4th Ed., New York, McGraw-Hill, 1977.

Wismar B.L., Ackerman, G.A.: *A Visual Approach to Histology.* Philadelphia, Davis Co., 1970.

Zamboni L.: *Fine Morphology of Mammalian Fertilization.* New York/London, Harper & Row Publishers, 1971.

Index

Page	Line	Errata	Corrige
opposite p. 1	5	membrane plasmique	Plasma membrane
2	22	Plate 1.8	Plate 1.9
70	43	Plate 4.1	Plate 3.1
89	diagram	muscle squelettique	skeletal muscle
90	13	Plate 4.3	Plate 4.8
108	running-Plate	Plate 3.4	Plate 5.5.
163	28	see p. 183	see p. 182
171	27	Plate 8.29 A	Plate 8.30 A
172	20	see p. 183	see p. 182
175	10	see p. 183	see p. 182
175	28	see p. 183	see p. 182
182	31	Plate 8.5	Plate 8.57
182	44	Plate 8.32 B	Plate 8.31 B

Finito di stampare nel mese di dicembre 1989
presso le officine della LITOSTAMPA ISTITUTO GRAFICO - Gorle (Bg)
per conto della PICCIN NUOVA LIBRARIA s.p.a. - Padova (Italy)